Clinical Tests of
Respiratory Function

Clinical Tests of Respiratory Function

THIRD EDITION

Professor G. John Gibson, BSc, MD, FRCP, FRCPEd
Consultant Physician, Freeman Hospital and
Professor of Respiratory Medicine,
Newcastle University,
Newcastle upon Tyne, UK

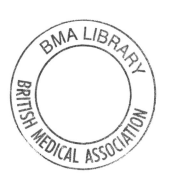

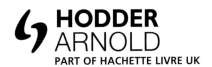

HODDER
ARNOLD
PART OF HACHETTE LIVRE UK

First published in Great Britain in 1984 by Macmillan
Second edition 1996, Chapman & Hall
This third edition published in 2009 by
Hodder Arnold, an imprint of Hodder Education, part of
Hachette Livre UK, 338 Euston Road, London NW1 3BH

http://www.hoddereducation.com

Hachette Livre UK's policy is to use papers that are natural, renewable and
recyclable products and made from wood grown in sustainable forests.
The logging and manufacturing processes are expected to conform to
the environmental regulations of the country of origin.

Whilst the advice and information in this book are believed to be true and
accurate at the date of going to press, neither the author nor the publisher
can accept any legal responsibility or liability for any errors or omissions that
may be made. In particular (but without limiting the generality of the preceding
disclaimer) every effort has been made to check drug dosages; however it is still
possible that errors have been missed. Furthermore, dosage schedules are constantly
being revised and new side-effects recognized. For these reasons the reader is strongly
urged to consult the drug companies' printed instructions before administering any
of the drugs recommended in this book.

British Library Cataloguing in Publication Data
A catalogue record for this book is available from the British Library

Library of Congress Cataloging-in-Publication Data
A catalog record for this book is available from the Library of Congress

ISBN-13   978-0-340-92561-4

1 2 3 4 5 6 7 8 9 10

Commissioning Editor: Philip Shaw
Project Editor: Amy Mulick
Production Controller: Karen Tate
Cover Designer: Laura DeGrasse

Typeset in 9.5/12 Berling by Charon Tec Ltd., A Macmillan Company. (www.macmillansolutions.com)
Printed and bound in Spain

Contents

PART D   Interpretation of respiratory function tests

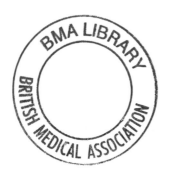

Preface

In the 25 years since the first edition of this book, respiratory function tests have become more integrated within the clinical practice of respiratory medicine, though perhaps not always with the discrimination desirable. Technological advances and computerization have brought great benefits in terms of convenience and accuracy, but there is a downside, with some erosion of technical skills and less accessible raw measurements. The need to understand the basis of the tests in order to use them optimally has not diminished.

A great fillip to the discipline has been the increasing recognition of sleep-disordered breathing and the explosive expansion of respiratory measurements during sleep. At the same time, measurements on exercise have become more generally available and also better standardized. Although sleep and exercise measurements are both covered more comprehensively in monographs dedicated specifically to them, their increasing importance in respiratory function testing is reflected by more extensive coverage in this edition. Even in traditional areas, such as asthma and chronic airways disease, where functional measurements are well established, better understanding of pathophysiology and improvements in technology have expanded their rational application.

The aims of the book are essentially unchanged – to explain the pathophysiology underlying the most useful tests of respiratory function in disease, at rest, during exercise and during sleep; to describe the abnormalities seen both in respiratory and non-respiratory disease; and to review the value and interpretation of the measurements in clinical practice. Many recent references have been added but, inevitably, the choice is selective and relevant earlier references have been retained, not least because reviewing the recent literature shows that reinvention of the wheel is not uncommon.

GJ Gibson
Newcastle upon Tyne, 2008

Preface to the first edition

Tests of respiratory function have been available for clinical use for about 30 years but they are still not fully integrated in the mainstream of clinical medicine. I think they are often ill understood and therefore frequently misused, or, more importantly, not used when they should be. The main aim of this book is to narrow the divide between respiratory physiology and the lung function laboratory on the one hand, and the bedside or outpatient clinic on the other. To a large extent, the failure to apply the tests appropriately stems from the misguided feeling that complicated laboratory-based measurements are needed, when, in fact, simple tests used in the ward or clinic are often of much greater value. To many the jargon and hieroglyphics of respiratory physiology are undoubtedly inhibiting and, it must be admitted, respiratory physiologists have themselves been to blame for perpetuating the mystique of their subject and often for failing to promote a pragmatic approach which can be routinely applied to clinical situations. The more tests used and the more indices recorded, the more superficially impressive (and perhaps the more lucrative) is the report on an individual patient; the disadvantages of this approach are that it dilutes the clinical relevance of the information and may assault the comprehension of its recipient.

I hope this book will be of value to respiratory physicians in practice and in training, and particularly to those involved in the interpretation of the commonly performed tests of respiratory function. The tests described are conventional measurements of function of the 'whole organ'; tests of respiratory function in the broadest sense might also include biochemical and subcellular techniques applied to bronchial secretions, lung tissue or fluid lavaged from the lung, as well as studies of pulmonary metabolism and of the way drugs are handled by the lung. All these are expanding fields but so far none has generated a widely applicable clinical test.

This book is not primarily a laboratory manual with a detailed technical account of the tests, nor does it give comprehensive normal or reference values as these are fully covered elsewhere, notably by Cotes. The choice of tests included is a personal one – I did not set out to cover every conceivable test, but I have concentrated on those that I find to be of value in assessing the severity of a functional disturbance, in elucidating its mechanism, in differential diagnosis and in following responses to treatment. I have included a few tests that are of doubtful clinical applicability (e.g. the D_m and V_c components of the CO diffusing capacity), or are too demanding of technology for widespread use (e.g. the multiple inert gas technique of Wagner and West), where these aid the understanding or interpretation of simpler tests. I must also admit that occasionally the criterion for inclusion of an unusual feature or piece of information has been simply that I find it interesting. In many situations the exact pathogenesis of abnormalities of respiratory function tests is ill understood, but where specific mechanisms are established or likely, I have tried to explain these, with the philosophy that sensible application of the tests is more likely to result from understanding or from a questioning attitude than from ignorance or unwarranted assumptions.

GJ Gibson
Newcastle upon Tyne, 1983

PART A

THE TESTS AND THEIR PHYSIOLOGICAL BASIS

Respiratory Mechanics

1.1 MECHANICS OF INSPIRATION AND EXPIRATION

1.1.1 Elasticity of lungs and chest wall

Both the lungs and the surrounding chest wall are elastic structures, i.e. they tend to return to their previous configuration when a distending force is removed. At the end of a quiet expiration in a normal subject, the volume of the lungs (functional residual capacity, FRC) represents the mechanically 'neutral' position of the respiratory system as a whole. The respiratory muscles are relaxed and there is no net force acting across the combined lungs and chest well, i.e. the pressure within the alveoli is the same as the external atmospheric pressure. There is, however, a balance of passive forces acting across the lungs and chest wall individually. Functional residual capacity corresponds to the neutral (relaxed) position of the overall respiratory system provided that the lungs and chest wall are coupled together, but neither component is at its own unstressed neutral volume. When a surgeon opens the chest or if a pneumothorax occurs, the lungs collapse due to their inward (positive) recoil and the ribs spring apart because at FRC the recoil of the chest wall is outwards (negative). The introduction of air into the pleural space thus uncouples the lungs from the chest wall and allows each to approach its own neutral volume. Functional residual capacity is the volume adopted by the relaxed intact respiratory system

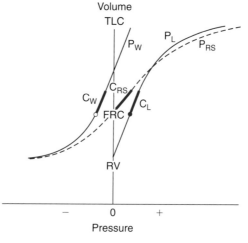

Figure 1.1 'Rahn diagram',[1] showing the static pressure–volume relations of the lungs (lung recoil pressure, P_L), chest wall (chest wall recoil pressure, P_W) and total respiratory system (recoil pressure of the total respiratory system, P_{RS}) in a normal subject. The approximate range of tidal breathing is indicated by heavy lines, the slopes of which represent compliance of the total respiratory system (C_{RS}), lungs (C_L) and chest wall (C_W). See text for further explanation.

FRC, functional residual capacity; RV, residual volume.

because inward recoil of the lungs is exactly balanced by outward recoil of the chest wall.

The interrelations can be visualized using the static pressure–volume (PV) curves of the lungs, chest wall and their combination, the total respiratory system (Fig. 1.1). The recoil pressure of the total respiratory system (P_{RS}) is simply the algebraic sum of the recoil pressures of its components, the lungs (P_L) and chest wall (P_W), i.e.

$$P_{RS} = P_L + P_W \qquad (1.1)$$

The 'chest wall' in this context includes both the ribcage and the abdomen, as the latter is displaced by descent of the diaphragm with each inspiration.

At FRC, P_{RS} is zero and therefore $P_L = -P_W$. Below FRC, P_W is responsible for the increasingly negative value of P_{RS}; this results mainly from the passive downward recoil of the stretched diaphragm, which is forced progressively upwards at lower lung volumes. At high volumes P_L is the main contributor to P_{RS}, but above its own neutral position (i.e. where $P_W = 0$) the chest wall also has a positive (inward) recoil. The compliance of the lungs (C_L), which is change in volume divided by the change in transpulmonary pressure, can be visualized as the slope of the pressure–volume curve. Usually this is measured over the approximate range of tidal breathing (e.g. between FRC and FRC + 0.5 L, indicated by heavy lines in Fig. 1.1). The compliance of the total respiratory system (C_{RS}) is less than that of each of its components (C_L, C_W); the lungs and chest wall share a common volume change (ΔV), while the change in distending pressure applied across the total system (ΔP_{RS}) is the sum of the pressures applied across the lungs (ΔP_L) and chest wall (ΔP_W) individually, so that:

$$\frac{\Delta P_{RS}}{\Delta V} = \frac{\Delta P_L}{\Delta V} + \frac{\Delta P_W}{\Delta V}$$

that is:

$$\frac{1}{C_{RS}} = \frac{1}{C_L} + \frac{1}{C_W} \qquad (1.2)$$

The important interrelations between the pressures acting on the respiratory system are illustrated in Fig. 1.2. Across the lungs, the inward pressure of elastic recoil (P_L) is balanced by an equal and opposite net distending pressure, which is the difference between the pressure at the pleural surface (P_{pl}) and in the alveoli (P_{alv}), i.e.

$$P_L = -(P_{pl} - P_{alv}) = P_{alv} - P_{pl}$$

or

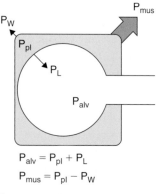

$$P_{alv} = P_{pl} + P_L$$
$$P_{mus} = P_{pl} - P_W$$

Figure 1.2 Pressures acting on the respiratory system. See text for further explanation.

P_{alv}, alveolar gas pressure; P_L, lung recoil pressure; P_{mus}, net pressure generated by respiratory muscles; P_{pl}, plural surface pressure; P_W, chest wall recoil pressure.

$$P_{alv} = P_{pl} + P_L \qquad (1.3)$$

Similarly, across the chest wall its passive recoil pressure (P_W) is balanced by a net distending pressure, which is the difference between the pressure resulting from muscle contraction (P_{mus}) and pleural pressure, i.e.

$$P_W = -(P_{mus} - P_{pl}) = P_{pl} - P_{mus}$$

or

$$P_{mus} = P_{pl} - P_W \qquad (1.4)$$

By a similar argument, the recoil pressure of the total respiratory system (P_{RS}) is balanced by the difference between P_{mus} and alveolar pressure, i.e.

$$P_{RS} = -(P_{mus} - P_{alv}) = P_{alv} - P_{mus}$$

or

$$P_{mus} = P_{alv} - P_{RS} \qquad (1.5)$$

Note that P_W may be positive (acting inwards) or negative (acting outwards), as also may P_{mus} (i.e. expiratory or inspiratory): with proper attention to sign, Equations 1.4 and 1.5 still apply.

1.1.2 Mechanics of normal inspiration and expiration

At the start of a normal inspiration, muscle contraction exerts a 'pull' on the chest wall, consequently lowering pleural pressure surrounding the lungs and also alveolar pressure within the lungs. The pressure applied by the inspiratory muscles is used mainly to overcome two types of force, elastic and resistive. Elastic forces are related to change in volume, and resistive forces to flow (change in volume per unit time, dV/dt or $\dot{V}$). In addition, a small proportion of the pressure applied is dissipated in overcoming a third type of force caused by inertia, i.e. the force required to initiate airflow, which depends on acceleration of gas and tissue (change in flow per unit time, d^2V/dt^2 or $\ddot{V}$). The pressure required is, however, usually small and for most purposes can be ignored.

Elastic and resistive forces relate to different physical properties of the respiratory system and are also determined at different sites, the former predominantly by the alveoli and chest wall and the latter by the airways. Although the alveoli themselves have a flow resistance ('tissue resistance') and, in addition, the airways are elastic, quantitatively these effects are small. Consequently, the mechanical performance of the respiratory system can conveniently be abbreviated to a description of the elastic properties of the lungs and chest wall and the resistance of the airways.

The sequence of events during a normal breathing cycle is illustrated in Fig. 1.3. At end expiration (Fig. 1.3a), lung recoil pressure is approximately 5 cmH$_2$O (inwards, therefore expiratory and by convention positive) and chest wall recoil pressure is equal and opposite (outwards, therefore inspiratory and by convention negative). This balance produces a pleural pressure at FRC of about -5 cmH$_2$O and alveolar pressure ($P_{pl} + P_L$) is zero, i.e. atmospheric, so no air is flowing. Inspiratory muscle contraction gives an additional outward force (P_{mus}, negative because inspiratory), which is transmitted via the pleural space to the alveoli, where the pressure becomes subatmospheric, generating a pressure gradient between the alveoli and the mouth and consequent inspiratory airflow. Figure 1.3b shows the situation at approximately mid-inspiration; the pressure of -5 cmH$_2$O generated by the inspiratory muscles has been used partly to overcome the greater inward recoil of the expanding lung, with the remainder seen as the subatmospheric P_{alv}. At end inspiration (Fig. 1.3c), recoil of both the chest wall and lungs is more positive and, since P_{alv} is once more zero, airflow has ceased and all the actively applied pressure is being

used to overcome elastic forces and maintain the increased volume of the lungs and chest wall. Expiration begins once the inspiratory muscles start to relax. Normal expiration at rest is usually described as 'passive' as the expiratory muscles do not contract. In fact the converse is true: *inspiratory* activity continues during most of expiration and acts as a brake on expiratory flow. Figure 1.3d shows the position at mid-expiration, with the lungs and chest wall having regained the same volume as in Fig.1.3b; slightly less inspiratory muscle activity than at the same volume during inspiration results in a supra-atmospheric alveolar pressure and expiratory flow.

Figure 1.3 also illustrates how, during quiet breathing in a normal subject, more of the pressure generated by inspiratory muscle contraction is dissipated in overcoming elastic forces than is needed to produce airflow.

1.1.3 Mechanics of inspiration and expiration in disease

The effects of the major types of mechanical abnormality found in disease are modelled in a similar fashion in Figs 1.4–1.6. Each starts from the same balance of pressures at FRC and assumes a similar tidal volume change as in the healthy subject (Fig. 1.3); the likely differences in absolute lung volumes are ignored.

Figure 1.4 shows an example where airway resistance is increased by disease narrowing the airways. If we assume no change in elastic properties, then the situations at end expiration and end inspiration (where $P_{alv} = 0$ and there is no flow) are similar to the normal. However, when air is flowing (Fig. 1.4b,d), larger swings of pleural and alveolar pressures are necessary to produce a normal flow through the narrowed airway. Greater inspiratory muscle contraction is therefore seen (compare Fig. 1.4b with Fig. 1.3b) and there may be less post-inspiratory braking (compare Fig. 1.4d with Fig. 1.3d); the plot of pleural pressure against volume during tidal breathing shows much wider 'looping' than normal (compare Fig. 1.4e with Fig. 1.3e). This is an index of the greater work necessary to overcome the increased airway resistance.

Figures 1.5 and 1.6 show the effects of 'stiffening' the lungs and chest wall respectively, with a reduction in the compliance of each by 50 per cent. (This

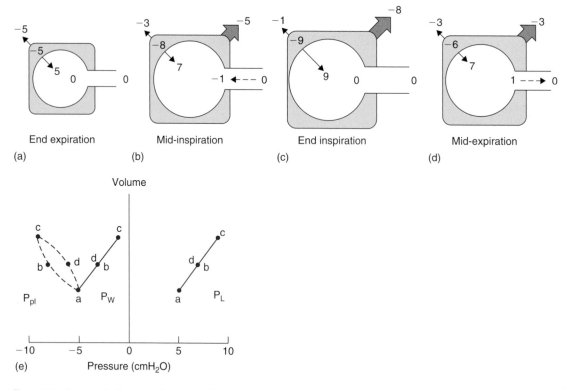

End expiration   Mid-inspiration   End inspiration   Mid-expiration
(a)   (b)   (c)   (d)

Figure 1.3 Schematic diagram of pressure relations at various stages of the tidal breathing cycle in a normal subject. The pressures recorded (cf. Fig. 1.2 and Equations 1.3–1.5) represent values in cmH_2O of elastic recoil of the lungs and chest wall (thin arrows), the pressure resulting from contraction of the respiratory muscles (broad arrow), alveolar pressure, pressure at the mouth (always zero) and pressure at the pleural surface between the lungs and chest wall (P_{pl}). Broken arrows show the direction of the airflow, if any. The first four diagrams illustrate the pressures prevailing at end expiration (i.e. functional residual capacity, FRC) (a), mid-inspiration (b), end inspiration (c) and mid-expiration (d); (b) and (d) represent the same lung volume. (e) The corresponding pressure–volume (PV) relations, with closed circles representing the volumes illustrated in (a–d); lung recoil pressure (P_L) and chest wall recoil pressure (P_W) describe the static PV curves of the lungs and chest wall, respectively (hysteresis is ignored). The loop indicated by the broken line represents the dynamic relation between pleural pressure and volume during the breath. See text for further explanation.

results in a similar reduction in compliance of the total respiratory system of 33%.) Comparing Figs 1.5 and 1.6 with Fig. 1.3 shows that more inspiratory muscle activity is necessary throughout inspiration to overcome the stiffer tissues; in Fig. 1.5 the reduced compliance is reflected in greater values of lung recoil pressure and in Fig.1.6 in greater inward recoil (or less outward recoil) of the chest wall. With 'stiff' (low compliance) lungs during expiration, the greater recoil (Fig. 1.5d) compared with normal results in a higher pressure driving expiration.

The 'purist' approach to the characterization of the mechanical performance of the respiratory system would therefore be to measure the elastic properties of the chest wall, the elastic properties of the lungs and the resistance of the airways. However, the first is difficult, if not impossible, in the conscious subject; the second is uncomfortable and usually unnecessary in clinical practice; the third can be technically demanding and may not necessarily give the most appropriate information. Consequently, neither compliance nor airway resistance is measured directly in routine practice in most lung function laboratories. The pragmatic approach is to assess the distensibility of the lungs by measurements of lung volume, and airway calibre by tests of maximum flow during a forced expiration. The justification for the use of these technically simpler measurements is outlined

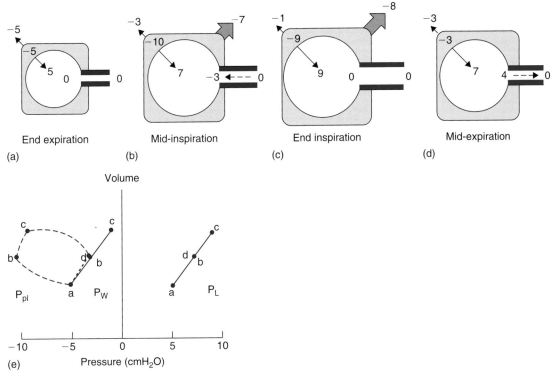

Figure 1.4 Schematic diagram of pressure relations at various stages of the tidal breathing cycle in a subject with increased airway resistance. Conventions are as in Fig. 1.3. There are no changes in the elastic properties of the lungs or chest wall, so the pressures prevailing at end expiration (a) and end inspiration (c) are identical to those in the normal subject in Fig. 1.3. The increased airway resistance demands larger than normal swings in alveolar pressure to maintain the same ventilation; a more negative pressure is applied by the inspiratory muscles during inspiratory flow (b), and it is assumed that no braking occurs during expiration (d). These differences are reflected in greater swings in pleural pressure and much wider looping of the relation between pleural surface pressure (P_{pl}) and volume (e).

P_L, lung recoil pressure; P_W, chest wall recoil pressure.

below, after a brief discussion of the determinants and implications of the 'purer' measurements.

1.2 MEASUREMENTS OF DISTENSIBILITY OF THE LUNGS AND CHEST WALL

The elastic properties of the lungs and chest wall are described by their individual static pressure–volume relationships, as illustrated by the 'Rahn diagram' (Fig. 1.1).[1] The distensibility of each alone can be assessed by relating volume change to static transpulmonary or passive transthoracic pressure respectively. 'Partitioning' of the pressure across the respiratory system in this way requires estimation of pleural pressure.

Note that when, during positive pressure inflation of a patient's lungs, the anaesthetist measures compliance or 'stiffness', he is usually assessing the compliance of the lungs and chest wall (C_{RS}) together. This is inevitably less than that of the lungs alone, because of the additional pressure that has to be exerted in order to distend the chest wall; however, in most pathological conditions (apart from skeletal abnormalities), reduced C_{RS} is due to reduced lung compliance.

1.2.1 Lung pressure–volume curves in health and disease

During inflation the alveoli behave like balloons, in that they become progressively more difficult to inflate as they reach their full capacity. Hence, the

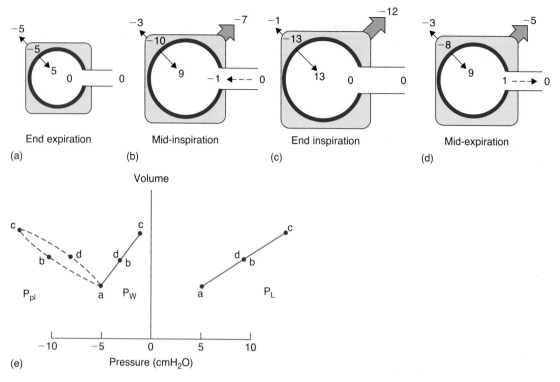

Figure 1.5 Schematic diagram of pressure relationships at various stages of the tidal breathing cycle in a subject with abnormally stiff lungs. Conventions are as in Fig. 1.3. The elastic properties of the chest wall and the airway resistance are normal and it is assumed that the pressures at functional residual capacity (FRC) (a) are unchanged. Lung compliance is reduced by 50 per cent compared with the normal subject in Fig. 1.3, so that, for the same tidal volume, lung recoil pressure increases by twice the normal amount between end expiration and end inspiration (c) (i.e. from 5 cmH$_2$O to 13 cmH$_2$O, compared with 5 cmH$_2$O to 9 cmH$_2$O in Fig. 1.3). More inspiratory muscle effort is required both during inspiration (b) and at the end of inspiration (c). Whether expiratory braking (d) is similar to normal is not clear. The peak-to-peak swings of pleural surface pressure (P$_{pl}$) are greater than normal but, since airway resistance is normal, the pressure–volume loop is narrow (e).

P$_L$, lung recoil pressure; P$_W$, chest wall recoil pressure.

elastic recoil pressure of the lungs becomes disproportionately large at higher lung volumes. Consequently the relation between lung recoil pressure and volume is curvilinear, with the compliance of the lungs falling (its reciprocal, elastance or 'stiffness', increases) at high volumes (Fig. 1.1). Also, at high lung volumes the efficiency of the inspiratory muscles becomes progressively less because, as with any muscle, the associated reduction in fibre length reduces their capacity to generate force. Full inflation (i.e. total lung capacity, TLC) is achieved when the most negative pleural pressure that can be developed by inspiratory muscle contraction balances the lung recoil pressure. Clearly, the magnitude of this pleural pressure is dependent on the strength

of the inspiratory muscles. At high volumes some muscular effort is also needed to distend the chest wall (Fig. 1.7a). If the muscles are weak (Fig. 1.7b), less pressure can be applied to the lungs and chest wall, so their expansion is incomplete and their recoil pressures at full inflation are less than normal. If the chest wall is abnormally stiff (Fig. 1.7c), its distension requires a larger proportion of the force applied, attenuating the fall in pleural pressure and thus preventing complete expansion of the lungs. Again, therefore, lung recoil pressure at TLC is less than normal. If the lungs themselves are abnormally stiff (e.g. in pulmonary fibrosis) (Fig. 1.7d), the balance of distending and recoiling pressures is again reached at a lower than normal TLC, but in this case

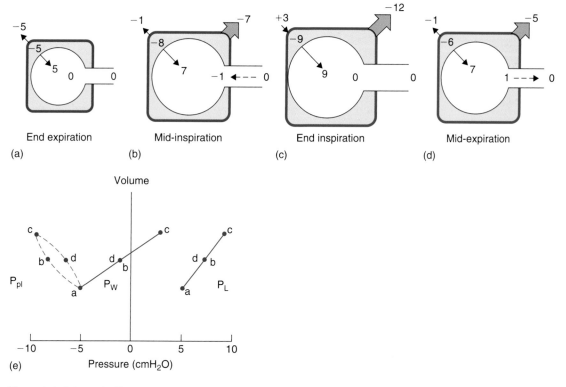

Figure 1.6 Schematic diagram of pressure relationships at various stages of the tidal breathing cycle in a subject with an abnormally stiff chest wall. Conventions are as in Fig. 1.3. The elastic properties of the lungs and the airway resistance are normal and it is assumed that pressures at functional residual capacity (FRC) (a) are normal. The compliance of the chest wall is reduced by 50 per cent compared with the normal subject in Fig. 1.3. As a result, the chest wall recoil for the same tidal volume increases by twice the normal amount between end expiration and end inspiration (c) (i.e. from $-5\,cmH_2O$ to $+3\,cmH_2O$, compared with $-5\,cmH_2O$ to $-1\,cmH_2O$ in Fig. 1.3). As with stiffening of the lungs (Fig. 1.5), greater inspiratory muscle effort is required throughout inspiration but, since this is used to overcome the stiffness of the chest wall, it is not in this case reflected in abnormal swings of pleural pressure (P_{pl}). Again, the extent of expiratory braking (d) is uncertain.

P_L, lung recoil pressure; P_W, chest wall recoil pressure.

lung recoil pressure at TLC is greater than normal because at this lower volume the inspiratory muscles are operating with a better mechanical advantage, such that a maximum effort results in a pleural pressure that is more negative than could be achieved at a normal TLC.

In the converse situation, where the distensibility of the lungs is greater than normal (e.g. in emphysema) (Fig. 1.7e), TLC increases to the point where again there is a balance between inspiratory muscle 'pull' and recoil of the chest wall and lungs. This is reached at a larger TLC because of the considerable diminution of lung recoil pressure in emphysema. It is important to note that in the models shown in Fig. 1.7 the effect of changing only one variable at a

time (active pressure generated by the inspiratory muscles, passive recoil of the lungs or chest wall) has been explored, ignoring any compensatory changes such as undoubtedly occur in disease.

The PV curve of the lungs is the sum on the volume axis of the PV curves of millions of alveoli plus the alveolar ducts and terminal bronchioles and even a small contribution from the conducting airways. At a particular overall lung volume, different alveoli may be at different points on their individual PV curves because of regional differences in pleural pressure induced by gravity (see below). Consequently, at an equivalent lung volume during inspiration and expiration, individual lung units are likely to be contributing to the overall volume in

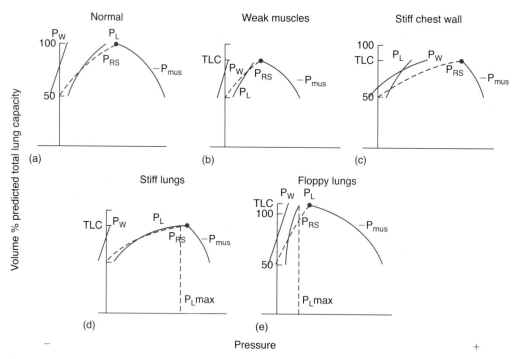

Figure 1.7 Determinants of total lung capacity (TLC) illustrated by pressure–volume relations. (a) In a normal subject TLC is reached when the net pressure generated by the respiratory muscles (P_{mus}) is balanced by the recoil of the respiratory system (P_{RS}). At full inflation with the glottis open, alveolar pressure is zero, and therefore, from Equation 1.5, $P_{RS} = -P_{mus}$. The determinants of TLC are therefore conveniently explored by plotting the mirror image of the curve relating P_{mus} to lung volume on the Rahn diagram. (b) If the inspiratory muscles are weak, P_{mus} is less negative, and the balance $P_{RS} = -P_{mus}$ is reached below the normal TLC. The static pressure–volume curves are therefore truncated, and at the reduced TLC the values of P_{RS} and of maximum lung recoil pressure (P_{L}max – dotted vertical line) are less than normal. (c) If the chest wall is abnormally stiff, chest wall recoil pressure (P_{W}) and therefore P_{RS} are increased and again the balance $P_{RS} = -P_{mus}$ is reached at an abnormally low volume. P_{L}max is less than normal. (d) If the lungs are abnormally stiff, P_{L} and therefore P_{RS} are increased, but in this case P_{L}max is supernormal; the inspiratory muscles at the smaller lung volume are operating at a more favourable length and are able to generate a more negative inspiratory pressure than they can at a normal TLC. (e) If the distensibility of the lungs is increased, P_{L} and therefore P_{RS} are reduced, and the balance $P_{RS} = -P_{mus}$ is reached at a volume above the normal TLC. P_{L}max is below normal.

different proportions. Add to this the fact that the lung recoil pressure measured arises both from tissue elements in the alveolar walls and from the surface film lining the alveoli, and it is, perhaps, surprising that the overall pressure–volume relation of the lungs can be described by a smooth reproducible curve.

1.2.2 Measurement of the lung pressure–volume curve

Construction of the static PV curve of the lungs requires measurements of change in lung volume and the pressure difference between alveoli and pleural surface during breath holding (since, from

Equation 1.3, $P_{L} = P_{alv} - P_{pl}$). The volume change is easily measured by a spirometer or, alternatively, the subject may be seated within a volume displacement body plethysmograph (see below); the transpulmonary (mouth–pleural) pressure can be obtained by measuring oesophageal pressure during breath-holding. A small balloon-tipped catheter or miniature pressure transducer is introduced into the lower third of the oesophagus, usually via the nose. If a balloon is used, a volume of air is introduced that is neither too large to distend the oesophagus nor too small to cause the balloon itself to develop a negative recoil;[2] in practice this is between 0.2 mL and 0.5 mL. The position of the pressure recording device is adjusted up and down usually by trial and error to give the most negative value of pressure at FRC. Alternatively, the depth may be standardized in relation to the subject's height; the data of Zapletal *et al.* suggest positioning the tip of a 10-cm balloon at a depth of (height/5 + 9) cm from the nostril.[3]

The subject is asked to inspire fully and hold his breath at full inflation while the pressure signal stabilizes; the subject then breathes out decrements of volume, holding the breath for 1–2 s at each volume (Fig. 1.8a); if the measurements are made using a spirometer rather than a plethysmograph, the subject should maintain an inspiratory effort during each breath hold. If the subject is allowed to relax (e.g. against a shutter), a correction to the volume is necessary because of the small reduction in lung volume associated with the positive alveolar pressure during relaxation (Boyle's law). A variable-volume plethysmograph (see Section 1.3) has the advantage that this small volume change is measured directly and the true change in thoracic gas volume is obtained. To measure lung recoil pressure at TLC a sustained inspiratory effort is essential because, once the subject relaxes, the resulting positive alveolar pressure reduces the volume of gas in the lungs to a level slightly below TLC and consequently lung recoil pressure is less. The volume change resulting from relaxation is admittedly small: even at full inflation, where the effect is greatest, it amounts to only a small proportion of the lung volume. (For example, if respiratory system recoil at TLC is 40 cmH_2O and atmospheric pressure is 1000 cmH_2O, the absolute alveolar pressure increases during relaxation from 1000 cmH_2O to 1040 cmH_2O, i.e. by 4%, and therefore, according to Boyle's law, lung volume declines by 4%.) But, because of the shape of the PV curve of the lungs, even this small decrement of volume close to full inflation can appreciably reduce the maximum recoil pressure. Thus, in the example shown in Fig. 1.8b, 4 per cent gas compression at TLC would imply a reduction in volume of only 0.3 L but a reduction in recoil pressure of approximately 12 cmH_2O.

Measurements are made during interrupted expiration, usually over the volume range from TLC to FRC as illustrated in Fig. 1.8. Below FRC, the PV relationship deviates from a monophasic curve as small airways close progressively at low lung volumes during deflation.[4] Consequently, the alveoli that these airways subtend no longer contribute to volume change, so that the overall lung compliance falls and the PV curve takes on a sigmoid shape. This appearance is more marked if measurements are made during *inspiration* starting from low volumes (see below). Care needs to be taken in interpretation of oesophageal pressure at low lung volumes as it may be subject to artefacts due to compression of the oesophagus by mediastinal structures.[5]

A line can be fitted by eye to PV data obtained during interrupted expiration, with the static compliance of the lungs estimated by approximating the curve over the tidal breathing range (e.g. FRC to FRC + 0.5 L) to a straight line and measuring its slope. Alternatively, recoil pressures at standard lung volumes (e.g. 60%, 90% TLC) are measured or the whole curve is compared with a normal reference range.[6,7]

Variability of the PV curve between normal individuals is due in part to differences in the size of the lungs, which, in turn, are probably due mainly to variation in alveolar number. The variability can be reduced by expressing lung volume as a percentage of either the predicted or actual TLC. The former aims to take account only of body size (which is an important determinant of TLC); the latter takes account also of variation in size of the lungs. In normal subjects the distinction usually matters little. However, it is more important in disease, when expressing lung volume as 'per cent predicted TLC' is usually the more relevant since it allows comparison between subjects of different body size, without concealing any information related to differences in lung size caused by disease. For the same reason, it may be more appropriate to express the compliance not as litres per cmH_2O but as per cent predicted TLC per cmH_2O. As an approximation, the average normal value is about 4 per cent predicted TLC cmH_2O^{-1}.[8]

Because of the problems of size correction of a curvilinear relationship, various mathematical models have been fitted to the overall curve. The most successful is a monoexponential function; this usually fits the data well, at least over the volume range TLC to FRC. The most useful parameter of such a monoexponential function is the volume-independent shape factor, K (Fig. 1.9).[9]

The PV relationship is dependent on the preceding breathing pattern ('volume history'); conventionally, the expiratory curve is recorded after two or three full inspirations to distend the lungs,

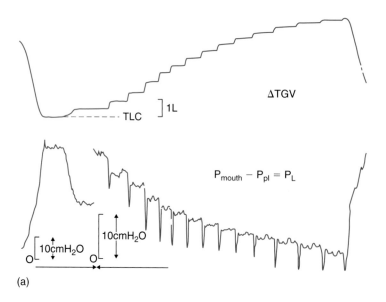

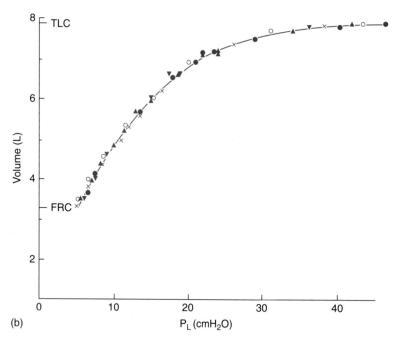

Figure 1.8 Construction of static pressure–volume (PV) curve of the lungs. (a) Record of volume expired (upper trace) and transpulmonary pressure ($P_{mouth} - P_{pl}$) during interrupted expiration. During breath-holding, alveolar pressure (P_{alv}) equals mouth pressure (P_{mouth}), therefore: $P_{mouth} - P_{pl} = P_{alv} - P_{pl} = P_L$ (Equation 1.3). From the plateau values of volume and pressure, the static expiratory PV curve is constructed. (b) Diagram showing such a curve drawn by eye through points recorded from five separate deflation manoeuvres from total lung capacity (TLC) to functional residual capacity (FRC).

P_L, lung recoil pressure; P_{pl}, pleural surface pressure.

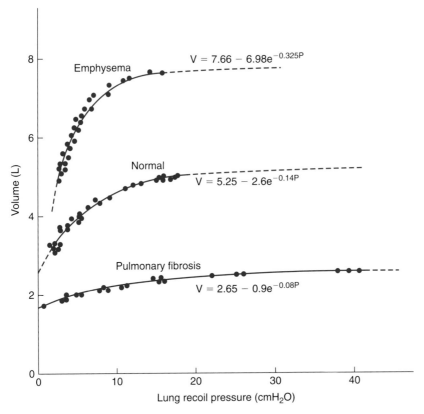

Figure 1.9 Monoexponential functions fitted mathematically to pressure–volume (PV) curves from a normal subject (middle curve) and patients with emphysema (upper curve) and pulmonary fibrosis (lower curve). The fitted function is of the form $V = V_{max} - Ae^{-KP}$, where V_{max} is the asymptotic extrapolated 'maximum' volume at $P = \infty$, A is a constant related to the intercept of the curve on the volume axis and K is a volume-independent shape factor. K is characteristically increased in emphysema and is reduced in some patients with pulmonary fibrosis. Values of K in the examples shown are $0.14\,cmH_2O^{-1}$, $0.325\,cmH_2O^{-1}$ and $0.08\,cmH_2O^{-1}$ in normal, emphysema and pulmonary fibrosis, respectively.

ensuring that the maximum number of alveoli are functioning and contributing to the measurement.

1.2.3 Inspiratory and quasistatic pressure–volume curves of lungs

If measurements are made during inspiration rather than expiration, the recoil pressure measured at a given lung volume is rather greater (Fig. 1.10). The difference is due partly to hysteresis of alveolar tissue, but quantitatively more important is the effect of different numbers of lung units contributing to a given lung volume during expiration and inspiration. During expiration some small airways close (see Chapter 2, Section 2.1.10), and

during the subsequent inspiration they reopen only when a critical opening pressure is reached; the alveoli subtended by these airways therefore make no contribution to the overall volume change until airway opening occurs. Hence, on inspiration, a given lung volume is likely to imply a smaller number of more distended (and therefore less compliant) alveoli than on expiration.

The full expiratory and inspiratory PV curve of the lung can also be constructed by recording pleural pressure during continuous slow expiration and inspiration.[4] With care the relationship obtained (quasistatic PV curve) closely approximates that constructed by fitting curves to points measured during stepwise interruption of airflow.

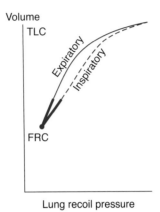

Figure 1.10 Theoretical static pressure–volume (PV) curve of the lung obtained during interrupted expiration (solid line) and interrupted inspiration (broken line) between functional residual capacity (FRC) and total lung capacity (TLC). The inspiratory curve is displaced to higher recoil pressures and the compliance in the tidal range (heavy lines) is lower on inspiration.

1.2.4 Clinical use of static pressure–volume curves

Pressure–volume curves are rarely measured nowadays in routine assessment of patients in the clinical lung function laboratory, although they are often applied in research studies of detailed lung mechanics. In recent years there has, however, been a resurgence of interest in their clinical value in patients with severe lung disease such as the acute respiratory distress syndrome (ARDS), who require positive pressure ventilation. In this condition many alveoli are filled with fluid, airway closure occurs more readily and the small airways have abnormally large opening pressures, exaggerating the difference between expiratory and inspiratory PV curves and requiring high ventilator pressures to maintain gas exchange. Some ventilators can be programmed to derive static or quasi-static PV curves of the respiratory system in patients undergoing positive-pressure ventilation, with the results used as a guide to ventilator management (see Chapter 13, Section 13.5).[10]

1.2.5 Dynamic lung compliance

Conventionally, the PV curve of the lungs is plotted with a positive recoil pressure (Rahn diagram, Fig. 1.1), but for some purposes the mirror image curve (Campbell diagram),[11] where pleural pressure during breath-holding is plotted against lung volume, is more useful (Fig. 1.11). Visualizing PV relationships in this way allows comparison between the pleural pressure developed statically during breath-holding and dynamically during breathing. In theory, the former is overcoming only static forces, while the latter has to overcome both elastic and resistive forces. In the early twentieth century the Swiss physiologist Rohrer analysed theoretically the elastic and resistive forces involved in breathing; his compatriots Neergaard and Wirz extended his work by suggesting that measuring pleural pressure at the points of zero airflow, i.e. end inspiration and end expiration, would eliminate the contribution of flow-resistive forces, so that lung distensibility alone could be assessed during tidal breathing. On a plot of pleural pressure against volume during tidal breathing (Fig. 1.11), the slope of the line joining the volume extremes (where flow is assumed to be zero) is known as the dynamic compliance of the lungs. In normal subjects dynamic compliance is slightly less than compliance measured during interrupted expiration,[7] and it is usually closer to the static inspiratory compliance. In diseased lungs, however, the static and dynamic measurements may diverge markedly. Because the damage caused by most diseases is not uniform throughout the lungs, cessation of airflow at the mouth does not coincide with cessation of airflow within the lungs. Redistribution of air, or *Pendelluft*, continues in the lungs after flow has ceased (or even reversed) at the mouth. As a result some of the pleural pressure measured when airflow has ceased at the mouth (and therefore apparently overcoming elastic forces) is actually being dissipated against resistive forces. Thus, the 'elastic' pressure is overestimated and the true compliance of the lungs is underestimated. Consequently in diseased lungs the dynamic compliance falls as the frequency of breathing increases. Paradoxically, for an apparent index of lung elasticity, this 'frequency dependence of dynamic compliance' is sometimes used as a test for early disease of the peripheral airways.[12]

1.2.6 Elastic properties of the chest wall

The PV curve of the chest wall of normal subjects is approximately linear between FRC and TLC, with chest wall recoil negative (i.e. outward) at FRC and positive at TLC (Fig. 1.1). At full inflation the recoil

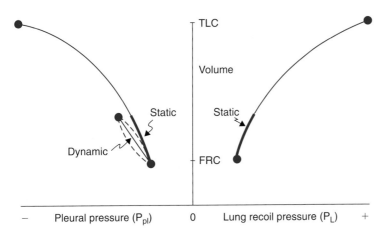

Figure 1.11 Static pressure–volume (PV) curve of the lungs (right-hand panel) with mirror-image curve representing pleural pressure (P_{pl}) during breath-holding at various lung volumes (left-hand panel). The loop indicated by the broken line represents pleural pressure during a tidal breath, and the slope of the line joining points of zero airflow represents 'dynamic lung compliance', which is usually less than static compliance measured during interrupted expiration.

P_L, lung recoil pressure.

of the total respiratory system is determined mainly by the elastic recoil of the lungs, which, numerically, normally greatly exceeds the recoil of the chest wall. At decreasing volumes below FRC the chest wall resists deflation more and more markedly, i.e. chest wall compliance declines progressively and consequently its recoil becomes very negative. Transdiaphragmatic pressure (P_{di}) measurements show that this outward recoil at low volumes is due to downward (caudal) recoil of the diaphragm, which is stretched by the abdominal (expiratory) muscles contracting to reduce volume below FRC.[13]

In the conscious subject the PV curve of the chest wall is difficult to construct reliably. In principle it can be obtained by measuring oesophageal pressure during relaxation against a closed airway during stepwise inflation or deflation, but complete relaxation is difficult to ensure. An alternative technique, which requires less cooperation from the subject, is that of Heaf and Prime, where measurements of mouth and oesophageal pressures are made during breathing against positive and negative pressures applied at the mouth to produce shifts in end expiratory thoracic volume.[14] In practice, consistent measurements of the compliance of the chest wall are difficult to achieve, even in trained subjects; measurements made in the conscious subject differ from those under general anaesthesia and muscle paralysis, because normal muscle tone contributes to the 'passive' recoil pressure of the chest wall.[15]

In disease, alterations in lung (or chest wall) compliance are usually mirrored by changes in lung volume and, in particular, total lung capacity: 'stiff' lungs are usually small, and 'floppy' lungs usually large (Fig. 1.7). Consequently, the need for direct PV measurements can usually be obviated by measurement of vital capacity (VC) and TLC.

1.3 MEASUREMENTS OF LUNG VOLUME AND ITS SUBDIVISIONS

The classical subdivisions of lung volume are illustrated in Fig. 1.12.

1.3.1 Spirometers

In general, measurement of the volume of air inspired or expired may be required for two very different purposes: either continuous monitoring of ventilation over a period of time, or single manoeuvres such as forced expiration. A spirometer measures the volumes of air inspired and expired but is not able to measure the absolute volume of air in the lungs.

The traditional water-filled spirometer comprises a cylinder inverted in a trough of water (Fig. 1.13a). The level of the cylinder is determined by the volume of air within, and this varies as the subject breathes in and out. It was derived from the gas holder or 'gazometer' used by the pioneering

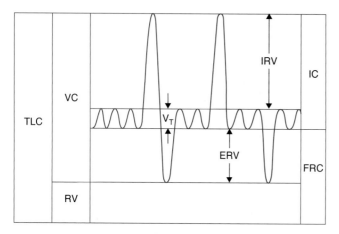

Figure 1.12 Classical subdivisions of lung volume, showing tidal breathing, full inspiration to total lung capacity (TLC), and full expiration to residual volume (RV).

ERV, expiratory reserve volume (FRC − RV); FRC, functional residual capacity; IC, inspiratory capacity (TLC − FRC); IRV, inspiratory reserve volume (IC − V_T); V_T, tidal volume.

chemists of the eighteenth century such as Priestley and Lavoisier and was refined as a spirometer for general use in human subjects by Hutchinson in the mid-nineteenth century.[16] The size of a water-filled spirometer depends on its purpose; most commonly its capacity is about 11 L, but a very large version (Tissot), used for collecting expired air over several minutes, may contain up to 100 L of gas. The movement of the air-containing cylinder is registered by a pen on a revolving kymograph. A variant is the Krogh spirometer, in which the gas is collected in a wedge-shaped bell, pivoted along one edge, with the angular displacement of the bell recorded by a suitable transducer.

The classical water-containing spirometer was largely replaced by 'dry' instruments such as the bellows spirometer (e.g. the 'Vitalograph') (Fig. 1.13b) or the 'rolling seal' spirometer, which consists of a piston moving along a large-bore drum (Fig. 1.13c). More commonly nowadays, devices that measure flow are used, with volume derived by electrical integration of the flow measured at the mouth. The principle underlying the pneumotachograph (Fig. 1.14a) is the physical equivalent of Ohm's Law in an electrical circuit:

Flow = pressure difference/resistance

(Compare with current (I) = potential difference (E or V)/resistance (R).)

Hence, if the resistance of the instrument is known and the pressure drop across it is measured by a suitable pressure transducer, flow is readily obtained; electrical integration of the flow signal with respect to time then gives the volume inspired or expired. Other types of portable spirometer include rotating-vane, heated-wire and fixed-orifice devices.

1.3.2   Whole-body plethysmograph

The whole-body plethysmograph has several uses but most commonly it is used for measurement of the absolute volume of gas in the lungs, from which the various subdivisions of lung volume can be derived (Fig. 1.12). In the most commonly used type, the constant volume plethysmograph (Fig. 1.15a), described by DuBois and colleagues,[17] the subject is completely enclosed in a rigid air-tight chamber. A pneumotachograph at the mouth measures airflow and a shutter is used to close the airway as required. The basic principle on which the plethysmograph operates is that stated by Boyle's law: at constant temperature, the pressure exerted by a gas is inversely proportional to its volume ($P \times V$ is constant or $P_1V_1 = P_2V_2$). Plethysmography utilizes the fact that, during breathing, changes in lung volume occur for two reasons. The more obvious is the mass movement of molecules of gas into and out of the lungs.

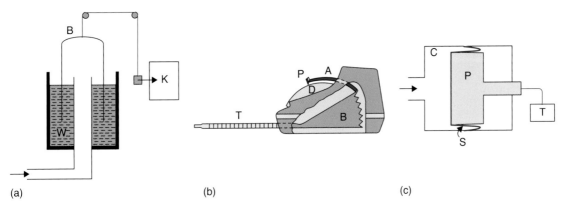

Figure 1.13 Spirometers that measure volume directly: (a) water-filled spirometer comprising a lightweight counterbalanced bell (B) inverted over water (W) and attached to a direct writing pen and kymograph (K) via a pulley system. (b) 'Vitalograph'-type wedge spirometer sealed by bellows (B). Expansion of the bellows produced by forceful expiration via tube (T) is recorded by arm (A) attached to pen (P), which moves across paper on drum (D). (c) Rolling-seal spirometer comprising a wide-bore cylinder (C) along which a piston (P) travels. The piston is attached around the internal circumference of the cylinder by a thin flexible rolling seal (S), which reduces the resistance to movement of the piston. A transducer (T) measures the linear displacement of the piston, which is proportional to volume change.

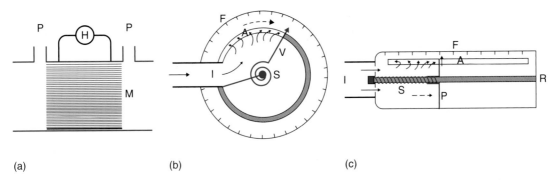

Figure 1.14 (a) Fleisch pneumotachograph. The resistance of the delicate wire mesh (M) is effectively constant over the working range of the instrument. Pressure difference is measured between either end of the mesh (P) by a differential transducer. Flow is calculated by application of Ohm's law or is calibrated directly. A heater coil (H) may be used to maintain body temperature pressure saturated (BTPS) conditions by heating the instrument to 37°C. (b) Original Wright peak flow meter. Air is forcibly expired through a radial inlet (I) and escapes via an aperture (A) opened by radial motion of a pivoted vane (V). Motion of the vane is opposed by a spring (S). The aperture is uncovered and movement of the vane is proportional to the peak expiratory flow (PEF) indicated by the pointer on the calibrated scale of flow (F). Solid arrows indicate the direction of airflow and the broken arrow indicates the motion of the vane. (c) Mini Wright peak flow meter. Air is forcibly expired into a cylinder and escapes via a longitudinal aperture (A) opened by motion of a lightweight piston (P) along a central rod (R). Motion of the piston is opposed by a spring (S). As the piston travels, the aperture is uncovered in proportion to the PEF and the piston moves a small pointer along the calibrated scale of flow (F). Solid arrows indicate the direction of airflow and the broken arrow indicates the motion of the piston.

In addition, however, because during inspiration alveolar pressure is inevitably slightly less than atmospheric pressure, and during expiration slightly greater than atmospheric pressure, there is alternating rarefaction and compression of intrathoracic gas. Bulk movement of gas is quantitatively much the more important during normal breathing, but if breathing efforts continue against a closed airway the second mechanism still operates and its magnitude can be quantified by the accompanying reciprocal changes in pressure within the rigid box. These pressure changes are utilized in the measurement of absolute thoracic gas volume (see below).

The second type of whole-body plethysmograph is the variable volume or volume displacement instrument (Fig. 1.15b,c).[18,19] Here the subject breathes in and out from the surrounding atmosphere rather than from the box itself, and the instrument allows continuous recording of the accompanying changes in thoracic volume. The plethysmograph therefore acts essentially as a spirometer, but measuring changes in thoracic gas volume rather than volume expired. The information obtained differs from that recorded with a conventional spirometer as chest movements include volume changes resulting from rarefaction (during inspiration) and compression (during expiration) of thoracic gas, in addition to the volumes inspired and expired. In the original instrument described by Mead,[18] volume is displaced into and out of a lightweight water-filled wedge (Krogh) spirometer (Fig. 1.15b). An alternative (Fig. 1.15c), which is more commonly used, is to incorporate a pneumotachograph into the wall of the box, across which flow is measured and electrically integrated to give the change in thoracic volume.[19]

1.3.3   Measurement of lung volumes by plethysmography

For measurement of absolute lung volume by plethysmography, either a constant-volume[17] (Fig. 1.15a) or variable-volume[18,19] (Fig. 1.15b,c) instrument can be used. The former is more commonly employed, but the principle is easier to appreciate by considering the variable volume instrument.

A shutter in the mouthpiece is closed transiently, usually at end tidal expiration (FRC), and the subject is asked to make inspiratory and expiratory efforts against it. Bulk movement of gas into and out of the lungs is thus prevented, but during inspiratory efforts the negative (i.e. subatmospheric) alveolar pressure produces slight rarefaction of alveolar gas so that thoracic volume increases a little, displacing a volume (ΔV) of gas into the box spirometer or through the flow screen. From Boyle's law ($P_1 V_1 = P_2 V_2$), at any instant during an inspiratory effort against the shutter, the original thoracic gas volume (V) is related to the degree of rarefaction (ΔV) and to the accompanying fall in alveolar pressure (ΔP) as follows:

$$P_1 V_1 = (P_1 - \Delta P)(V_1 + \Delta V)$$

where P_1 is barometric pressure. Therefore, by expansion of the brackets:

$$P_1 V_1 = P_1 V_1 - V_1 \Delta P + P_1 \Delta V - \Delta P \Delta V$$

Since ΔP and ΔV are both very small, their product can be ignored, and therefore:

$$V_1 = P_1 (\Delta V / \Delta P) \qquad (1.6)$$

With the shutter closed, it is assumed that no airflow is occurring during panting efforts; consequently, in this situation (unlike during breathing), the change in alveolar pressure equals the change in pressure at the mouth, where it is measured by a suitable transducer; ΔV is measured directly by the plethysmograph as the displaced volume. Mouth pressure (i.e. alveolar pressure, provided the shutter is closed) is displayed against ΔV on a visual display unit (VDU), and the slope of the resulting line ($\Delta V / \Delta P$) is substituted in Equation 1.6. As soon as the shutter opens, the subject is asked to inspire fully to TLC, and this volume is added to the measured thoracic gas volume (TGV) to give total lung capacity. Subtraction of VC then gives residual volume (RV).

With a constant-volume plethysmograph (Fig. 1.16),[17] ΔV is not measured directly but is reflected by changes in box pressure since the rarefaction of thoracic gas accompanying an inspiratory effort against a closed airway produces a proportional rise in pressure within the rigid box. The pressure change is calibrated in terms of the change in lung volume by introducing a known volume of gas, usually from a small pump, while the subject sits inside the plethysmograph holding his breath.

The whole-body plethysmograph measures all thoracic gas and, indeed, all gas within the body that shares the pressure changes resulting from breathing efforts. This would include an emphysematous bulla, a pneumothorax and, possibly, abdominal gas. The possible contribution of the latter is complex as it depends not only on the volume of gas below the diaphragm but also on the breathing pattern that the subject adopts during the measurement (Fig. 1.17). If inspiratory efforts are made mainly with the diaphragm, abdominal pressure increases as pleural pressure becomes more negative; but if the subject

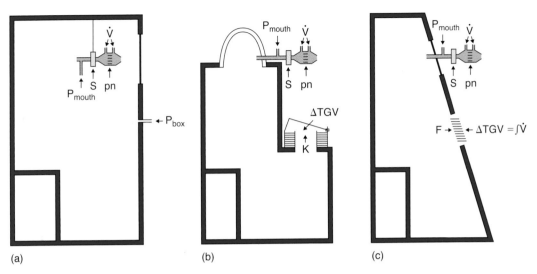

(a)   (b)   (c)

Figure 1.15 Three types of whole-body plethysmograph. (a) Constant-volume plethysmograph: the subject is completely enclosed and breathes in and out *from the box*. Mouth pressure (P_{mouth}) and box pressure (P_{box}) are measured by individual transducers, and the mouthpiece is attached to a shutter assembly (S) and pneumotachograph (pn) across which flow ($\dot{V}$) is measured by a third transducer. (b) Variable-volume box with Krogh water-filled spirometer (K): the mouthpiece is connected to the exterior and attached to a shutter (S) and pneumotachograph (pn). As the subject inspires air *from outside the box*, the subject's thoracic expansion (ΔTGV) displaces an equal volume of air (at body temperature pressure saturated, BTPS) into the low-impedance spirometer. (c) Variable-volume box with flow screen (F): similar to (b), except that ΔTGV (BTPS) is obtained by integration of flow across the flow screen (a second pneumotachograph) in the wall of the box.

TGV, thoracic gas volume.

uses the intercostal or accessory muscles relatively more than the diaphragm, the abdominal pressure largely follows pleural pressure. In the former case, compression of abdominal gas occurs, which to a minor extent would offset the rarefaction of thoracic gas, while in the latter situation, gas both above and below the diaphragm is rarefied. The former will therefore lead to slight underestimation, and the latter to slight overestimation, of the volume of thoracic gas. The effect is small because the volume of abdominal gas is small relative to thoracic gas; most subjects pant predominantly with the ribcage muscles so that the net effect is usually overestimation of TGV by 200–300 mL.[20]

A potentially more important error can occur in patients with airway obstruction, in whom changes in mouth pressure during panting against a shutter may be less than changes in alveolar pressure. If the airway resistance is high, there is an inevitable slight delay in equilibration of alveolar and mouth pressures during this manoeuvre such that they become out of phase with each other; the consequent underestimation of change in alveolar pressure

during panting against a shutter results in overestimation of thoracic gas volume (Fig. 1.18).[21,22] This artefact is greater the narrower the airways, the more compliant the upper airway and the more rapidly the subject pants. It can be largely negated, even in patients with airway obstruction, by the subject supporting the cheeks and floor of the mouth with his hands (reducing the compliance of the mouth and pharynx) and by panting gently and slowly, with a frequency of less than 1 Hz (allowing more time for mouth and alveolar pressures to equalize, thereby minimizing the phase difference between the two measurements).

1.3.4 Measurement of lung volumes by inert gas dilution

To estimate lung volumes by the closed circuit inert gas method,[23] the subject rebreathes a gas mixture containing a measured concentration of an inert gas, usually helium (Fig. 1.19). The gas gradually equilibrates with the resident gas in the lungs, and the helium concentration falls progressively, and

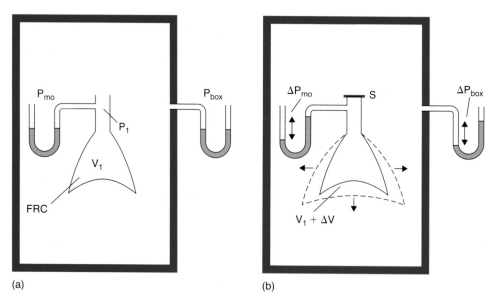

(a)   (b)

Figure 1.16 Measurement of thoracic gas volume (TGV) using a constant-volume plethysmograph. (a) Conditions during breath-holding with open airway at lung volume V_1 (e.g. functional residual capacity, FRC), at which alveolar pressure is atmospheric; mouth pressure (P_{mo}) and box pressure (P_{box}) are also atmospheric. (b) Situation during a gentle inspiratory effort against a shutter (S), which has been closed at the mouth; alveolar pressure is now subatmospheric, as registered by manometer recording P_{mo} on the patient side of the shutter. Rarefaction of intrathoracic gas produces a small increase (ΔV) in lung volume, which causes a predictable increase in P_{box}. See text for further amplification.

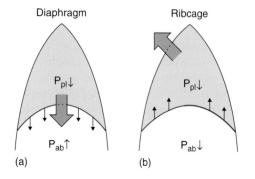

Figure 1.17 Effects of panting with different inspiratory muscles on estimates of thoracic gas volume (TGV). If the diaphragm alone is used (a), abdominal pressure (P_{ab}) increases as pleural surface pressure (P_{pl}) decreases; therefore abdominal gas is compressed as thoracic gas is rarefied and TGV is underestimated. If the ribcage muscles (inspiratory intercostals ± accessory muscles) predominate (b), both P_{ab} and P_{pl} decrease with inspiratory efforts, so that both thoracic and abdominal gas are rarefied and TGV is overestimated.

stabilizes once mixing is complete. The circuit includes a spirometer and helium analyser; carbon dioxide (CO_2) is absorbed from the circuit to prevent stimulation of breathing, and oxygen has to be

added continuously to keep the total volume of gas (breathing circuit plus subject's lungs) constant. The subject is usually switched in at the end of a normal expiration (FRC) and the spirometer record is monitored continuously so that sufficient oxygen can be added to maintain a stable end expiratory volume. It is recommended that the subject continues until the helium concentration falls by no more than 0.02 per cent over a 30-s period.[24] At the end of the procedure the subject takes a full inspiration and the measured inspiratory capacity is added to the FRC to give TLC, followed by a VC expiration to give RV. In a normal subject, mixing is effectively complete and a stable helium concentration achieved in 5–10 min. In patients with airway disease, mixing is much slower and the end point may be somewhat arbitrary.

In normal subjects, plethysmographic and dilutional estimates of TLC are very close, but large differences can be seen in patients with airway disease. A bulla represents an extreme cause of such discrepancies, since most bullae are virtually unventilated, but all patients with significant airflow obstruction have some areas of lung where ventilation is very slow; this is the most common

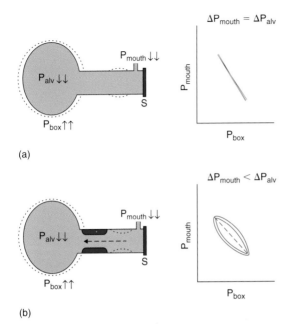

$$\Delta P_{mouth} = \Delta P_{alv}$$

$$\Delta P_{mouth} < \Delta P_{alv}$$

(a)

(b)

Figure 1.18 Potential overestimation of thoracic gas volume by plethysmography. (a) In a normal subject, the fall in alveolar pressure (P_{alv}) during an inspiratory effort against the shutter (S) occurs almost simultaneously with an equivalent fall in mouth pressure (P_{mouth}), so that the plot of P_{mouth} against box pressure (p_{box}) is a straight line. (b) With a high airway resistance, there is a time delay (phase difference) between changes in P_{alv} and P_{mouth}, so that the plot of P_{mouth} against P_{box} shows looping, as the change in P_{mouth} underestimates the change in P_{alv}. Applying Boyle's law using P_{mouth} as the index of P_{alv} in this situation results in overestimation of lung volume. The artefact is increased at higher panting frequencies and with a more compliant upper airway.

cause of differences between the results of the helium dilution and plethysmographic techniques. Both the potential overestimation of TGV by plethysmography and the almost inevitable under-estimation by helium dilution are a consequence of the same pathological changes, i.e. generalized airway narrowing and the resulting uneven distribution of inspired gas.

Even simpler is estimation of lung volume by dilution of inert gas during a single breath that is held at full inflation for a standard period. Such an estimate is obtained during measurement of single breath diffusing capacity (transfer factor) for carbon monoxide (see Chapter 3, Section 3.1). This 'alveolar volume' (V_A) is close to TLC in healthy lungs, but in airway disease the reservations relating to the rebreathing estimate apply even more strongly to V_A, which underestimates TLC to a greater extent.

1.3.5 Measurement of lung volumes using imaging techniques

Another approach to measurement of lung volumes is the use of radiographic imaging. Total lung capacity can be estimated using good-quality posteroanterior and lateral radiographs taken at full inspiration with a standard target–film distance of 2 m: using hard copy films the lung field is divided into a series of elliptical 'slices', the volumes of which are calculated from measurements made in three dimensions.[25] The volume of the heart is calculated and subtracted and assumptions are made about volumes of tissue and blood. Good concordance with plethysmographic estimates can be obtained in normal subjects, but the validity of the technique in diseased lungs is less certain. Use of digitizing computer techniques relieves the tedium of the calculations.[26] More recently, computer programs have been developed for calculation of lung volumes from helical computed tomography (CT) scans. Comparison with plethysmographic measurements of TLC shows good correlation but consistent underestimation by about 12 per cent, attributable mainly to the different postures (supine and upright respectively) in which CT scanning and plethysmography are performed.[27] The CT method has the advantage that the volume of each lung individually is readily obtainable.[28]

1.4 MEASUREMENTS OF VENTILATION

Measurements of minute ventilation are commonly made during both metabolic investigation and exercise testing. The classic methods include use of a large water-filled spirometer or measuring the volume of gas breathed via a dry gas meter or expired into a Douglas bag over a defined period. These methods have largely been replaced by integration of airflow, employing similar technology to that utilized by modern spirometers. However, all have the disadvantage that the application of a mouthpiece, facemask or other interface can change the breathing pattern and increase resting ventilation.[29]

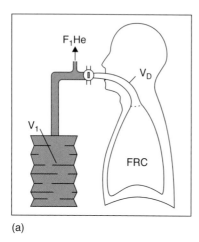 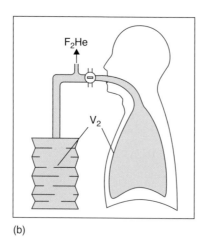

(a)   (b)

Figure 1.19 Closed-circuit inert gas method for measuring lung volumes. (a) The subject is attached to a reservoir circuit of volume V_1, containing gas with initial helium concentration F_1He. (b) After rebreathing and equilibration, the concentration of helium falls to F_2He and the new volume (V_2) in which it is diluted equals the sum of the circuit, V_1 and the lung volume (usually functional residual capacity, FRC) at which the subject was connected. The two helium concentrations are measured and, together with the volume of the circuit, are used to calculate lung volume. V_D, dead space.

Breathing tends to become more regular and the increase in ventilation is due mainly to an increase in tidal volume, associated with a switch from nasal to mouth-breathing.[30] These effects can be avoided by various non-invasive external measurements of chest wall movement, such as are widely applied for medium-term monitoring, e.g. during sleep. The types of device utilized are listed in Table 1.1. The simplest is a stethograph: this measures ribcage circumference but gives very incomplete information as, functionally, the 'chest wall' comprises not only the ribcage but also the diaphragm and abdomen, the motion of which contributes to enlargement of the thoracic cavity.

Other devices of varying sophistication have been developed to monitor ventilation semi-quantitatively. Accurate estimation is possible in normal subjects from external recordings of both ribcage and abdominal movement using the principle developed by Konno and Mead.[31] They showed that the total displacement of the chest wall could be measured by summing the volume changes of the two compartments. In normal subjects during tidal breathing these are related almost linearly to changes in their anteroposterior (AP) diameters. The AP diameters can be measured by two pairs of small electromagnets (magnetometers) (Fig. 1.20). Their signals are calibrated

in terms of relative volume change by an 'isovolume' manoeuvre, in which the subject with closed mouth and wearing a noseclip makes gentle breathing efforts, shifting volume back and forth between ribcage and abdomen. For accurate results the posture needs to be unchanging and, to avoid problems of gas compression and distortions of shape, the efforts are kept small. Ribcage and abdominal dimensions are displayed on a VDU in x–y mode and, since the total thoracic gas volume is virtually constant during the manoeuvre, adjustment of the amplifier gains to give an angle of 45 degrees (i.e. a slope of −1) allows immediate calibration in terms of the relative volume change of the two compartments (Fig. 1.21). Calibration in terms of absolute volume may then be achieved by comparison of the summed signal with that recorded by a spirometer.

A similar isovolume calibration can be performed when using other external devices such as the respiratory inductance plethysmograph (RIP), but here the relationship established is between cross-sectional area and volume, rather than between diameter and volume (Fig. 1.20). Alternatively, calibration can be performed by utilizing the effect of change in posture. The contributions of abdominal and ribcage movement to the overall tidal volume normally change with posture, such that, in the supine

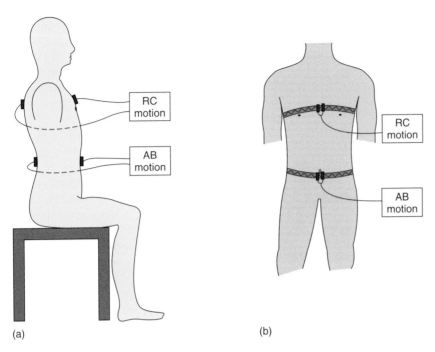

(a)

(b)

Figure 1.20 Measurement of chest wall motion by (a) magnetometers that record anteroposterior (AP) diameter and (b) inductance coils to measure cross-sectional areas of ribcage (RC) and abdomen (AB).

Table 1.1 Measurement of ventilation from external dimensions

Technique	Measurements
Magnetometry	AP diameter
Stethography	Circumference
Respiratory inductance plethysmography	Cross-sectional area
Optoelectronic plethysmography	Volume

AP, anteroposterior.

position, motion of the abdomen is relatively greater than when the subject is upright. To calculate the tidal volume from the two cross-sectional areas requires two calibration factors that relate the volume change of each individual compartment to its change in area. If measurements are made in two postures and compared with a spirometer signal, this produces two simultaneous equations, the solution of which should provide the two unknown calibration factors. This method is, however, open to the objection that the calibration factors themselves vary with posture. Other methods that can be applied for either magnetometers[32] or the inductance plethysmograph[33] utilize the natural breath-to-breath variation in a single posture; using a computer, the volume recorded at the mouth (with a spirometer or by integration of airflow) is compared with the signals from ribcage and abdominal motion for each of several breaths, in order to derive best-fit calibration factors, which are then applied to measure ventilation. Equally accurate results have been reported in lean, healthy subjects using standard ratios of the gains of ribcage and abdominal dimensional changes to calculate ventilation.[34] A portable version of the respiratory inductance plethysmograph suitable for use during exercise has been reported to give promising results.[35] Methods based on only one or two dimensions to represent volume changes are likely to be less accurate in patients with lung disease in whom chest wall motion can be complex and distorted. Much more detailed information is available with the technique of 'optoelectronic plethysmography'.[36] This utilizes a large number (more than 80) of small reflective

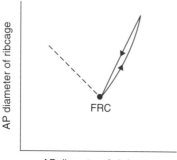

Figure 1.21 Anteroposterior (AP) diameter of ribcage plotted against AP diameter of abdomen – the so-called Konno–Mead display.[31] During tidal breathing (solid line) the two components of the chest wall move together, but slight looping may be seen. During an isovolume manoeuvre (broken line) they are out of phase. Adjustment of the amplifier gains to give a slope of −1 (i.e. an angle of 45°) allows calibration of relative linear dimensions in terms of volume change.

FRC, functional residual capacity.

markers on the anterior and posterior surfaces of the trunk, from which light is reflected from an infrared source to television (TV) cameras linked to a computer (Fig. 1.22). The computer program uses the three-dimensional coordinates of the markers to calculate the chest wall surface area by triangulation and hence derives changes in overall chest wall and compartmental volumes. Studies to date report good accuracy, even in patients with a distorted chest wall due to pulmonary hyperinflation.

1.5 RESPIRATORY MUSCLE FUNCTION

1.5.1 Actions of the respiratory muscles

The major inspiratory muscle is the diaphragm, which forms a musculotendinous partition between the thoracic and abdominal cavities. Its geometry is quite complex. Goldman and Mead pointed out that during tidal breathing there exists a large circumferential surface below the lungs where the superior surface of the diaphragm and the inner surface of the ribcage are in intimate contact (Fig. 1.23).[37] With a moment's thought, this important point is self-evident, but the significance of this 'zone of apposition' had not

previously been appreciated. During inspiration the diaphragmatic muscle fibres shorten and the diaphragm as a whole moves caudally in piston-like fashion. The zone of apposition therefore acts as a reserve of intrathoracic surface, diminishing as lung volume increases. It is greater in the supine position where FRC is smaller.

As the diaphragm contracts it lowers pleural pressure and increases abdominal pressure. The reduction in pleural pressure produces an inflationary effect on the lungs. The effect on the ribcage of lowering P_{pl}, however, would be deflationary unless other effects were operative. The complex arrangement of the diaphragm ensures that this deflationary tendency is more than outweighed by the inflationary effect of increasing abdominal pressure (via the zone of apposition) and by a further inflationary effect consequent on the insertions of the diaphragm in the lower ribs (Fig. 1.24). Electromyography (EMG) during quiet tidal breathing shows that phasic inspiratory activity is present also in the inspiratory intercostal, parasternal and scalene muscles.[38] Formerly regarded as 'accessory' inspiratory muscles, these are more appropriately regarded as primary muscles of inspiration. During deeper or more forceful inspiration, other (truly accessory) muscles become active, the most important being the sternomastoids. In disease, where the load on the inspiratory muscles is increased, the accessory muscles are more active and contract even during resting tidal inspiration.

The main expiratory muscles are the muscles of the abdominal wall. In normal subjects they are inactive during tidal breathing but expiratory EMG activity is detectable in some patients with chronic lung disease, most notably in the deepest muscle layer, the transversus abdominis.[39] In healthy subjects they become active during exercise; their other important respiratory function is the generation of large positive intrathoracic pressures during coughing.

1.5.2 Volitional tests

Although assessment of the passive static mechanical properties of the chest wall is difficult and of limited value, simple measurements of maximum static performance are easily applied and often useful.

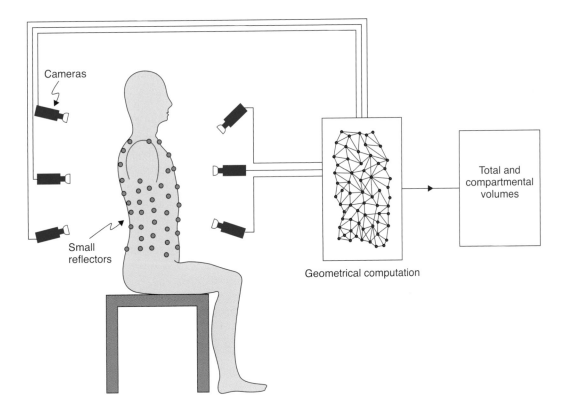

Figure 1.22 Optoelectronic plethysmography. Light shone on a number of small reflective markers attached to the trunk is detected by an array of cameras and fed to a computer, which reconstructs a three-dimensional model of the chest wall (ribcage and abdominal) shape and motion by triangulation.

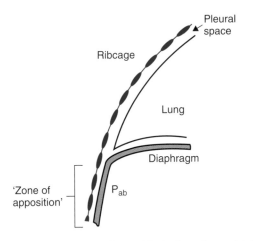

Figure 1.23 'Zone of apposition' where the parietal pleura lining the internal surface of the ribcage is in contact with the parietal pleura lining the thoracic surface of the diaphragm. This zone provides a reserve of surface to allow lung expansion. Abdominal pressure (P_{ab}) has an important influence on ribcage expansion because of this area of contact.

1.5.2.1 Maximum static respiratory pressures

At the simplest level, respiratory muscle power can be assessed by having the subject blow forcefully against a column of mercury, the height of which registers the maximum expiratory pressure. In practice, a simple pressure transducer is more convenient. Rohrer[40] and later Rahn et al.[1] made systematic measurements of maximum static expiratory and inspiratory pressures at different lung volumes, and showed that the highest expiratory pressures were recorded close to TLC and the most negative inspiratory pressures at low volumes (Fig. 1.25). This corresponds to the predicted consequences of the length–tension properties of the respiratory muscles, since at TLC the expiratory muscles are at their greatest (i.e. optimal) length, but the inspiratory muscles are at their shortest, while the converse applies at volumes close to RV.

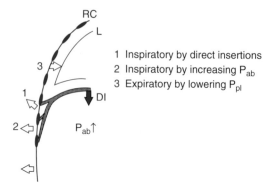

1 Inspiratory by direct insertions
2 Inspiratory by increasing P_{ab}
3 Expiratory by lowering P_{pl}

Figure 1.24 Actions of the diaphragm (DI) on the chest wall of a normal subject: the lower ribcage (RC) is expanded (1) by direct insertions of the diaphragm into the lower ribs and (2) by increasing abdominal pressure (P_{ab}) via the zone of apposition. These effects are partly offset by (3) the deflating effect of increasingly negative pleural pressure as the diaphragm contracts.

L, lung.

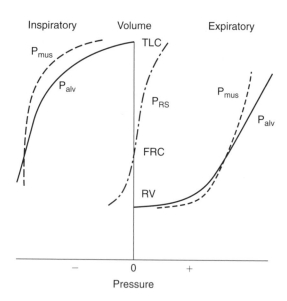

Figure 1.25 Maximum pressures developed by the respiratory system (after Rohrer[40]). Solid lines represent the alveolar pressure (P_{alv}) recorded at various lung volumes during a series of maximum static inspiratory (left) and expiratory (right) efforts. Measurements are made with a closed (or almost closed) airway, in which case P_{alv} can be measured at the mouth. The dotted and dashed line represents the recoil pressure of the total respiratory system (P_{RS}) measured during relaxation (cf. Fig. 1.1). The net pressure generated by the respiratory muscles (P_{mus}, dashed line) can be calculated since $P_{mus} = P_{alv} - P_{RS}$ (Equation 1.5).

FRC, functional residual capacity; RV, residual volume; TLC, total lung capacity.

Maximum static pressure measured at the mouth is the same as alveolar pressure, provided that the glottis is open. Conventionally, maximum static pressures are recorded as the values sustained for at least 1 s. Maximum expiratory efforts are performed against a closed, or virtually closed, airway after a full inspiration, and maximum inspiratory pressures after full expiration, i.e. close to TLC and RV respectively. The pressure recorded at the mouth includes a contribution (minor in normal subjects) from the passive recoil of the respiratory system but mainly reflects the net pressure resulting from contraction of the respiratory muscles – agonists and antagonists combined. Strictly, to assess the power of the respiratory muscles per se, measurements at FRC would be more appropriate, as passive recoil of the respiratory system is then zero, but most series of reference values report measurements made at the volume extremes.

1.5.2.2 Assessment of diaphragmatic function

The contribution of the diaphragm alone can be assessed by direct measurement of P_{di} using small balloons or transducers in the oesophagus and stomach.[41,42] Measurements made during various manoeuvres show that the diaphragm may not necessarily contract maximally, even during the most

forceful voluntary inspiratory efforts.[41,43,44] The diaphragm has a unique dual role at the boundary of the thorax and abdomen, acting agonistically with the ribcage muscles in the generation of negative intrathoracic pressures and with the abdominal wall muscles in the generation of positive abdominal pressures, e.g. during defecation or parturition. In some normal subjects the greatest P_{di} during maximum efforts is achieved during such expulsive rather than inspiratory manoeuvres.[41] Many subjects can be trained to produce even greater pressures during efforts that combine features of both manoeuvres.[43] Such 'gymnastics' are, however, not appropriate in clinical testing and often result in less negative pleural pressures than do more natural inspiratory manoeuvres.[44]

In individuals with bilateral diaphragmatic weakness, the VC is markedly less in the supine (or near-supine) posture than when upright, because of the effect of gravity on the abdominal contents. In most healthy subjects VC falls by about 10 per cent on assuming the supine position. A supine fall of more than 30 per cent of the upright value usually implies severe diaphragmatic weakness.[42]

1.5.2.3 Sniff and cough pressures

An alternative to maximum static inspiratory pressure is measurement during a forceful sniff, which most individuals find easier to perform. Initially this was proposed with measurement of P_{di} (sniff P_{di}) as a specific test of diaphragmatic function.[45] Subsequently it was used with oesophageal pressure and most commonly now with measurement of nasal pressure – the sniff nasal inspiratory pressure (SNIP).[46] Measurements are made via a catheter wedged in one nostril while the subject sniffs through the other unoccluded nostril (Fig. 1.26). The pressure recorded reflects that in the nasopharynx, which, in turn, in most subjects approximates alveolar pressure. SNIP will, however, underestimate intrathoracic pressure if the nose is severely obstructed or in patients with generalized airway narrowing such as asthma or chronic obstructive pulmonary disease (COPD).[47] Several practice efforts are likely to be needed.[48] Although most patients find the forceful sniff easier to master than a maximum static inspiratory effort, in some the converse is true. In clinical testing, good practice is to have the subject attempt both and to accept the numerically higher value as the more valid inspiratory measurement for that individual.

Unfortunately, there is no equivalent to the forceful sniff for simple assessment of expiratory muscle strength. To use the obvious option, a forceful cough, requires measurement of abdominal or oesophageal pressure, since coughing is accompanied by closure of the glottis as the expiratory pressure is developed. Abdominal (gastric) pressure gives a more accurate assessment than oesophageal pressure as the latter tends to be rather lower, due to the development of a transdiaphragmatic pressure by active contraction or passive stretching (or both) during coughing.[49]

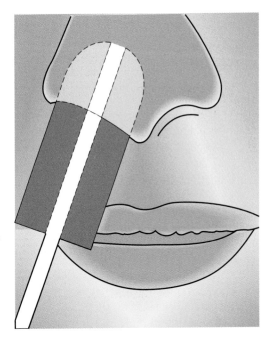

Figure 1.26 Sniff nasal inspiratory pressure measured by a transducer attached to a catheter lodged in one nostril while the subject makes a forceful sniff via the other (patent) nostril.

1.5.2.4 Clinical use of volitional tests

All the tests discussed so far are, by definition, strictly effort-dependent. Consequently, they are very useful for excluding significant respiratory muscle weakness but sometimes less satisfactory for confirming it, as the measurements are not fail-safe and apparently impaired values may be due to inadequate technique or poor motivation as well as to disease. Where they score is in the simplicity and wide availability of the technology required. When interpreted in the appropriate clinical context they suffice in most cases. The non-volitional techniques discussed below involve more complex equipment and greater expertise, which are available in only a few centres.

1.5.3 Non-volitional tests

1.5.3.1 Electrical and magnetic stimulation

The electrical activity of many individual respiratory muscles can be recorded using either surface or needle electrodes. Additionally, the diaphragmatic signal is recordable with an oesophageal electrode.[42] The method originally described used electrical stimulation of the phrenic nerves in the neck with recording of the diaphragmatic EMG to calculate phrenic nerve conduction time, the amplitude of the EMG response or the pressure generated by stimulated diaphragmatic contraction.[50,51] Magnetic stimulation offers several advantages (Table 1.2) and has superseded electrical stimulation in many centres.[52] Magnetic stimulation of the phrenic nerves can be performed either with a single coil placed over the lower cervical spine or by unilateral or bilateral stimulation with smaller figure-of-eight coils over the anterolateral surface of the neck. The latter produces more specific stimulation of the phrenic nerves with less contamination by activation of other nerves and muscles. If magnetic stimulation is used to measure phrenic nerve conduction time, anterolateral stimulation is preferable to cervical, and oesophageal recording gives the most reliable results.[53] The compound muscle action potential can also be quantified using oesophageal electrodes; it is absent or its amplitude is markedly reduced in patients with diaphragmatic paralysis or weakness.[54] Surface recording is more problematic as the optimal site varies between individuals.[55]

Phrenic nerve stimulation is frequently combined with measurement of the pressure generated by the resulting brief diaphragmatic contraction. This value ('twitch' P_{di}) is considerably less than that recorded during a maximum voluntary contraction, such as a sniff; a value less than $15 \, cmH_2O$ is suggestive of diaphragmatic dysfunction.[42] Similar information can be obtained with a single balloon-catheter system or miniature transducer measuring oesophageal

pressure or, in principle, by measuring mouth pressure.[56] Although the latter technique has been used successfully to demonstrate diaphragmatic weakness,[57] not all have found it reliable,[58] and using mouth pressure as a guide to pleural or transdiaphragmatic pressure is not valid in patients with generalized airway obstruction as the signal is delayed and damped by slow transmission of pressure from the lungs to the mouth.[59]

The expiratory abdominal muscles can be stimulated directly by electrical techniques or magnetically via the relevant nerve roots by placing the stimulator over the lower dorsal spine. The former has been used in detailed analyses of the actions of individual abdominal muscles and the latter as a non-volitional test of expiratory muscle function.[60]

1.5.3.2 Clinical use of non-volitional tests

In general, non-volitional tests of respiratory muscle function are of greatest value when there is uncertainty regarding the interpretation of apparently impaired function after volitional testing and in patients who are unable to cooperate as, for example, in the intensive care setting. They may also help in distinguishing diaphragmatic weakness due to upper and lower motor neuron lesions, as in the former a disproportionate reduction in P_{di} during voluntary manoeuvres would be expected.

Using cranial magnetic stimulation to study the central nervous system pathways of respiratory control is an active area of research, and measurement of central nerve conduction time may prove of value in investigating respiratory muscle dysfunction due to diseases, such as multiple sclerosis, which can affect the upper motor neurons.[42]

Table 1.2 Comparison of electrical and magnetic phrenic nerve stimulation

	Electrical	Magnetic
Technical difficulty	Can be difficult to locate nerves	Easy
Discomfort	Uncomfortable	Much less uncomfortable
Reliability	Not fail-safe	Reliable
Specificity	High	More contamination (anterolateral stimulation more specific)
Twitch pressure	Reflects diaphragm in isolation	Slightly greater because some agonist action
Equipment cost	Modest	Expensive

1.5.4 Respiratory muscle endurance and fatigue

1.5.4.1 Endurance

Muscle endurance defines the ability of a muscle to sustain a task over time. In qualitative terms this is related to the ability of the muscle to resist fatigue. Muscle endurance is related to strength, but additional factors such as the supply of oxygen to the muscle are also relevant.

Traditionally the overall endurance of the respiratory system is measured by comparing the maximum ventilation sustainable on exercise with the maximum voluntary ventilation measured over a short period at rest ('sprint MVV').[42] In practice, however, this method has limited applicability in clinical investigation. The maximum voluntary ventilation itself is not a specific index of muscle endurance as it depends additionally on lung and chest wall mechanics.

More specific information can be obtained by measuring the pressure-time product, which is the average pressure developed by a muscle or muscles under loaded conditions multiplied by the time for which the pressure can be sustained. The pressure chosen (e.g. mouth, transpulmonary, transdiaphragmatic) depends on which muscle(s) (usually inspiratory) are being assessed. The pressure can be expressed as a fraction of the relevant maximum inspiratory pressure to give the pressure-time index (PTI), also known (less correctly) as the tension-time index (TTI). It has been shown that values of this index for the diaphragm below 0.18 are unlikely to result in fatigue in healthy subjects.[42]

Respiratory muscle endurance is most often assessed with the subject breathing via an external added load, usually either an orifice-type resistance[61] or a valve in the inspiratory circuit that requires the development of a threshold pressure at the beginning of each inspiration.[62] The possible indices of endurance include the duration for which a subject can tolerate the load and the maximum sustainable inspiratory pressure (which can be expressed as a proportion of maximum static inspiratory alveolar pressure, $P_I$max).[42] In one device the size of the threshold load can be adjusted by adding weights to a plunger, which provides the inspiratory valve.[63]

Although not widely applied, such devices have been used in studies of inspiratory muscle training and rehabilitation in patients with chronic lung disease.

1.5.4.2 Respiratory muscle fatigue

The attractive concept of fatigue of the respiratory muscles as a cause of respiratory failure has generated many studies over the years.[64] These have highlighted the importance of respiratory muscle dysfunction in many conditions where the muscles themselves are diseased, where their normal function is compromised by abnormal ventilatory mechanics, where the 'load' against which they have to work is increased, or where varying combinations of these factors operate.

Muscle fatigue, in this context, is defined as a loss in the capacity for developing force and/or velocity of a muscle, resulting from muscle activity under load and that is reversible by rest.[65] The last point is important as it distinguishes fatigue from weakness. To be useful, a clinical test of fatigue or 'pre-fatigue' needs to be sufficiently sensitive to detect the 'prodromal' phase before a muscle fails as a generator of force so that, where possible, appropriate therapeutic steps can be taken to forestall power failure. The precise point at which incipient fatigue develops in an individual, and the most appropriate clinical test(s) for its detection, have remained elusive. Although the concept remains attractive, the clinical value of most of the techniques described is doubtful. It is important to note that fatigue is not necessarily located peripherally in the neuromuscular apparatus: the phenomenon of 'central fatigue', in which the neural drive to the respiratory muscles declines in the face of a potentially damaging load may be more important than peripheral fatigue as a mechanism of protecting the muscles from the adverse effects of prolonged forceful contractions.

Both EMG and mechanical indices have been proposed for the early recognition of fatigue; the techniques have mostly been applied before and after breathing against a 'fatiguing' load such as a very high external resistance:

• *Response to electrical stimulation:* The standard method for assessing the fatiguability of limb muscles is measurement of the force of contraction resulting from stimulation at increasing frequency. This approach has been used successfully with the sternomastoid muscle to construct a frequency–force relationship.[66] With the diaphragm, the pressure (P_{di}) response to phrenic nerve stimulation can be measured and a frequency–pressure curve constructed.[67] In fatigued healthy subjects the characteristic finding is of rapid recovery of the response to high-frequency stimulation and markedly delayed response to lower-frequency stimulation – the phenomenon of 'low-frequency fatigue'; this can be quantitated as a fall in the ratio of responses to stimulation frequencies of 20 Hz and 50 Hz (20:50 ratio).

- *Spectral analysis of EMG:* Fatigue is associated with a change in the frequency spectrum of the EMG during spontaneous breathing. There is an increase in amplitude of lower-frequency components and a decrease in amplitude at higher frequencies. This can be quantitated by calculating the ratio of the amplitudes of signals over arbitrary ranges of higher and lower frequencies ('high/low ratio').[68] Unlike low-frequency fatigue (which is recorded in response to stimulated contraction), the high/low ratio is rapidly restored to normal during recovery and may therefore be less sensitive.[69] It has not been widely accepted as a specific index of fatigue.[65]

- *Maximum relaxation rate:* Fatigued muscle relaxes abnormally slowly. Relaxation of the diaphragm can be quantified from the decline in P_{di} after a brief contraction, by calculating either the maximum relaxation rate (MRR) or the time constant of relaxation assuming a monoexponential decay. The MRR of P_{di} is similar following maximal voluntary sniffs and phrenic nerve stimulation.[70] In normal subjects the decline in pressure can be followed more simply by measurements in the mouth or nostril.[71] As with absolute pressures, however, the MRR measured proximally is unreliable as a guide to changes in intrathoracic pressure in patients with abnormal pulmonary mechanics. The relaxation rate has been shown to slow after potentially fatiguing exercise in patients

with COPD,[72] but the relation between slowed relaxation and force loss during fatigue is unclear.[42]

1.6 AIRWAY FUNCTION

The measurements discussed so far are obtained under static conditions, but when air flows pressure is also dissipated in overcoming the resistance of the airways through which the gas molecules travel.

1.6.1 Sources of respiratory resistance

This airway resistance is of two main types: the most obvious is that due to friction, both between gas molecules and between the gas and the airway wall. There is, however, an additional component that results from convective acceleration of gas molecules. This is due to the pressure required to increase the linear velocity of gas molecules flowing from airways of greater to lesser overall cross-sectional area: since bulk gas flow (i.e. the volume of gas per second) is the same throughout the tracheobronchial system, individual molecules move with greater velocity through airways in which the overall cross-sectional area is less. The complex system of branching tubes that comprises the normal airway increases in total cross-sectional area from trachea to respiratory bronchioles; although individual airways narrow progressively towards the alveoli, the increase in airway numbers with each generation outweighs this. For this reason, the major site of resistance to airflow during quiet breathing in a normal subject is in the central airway, in the larynx and in the nose. Consequently, during expiration, the linear velocity of individual gas molecules increases as they move centrally.

The magnitude of the frictional resistance depends on whether the flow is mainly streamlined (laminar) or turbulent. The balance between the two at various levels of the tracheobronchial tree in turn depends on the dimensions and irregularities of the airways, the rate of airflow and the physical properties of the gas being breathed. In general, airflow in the upper airway, trachea and larger bronchi is more turbulent particularly at higher flows, whereas in the peripheral airways during quiet breathing it is more nearly laminar except near bifurcations. With laminar flow, airway resistance is very dependent on gas viscosity (an index of how strongly gas molecules adhere to each other), whereas resistance to turbulent flow depends more on the density of the gas breathed; for this reason, a low-density gas mixture such as heliox, in which nitrogen is replaced by helium, reduces the resistance most markedly in the larger, more central airways. Similarly, maximum expiratory flow, particularly at higher lung volumes, increases at altitude due to less resistance to turbulent flow consequent on the lower density of inspired air at lower barometric pressure.

Lung tissue and the chest wall also display resistance to motion; in most situations and conditions this is much less than airway resistance, and in clinical testing is rarely measured per se. Lung tissue and chest wall resistance is, however, included in the measurements obtained using some techniques (see below).

1.6.2 Nasal resistance

Quantitation of the flow resistance of the nose has attracted much less interest than the remainder of the airway, but several methods are available for its measurement. Nasal airway resistance (R_{na}) is usually distributed unequally between the two nostrils in parallel and the distribution varies within an individual over a few hours (the 'nasal cycle'). This within-subject variation needs to be borne in mind when measurements of R_{na} are made, e.g. in assessment of structural abnormalities, in evaluating the treatment of rhinitis and in nasal challenge testing. The main differences between the various methods for measuring R_{na} relate to whether measurements are made during normal breathing ('active' rhinomanometry) or during breath-holding with an external flow source ('passive' rhinomanometry).

In active posterior rhinomanometry, pressure is recorded under the palate via a tube, around which the lips are tightly closed; the tube is incorporated in a tightly fitting facemask connected to a pneumotachograph. This method gives total R_{na} directly but requires considerable cooperation from the subject.

In active or passive anterior rhinomanometry, measurements are made in each nostril separately, with pressure recorded from the contralateral occluded nostril. These techniques suffer from the disadvantage that the intubation itself can affect R_{na}.

Other methods for measuring R_{na} include oscillometric and interrupter techniques similar to those described below for total airway resistance (see Sections 1.6.4.2 and 1.6.4.4).[73] Measurements of maximum flow via the nose can also be used, particularly peak inspiratory nasal flow;[74] this is relatively independent of effort as dynamic narrowing of the anterior nares during forceful inspiration provides a flow-limiting mechanism, a situation analogous to dynamic narrowing of the intrathoracic airways during forced expiration (see Section 1.6.4).

Because the relation between pressure and flow through the nose is non-linear, R_{na} varies with pressure. Results are, therefore, usually standardized by expressing the value at a specific pressure – usually either 150 Pa for unilateral measurements or 75 Pa for bilateral measurements.

An alternative approach to assessment of nasal potency is by reflection of acoustic stimuli applied at the nostrils to measure nasal volume or to identify sites of narrowing.[75] Acoustic rhinometry gives structural information rather than the functional information obtained by measuring nasal resistance. The two are not necessarily closely related, and the techniques should be regarded as complementary.

1.6.3 Determinants of overall airway resistance

The larger airways are supported by cartilaginous rings but these are incomplete posteriorly, where appreciable changes in calibre can occur by invagination of the posterior membrane. The smaller airways have less cartilage and are more susceptible to compressing and distending forces, as well as changing calibre with contraction of the smooth muscle in their walls. The larger intrathoracic airways are surrounded by pleural pressure, while the intrapulmonary airways are supported by the surrounding alveoli, which are attached to their outer layer. These factors, together with the passive elasticity of the airways, determine the increasing calibre and declining airway resistance as lung volume increases (Fig. 1.27). Because the relation of airway resistance to volume approximates to a hyperbola, its reciprocal, airway conductance (G_{AW}), has an approximately straight-line relation to lung volume. The variation of airway conductance with lung volume can largely be removed if conductance is divided by the thoracic gas volume at which it is measured, to

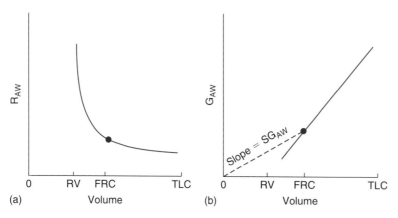

Figure 1.27 Variation of airway resistance (R_{AW}) with lung volume (a). In a normal subject, R_{AW} increases considerably below functional residual capacity (FRC). The relation of R_{AW} to volume is approximately hyperbolic and therefore its reciprocal, airway conductance (G_{AW}), shows a linear relation to volume (b). Specific conductance (SG_{AW}) does not completely remove the effect of lung volume, since the G_{AW}–volume plot usually does not pass through the origin.

RV, residual volume; TLC, total lung capacity.

give specific airway conductance (SG_{AW}). Strictly, however, SG_{AW} is completely independent of lung volume only if the plot of airway conductance to volume passes through the origin (which is usually not the case – see Fig. 1.27). Alternatively, R_{AW} can be multiplied by volume to give specific airway resistance (the reciprocal of SG_{AW}).

In addition to passive forces, bronchial calibre is dependent also on the tone of the bronchial smooth muscle, which is under the control of the parasympathetic nervous system. Evidence in humans suggests no direct innervation of bronchial muscle by the sympathetic nervous system,[76] although β-adrenoceptors are present in normal airways and can be stimulated pharmacologically. Thus, even in healthy individuals, a parasympathetic antagonist (e.g. atropine) produces a measurable decrease in airway resistance, whereas a β-sympathetic antagonist has no effect as long as the subject is in a resting unstressed state. Smooth muscle tone exerts an important influence on measurements of airway resistance; in normal subjects, when tone and therefore airway resistance are increased by inhalation of a bronchial irritant, it can transiently be reduced by a full inspiration.[77] Reduction in airway resistance is also demonstrable with hypercapnia, both in normal subjects and in those with airway disease.[78] Hypocapnia has little effect in normal subjects but increases airway resistance, presumably by bronchoconstriction, in subjects with asthma.[79] The reported effects of hypoxia (low inspired P_{O_2}) have

been variable: some studies report a reduction in airway resistance,[78] while most suggest a bronchoconstrictor response.[80]

The approximate distribution of airway resistance in a normal subject during quiet breathing is shown in Fig. 1.28, which emphasizes that most of the resistance to airflow resides in the larger, more central airways. 'Small' airways are usually defined as those with a diameter of less than 2 mm and are approximately equivalent to airways distal to the ninth generation; in healthy subjects, because of the large total cross-sectional area of the airways at this level, they account for only a small proportion of the overall resistance. An important corollary is that extensive disease can be present in the more peripheral smaller airways before an increase in total airway resistance is detectable.

1.6.4 Measurement of airway resistance

For the quantitation of airway resistance, the basic measurements required are the pressure difference between the mouth and alveoli and the flow. The latter can readily be measured at the mouth, but problems can arise if the subject breathes a gas of different density compared with that of air at sea level (e.g. air at altitude or heliox). This alters the resistance of a pneumotachograph, which needs to be calibrated using a gas of comparable density. It is more difficult to measure alveolar pressure, and most of the

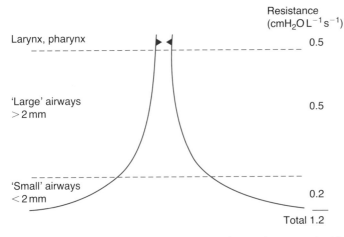

Figure 1.28 Average distribution of airway resistance in a normal subject during quiet breathing. The 'trumpet' shape of the airway represents the great increase in total cross-sectional area as the alveoli are approached and accounts for the very low resistance of peripheral airways.

Table 1.3 Comparison of techniques for measuring respiratory resistance

	Resistances included	Equipment cost	Cooperation required	Breathing pattern	Discomfort
Pleural pressure measurement	aw, t	Low	High	Tidal	Significant
Interrupter	aw, t, cw	Modest	Little	Tidal	Little
Plethysmography	aw	High	High	Panting (tidal)	Little
Forced oscillation	aw, t, cw	Modest	Little	Tidal	Little

aw, airway; cw, chest wall; t, lung tissue.

techniques that have been developed for measurement of airway resistance are aimed at circumventing this problem (Table 1.3).

1.6.4.1 Pleural pressure method

The classic method of Mead and Whittenberger uses continuous measurement of pleural (oesophageal) pressure from which alveolar pressure is derived (Equation 1.3).[81] This is used for research purposes but is too cumbersome and invasive for clinical use.

1.6.4.2 Interrupter method

In the interrupter method developed originally by Clements et al.,[82] airflow is repeatedly interrupted for brief periods, during which mouth pressure is measured as an index of alveolar pressure; resistance is calculated using the flow measured immediately before interruption. Equalization of alveolar and mouth pressures during interruption

is, however, not instantaneous and the time lag increases as resistance increases, with the result that it is progressively underestimated as airway narrowing becomes more severe. Despite these caveats, the technique, which requires little cooperation from the subject, has been found to be of value, particularly in children in whom other methods are more difficult to use.[83,84]

1.6.4.3 Plethysmographic method

In clinical testing in adults the most commonly applied method of measuring R_{AW} is by plethysmography, for which a constant-volume body box is usually used.[85] The seated subject (Fig. 1.15a) breathes through a pneumotachograph, and measurements of flow ($\dot{V}$) and box pressure (P_{box}) are displayed in x–y mode on a VDU. A shutter at the mouth is then closed and the subject is asked to continue making gentle respiratory efforts during which mouth pressure (now assumed to equal P_{alv} since no air is flowing) is displayed against P_{box}. Multiplication of the slopes of these two relationships gives airway resistance as the P_{box} term cancels out:

$$\frac{P_{box}}{\dot{V}} \times \frac{P_{alv}}{P_{box}} = \frac{P_{alv}}{\dot{V}} = R_{AW} \qquad (1.7)$$

It should be emphasized that the measurement is made during airflow; closure of the shutter is merely a calibration device that allows expression of P_{box} in terms of P_{alv}. Closure of the shutter also allows simultaneous measurement of thoracic gas volume (see Section 1.3.3) and hence calculation of specific airway conductance.

The potential error that can cause overestimation of plethysmographic lung volumes[21,22] can similarly lead to overestimation of airway conductance (underestimation of airway resistance) in patients with airflow obstruction. This occurs if the change in mouth pressure underestimates change in alveolar pressure. However, since G_{AW} and TGV are affected to the same degree, SG_{AW} is unaffected. As discussed in Section 1.3.3, this artefact is minimized by having the subject pant relatively slowly ($<1\,Hz$) and support the cheeks with the hands. Box pressure can be used as a function of alveolar pressure during panting only if no changes occur due to temperature or humidity of the gas. To circumvent these effects it is recommended that the pneumotachograph is heated to $37°C$ and the subject pants very shallowly, with the aim of limiting the front of gas moving in and out to the pneumotachograph itself. Sometimes plethysmographic measurements of R_{AW} are made during tidal breathing, in which case temperature problems are avoided by having the subject breathe from a separate bag of warmed air within the box. A further advantage of panting is that the vocal cords are abducted, which in normal subjects minimizes the contribution of the larynx to the total airway resistance.[86] However, this may not apply in patients with generalized airway obstruction.[87]

1.6.4.4 Forced oscillation method

If sinusoidal oscillations of flow (such as from a loudspeaker) are superimposed on a subject's normal tidal flow, the resulting pressure and flow profiles can be processed to measure respiratory impedance (Z_{RS}) and thus analyse the mechanical behaviour of the respiratory system.[88] Usually, the oscillating signal is applied at the mouth via a mouthpiece (to measure 'input impedance'), but it can also be applied to the chest wall (to measure 'transfer impedance').

As discussed in Section 1.2, the overall impedance of the respiratory system comprises functions of volume (compliance), flow (resistance) and acceleration (inertance). However, the relationship between pressures applied to overcome each of these differs importantly in the time domain. In simple terms, if we consider a tidal inspiration, the pressure overcoming inertial forces is applied *before* the breath (as it is used to accelerate gas and tissues) and that applied to overcome elastic forces maintains thoracic volume *after* the breath; in this simple analysis the only pressure applied *synchronously* with the breath is that overcoming resistive forces. For the measurement of resistance, only the pressure related to flow is required and the impedances due to elastic and inertial properties are considered together as their sum, known as 'reactance' (X_{RS}). With sinusoidal flow the latter two impedances are 180 degrees out of phase with each other; at low-oscillation frequencies elastic impedance is relatively greater, while at high frequencies inertial impedance dominates. At one particular frequency, the resonant frequency, they are equal and opposite and cancel each other out, i.e. reactance is zero. At the resonant frequency, pressure and flow are completely in phase and the respiratory resistance is directly measurable.

Forced oscillation is usually performed at a number of frequencies simultaneously with values for resistance (R_{RS}) and reactance (X_{RS}) of the respiratory system derived by spectral (frequency domain) analysis of the continuous relationship between the pressure applied and airflow measured at the mouth. The frequency range employed is usually between about $2\,Hz$ and $30\,Hz$. In patients with generalized airway obstruction, R_{RS} is increased at all frequencies and resonant frequency is also increased (Fig. 1.29). Oscillations at high frequencies are transmitted less well to the smaller peripheral airways but abnormal measurements at lower frequencies, below the resonant frequency, are likely to reflect narrowing of these airways.[89]

Subjects should avoid flexing the neck and the cheeks and floor of the mouth should be supported (as for plethysmography), otherwise part of the superimposed flow is dissipated in oscillation of the compliant upper airway. The technique can be applied during sleep, anaesthesia and assisted ventilation; it also has the advantages that measurements are made during quiet breathing and the equipment is portable.

1.6.5 Determinants of maximum flow

The measurements of airway resistance described above are all performed during breathing with low pressures and flows; they therefore assess the dimensions of the airways in their relatively unstressed state. (Ideally, the measurements would be made with zero airflow, but this is an unreal aim.) Inevitably, once airflow occurs, pressure differences arise across the airway wall and the potential exists for additional dynamic effects on airway calibre due to distending or compressing forces. These are seen to greatest effect during forced expiration, which forms the basis of most clinical assessments of airway function.

1.6.5.1 Isovolume pressure–flow curves

The easiest starting point for considering the complexities of the deceptively simple forced expiratory manoeuvre is with the relation between driving pressure and flow – the so-called isovolume pressure–flow (IVPF) relationship originally analysed by Fry and Hyatt.[90] To construct such a curve the subject has to perform a series of expiratory manoeuvres from full inflation with varying degrees of effort, and at a specific constant lung volume the relation between the alveolar pressures generated and the resulting instantaneous expiratory flows is examined. Alveolar pressure is calculated from pleural (oesophageal) and lung recoil pressures (Equation 1.3). Each expiratory effort produces one point on the IVPF curve; a model curve for a normal subject at 50 per cent of VC is shown in Fig. 1.30. As the effort increases, so does the flow, but the increments of flow decline progressively until a maximum value is achieved; beyond a certain pressure greater effort fails to increase flow. Figure 1.30 also shows likely intrathoracic pressure relations at selected points on the curve – in simple terms expiratory efforts exceeding a certain level are wasteful, in that larger pressures applied in the alveoli are met by

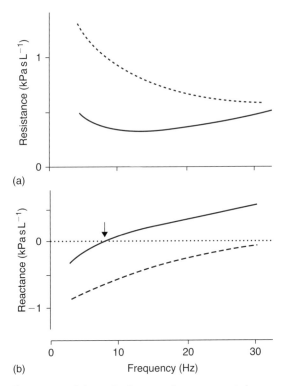

(a)

(b)

Figure 1.29 Schematic diagram of measurements by forced oscillation at several different frequencies in a healthy subject (solid lines) and a patient with chronic obstructive pulmonary disease (COPD) (broken lines). Resistance (a) is increased and more frequency-dependent in the patient, while reactance (b) is less; the arrow represents resonant frequency, which is also increased in the patient. Redrawn from ref. 88.

greater compressing forces across the intrathoracic airways, with the net effect of no increase in flow.

1.6.5.2 Equal pressure point analysis

During normal breathing, or with only gentle expiratory efforts, pleural pressure remains subatmospheric and consequently there is a net distending force across the airway. With a further increase in expiratory effort, pleural pressure becomes supra-atmospheric and, as the driving alveolar pressure is dissipated along the airways, points are reached where the intra- and extrabronchial pressures are equal. These are the equal pressure points (EPPs) as defined in the model of events during forced expiration by Mead et al.[91]

'Downstream' from the EPPs in this model there is a tendency for dynamic compression and

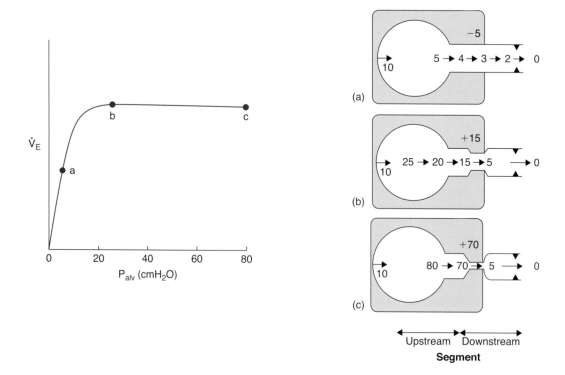

Figure 1.30 (Left): Schematic expiratory isovolume pressure–flow curve of a normal subject at approximately 50 per cent vital capacity (VC). Provided that a minimum driving pressure is generated, expiratory flow becomes independent of the pressure applied. (Right): The likely prevailing pressures with various efforts (conventions as in Fig. 1.3). At this volume, lung recoil pressure (P_L, represented by an arrow) is assumed to be $10\,cmH_2O$ and alveolar gas pressure (P_{alv}) is calculated as $P_{pl} + P_L$ (Equation 2.3). At (a) a small expiratory effort produces an alveolar pressure of $5\,cmH_2O$ but, since pleural pressure (P_{pl}) remains subatmospheric, the net transmural pressure acting across the intrathoracic airway favours expansion rather than compression. With an increase in effort, P_{pl} becomes positive and the conditions exist where P_{pl} may exceed the pressure within the airway. Once the pressure in the intrathoracic airway falls below the surrounding P_{pl} (b), there is a tendency for the airway to narrow. As the effort increases further, this dynamic compression becomes more marked and greater force is met by greater resistance, with the result that flow remains virtually constant (c).

$\dot{V}_E$, expiratory flow.

consequent flow limitation to occur. In healthy individuals, over much of the VC range, EPPs during forced expiration develop in the lobar or segmental bronchi, but at low volumes EPPs migrate upstream so that at these volumes the smaller airways become more important in the determination of maximum expiratory flow. The EPPs and sites of flow limitation during forced expiration are not necessarily identical, however; their relation depends also on the properties of the airway wall, degree of muscle tone, etc. In the equal pressure point analysis,[91] the total airway from alveolus to mouth is

considered during forced expiration to comprise only two segments defined by the EPPs. The advantage of this model is to simplify consideration of the factors determining maximum expiratory flow, as the mechanical conditions in the 'upstream' segment (i.e. from alveoli to EPPs) can be simply defined. In brief, since by definition the intra-airway pressure at the EPPs equals P_{pl}, the driving pressure along the upstream segment is $(P_{alv} - P_{pl})$. From Equation 1.3, this equals lung recoil pressure. Therefore, once sufficient expiratory effort is applied for EPP conditions to be established at a given lung volume, both the flow and the driving pressure along the upstream segment at that volume are fixed. The resistance of this upstream segment during forced expiration (R_{us}) is therefore given by:

$$R_{us} = \frac{P_L}{\dot{V}_E max} \qquad (1.8)$$

Measurements of R_{us} have been used in research studies as an index of the function of the smaller airways. Although both $\dot{V}_E max$ and P_L decline as volume decreases, the value of R_{us} is relatively independent of volume over a fairly wide range.

If an airway were to close because of dynamic compression during forced expiration, the pressure immediately upstream (i.e. on the alveolar side) of the occluded segment would rapidly equalize with alveolar pressure; since this is always greater than the surrounding pleural pressure, there would then be a net force across the occluded airway tending to reopen it. This is clearly an unstable situation and the resulting oscillation of half-open airways accounts for the wheeze that can be heard, even in normal subjects, during forced expiratory manoeuvres.

1.6.5.3 Starling resistor model of forced expiration

In an alternative analysis of forced expiration proposed by Pride et al., account is taken additionally of the compressibility of the airway itself over the segment where dynamic narrowing occurs.[92] Pride and colleagues likened the situation of the 'floppy' tube (the airway) exposed to a positive surrounding pressure to a 'Starling resistor', in which flow along the tube is determined not by the difference between inlet and outlet pressures but by the difference between inlet and surrounding pressure. As a result, changes in the downstream pressure do not influence the flow.

1.6.5.4 Wave speed analysis of forced expiration

A more recent analysis of the mechanism of flow limitation during forced expiration involves consideration of the speed of wave propagation along the airway.[93] The analysis predicts that the 'choke point' that limits flow in an elastic tube occurs where the

local velocity of flow of fluid (in this case expired air) reaches the speed of propagation of the pressure wave (which is analogous to the pulse wave of arterial blood flow). The latter depends on the compliance or stiffness of the airway wall. This mechanism of flow limitation is particularly relevant at high lung volumes, close to full inflation. Study of both healthy and asthmatic individuals has shown that peak expiratory flow (PEF) is probably limited by such a mechanism.[94] At lower lung volumes, both wave speed limitation and dynamic compression in smaller airways are likely to contribute in determining maximum expiratory flow.

The model IVPF curve with a plateau of $\dot{V}$ illustrated in Fig. 1.30 does not apply to all subjects. Maximum expiratory flow may be more effort-dependent than previously appreciated, as some healthy subjects show 'positive effort dependence' of $\dot{V}_E max$ at lung volumes between 50 and 80 per cent of VC.[95] This phenomenon has been related to distorting effects of the high intrathoracic pressure on wave speed propagation in the central airway, which in turn affects the site of the choke point and the consequent maximum flow. The magnitude of 'positive effort dependence' is, however, not large and does not detract from the strength of tests of forced expiration, which in clinical practice are relatively independent of effort.

1.6.5.5 Forced inspiration

Less attention has been paid to forceful inspiration as the conditions for dynamic compression generally do not apply with inspiratory efforts. However, a corresponding IVPF curve can be constructed during inspiratory manoeuvres of varying effort (Fig. 1.31). The relation is curvilinear but inspiratory flow does not reach a plateau, and at all lung volumes it continues to increase with increasing effort. Maximum inspiratory flow at a given volume is dependent on airway calibre and on the strength and speed of shortening of the inspiratory muscles.

1.6.5.6 Maximum flow volume curves

An infinite number of expiratory and inspiratory IVPF curves can in theory be constructed for the infinite number of lung volumes encompassed by the VC. Figure 1.32 shows examples in a model normal subject at four different volumes. The

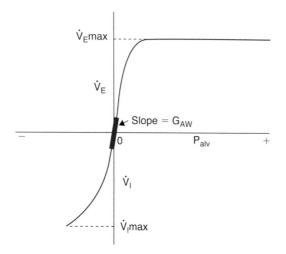

Figure 1.31 Schematic expiratory and inspiratory isovolume pressure–flow (IVPF) curves at 50 per cent vital capacity (VC). The slope of the curve close to zero pressure represents airway conductance (G_{AW}, $\Delta\dot{V}/\Delta P$). Maximum expiratory flow ($\dot{V}_E$ max) is relatively independent of effort but, since no plateau of inspiratory flow occurs, maximum inspiratory flow ($\dot{V}_I$ max) is totally effort-dependent.

P_{alv}, alveolar gas pressure; $\dot{V}_E$, expiratory flow; $\dot{V}_I$, inspiratory flow.

larger the lung volume, the higher the maximum expiratory flow that can be generated and, in general, the greater the pressure necessary to produce that maximum flow; at volumes close to full inflation, effort dependence is more pronounced.

The IVPF curve, although of much theoretical interest, is of no practical value. The maximum flow–volume curve, however, is much more familiar and easily obtainable. The maximum expiratory flow–volume (MEFV) curve describes the flow maxima throughout the VC and is obtained in a single forced expiratory manoeuvre. Its relation to the IVPF curve is illustrated in Fig. 1.32. During a continuous forced expiration initiated from TLC, flow rises rapidly to a peak value and then declines progressively. The peak is usually slightly higher than the PEF measured with a simple peak flow meter (Fig. 1.14a,b), since the latter has to be sustained for 10 ms to be registered. The corresponding

maximum inspiratory flow–volume (MIFV) curve is obtained by the subject inspiring forcefully after a full expiration to RV. Its appearance is more symmetrical, with peak inspiratory flow (PIF) seen approximately in the middle of the VC.

Numerous indices can be obtained from flow–volume curves, most commonly maximum expiratory flows* at standard lung volumes (25%, 50%, 75% VC, etc.). The general contour of the curves should also be examined, particularly in relation to identifying the possible presence of localized narrowing of the central airway (see below).

Variation in the pattern of emptying of different lung units alters the shape of the expiratory curve; the commonest pattern is the development of a concavity (convexity to the volume axis). The slope of the downstroke of the MEFV curve has units of time^{-1} (i.e. litres per second divided by litres), and the shorter the time of lung emptying, the steeper the slope. In theory, the rate of emptying of a single lung unit (airway plus the alveoli it subtends) depends on the resistance and compliance of the unit (strictly the product $R \times C$, which is analogous to the time constant of an electrical circuit). A low resistance or low compliance encourages rapid emptying, whereas high resistance or high compliance delays emptying. The effect of combining a slowly emptying with a rapidly emptying lung unit is modelled in Fig. 1.33. The resulting combined flow–volume curve shows a marked concavity, due to the slower emptying unit contributing relatively more to the latter part of expiration. This example is an extreme model of the consequences of diffuse intrathoracic airway obstruction in which a wide range of emptying rates occurs. Note, however, that curvilinearity is not necessarily diagnostic of *pathological* airway narrowing, as this pattern is essentially an exaggeration of the appearances seen with healthy ageing (see Chapter 8).

Maximum flow–volume curves can be recorded in either of two ways, depending on whether the volume signal is derived from gas expired at the mouth (the more common method) or from change in thoracic gas volume. To record the latter, the subject needs to be seated in a variable-volume

*Now known as forced expiratory flow at specific per cent VC *expired*, e.g. FEF_{25}, FEF_{50}, FEF_{75}; these are equivalent to the previous indices, maximum expiratory flows at specific per cent VC *remaining* in the lung, i.e. MEF_{75}, MEF_{50}, MEF_{25} respectively (or $\dot{V}_E max_{75}$, etc.).

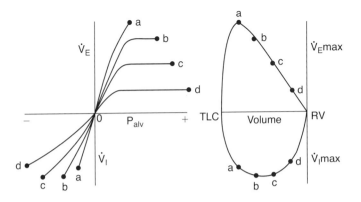

Figure 1.32 Relation between isovolume pressure–flow (IVPF) curves **(Left)** and maximum flow–volume (MEFV, MIFV) curves **(Right)**. A family of four IVPF curves at declining volumes a, b, c and d is illustrated. At volume a, close to total lung capacity (TLC), no plateau of expiratory flow is seen and maximum expiratory flow ($\dot{V}_E$max) is totally effort-dependent. At lower volumes, expiratory flow maxima occur, corresponding to $\dot{V}_E$max values at those volumes on the MEFV curve, which is recorded during a single forced expiration from full inflation. The corresponding flow maxima on inspiration are totally effort-dependent and are shown at the same volumes a, b, c and d.

P_{alv}, alveolar gas pressure; RV, residual volume; $\dot{V}_I$, inspiratory flow.

plethysmograph, which, in addition to the volume expired, also records the reduction due to compression of thoracic gas consequent on the markedly positive alveolar pressure (Boyle's law). Examples of model curves recorded by both methods are illustrated in Fig. 1.34; the difference in a normal subject is small but in patients with severe airway obstruction it can be pronounced.[96] For detailed analyses of pulmonary mechanics it is preferable to record change in thoracic gas volume, since this can be related directly to lung recoil pressure, but most clinical measurements use expired volume.

Airflow resistance can be increased artificially by adding a simple resistance (e.g. a narrow orifice) at the mouth through which the subject breathes. The effects of this on the maximum flow–volume curve of a normal subject are very different from the pattern seen in patients with diffuse intrathoracic airway narrowing. In the artificial situation (Fig. 1.35), there is a reduction of maximum expiratory flow at high lung volumes (including peak flow) and of maximum inspiratory flow throughout the volume range. The flow rates that are most affected, therefore, are those most dependent on effort, and the net result is similar to a graded reduction in the effort applied. In this situation the additional

resistance is in series with the subject's natural airway resistance. The IVPF curves in Fig. 1.35 show the consequence for airflow. During the forced manoeuvre some of the applied pressure is now dissipated in overcoming the additional resistance and less of the driving (alveolar) pressure is available to overcome the innate resistance of the airways. At low lung volumes, however, flow is unaffected because at these volumes maximum flow is less effort-dependent and normally the large alveolar pressure developed during forced expiration is dissipated in dynamic compression of intrathoracic airways. By contrast, at higher volumes on expiration, and throughout forced inspiration, the effect of an added resistance is clearly seen as a reduced flow. Although breathing through an artificial resistance at the mouth has been used in attempts to mimic the mechanical effects of the common forms of airflow obstruction, the effect is clearly quite different; the appropriate parallel is with the rarer (but nonetheless important) extrathoracic airway obstruction seen with constricting lesions in the larynx or trachea (see Chapter 12, Section 12.1.2.2).

Another feature, sometimes seen on maximum flow–volume curves, is oscillation of flow giving a so-called 'sawtooth pattern' (Fig. 1.36). In the earlier literature this was ignored or dismissed as

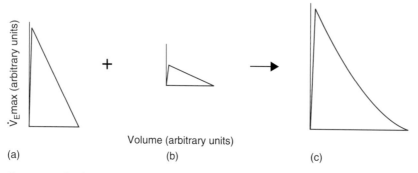

Figure 1.33 (a,b) Maximum expiratory flow–volume curves of two theoretical lung units with different rates of emptying. When these empty in parallel, the combined flow–volume curve (c) is curvilinear because the rapidly emptying unit contributes relatively more to the overall expired volume in the earliest part of expiration. (The curves have been constructed by assuming that emptying of each unit is monoexponential; they contribute equal volumes but the time constant of (b) is five times longer than that of (a).)

$\dot{V}_E$max, maximum expiratory flow.

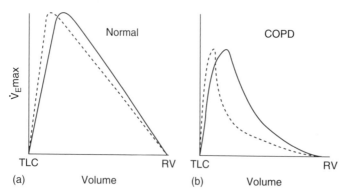

Figure 1.34 Maximum expiratory flow–volume curves obtained by measuring flow at the mouth and either change in thoracic gas volume (TGV) (solid line) or volume expired (broken line) in (a) a normal subject and (b) a patient with diffuse airway obstruction (chronic obstructive pulmonary disease, COPD). The decline of TGV results from both expiration and gas compression and is therefore greater in early expiration than the change in expired volume. Little difference is apparent in the normal subject but a large difference is seen with airway obstruction and hyperinflation as the volume of gas compressed is greatly increased.

RV, residual volume; TLC, total lung capacity; $\dot{V}_E$ max, maximum expiratory flow.

instrumental noise, but it is now well recognized as a pathophysiological phenomenon. It usually signifies instability of the upper airway, with consequent fluctuation of airway calibre; less commonly it may reflect fluctuation of the driving pressure. This appearance has been described in some patients with the obstructive sleep apnoea syndrome (see Chapter 18, Section 18.2.4.3), but it is not specific for this condition and it is also seen in snorers without sleep apnoea, in some subjects with structural upper airway obstruction, after thermal injury to the airway, in people with neuromuscular conditions causing bulbar weakness and in those with extrapyramidal disorders.[97]

1.6.5.7 Partial flow volume curves

At a given lung volume in a normal subject maximum expiratory flow is dependent on the effective driving pressure and the calibre of the airways. The

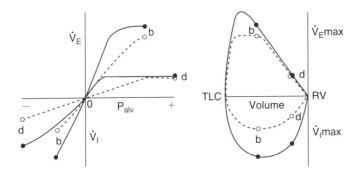

Figure 1.35 Isovolume pressure–flow (IVPF), maximum expiratory flow–volume (MEFV) and maximum inspiratory flow–volume (MIFV) curves when an artificial resistance is added at the mouth (broken lines). The solid lines correspond to the normal relationships illustrated in Fig. 1.32, but only volumes b and d are shown for clarity. The effect of the artificial resistance added in series is to reduce the pressure drop along the natural airway. With gentle efforts the total resistance of the two in series is increased, i.e. conductance is reduced, and therefore the slopes of the IVPF curves near zero pressure are reduced. Maximum inspiratory flow ($\dot{V}_I$ max) is reduced at all volumes, as is maximum expiratory flow ($\dot{V}_E$ max) at high volumes. At lower volumes, however, the reduction in the pressure that is applied along the natural airway has no effect on $\dot{V}_E$ max but reduces the extent of dynamic compression.

former is a function of lung recoil pressure and the latter depends on the degree of bronchomotor tone; both factors can vary with the immediately preceding breathing pattern ('volume history'). In normal subjects a preceding full inspiration minimizes both lung recoil pressure at a given volume and bronchomotor tone, factors that potentially have opposite influences on the flow developed during a subsequent forced expiration. Recording flow–volume curves with initiation of forced expiration from lung volumes below full inflation is therefore sometimes used to allow the influence of bronchomotor tone to be assessed. Such partial expiratory flow–volume (PEFV) curves (Fig. 1.37) have been used to assess the effect of bronchodilator drugs in normal subjects,[98] as the size of the signal obtainable from MEFV curves is limited by abolition of tone consequent on full inspiration.

1.6.5.8 Expiratory flow limitation during tidal breathing

In healthy subjects maximum expiratory and inspiratory flows greatly exceed those developed during resting tidal breathing, although during maximal exercise the greater flows may approach maxima, particularly towards the end of expiration. In patients with advanced airway obstruction, the flow

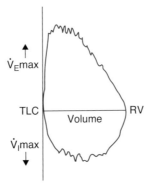

Figure 1.36 Maximum expiratory flow–volume (MEFV) and maximum inspiratory flow–volume (MIFV) curves showing 'sawtooth' oscillations of flow.

RV, residual volume; TLC, total lung capacity; $\dot{V}_E$ max, maximum expiratory flow; $\dot{V}_I$ max, maximum inspiratory flow.

reserve is greatly diminished, especially on expiration, and tidal expiratory flow may be limited, even at rest. A 'physiological' response to this situation is for the patient to adopt a higher-volume breathing range, as increasing end inspiratory and end expiratory volumes allows greater expiratory flows to be developed. This occurs at rest, with a further acute volume rise during exercise (dynamic hyperinflation) – but at the cost of both an increased elastic

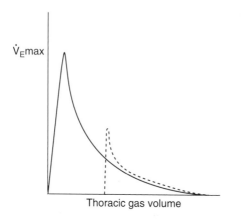

Figure 1.37 Maximum (solid line) and partial (broken line) expiratory flow–volume (MEFV, PEFV) curves in a patient with airflow obstruction. The initial peak of the PEFV curve mainly reflects emptying of the conducting airways.

$\dot{V}_E$ max, maximum expiratory flow.

load on the inspiratory muscles and a reduction in their efficiency (see Chapter 9, Section 9.11.2). Resting tidal expiratory flow limitation was originally recognized by superimposing a tidal flow volume curve on the MEFV curve.[99] However, comparison of tidal and maximum expiratory flow at what appear to be identical lung volumes is often invalid for several reasons: as explained above, use of iso expired volume as the reference for comparison is likely to be inappropriate, especially in this population of patients in whom change in expired volume is likely to be very different from change in absolute lung volume, due to the exaggerated effects of gas compression. Furthermore, the flow recorded is dependent on the volume and time history preceding the manoeuvre, i.e. the effect on airway calibre of a preceding full inflation, the time taken over the inspiration and the time for which it was held before expiration.[100] An alternative, and more valid, method for detection of tidal expiratory flow limitation is to apply a negative (suction) pressure transiently at the mouth during tidal expiration.[101] Normally, this should generate a transient increase in expiratory flow; if it fails to do so, it is concluded that flow limitation is present (Fig. 1.38). An alternative way of demonstrating the same phenomenon is by manual compression of the abdominal wall during tidal expiration.[102] Normally this results in an increase in flow and, if it fails to do so, it is assumed that flow limitation is present.

1.6.5.9 Simple spirometric indices

Historically, measurements obtained during forced expiration were used as an indirect guide to the maximum breathing capacity, i.e. the largest volume of air that a subject can shift per minute. As with other tests, such as the CO diffusing capacity, however, the indirect index has proved of more clinical value than the original measurement. The forced expiratory volume in 1s (FEV_1) is not immediately evident on a curve relating maximum flow to volume, but many automated spirometers indicate it by marking the volume expired after 1s. In effect, the FEV_1 integrates the maximum flow over a large part of the VC (>70% in normal subjects).

The simplest and most practicable guide to the presence of airflow limitation is the ratio of the FEV_1 to the VC or forced vital capacity (FVC).[103,104] Opinions differ as to whether the FEV_1 should be related to the FVC measured in the same manoeuvre, or to the true VC, which was defined by Hutchinson in 1846 as 'the greatest voluntary expiration following the deepest inspiration'.[105] Occasionally the VC measured on inspiration from RV may give the largest value. In normal subjects it matters little which is used, but in patients with airflow obstruction the FVC frequently falls short of the more relaxed measurement,[106] partly as a result of the associated compression of thoracic gas, possibly because of greater airway closure during the more forced manoeuvre and often simply because a patient with severe airway narrowing cannot sustain the very prolonged forced expiration required. Use of the ratio of FEV_1 to FVC may therefore sometimes obscure the presence of an obstructive ventilatory defect. Some laboratories report both a forced and a 'relaxed' VC, but this gives rise to occasional nonsensical reports where the FVC is allegedly greater than the VC (which, by definition, cannot be the case). Latest guidance (which accords with my own prejudice) is that, for classification of ventilatory defects, the maximum VC measured, whether forced or relaxed, is the most useful to report and to relate to the FEV_1.[107]

Of the timed indices derived from forced expiration, FEV_1 is much the most popular, but $FEV_{0.5}$ and $FEV_{0.75}$ have been used widely in children as children normally have very rapid lung emptying, so that FEV_1 may be too close to VC for it to be discriminatory (i.e. FEV_1/VC may approach 100

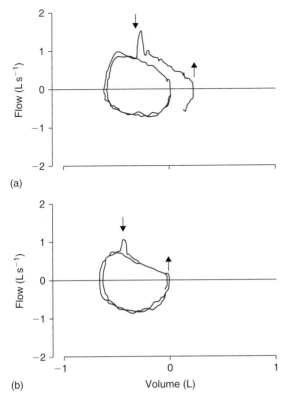

(a)

(b)

Volume (L)

Figure 1.38 Detection of flow limitation during tidal breathing. Tidal flow–volume loops recorded from a patient with (a) and without (b) expiratory flow limitation; negative pressure has been applied at the mouth during expiration between the arrows. In (a) there is an increase in expiratory flow throughout the period of negative pressure application, while in (b) only a transient increase due to emptying of the upper airway is seen. From ref. 101.

per cent). Latterly, FEV_6 has been proposed as a useful index, but for use in the denominator rather than the numerator of this ratio,[108] on the grounds that measuring FVC in patients with airway obstruction may require an exhausting maximal expiration that can take 15 s or more. Use of FEV_6 and FEV_1/FEV_6 is currently being promoted particularly for epidemiological and workplace studies where large numbers of measurements are required,[109] but some have found the resulting frequency of misclassification of patients to be unacceptable.[110]

A further measurement sometimes taken from the forced expiratory spirogram was formerly known as the maximum mid-expiratory flow (MMF)[111] and

is now known as the forced expiratory flow between 25 and 75 per cent of the FVC (FEF_{25-75}). This represents the average maximum flow over the middle two quarters of the FVC but, unlike flow at one specific lung volume, it is easily obtained from the spirogram relating volume to time (Fig. 1.39a). It has the theoretical advantage of avoiding measurement during the most effort-dependent first quarter of the FVC. It is obtained routinely in many laboratories in North America but has not generated as much enthusiasm in Europe. Its very wide variability among normal subjects limits its usefulness, and its early promise as a specific test for 'small airway' disease[112] has not stood the test of time. Its value is very dependent on VC and therefore it falls with both airway obstruction and restriction of lung volumes. Its specificity can be increased (like that of the FEV_1) by expressing it as a ratio in proportion to VC.

1.6.5.10 Forced expiratory measurements in the time domain

As an alternative to measurements of volume or flow, the third variable, time, has the advantage of focusing on the terminal phase of forced expiration, which is most relevant for evaluating the earliest effects of airway disease.

The mathematical technique of moments analysis can be applied to the forced expiratory spirogram to calculate various time domain indices such as the mean transit time for gas molecules to pass from the alveoli to the mouth.[113,114] As discussed above, the rate of emptying of some lung units may be very slow and, if their contribution to the overall lung volume is small, their effect will not readily be detected in terms of volume or flow. Transit time analysis is a detailed mathematical corollary of the well-known physical sign of airway obstruction, prolongation of the forced expiratory time. The mathematical distribution of the transit times of gas molecules to pass from alveoli to mouth can be expressed in terms of the mean value, the coefficient of variation of the values and the 'index of skewness' of the distribution. The mean transit time, or 'first moment', is given by the 'centre of gravity' of the volume–time curve (Fig. 1.39b); the other two parameters are derived from higher 'moments' of the curve, and each gives progressively greater weight to those lung units that empty most slowly.

1.6.6 Interrelation of tests of airway function

Airway conductance ($\dot{V}/P_{alv}$), as conventionally measured with small efforts and low flows, can be visualized on the IVPF curve as its slope near the origin (see Fig. 1.31). With greater applied efforts, conductance would be represented graphically by the slope of a line joining the relevant point on the curve to the origin, and its value therefore falls (resistance increases) as the effort increases. Clearly, therefore, attempts to quantitate the resistance of the whole airway during forced expiration are meaningless, since once maximum expiratory flow is achieved the calculated value becomes arbitrarily dependent on the driving pressure.

The question of the 'best' test for assessing the severity of airway obstruction is somewhat controversial. To the purist, R_{AW} would seem the obvious solution but this measurement has certain disadvantages, even apart from the practicalities of its measurement. First, it is usually measured using a technique aimed at minimizing dynamic changes – but in patients with generalized airflow obstruction, pathological changes in the airway walls alter their dynamic behaviour, and increased collapsibility or compressibility is an important contributor to the narrowing. Secondly, R_{AW}, as measured conventionally, is dominated, at least in normal subjects, by the calibre of the larger airways. Measurements of R_{AW} or SG_{AW} should not, however, be regarded as dependent solely on the larger airways, because once the resistance of the small airways increases sufficiently to produce symptoms, the overall airway resistance will show a measurable increase. In symptomatic patients the FEV_1 is also likely to be reduced, but, again, it is not very sensitive to early changes in small airways. The anticipated greater sensitivities of FEF_{25-75}, $\dot{V}_E max$ at small lung volumes, frequency dependence of compliance and mean transit time are often outweighed by their greater variability, both within and between subjects, when compared with FEV_1. Other methods of potential value for detection of early narrowing of the peripheral airways include measurements

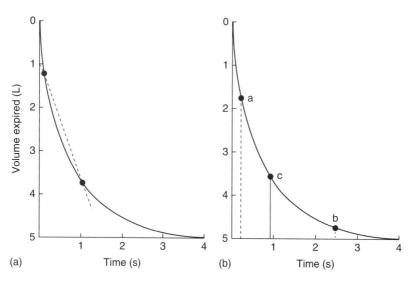

(a)   Time (s)   (b)   Time (s)

Figure 1.39 Record of expired volume against time during a forced expiration. (a) Diagram showing measurement of forced expiratory flow between 25 and 75 per cent of the forced vital capacity (FVC), or FEF_{25-75}, represented by the slope of the broken line joining points at 25 per cent and 75 per cent of expired vital capacity. In this example the FEF_{25-75} is 2.7 L.s^{-1}. (b) Illustration of mean transit time analysis. Gas molecules expired early have a short transit time from alveoli to the mouth (e.g. 0.2 s at point a), whereas later in the breath the transit time is longer (e.g. 2.5 s at point b). The mean transit time c is given by dividing the integrated area under the curve by the FVC and the measurement is weighted in favour of the most slowly emptying alveoli.

using forced oscillation at low frequencies[89] and indices of gas exchange. These are discussed in more detail in relation to early detection of chronic obstructive pulmonary disease in Chapter 9 (see Section 9.12.2).

Inspection of the IVPF curve (see Fig. 1.31) shows that there is no reason a priori why there should be a close relation between, on the one hand, airway resistance or conductance measured with gentle efforts at low flow and, on the other hand, tests based on forced expiration. In patients with diffuse airway narrowing, however, the two types of measurement tend to move in the same direction so that in disease there are weak correlations between FEV_1 and plethysmographic[115] or oscillometric[116] measurements of airway resistance.

1.6.7 Bronchodilator testing

A common situation where sequential measurements of airway function are desired is in assessing the effects of bronchodilator drugs. In patients with established airway obstruction, either SG_{AW} or forced expiratory tests can be used. The changes in each would not be expected to be related linearly, however, so any attempt to equate differential proportional changes with the relative effects of a drug on 'large' or 'small' airways is fraught with danger. During forced expiration the largest proportional differences are often found with $V_E max$ at small lung volumes, but changes in the VC or absolute thoracic gas volume need to be taken into account for a full interpretation of such changes. In practice, despite its theoretical disadvantages, the FEV_1 has been the most frequently used measurement for assessing bronchodilator responses in patients with airflow limitation. Various arbitrary increases either as absolute volume or as per cent change, or both (e.g. >12% and >200 mL) have been recommended for identifying a 'significant' response,[107] but their clinical value is very limited. In patients with more severe airway obstruction (e.g. due to COPD), however, symptomatic benefit from bronchodilators relates more closely to reduced static and dynamic hyperinflation consequent on dilatation of small airways (see Chapter 9, Section 9.11.5).

In normal subjects, the size of a bronchodilator signal is very limited if FEV_1 is used, as FEV_1 pre-bronchodilator is already a high proportion of the VC; in this situation, measurement of SG_{AW} has a distinct advantage as changes of twofold or more can be seen in normal subjects after a bronchodilator, and dose–response relationships can be assessed more easily.

1.6.8 Tests of airway responsiveness

1.6.8.1 Direct and indirect stimuli

Tests of airway responsiveness have developed mainly from the recognition that individuals with asthma show unusually large bronchoconstrictor responses (airway hyperresponsiveness) to a variety of inhaled agents. Some of the commoner agents used in challenge testing are listed in Table 1.4. Some, in particular histamine and methacholine, provoke bronchoconstriction by a direct stimulatory effect on airway smooth muscle. Those agents that act indirectly, on the other hand, do so via an effect on other cells in the airway, such as inflammatory cells, epithelial cells and nerves.[117,118] Some challenges, e.g. with occupational agents or lysine aspirin, are used only in selected individuals in whom specific sensitivity is suspected and by laboratories with particular interest and expertise in the relevant area. Other indirect challenges, such as with adenosine, have largely been confined to research studies. Histamine and methacholine challenges, however, are performed widely and safely in clinical testing. Preference in most laboratories has moved towards methacholine, mainly because its fewer side effects allow higher concentrations to be used in incremental testing.

1.6.8.2 Methods for measuring airway responsiveness

Detailed guidelines on indications and procedures have been published by both the European Respiratory Society[119] and the American Thoracic Society (ATS).[120] For methacholine challenge, three main protocols are in use, each involving incremental dosing according to standard schedules. In the tidal breathing method,[121] the subject breathes as normally as possible while the solution is nebulized continuously for 2 min. The response is measured 30 s and 90 s after nebulization of the first (weakest) concentration; if a predefined fall in the index being measured has not been achieved,

Table 1.4 Agents used for inhalation challenge testing[117,118]

Directly acting	Indirectly acting
Methacholine	**Specific:**
Histamine	Allergen/occupational agents
	Lysine aspirin
	Non-specific:
	Exercise
	Isocapnic hyperventilation
	Osmotic stimuli:
	Hypertonic saline
	Mannitol
	Distilled water ('fog')
	Adenosine

the next highest concentration is nebulized for 2 min, starting 5 min after the first. The procedure is repeated until a predefined functional threshold is reached or until the highest concentration has been nebulized. In the other two methods, the subject takes a sequence of five full inhalations of each methacholine concentration, again starting with the most dilute and delivered either by a dosimeter[122] or from a series of handheld bulb nebulizers.[123] The recommended time sequence for the measurements and the intervals between nebulization are similar to those for the tidal breathing method. As originally described, doubling concentrations of methacholine were used but more recently the ATS recommended using quadrupling doses.[120] This halves the maximum number of steps involved (from ten to five) and thus reduces the cumulative dose.

The response to challenge can be measured in a number of ways. Much the commonest is the PC_{20}, the lowest concentration of methacholine provoking a reduction below the baseline FEV_1 of 20 per cent. Sometimes, especially in epidemiological studies where many non-asthmatic (and therefore less sensitive) individuals are included, an earlier response threshold (e.g. PC_{15} or even PC_{10}) is used. Less commonly, the estimated dose of methacholine (in micrograms) producing a similar fall in FEV_1 is quoted as PD_{20}, etc. The PC_{20} obtained may differ between the tidal breathing and deep inhalation methods.[124]

Other measurements can be substituted for FEV_1, such as SG_{AW} or resistance measured by forced oscillation. These have the theoretical advantage of avoiding full inspiration, which may

itself diminish the increased bronchial muscle tone resulting from the challenge. Resistance/conductance measurements may also give a numerically bigger signal in less sensitive (e.g. non-asthmatic) subjects, but these advantages are often negated by their greater intrinsic variability. Because of this variability, the threshold reduction for identifying a response in terms of SG_{AW} is set at a greater percentage level (e.g. a reduction variously between 35 per cent and 50 per cent below baseline).

Other approaches to assessing responses to challenge may have advantages over PC_{20}. The overall dose–response relationship to histamine or methacholine normally has a sigmoid shape and can be defined in terms of a threshold (sensitivity), slope (reactivity) and maximal response plateau. The last is seen in healthy subjects and some subjects with asthma; its apparent absence in other asthmatic individuals has potentially important clinical implications (see Chapter 11, Section 11.3.2).[125] In effect, the PC_{20} FEV_1 combines elements of sensitivity and reactivity and, for reasons of convenience, is much the commonest index used in clinical testing. Repeatability of PC $(D)_{20}$, however, is only modest, with a within-subject standard deviation of about 1.0 doubling doses,[126] and this needs to be taken into account when repeat measurements are compared.

1.6.8.3 Interpretation of bronchial challenge tests

A potential problem of interpreting the response to challenge testing is the influence of pre-challenge airway calibre. Geometry dictates that, for a given stimulus, a larger effect would be anticipated in an airway that was already narrowed.[127] The resistance of a tube is inversely proportional to the fourth power of its radius, and therefore a given reduction in bronchial muscle length will produce a much larger increase in the resistance of a smaller tube. Second, if the initial bronchial tone is abnormally high, the smooth muscle is likely to be operating on a steeper portion of its stimulus–response curve, which will amplify the geometrical effect (Fig. 1.40). A characteristic of asthma is that hyperresponsiveness is disproportionate to any reduction in airway calibre, with no clear relationship between bronchial responsiveness and baseline function.[128] Such a 'baseline effect' is, however, clearly evident in COPD[129] and also in cross-sectional epidemiological studies of randomly selected populations, which show increasing airway responsiveness as FEV_1 (% predicted) declines.[130] Whether, in the general population, greater airway responsiveness results in poorer function or vice versa remains conjectural.

1.7 OBSTRUCTIVE AND RESTRICTIVE VENTILATORY DEFECTS

These widely used terms date from the classical analyses of patterns of pulmonary insufficiency by Baldwin *et al.*[131] Conceptually, it is easy to distinguish abnormalities that relate predominantly to the airways and impede flow (obstructive defect) from abnormalities that affect the lung tissue, chest wall or respiratory muscles and prevent normal lung expansion (restrictive defect). Sometimes, a reduction in VC in the absence of any measurements of absolute lung volumes is described as a restrictive defect – but this is unhelpful as most patients with moderate or severe airflow obstruction show some reduction in VC. Use of spirometry alone to identify patients with a restrictive ventilatory defect results in frequent misclassification[132] and the term should be confined to patients with a demonstrable reduction in TLC. A reduced TLC is almost always accompanied by a reduced VC. With intrapulmonary restriction the RV is usually normal or slightly reduced so that the RV/TLC ratio may be high. A less common, but well recognized, pattern is that of isolated reduction of RV with values of VC and TLC that are both within the limits of normal. This has been observed in various pathological conditions, including cardiac failure, sarcoidosis and skeletal deformities.[133] With extrapulmonary restriction, particularly if caused by respiratory muscle weakness, the RV may be increased. With restrictive defects, the FEV_1 and VC are usually decreased in approximate proportions to each other; sometimes the FEV_1/VC is actually greater than normal, but in practice this is difficult to detect since it cannot exceed 100 per cent.

The hallmark of an obstructive defect is evidence of airway narrowing – this may be suggested by an increased airway resistance but this (or its reciprocal conductance) should always be related to lung volume. More usually, classification is based on a reduced ratio of FEV_1 to VC. Sometimes a value below 70 per cent in older subjects or below 75 per cent in younger subjects is used as the criterion for the presence of clinically significant airway narrowing, but comparison of the ratio with relevant age-related norms is more appropriate. Use of the FEV_1/VC ratio is satisfactory in most situations, with the exception of narrowing of the central airway to which the FEV_1 is poorly sensitive. In established diffuse airway disease, reliance should not be placed on the ratio as a guide to severity of airway obstruction as this can be very misleading: for example, it is not uncommon to see a greater increase in VC than in FEV_1 (i.e. a fall in the FEV_1/VC ratio) during improvement in a patient's clinical state (e.g. during recovery from asthma, after a bronchodilator in emphysema). For assessment of the severity of airway narrowing, the FEV_1 in relation to the predicted value is therefore usually the best criterion.

As mentioned above, in patients with diffuse airway narrowing, a reduced FEV_1 and FEV_1/VC is often associated with some reduction of the VC and usually with an increase in RV, in RV/TLC and in TLC itself. Although often used as an index of airway narrowing, the FEF_{25-75} is less specific as it varies with both the VC and the FEV_1/VC ratio. If VC changes, the measurement is made over a different absolute volume range, which complicates interpretation.[134]

Further problems arise with the fairly common finding of a mixed obstructive and restrictive defect: the problems are, first, the recognition of both an airway and an alveolar (or chest wall) component and, second, the decision as to whether the changes are attributable to a single disease or, perhaps more commonly, to different pathological processes, the respective contributions of which may require quantitation. In a patient with an otherwise typical restrictive ventilatory defect, a reduced FEV_1/(F)VC definitely signifies an airway component (especially since many such patients would normally be expected to have an increased FEV_1/VC), but a rise in RV is less specific for airway pathology since it also occurs with cardiac disease and muscle weakness.

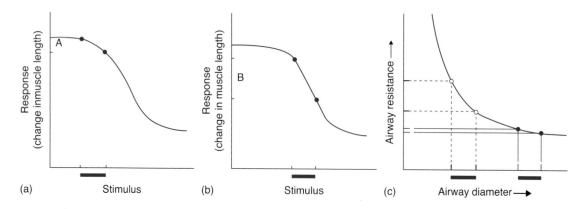

Figure 1.40 Geometric factors that may affect assessment of bronchial reactivity (after Benson[127]). (a,b) The stimulus–response relationship for bronchial smooth muscle is shown schematically; if a stimulus is applied when the muscle is relaxed (a), a small response (A) occurs, but if the same stimulus is applied when the muscle is partly contracted (b), the relationship is steeper and a greater reduction in muscle length (B) is seen. (c) The curvilinear fourth-power relation between airway resistance and diameter implies that a given reduction in airway diameter produces a greater increase in resistance when the starting diameter is less.

A not uncommon pattern in a patient with mixed pathology is to find spirometric evidence of airflow obstruction (low FEV_1/VC ratio), together with a reduced VC, a raised RV and a normal TLC. The last may result from a balance of opposing influences, with lung fibrosis (or other alveolar pathology) tending to shrink the lungs, and airway obstruction tending to produce hyperinflation. Such a situation is exemplified by a study of patients with asbestosis who also had airway disease.[135] It would be very convenient for those reporting lung function tests to have a word for 'the TLC is not as high as expected for this level of airflow obstruction, suggesting that there may in addition be a pathological process tending to produce a restrictive defect', but unfortunately no simple term for this pattern exists.

REFERENCES

1 Rahn H, Otis AB, Chadwick LE, Fenn WO. The pressure–volume diagram of the thorax and lung. *Am J Physiol* 1946; **146**: 161–78.

2 Milic Emili J, Mead J, Turner JM, Glauser EM. Improved technique for estimating pleural pressure from oesophageal balloons. *J Appl Physiol* 1964; **19**: 207–11.

3 Zapletal A, Paul T, Samanek M. Pulmonary elasticity in children and adolescents. *J Appl Physiol* 1976; **40**: 953–61.

4 Ingram RH, O'Cain CF, Fridy WW. Simultaneous quasi-static lung pressure–volume curves and 'closing volume' measurements. *J Appl Physiol* 1974; **36**: 135–41.

5 Knowles JH, Hong SK, Rahn, H. Possible errors using oesophageal balloons in determination of pressure–volume characteristics of the lung and thoracic cage. *J Appl Physiol* 1959; **14**: 525–30.

6 Quanjer PH. Standardized lung function testing. *Clin Respir Physiol* 1983; **19** (suppl. 5): 28–32.

7 Galetke W, Feier C, Muth T, *et al*. Reference values for dynamic and static pulmonary compliance in men. *Respir Med* 2007; **101**: 1783–9.

8 Yernault JC, Baran D, Englert M. Effect of growth and aging on the static mechanical lung properties. *Bull Eur Physiopathol Resp* 1977; **13**: 777–88.

9 Gibson GJ, Pride NB, Davis J, Schroter RC. Exponential description of the static pressure–volume curve of normal and diseased lungs. *Am Rev Respir Dis* 1979; **120**: 799–811.

10 Jonson B, Svantesson C. Elastic pressure–volume curves: what information do they convey? *Thorax* 1999; **54**: 82–7.

11 Campbell EJM. *The Respiratory Muscles*, Lloyd-Luke, London, 1958.

12 Woolcock AJ, Vincent NJ, Macklem PT. Frequency dependence of compliance as a test for obstruction in the small airways. *J Clin Invest* 1969; **48**: 1097–106.

13 Agostoni E. Statics, in *The Respiratory Muscles*, 2nd edn (eds EJM Campbell, E Agostoni and J Newsom Davis), Lloyd-Luke, London, 1970, pp. 48–79.

14 Heaf PJD, Prime FJ. The compliance of the thorax in normal human subjects. *Clin Sci* 1956; **15**: 319–27.

15 De Troyer A, Bastenier-Geens. Effects of neuromuscular blockade on respiratory mechanics in conscious man. *J Appl Physiol* 1979; **47**: 1162–8.

16 Gibson GJ. Spirometry then and now. *Breathe* 2005; **1**: 206–16.

17 DuBois AB, Botelho SY, Bedell GN, *et al*. A rapid plethysmographic method for measuring thoracic gas volume. *J Clin Invest* 1956; **35**: 322–6.

18 Mead J. Volume displacement body plethysmograph for respiratory measurements in human subjects. *J Appl Physiol* 1960; **15**: 736–40.

19 Stanescu DC, de Sutter P, van de Woestijne KP. Pressure-corrected flow body plethysmograph. *Am Rev Respir Dis* 1972; **105**: 304–5.

20 Habib MP, Engel LA. Influence of the panting technique on the measurement of thoracic gas volume. *Am Rev Respir Dis* 1978; **117**: 265–71.

21 Stanescu DC, Rodenstein D, Caubergs M, van de Woestijne KP. Failure of body plethysmography in bronchial asthma. *J Appl Physiol* 1982; **52**: 939–48.

22 Rodenstein DO, Stanescu DC. Reassessment of lung volume measurement by helium dilution and by body plethysmography in chronic airflow obstruction. *Am Rev Respir Dis* 1982; **126**: 1040–44.

23 Meneely GR, Kaltreider NL. The volume of the lung determined by helium dilution. *J Clin Invest* 1949; **28**: 129–39.

24 Ferris B. Epidemiology standardization project: III. Recommended standardized procedures for pulmonary function testing. *Am Rev Respir Dis* 1978; **118** (suppl.): 78–9.

25 Barnhard HJ, Pierce JA, Joyce JW, Bates JH. Roentgenographic determination of total lung capacity. *Am J Med* 1960; **28**: 51–60.

26 Pierce RJ, Brown DJ, Holmes M, *et al*. Estimation of lung volumes from chest radiographs using shape information. *Thorax* 1979; **34**: 726–34.

27 Kanczor H-U, Heussel CP, Fischer B, *et al*. Assessment of lung volumes using helical CT at inspiration and expiration: comparison with pulmonary function tests. *Am J Roentgenol* 1998; **171**: 1091–5.

28 Brown MS, McNitt-Gray MF, Goldin JG, *et al*. Automated measurement of single and total lung volume from CT. *J Comput Assist Tomogr* 1999; **23**: 632.

29 Gilbert R, Auchincloss JH, Brodsky J. Changes in tidal volume, frequency and ventilation induced by their measurement. *J Appl Physiol* 1972; **33**: 252–4.

30 Rodenstein DO, Mercenier C, Stanescu DC. Influence of the respiratory route on the resting breathing pattern in humans. *Am Rev Respir Dis* 1985; **131**: 163–5.

31 Konno K, Mead J. Measurement of the separate volume changes of rib cage and abdomen during breathing. *J Appl Physiol* 1967; **22**: 407–22.

32 Stagg D, Goldman M, Newsom Davis J. Computer-aided measurement of breath volume and time components using magnetometers. *J Appl Physiol* 1978; **44**: 623–33.

33 Sackner MA, Watson H, Belsito AS, *et al*. Calibration of respiratory inductive plethysmograph during natural breathing. *J Appl Physiol* 1989; **66**: 410–20.

34 Banzett RB, Mahan ST, Garner DM, Brughera A, Loring SH. A simple and reliable method to calibrate respiratory magnetometers and Respitrace. *J Appl Physiol* 1995; **79**: 2169–76.

35 Clarenbach CF, Senn O, Brack T, Kohler M, Bloch KE. Monitoring of ventilation during exercise by a portable respiratory inductive plethysmograph. *Chest* 2005; **128**: 1282–90.

36 Cala SJ, Kenyon CM, Ferrigno G, *et al*. Chest wall and lung volume estimation by optical reflectance motion analysis. *J Appl Physiol* 1996; **81**: 2680–89.

37 Goldman MD, Mead J. Mechanical interaction between the diaphragm and rib cage. *J Appl Physiol* 1973; **35**: 197–204.

38 De Troyer A, Estenne M. Co-ordination between rib cage muscles and diaphragm during quiet breathing in humans. *J Appl Physiol* 1984; **57**: 899–906.

39 Ninane V, Rypens F, Yernault J-C, De Troyer A. Abdominal muscle use during breathing in patients with chronic airflow obstruction. *Am Rev Respir Dis* 1992; **146**: 16–21.

40 Rohrer F. Der Zusammenhang der Atemkräfte und ihre Abhängigkeit vom Dehnungszustand der Atmungsorgane. *Pflügers Arch ges Physiol* 1916; **165**: 419–44.

41 Agostoni E, Rahn H. Abdominal and thoracic pressures at different lung volumes. *J Appl Physiol* 1960; **15**: 1087–92.

42 American Thoracic Society/European Respiratory Society. ATS/ERS statement on respiratory muscle testing. *Am J Respir Crit Care Med* 2002; **166**: 518–624.

43 Gibson GJ, Clark E, Pride NB. Static transdiaphragmatic pressures in normal subjects and in patients with chronic hyperinflation. *Am Rev Respir Dis* 1981; **124**: 685–9.

44 De Troyer A, Estenne M. Limitations of measurement of transdiaphragmatic pressure in detecting diaphragmatic weakness. *Thorax* 1981; **36**: 169–74.

45 Miller JM, Moxham J, Green M. The maximal sniff in the assessment of diaphragm function in man. *Clin Sci* 1985; **69**: 91–6.

46 Heritier F, Rahm F, Pasehe P, Fitting JW. Sniff nasal inspiratory pressure: a non-invasive assessment of inspiratory muscle strength. *Am J Respir Crit Care Med* 1994; **150**: 1678–83.

47 Uldry C, Janssens JP, de Muralt B, Fitting JW. Sniff nasal inspiratory pressure in patients with chronic obstructive pulmonary disease. *Eur Respir J* 1997; **10**: 1292–6.

48 Lofaso F, Nicot F, Lejaille M, *et al.* Sniff nasal inspiratory pressure: what is the optimal number of sniffs? *Eur Respir J* 2006; **27**: 980–82.

49 Man WD-C, Kyroussis D, Fleming TA, *et al.* Cough gastric pressure and maximum expiratory mouth pressure in humans. *Am J Respir Crit Care Med* 2003; **168**: 714–17.

50 McKenzie DK, Gandevia SC. Phrenic nerve conduction times and twitch pressures of the human diaphragm. *J Appl Physiol* 1985; **58**: 1496–504.

51 Mier A, Brophy C, Moxham J, Green M. Phrenic nerve stimulation in normal subjects and in patients with diaphragmatic weakness. *Thorax* 1987; **42**: 885–8.

52 Similowski T, Fleury B, Launois S, *et al.* Cervical magnetic stimulation: a new painless method for bilateral phrenic nerve stimulation in conscious humans. *J Appl Physiol* 1989; **67**: 1311–18.

53 Luo YM, Johnson LC, Polkey MI, *et al.* Diaphragm electromyogram measured with unilateral magnetic stimulation. *Eur Respir J* 1999; **13**: 385–90.

54 Luo YM, Harris ML, Lyall RA, *et al.* Assessment of diaphragm paralysis with oesophageal electromyography and unilateral magnetic phrenic nerve stimulation. *Eur Respir J* 2000; **15**: 596–9.

55 Glerant JC, Mustfa N, Man WD, *et al.* Diaphragm electromyograms recorded from multiple surface electrodes following magnetic stimulation. *Eur Respir J* 2006; **27**: 334–42.

56 Yan S, Gauthier AP, Similowski T, Macklem PT, Bellemare F. Evaluation of human diaphragm contractility using mouth pressure twitches. *Am Rev Respir Dis* 1992; **145**: 1064–9.

57 Hughes PD, Polkey MI, Kyroussis, *et al.* Measurement of sniff nasal and diaphragm twitch mouth pressure in patients. *Thorax* 1998; **53**: 96–100.

58 Laghi F, Tobin MJ. Relationship between transdiaphragmatic and mouth twitch pressures at functional residual capacity. *Eur Respir J* 1997; **10**: 530–36.

59 Similowski T, Gauthier AP, Yan S, Machlem PT, Bellemare F. Assessment of diaphragm function using mouth pressure twitches in chronic obstructive pulmonary disease patients. *Am Rev Respir Dis* 1993; **147**: 850–56.

60 Kyroussis D, Polkey MI, Mills GH, *et al.* Stimulation of cough in man by magnetic stimulation of the thoracic nerve roots. *Am J Respir Crit Care Med* 1997; **156**: 1696–9.

61 McCool FD, McCann DR, Leith DE, Hoppin FG. Pressure–flow effects on endurance of inspiratory muscles. *J Appl Physiol* 1986; **60**: 299–303.

62 Nickerson BG, Keens TG. Measuring ventilatory muscle endurance in humans as sustainable inspiratory pressure. *J Appl Physiol* 1982; **52**: 768–72.

63 Eastwood PR, Hillman DR. A threshold loading device for testing of inspiratory muscle performance. *Eur Respir J* 1995; **8**: 463–6.

64 Macklem PT, Roussos CS. Respiratory muscle fatigue: a cause of respiratory failure? *Clin Sci* 1977; **53**: 419–22.

65 Respiratory Muscle Fatigue Workshop Group. Respiratory muscle fatigue. *Am Rev Respir Dis* 1990; **142**: 474–80.

66 Efthimiou J, Fleming J, Spiro SG. Sternomastoid muscle function and fatigue in breathless patients with severe respiratory disease. *Am Rev Respir Dis* 1987; **136**: 1099–105.

67 Moxham J, Morris ARJ, Spiro SG, Edwards RHT, Green M. Contractile properties and fatigue of the diaphragm in man. *Thorax* 1981; **36**: 164–8.

68 Gross D, Grassino A, Ross WRD, Macklem PT. Electromyogram pattern of diaphragmatic fatigue. *J Appl Physiol* 1979; **46**: 1–7.

69 Moxham J, Edwards RHT, Aubier M, *et al.* Changes in EMG power spectrum (high-to-low ratio) with force fatigue in humans. *J Appl Physiol* 1982; **53**: 1094–9.

70 Esau SA, Bye PTB, Pardy RL. Changes in rate of relaxation of sniffs with diaphragmatic fatigue in humans. *J Appl Physiol* 1983; **55**: 731–5.

71 Kyroussis D, Mills G, Hannegard CH, *et al.* Inspiratory muscle relaxation rate assessed from sniff nasal pressure. *Thorax* 1994; **49**: 1127–33.

72 Kyroussis D, Polkey MI, Keilty SEJ, *et al.* Exhaustive exercise slows inspiratory muscle relaxation rate in chronic obstructive pulmonary disease. *Am J Respir Crit Care Med* 1996; **153**: 787–93.

73 Eiser N. The hitch-hiker's guide to nasal patency. *Respir Med* 1990; **84**: 179–83.

74 Pertuze J, Watson A, Pride NB. Maximum airflow through the nose in humans. *J Appl Physiol* 1991; **70**: 1369–76.

75 Hilbert O, Pedersen OF. Acoustic rhinometry: recommendations for technical specifications and standard operating procedures. *Rhinology* 2000; **16** (suppl.): 3–17.

76 Richardson J, Beland J. Non-adrenergic inhibitory nervous system in human airways. *J Appl Physiol* 1976; **41**: 764–71.

77 Nadel JA, Tierney DF. Effect of a previous deep inspiration on airway resistance in man. *J Appl Physiol* 1961; **16**: 717–19.

78 Parsons PE, Grunstein MM, Fernandez E. The effects of acute hypoxia and hypercapnia on pulmonary mechanics in normal subjects and patients with chronic pulmonary disease. *Chest* 1989; **96**: 96–101.

79 Van Den Elshout FJJ, Van Herwaarden CLA, Folgering HTM. Effects of hypercapnia and hypocapnia on respiratory resistance in normal and asthmatic subjects. *Thorax* 1991; **46**: 28–32.

80 Dagg KD, Thomson LJ, Clayton RA, Ramsay SG, Thomson NC. Effect of acute alterations in inspired oxygen tension on methacholine induced bronchoconstriction in patients with asthma. *Thorax* 1997; **52**: 453–7.

81 Mead J, Whittenberger JL. Physical properties of human lungs measured during spontaneous respiration. *J Appl Physiol* 1953; **5**: 779–96.

82 Clements JA, Sharp JT, Johnson RP, Elam JO. Estimation of pulmonary resistance by repetitive interruption of airflow. *J Clin Invest* 1959; **38**: 1262–70.

83 Merkus PJ, Mijnsbergen JY, Hop WC, de Jongste JC. Interrupter resistance in preschool children: measurement characteristics and reference values. *Am J Respir Crit Care Med* 2001; **163**: 1350–55.

84 Sly PD, Lombardi E. Measurement of lung function in preschool children using the interrupter technique. *Thorax* 2003; **58**: 742–4.

85 DuBois AB, Botelho SY, Comroe JH. A new method for measuring airway resistance in man using a body plethysmograph. *J Clin Invest* 1956; **35**: 327–32.

86 Stanescu DC, Pattijn J, Clément J, van de Woestijne KP. Glottis opening and airway resistance. *J Appl Physiol* 1972; **32**: 460–66.

87 Higenbottam T, Payne J. Glottis narrowing in lung disease. *Am Rev Respir Dis* 1982; **125**: 746–50.

88 Oostveen E, MacLeod D, Lorino H, *et al.* The forced oscillation technique in clinical practice: methodology, recommendations and future developments. *Eur Respir J* 2003; **22**: 1026–41.

89 Goldman MD, Saadeh C, Ross D. Clinical applications of forced oscillation to assess peripheral airway function. *Respir Physiol Neurobiol* 2005; **148**: 179–94.

90 Fry DL, Hyatt RE. Pulmonary mechanics: a unified analysis of the relationship between pressure, volume and gas flow in the lungs of normal and diseased subjects. *Am J Med* 1960; **29**: 672–89.

91 Mead J, Turner JM, Macklem PT, Little JB. Significance of the relationship between lung recoil and maximum expiratory flow. *J Appl Physiol* 1967; **22**: 95–108.

92 Pride NB, Permutt S, Riley RL, Bromberger-Barnea B. Determinants of maximal expiratory flow from the lungs. *J Appl Physiol* 1967; **23**: 646–62.

93 Dawson SV, Elliott E. Wave-speed limitation on expiratory flow: a unifying concept. *J Appl Physiol* 1977; **43**: 498–515.

94 Pedersen OF, Brackel HJ, Bogaard JM, Kerrebijn KF. Wave-speed-determined flow limitation at peak flow in normal and asthmatic subjects. *J Appl Physiol* 1997; **83**: 1721–32.

95 Allen JL, Castile RG, Mead J. Positive effort dependence of maximal expiratory flow. *J Appl Physiol* 1987; **62**: 718–24.

96 Ingram RH, Schilder DP. Effect of gas compression on pulmonary pressure, flow and volume relationship. *J Appl Physiol* 1966; **21**: 1821–6.

97 Vincken WG, Cosio MG. Flow oscillations on the flow–volume loop: clinical and physiological implication. *Eur Respir J* 1989; **2**: 543–9.

98 Barnes PJ, Gribbin HR, Osmanliev D, Pride NB. Partial flow–volume curves to measure bronchodilator dose–response curves in normal humans. *J Appl Physiol* 1981; **50**: 1193–7.

99 Hyatt RE. The interrelationship of pressure, flow and volume during various respiratory manoeuvres in normal and emphysematous patients. *Am Rev Respir Dis* 1961; **83**: 676–83.

100 D'Angelo E, Prandi E, Milic-Emili J. Dependence of maximum flow–volume curves on time course of preceding inspiration. *J Appl Physiol* 1993; **75**: 1155–9.

101 Koulouris NG, Retsou S, Kosmas E, *et al.* Tidal expiratory flow limitation, dyspnoea and exercise capacity in patients with bilateral bronchiectasis. *Eur Respir J* 2003; **21**: 743–8.

102 Ninane V, Leduc D, Kafi SA, *et al.* Detection of expiratory flow limitation by manual compression of the abdominal wall. *Am J Respir Crit Care Med* 2001; **163**: 1326–30.

103 Tiffeneau R and Pinelli A. Air circulant et air captif dans l'exploration de la fonction ventilatrice pulmonaire. *Paris Med* 1947; **133**: 624–8.

104 Gaensler EA. Analysis of the ventilatory defect by timed capacity measurements. *Am Rev Tuberc* 1951; **64**: 256–78.

105 Hutchinson J. On the capacity of the lungs, and on the respiratory functions, with a view to establishing a precise and easy method of detecting disease by the spirometer. *Med Chir Trans* 1846; **29**: 137–252.

106 Gilson JC, Hugh Jones P. The measurement of the total lung volume and breathing capacity. *Clin Sci* 1949; **7**: 185–216.

107 Pellegrino R, Viegi G, Brusasco V, *et al.* Interpretative strategies for lung function testing. *Eur Respir J* 2005; **26**: 948–68.

108 Hankinson JL, Odencrantz JR, Fedan KB. Spirometric reference values from a sample of the general U.S. population. *Am J Respir Crit Care Med* 1999; **159**: 179–87.

109 Akpinar-Elci M, Fedan KB, Enright PL. FEV_6 as a surrogate for FVC in detecting airways obstruction and restriction in the workplace. *Eur Respir J* 2006; **27**: 374–7.

110 Hansen JE, Sun XG, Wasserman K. Should forced expiratory volume in six seconds replace forced vital capacity to detect airway obstruction? *Eur Respir J* 2006; **27**: 1244–50.

111 Leuallen EC, Fowler WS. Maximal midexpiratory flow. *Am Rev Tuberc* 1955; **72**: 783–800.

112 McFadden ER, Linden DA. A reduction in maximum mid-expiratory flow rate: a spirographic manifestation of small airway disease. *Am J Med* 1972; **52**: 725–37.

113 Permutt S, Menkes HA. Spirometry: analysis of forced expiration within the time domain, in *The Lung in the Transition Between Health and Disease* (eds P Macklem and S Permutt), Marcel Dekker, New York, 1979.

114 Pride NB. Analysis of forced expiration: a return to the recording spirometer? *Thorax* 1979; **34**: 144–7.

115 Guyatt AR, Alpers JH. Factors affecting airways conductance: a study of 752 working men. *J Appl Physiol* 1968; **24**: 310–16.

116 Wouters EFM, Mostert R, Polko AH, Visser BF. Forced expiratory flow and oscillometric impedance measurement in evaluating airway obstruction. *Respir Med* 1990; **84**: 205–9.

117 Joos GF, O'Connor B, Anderson SD, *et al.* Indirect airway challenges. *Eur Respir J* 2003; **21**: 1050–68.

118 Van Schoor J, Panwels R, Joos G. Indirect bronchial hyper-responsiveness: the coming of age of a specific group of bronchial challenges. *Clin Exp Allergy* 2005; **35**: 250–61.

119 Sterk PJ, Fabbri LM, Quanjer P, *et al.* Airway responsiveness: standardised challenge testing with pharmacological, physical and sensitising stimuli in adults. *Eur Respir J* 1993; **6** (suppl. 16): 53–83.

120 American Thoracic Society. Guidelines for methacholine and exercise challenge testing – 1999. *Am J Respir Crit Care Med* 2000; **161**: 309–29.

121 Hargreave FE, Ryan NC, Thomson P, *et al.* Bronchial responsiveness to histamine or methacholine in asthma: measurement and clinical significance. *J Allergy Clin Immunol* 1981; **68**: 347–55.

122 Rosenthal RR. Approved methodology for methacholine challenge. *Allergy Proc* 1989; **10**: 301–10.

123 Yan K, Salome C, Woolcock AJ. Rapid method for measurement of bronchial responsiveness. *Thorax* 1983; **38**: 760–65.

124 Allen ND, Davis ND, Hurst BE, Cockcroft DW. Difference between dosimeter and tidal breathing methacholine challenge: contributions of dose and deep inspiration bronchoprotection. *Chest* 2005; **128**: 4018–23.

125 Woolcock AJ, Salome CM, Yan K. The shape of the dose–response curve to histamine in asthmatic and normal subjects. *Am Rev Respir Dis* 1984; **130**: 71–5.

126 Chinn S, Schouten JP. Reproducibility of non-specific bronchial challenge in adults: implications for design, analysis and interpretation of clinical and epidemiological studies. *Thorax* 2005; **60**: 395–400.

127 Benson MK. Bronchial hyperreactivity. *Br J Dis Chest* 1975; **69**: 227–39.

128 Rubinfield AR, Pain MCF. Relationship between bronchial reactivity, airway calibre and severity of asthma. *Am Rev Respir Dis* 1977; **115**: 381–7.

129 Ramsdale EH, Morris MM, Roberts RS, Hargreave FE. Bronchial responsiveness to methacholine in chronic bronchitis: relationship to airflow obstruction and cold air responsiveness. *Thorax* 1984; **39**: 312–18.

130 Rijcken B, Schouten JP, Weiss ST, Speizer FE, van der Lende R. The relationship between airway responsiveness to histamine and pulmonary function level in a random population sample. *Am Rev Respir Dis* 1988; **137**: 826–32.

131 Baldwin E de F, Cournand A, Richards DW. Pulmonary insufficiency: I. Physiological classification, clinical methods of analysis, standard values in normal subjects. *Medicine (Baltimore)* 1948; **27**: 243–80.

132 Aaron SD, Dales RE, Cardinal P. How accurate is spirometry at predicting restrictive pulmonary impairment? *Chest* 1999; **115**: 869–73.

133 Owens MW, Kinasewitz GT, Anderson WM. Clinical significance of an isolated reduction in residual volume. *Am Rev Respir Dis* 1987; **136**: 1377–80.

134 Cockcroft DW, Berscheid BA. Volume adjustment of maximal mid-expiratory flow. *Chest* 1980; **78**: 595–600.

135 Barnhart S, Hudson LD, Mason SE, Pierson DJ, Rosenstock L. Total lung capacity: an insensitive measure of impairment in patients with asbestosis and chronic obstructive pulmonary disease? *Chest* 1988; **93**: 299–302.

Pulmonary Gas Exchange

2

The successful exchange of oxygen for carbon dioxide in the lungs depends on the integration of several physical and chemical processes. The importance of matching ventilation to perfusion and the capacity of the lungs for local adjustments has been recognized for 100 years and advances in technology have allowed increasingly detailed study. In diseased lungs 'compensatory' changes in local ventilation and/or perfusion often tend to minimize the functional consequences of structural damage.

The factors affecting pulmonary gas exchange are conveniently considered in three stages – ventilation, diffusion and perfusion. The bellows action of the thorax replenishes a proportion of the alveolar gas with fresh air during each breath; the result depends on the volume of gas in the lungs at the start of the breath (functional residual capacity, FRC), the size of the tidal volume and the efficiency with which these mix. Diffusion across the alveolar–capillary membrane, as conventionally assessed, includes not only the passage of gas molecules from alveoli into plasma but also diffusion across the red cell membrane and chemical combination of the gas with haemoglobin. The factors limiting the rate of uptake of a gas by the blood depend on the solubility and chemical combining properties of the gas. For example, for carbon monoxide (CO), haemoglobin has a high affinity and therefore combines with it with little rise in the partial pressure of CO in the blood ('back pressure'). Consequently, uptake of CO has little effect on the transfer of further CO molecules and its rate of uptake is therefore limited by diffusion rather than by perfusion. Haemoglobin combines less avidly with oxygen so that a back pressure rapidly builds up as the blood becomes saturated. Further uptake of oxygen then requires replenishment of red cells; consequently, oxygen uptake is dependent on both diffusion and perfusion. With a soluble gas that is inert (i.e. one that does not enter into chemical combination with haemoglobin), the rate of uptake is even more dependent on perfusion; such a gas can therefore be used to measure pulmonary blood flow (see Section 2.3). To assess the capacity of the lungs for gas diffusion, it is logical and convenient to use carbon monoxide (as discussed further in Chapter 3), while the efficiency of matching of ventilation and perfusion is better assessed by measuring arterial oxygenation (see Section 2.4).

2.1 PULMONARY VENTILATION

2.1.1 Convection and molecular diffusion

The passage of gas molecules between the mouth or nose and the proximal side of the alveolar membrane depends on two processes. Convection accounts for the larger proportion of the distance travelled, i.e. from the airway opening to approximately the respiratory bronchioles – this is the 'active' component of ventilation, where flow of gases is indiscriminate and determined by differences in total pressure. In the more distal pathways in the lungs, molecular diffusion takes over; here the movement of gases is effectively determined by gradients of their individual partial pressures and the diffusivity of the gas concerned. The two processes are not mutually exclusive: convective gradients also develop in the peripheral regions of the lungs, while in the more proximal airways some diffusion into and out of the main stream of convective airflow also occurs (a phenomenon known as 'Taylor dispersion'). A further minor factor promoting gas mixing is the 'churning' effect of cardiac contraction.

2.1.2 Dead space

The conducting airways, i.e. those in which no gas exchange is possible, constitute the anatomical dead space (about 150 mL in an adult). Any alveoli that have no perfusion also act as dead space. The physiological dead space comprises both of these plus a contribution from alveoli that have relatively more ventilation than perfusion. The size of the dead space can be calculated from the expired and alveolar CO_2 concentrations (F) or tensions (P) using the Bohr equation. The amount (volume) of CO_2 expired in each breath is calculated by multiplying the tidal volume (V_T) by the fractional concentration of CO_2 in expired air (F_ECO_2). The total volume of CO_2 expired with each breath comprises that expired from the dead space (V_D) (effectively zero since dead space by definition contains inspired air) and from the alveoli; the latter equals ($V_T - V_D$) multiplied by the fractional concentration of CO_2 in alveolar air (F_ACO_2), i.e.

$$V_T \times F_ECO_2 = (V_T - V_D) \times F_ACO_2$$

whence:

$$\frac{V_D}{V_T} = \frac{F_ACO_2 - F_ECO_2}{F_ACO_2}$$

or in terms of partial pressures:

$$\frac{V_D}{V_T} = \frac{P_ACO_2 - P_ECO_2}{P_ACO_2} \qquad (2.1)$$

The ratio V_D/V_T represents the proportion of each tidal breath that is wasted. Either the anatomical or the physiological dead space can be calculated, depending on the value of P_ACO_2 (alveolar gas tension of CO_2) used in Equation 2.1 (see Section 2.3).

Paradoxically, the physiological dead space is often more a test of inhomogeneous perfusion than of ventilation because alveoli with a dead-space-like effect (i.e. high ventilation/perfusion ratios) usually have impaired perfusion rather than excessive ventilation. An important consequence of the presence of a dead space is that the first 25 per cent or so of a normal tidal breath entering the alveoli is not fresh air but previously expired gas re-inspired from the dead space; the proportion is higher still in diseased lungs.

2.1.3 Effect of gravity on ventilation

Uneven distribution of ventilation is demonstrable in healthy subjects and is in part related to gravity-dependent regional differences (Fig. 2.1).[1,2] The size of the difference between the apex and the base of the lung depends on the absolute lung volume, the size of the tidal volume and the flow.[3,4] The effect of gravity has been explained using the simple analogy of a coiled spring in a gravitational field – the spring (or the lung) is distorted by its own weight, so that near the top the coils are further apart or the alveoli are relatively more distended. The shape of the

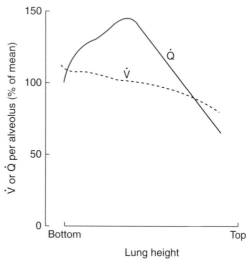

Figure 2.1 Regional distribution of ventilation and perfusion during tidal breathing in a healthy subject in the upright position. The distribution of ventilation (broken line) is for a normal-sized tidal breath from functional residual capacity (FRC) with a flow rate of 0.5 Ls^{-1} (based on ref 3). Over the upper two-thirds of the lung, relative perfusion (solid line) declines towards the apices more steeply than ventilation, but there is also a reduction at the lung bases (based on ref 4).

pressure–volume relationship of the lungs (Fig. 2.2) implies that the apical alveoli, which begin inspiration at a relatively large volume, are less compliant over the tidal range and therefore their proportion of the tidal volume is smaller than that received by the less distended and more compliant alveoli at the lung bases. This analogy gives only a partial explanation, as the weight of the abdominal contents is also a factor, without which the gravitational influence is considerably reduced.[5]

2.1.4 Effects of flow on distribution of ventilation

At higher flows, such as during exercise, regional differences in ventilation become less. Not only are the alveoli near the lung apices relatively more distended, but so also are their associated airways; consequently, the airway resistance in the upper zones is relatively low, the effect of which becomes more important with higher inspiratory flows. Another factor that may be important is differential activation of the respiratory muscles. During quiet breathing, the diaphragm is the main inspiratory muscle and it produces the largest changes in pleural pressure over the basal regions of the lungs;[6] when higher flows are required, activity of the inspiratory intercostal and accessory muscles increases and they produce a relatively greater change in pleural pressure distending the upper regions of the lungs, which would favour more even distribution of inspired air.

2.1.5 Effects of posture

In the recumbent posture, the gravitational gradient operates in the anteroposterior direction and again favours the more dependent parts of the lungs. There are important differences between the supine and prone postures, with more even distribution of ventilation prone than supine, an effect attributed to the influence of the heart and diaphragm. In the supine posture the anteriorly positioned and relatively mobile heart tends to compress the underlying lung, while when prone the heart is supported by the anterior chest wall.[7] In addition, the diaphragm moves to a higher (cephalad) position in the supine posture, compressing the lower lobes.

2.1.6 Intraregional inhomogeneity

Variation in the ventilation of different alveoli also occurs within lung regions, but the mechanisms are not fully understood. Two types of inhomogeneity are described (Fig. 2.3):[8] if diffusion of air along a

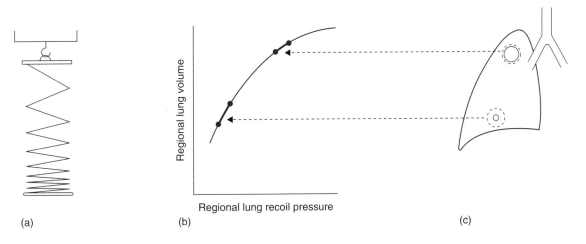

(a)   (b)   (c)

Regional lung volume

Regional lung recoil pressure

Figure 2.2 (a) Coiled spring or concertina suspended vertically, showing greater separation of the upper than the lower coils. The lung is similarly distorted by gravity so that, at a given lung volume, the alveoli near the apex are more distended than those near the base. Since the pressure–volume curves (b) of individual alveoli are similar, the larger upper alveoli are effectively stiffer and therefore (c) they receive less ventilation than basal alveoli during a normal tidal breath from end expiration (solid outlines) to end inspiration (broken outlines).

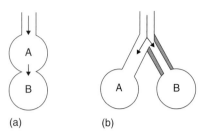

(a)   (b)

Figure 2.3 (a) Series or stratified inhomogeneity of ventilation; alveolus B receives less ventilation than the more proximal alveolus A. (b) Parallel inhomogeneity arising from local differences in mechanical properties. In this example, alveolus B receives less ventilation than A because the airway subtending B is narrower.

given pathway is incomplete during a breath, the more distal alveoli receive less ventilation than the more proximal alveoli – this represents 'series' or 'stratified' inhomogeneity. The second type is 'parallel' inhomogeneity, where alveoli are ventilated via parallel airways with differing mechanical characteristics – this is similar to the generation of regional differences considered above, but on a smaller, local scale. Ventilation can also occur via channels that bypass normal airways ('collateral' ventilation). Potential pathways include interalveolar pores (of Kohn), accessory bronchiole–alveolar communications and communications between respiratory bronchioles. The resistance of such pathways is usually high relative to that of the conventional airways, so that collateral ventilation is probably of little relevance in healthy lungs, but it may become important in disease.[9]

2.1.7 Washout tests for uneven ventilation

The overall uniformity and efficiency of ventilation can conveniently be assessed by simple tests in which the 'washout' of a gas is followed at the mouth, during either a period of tidal breathing or a single vital capacity exhalation. As originally described, both techniques utilize expired nitrogen, the concentration of which is recorded continuously after the subject has breathed pure oxygen. Later modifications to the multiple-breath method include the use of 21 per cent oxygen and 79 per cent argon (i.e. no nitrogen) to avoid the consequences of breathing 100 per cent oxygen over several minutes. In the single-breath technique, an

alternative to using nitrogen is to monitor the expired concentration of a bolus of inert gas (e.g. argon) inspired at residual volume (RV) at the beginning of the preceding full inspiration.

2.1.8 Multibreath washout tests

The multibreath technique originated with the work of Cournand et al.,[10] who showed that after 7 min of breathing pure oxygen the end tidal concentration of nitrogen normally fell to less than 2.5 per cent. They pointed out that this simple index of overall gas mixing was dependent on both the pattern of breathing and the lung volume (FRC) and that in hyperventilating subjects, where the washout rate was increased, abnormalities might be missed if measurements were made only after 7 min of 'washout'. This technique forms the basis of many subsequent studies using detailed analysis of washout curves. In principle, if gas mixing were perfect, the expired nitrogen concentration of a subject breathing pure oxygen would fall by the same proportion with each breath, i.e. the washout would be exponential. Plotting log N_2 concentration against time would then give a straight line (Fig. 2.4). In practice, in normal subjects the plot is usually slightly curvilinear (although in children it is more nearly rectilinear). In disease the curvilinearity is much more apparent (Fig. 2.4b). The curves can be analysed mathematically in terms of two or more 'compartments', but these rarely have any true anatomical correlates. In the diseased lung, where a wide variety of emptying patterns is found, the more compartments built in to the model, the more accurate the description of the washout pattern. In the analysis of multiple-breath washout curves, corrections can be made for variations of breathing pattern and FRC (e.g. by expressing the expired volume in terms of the number of 'turnovers' of FRC), and various indices based on the ventilation or turnovers to achieve reduction of the end tidal nitrogen concentration to a certain level have been described. Alternatively, moments analysis can be applied to the whole curve,[11] analogous to the moments analysis of the forced expiratory spirogram (see Chapter 1, Section 1.6.5.10); the first moment of the washout curve represents the 'centre of gravity' of the area under the curve, and successively higher moments, which are derived from power functions, further accentuate the tail of the curve. The various

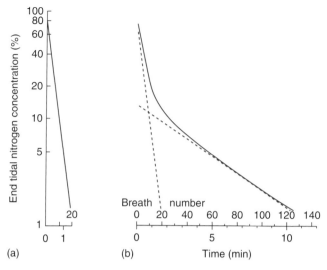

Figure 2.4 Multibreath nitrogen washout while breathing pure oxygen, with end tidal nitrogen concentration on a logarithmic scale plotted against time or breath number in (a) a normal subject and (b) a patient with generalized airway obstruction. Each subject is breathing with the same constant frequency. In the normal subject the washout of nitrogen is approximately exponential, so that the relationship plotted logarithmically is rectilinear. In the patient the rate of washout is much slower and cannot be described by a single exponential function. The curvilinear relationship can be approximated as the sum of two exponential functions (broken lines), which partition the lungs into theoretical rapidly and slowly emptying compartments.

derived indices offer a relatively sensitive method for detecting abnormalities in mild disease and are particularly valuable in children.[12]

2.1.9 Single-breath tests

The single-breath nitrogen test[13] is a simple, rapid method of assessing uneven ventilation. The subject inspires a vital capacity breath of pure oxygen from RV and then expires slowly, with the nitrogen concentration at the mouth recorded continuously. The type of record obtained is illustrated in Fig. 2.5. The originators of the test described three phases of the record of nitrogen concentration against expired volume. In the brief phase I the nitrogen concentration is zero, because initially the gas expired comes from the conducting airways, which contain pure oxygen. Phase II is also brief and represents the rapidly rising concentration as a mixture of dead space and alveolar gas is expired. Phase III, which occupies most of the expiration, is the 'alveolar plateau', which normally shows a very slowly rising concentration of nitrogen. A further terminal rise in nitrogen concentration (designated

phase IV) was defined subsequently.[14] Three main indices can be derived from the record of nitrogen concentration against time: the anatomical (or 'Fowler') dead space, the slope of the alveolar plateau, and the closing volume.

The anatomical dead space is rarely affected by disease, and it can be predicted from the subject's size (it approximates in millilitres the subject's bodyweight in pounds). Its measurement by Fowler's method assumes the presence of a 'front' of gas between the conducting airways and the gas-exchanging part of the lungs. If there were no gas mixing at the 'front', the expired nitrogen concentration would increase in a square-wave fashion as soon as the anatomical dead space had been expired (Fig. 2.6a). In reality some mixing occurs, which tends to blur the separation of dead space and alveolar gas; the graphical technique used to calculate the anatomical dead space is illustrated in Fig. 2.6b. The value calculated can vary, depending on technical factors: lengthening the breath-hold before the expiration reduces the calculated dead space, while increasing the inspired flow increases it. Both factors affect the position of the gas 'front' between the

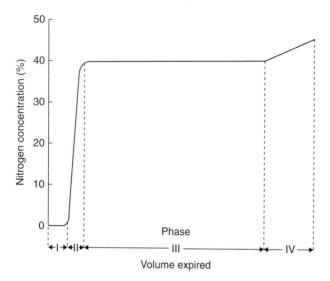

Figure 2.5 Single-breath nitrogen test with expired nitrogen concentration plotted against volume expired after a full inspiration of pure oxygen. Initially the expirate comes only from the anatomical dead space and contains pure oxygen (phase I); the nitrogen concentration then rises rapidly as a mixture of dead space and alveolar gas is expired (phase II), until an almost constant alveolar plateau is reached (phase III); towards the end of expiration the nitrogen concentration rises more sharply (phase IV).

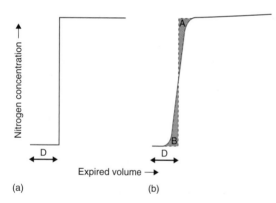

Figure 2.6 Single-breath nitrogen test as in Fig. 2.5. In the idealized situation (a), the size of the anatomical dead space (D) can be read directly on the expired volume scale. In the more realistic situation (b), the square wave is blunted as a mixture of dead space and alveolar gas is expired (phase II in Fig. 2.5). The anatomical dead space is calculated graphically by drawing a vertical line through phase II such that areas A and B are equal.

dead space and alveolar 'compartments': increased flow displaces it more distally, while initial breath-holding allows more time for diffusion and cardiogenic mixing to blur the front and move it proximally. Perhaps more surprisingly, the apparent size of the dead space depends on the gas used; it is greater with more dense gases, because with laminar flow a dense gas occupies the centre of the airstream and is carried deeper into the lungs so that its 'front' is more peripheral.[8] In practice the calculation of 'anatomical' dead space using this method is of theoretical rather than clinical interest.

The slope of phase III gives more relevant clinical information as it is a sensitive test of uneven ventilation. In simple terms, the gas concentration rises progressively because better-ventilated alveoli (with lower nitrogen concentrations) tend to empty before less well-ventilated alveoli. The measurement originally proposed was the slope over the half-litre between 750 mL and 1250 mL expired.[13] In young healthy subjects the average increase in nitrogen concentration over this volume range is about 0.7 per cent (i.e. 1.4% L^{-1}). As might be expected, the slope decreases if the breath is first held at end inspiration, as this results in better gas mixing.

2.1.10 Closing volume

The slope of phase III probably reflects mainly local inhomogeneity of ventilation, whereas phase IV is determined by gravity-dependent regional differences that result in an increasing contribution from

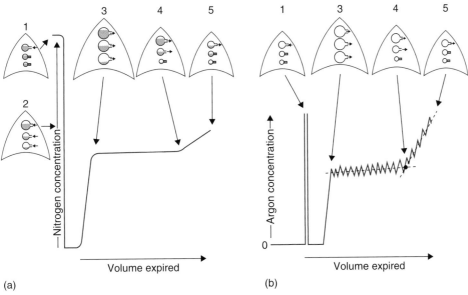

Figure 2.7 Two methods for estimating closing volume. Abscissa in each case records volume expired. (a) Single-breath nitrogen record, as in Fig. 2.5, with diagrams indicating alveolar size and airway patency at three levels in the lung; the shaded area within each alveolus represents the nitrogen concentration. Initially a full vital capacity of pure oxygen is inhaled from the residual volume (RV), and the nitrogen concentration at the mouth immediately falls to 0. At the start of inspiration (1) only the airways to the upper alveoli are patent but, because of the gradient of pleural pressure, the alveoli are already relatively well distended and therefore receive little oxygen. At mid-inspiration (2) all airways are patent but the lowermost alveoli receive the greatest ventilation and therefore by the end of inspiration these have the greatest oxygen (least nitrogen) concentration. In early expiration (3) all alveoli empty fairly evenly until, towards the end of expiration (4), progressive airway closure commences from the lung bases upwards. Since the basal alveoli (which have the greatest oxygen and least nitrogen concentrations) no longer contribute to the expirate, the nitrogen concentration at the mouth rises. The inflection on the record represents the volume at which closure of basal airways is first detectable (closing volume). At RV the more dependent airways are closed and the only alveoli contributing to the expirate in the final stages of expiration (5) are those near the lung apices, which received the least oxygen and therefore have the highest nitrogen concentration. (b) Record of argon concentration at the mouth during slow expiration from total lung capacity (TLC) after injection of a bolus of argon into the inspirate at RV. The bolus injected at the onset of inspiration (1) is distributed mainly to the uppermost alveoli, since the airways subtending the alveoli near the lung bases closed during the preceding expiration. Early in expiration (3) all alveoli empty fairly evenly and the expired argon concentration remains relatively constant until closure of basal airways (4) allows an increased contribution from the upper alveoli, which contain a higher argon concentration; progressive airway closure continues so that in the final stages of expiration (5) the alveoli contributing to the expirate are those that contain the highest concentration of argon. The oscillations on the record correspond to heart beats and are seen more readily with the greater amplification of the bolus technique compared with the resident gas (nitrogen) method.

the upper lobes as expiration proceeds. In the upright posture, closure of airways during expiration occurs first at the lung bases, rising progressively up the lung as RV is approached. The inflection on the expired nitrogen record at the onset of phase IV occurs because the more distended alveoli in the upper lung zones have received relatively less oxygen during the preceding inspiration; hence, they contribute a disproportionately large nitrogen concentration to the expirate once the airways supplying the basal alveoli start to close. The basal alveoli have lower nitrogen concentration due to their better ventilation with oxygen during the preceding inspiration (Fig. 2.7).

An alternative technique for measuring closing volume utilizes a bolus of an inert gas (xenon or argon) inspired at the start of the preceding full inspiration.[14] If such a bolus were to be inspired at FRC or above, it would be delivered preferentially to the lower zones of the lungs, as would be expected from the gravitational effects considered earlier. But if, in the upright posture, the bolus is inspired from RV, the pattern is very different, with preferential distribution to the apices and very little to the basal regions where the airways have closed during the preceding expiration. If, after a full inspiration, the expired concentration of the marker gas is now followed, a point of inflection is seen towards the end of expiration, at which its concentration rises abruptly. This is again the closing volume, i.e. the lung volume at which closure of dependent airways begins.

The term 'closing volume' (CV) usually refers to the difference in volume between the inflection point on the single breath recording (point of onset of phase IV) and residual volume, i.e. the volume expired during phase IV; this is usually expressed as a proportion of vital capacity (CV/VC). The term 'closing capacity' (CC) refers to the absolute volume at the point of inflection, i.e. CV + RV; it is often expressed as a proportion of total lung capacity (CC/TLC). Once clinically significant airflow obstruction develops, phase III becomes so steep that a phase IV may no longer be identifiable.

The rediscovery of the closing volume phenomenon in the 1960s rekindled interest in single-breath tests. They have been used, for example, in epidemiological studies for identifying early airway disease, but consistency of performance may be a problem in 'naive' subjects.[15]

2.2 LUNG PERFUSION

In an average-sized healthy individual the pulmonary vasculature receives approximately 6 L of blood each minute, but the volume of blood accessible for gas exchange at any instant is only 70–80 mL at rest, increasing to perhaps 150 mL on exercise. This represents the volume contained in the pulmonary capillaries within alveolar walls (the 'alveolar' vessels). The mechanics of pulmonary perfusion are less well studied than the equivalent basis of ventilation. It has been proposed that, rather than a system of branching tubes, the capillary bed is more accurately considered as two sheets of endothelial tissue separated by 'posts';[16] a useful analogy is with an underground carpark with a floor, ceiling and supporting posts.[17]

2.2.1 Gravitational effects on perfusion

In health, the effect of gravity on the distribution of perfusion is relatively greater than on ventilation (see Fig. 2.1). In the upright normal subject at rest there is very little perfusion of the lung apices because the relatively low pulmonary artery pressure developed at the hilum is insufficient to overcome the height of the lung. One important consequence of the situation of the pulmonary capillaries in the alveolar walls is that flow depends not only on the inlet and outflow pressures but also on the pressure of gas in the surrounding alveoli (Fig. 2.8).[18] If alveolar pressure exceeds local pulmonary arterial pressure, no blood flows; if alveolar pressure is less than arterial, but still greater than the pressure at the venous end of the capillary, the pressure governing flow is arterial minus alveolar rather than the usual difference between arterial and venous. If, however, alveolar pressure is less than venous, flow depends on the difference between arterial and venous pressures. All three of these situations are possible in the normal lung at different levels, and three zones, designated 1, 2 and 3, have been defined from above downwards (Fig. 2.8). The situation in zone 2, where alveolar rather than venous pressure represents the effective outflow pressure, is reminiscent of events in the airway during forced expiration, when the surrounding pleural pressure becomes an important determinant of airflow (see Chapter 1, Section 1.6.5.2). An increase in the driving (pulmonary arterial) pressure, as occurs during exercise, increases capillary blood volume by both greater distension of patent capillaries and recruitment of other vessels that were collapsed at lower perfusion pressures. The predictable gravity-dependent increasing perfusion down the lung may be reversed at the bases, especially at low lung volumes ('zone 4'). The mechanism may be narrowing of the extra-alveolar vessels consequent on the greater interstitial pressure at the lung bases.[17]

2.2.2 Pulmonary vascular tone

Pulmonary vessels react not only passively to the surrounding pressure but also actively to certain stimuli, of which local hypoxia appears to be the most potent, a response that helps to adjust local perfusion to local ventilation. Pulmonary vascular

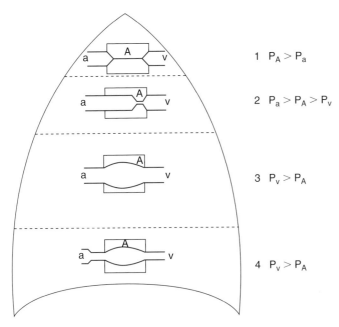

1 $P_A > P_a$

2 $P_a > P_A > P_v$

3 $P_v > P_A$

4 $P_v > P_A$

Figure 2.8 Effect of gravity on pulmonary perfusion in the upright lung. The lung may be considered as four distinct zones.[4] At rest there is little or no perfusion of apical alveoli (zone 1), because the pulmonary artery pressure is insufficient to overcome the hydrostatic pressure gradient due to gravity; the pressure (P_a) under which blood supplies the pulmonary capillaries is less than the surrounding alveolar pressure (P_A). Both P_a and the outflow pressure (P_v) increase down the lung and, once P_a exceeds P_A, flow occurs; if, however, P_v is less than P_A, the flow is determined not by the difference ($P_a - P_v$) but by ($P_a - P_A$), as in zone 2. Once P_v exceeds P_A (zone 3), the normal determinants of flow through a tube apply and ($P_a - P_v$) becomes the driving pressure. Perfusion therefore increases progressively down the lungs through zones 1 to 3, but at the lung bases flow is again reduced (zone 4) (cf. Fig. 2.1).

tone is also influenced by various endothelium-derived and circulating mediators.[19] Among the more important vasodilating factors are nitric oxide and prostacyclin. The pulmonary vessels are extensively innervated by autonomic nerves, but these probably have only a minor role in regulating vascular tone in humans.

2.2.3 Anatomical and physiological shunts

The analogue of the anatomical dead space is the 'anatomical shunt', i.e. the proportion of the cardiac output bypassing the lungs; normally this amounts to less than 5 per cent. The physiological dead space ('wasted ventilation') is analogous to the physiological shunt or venous admixture ('wasted perfusion'), which comprises the anatomical shunt through non-pulmonary vessels plus blood flow through any alveoli that are totally unventilated and a contribution from lung units with lower-than-average ventilation/perfusion ratios (see Section 2.4). Just as the

physiological dead space (paradoxically) gives information about the distribution of perfusion, so the physiological shunt largely assesses the distribution of ventilation.

2.2.4 Measurements of pulmonary blood flow

Total pulmonary blood flow can be measured by various techniques, e.g. dye dilution, thermodilution, Fick, etc., which are essentially the domain of the cardiologist and largely outside the scope of this brief review. With the Fick method, as practised at cardiac catheterization, the measurements required are the arterial and mixed venous (pulmonary arterial) oxygen content (concentration) and the overall oxygen consumption. The total pulmonary blood flow ($\dot{Q}_t$) is then given by:

$$\dot{Q}_t = \frac{\dot{V}O_2}{CaO_2 - C\overline{v}O_2} \tag{2.2}$$

where $\dot{Q}_t$ is total pulmonary blood flow, CaO_2 is arterial oxygen content, $C\bar{v}O_2$ is mixed venous oxygen content and $\dot{V}O_2$ is oxygen consumption.

An analogous equation can be written for CO_2 and is of relevance to respiratory laboratories because of the possibility of estimating mixed venous PCO_2 (and therefore CO_2 content) by rebreathing techniques (see Chapter 4). This is the 'indirect Fick' method, in which $\dot{Q}_t$ is calculated from:

$$\dot{Q}_t = \frac{\dot{V}CO_2}{C\bar{v}CO_2 - CaCO_2} \qquad (2.3)$$

where $C\bar{v}CO_2$ is mixed venous CO_2 content, $CaCO_2$ is arterial CO_2 content and $\dot{V}CO_2$ is CO_2 production.

At rest the accuracy of the CO_2 method is limited by the relatively small difference between $P\bar{v}CO_2$ and $PaCO_2$, but it has been used for estimating cardiac output during exercise when the venoarterial CO_2 difference widens appreciably.

Pulmonary blood flow can also be measured by inhalation of a highly soluble inert gas, as the rate of uptake of such a gas is a function of blood flow. In the original method of Krogh and Lindhard,[20] the subject takes a single maximal inspiration of a gas mixture containing nitrous oxide (N_2O) and then delivers two 'alveolar' samples separated by a period of breath-holding. The pulmonary blood flow is calculated from knowledge of the alveolar volume during the breath-hold, the change in N_2O concentration between the two samples and the solubility of N_2O. A later modification includes a second inert, but poorly soluble, gas.[21] The decay in the concentration of the soluble gas is analysed after collecting alveolar samples with varying breath-hold periods. In more recent methods, the concentration of a soluble gas is followed continuously during rebreathing[22] or during a single slow expiration,[23] and, by comparison with the concentration of the insoluble gas, the 'effective' pulmonary blood flow is calculated. All of these techniques are open to the objection that they are dependent on the distribution of ventilation as the soluble gas 'sees' flowing blood only in alveoli into which it is inspired. A different technique, developed by Lee and DuBois,[24] utilizes a constant-volume whole-body plethysmograph to record the contraction of thoracic gas volume as a soluble gas is absorbed by the pulmonary circulation; this method has been used to demonstrate the pulsatile nature of pulmonary capillary flow. Methods for studying the topographical distribution of lung perfusion are discussed in Section 2.4.

2.3 VENTILATION–PERFUSION RELATIONSHIPS

The net effects of uneven ventilation and perfusion are determined by variation in the balance of the two. The overall ratio of alveolar ventilation to perfusion (excluding the anatomical dead space) is usually about 0.9, but this can conceal a wide range of $\dot{V}_A/\dot{Q}$ ratios in individual alveoli ranging from 0 (unventilated alveoli, i.e. shunt) to infinity (unperfused alveoli, i.e. dead space).

The theoretical importance of this concept was appreciated long before techniques were available to demonstrate either the underlying mechanisms or their consequences. For example, Haldane in the early twentieth century reasoned that, whereas the effects of areas with high and low $\dot{V}_A/\dot{Q}$ on the carbon dioxide level of arterial blood might cancel each other, the situation with oxygen must be different because the shape of the oxygen dissociation curve implies that high $\dot{V}_A/\dot{Q}$ areas add very little extra oxygen to arterial blood and therefore are not able to compensate for the hypoxaemia resulting from low $\dot{V}_A/\dot{Q}$ areas.[25]

2.3.1 Oxygen–carbon dioxide diagram

As in the field of lung mechanics, a great stimulus to the understanding of $\dot{V}_A/\dot{Q}$ relationships came during the Second World War from the need to study the problems of aviators breathing hypoxic air at altitude. Two groups of researchers in the USA developed a theory and model of pulmonary gas exchange that analyses the effects of $\dot{V}_A/\dot{Q}$ mismatching and that, despite its limitations, still helps understanding of the concepts.[26–28] The analysis is represented graphically by the oxygen–carbon dioxide diagram, which relates the partial pressures of the two gases and examines all the possible combinations of PO_2 and PCO_2 in a lung supplied with inspired gas and pulmonary arterial blood of given compositions.[26]

The easiest starting point in this analysis is to consider what happens to PCO_2 and PO_2 as CO_2 is added

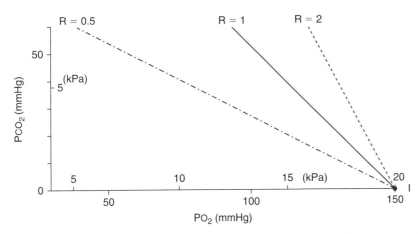

Figure 2.9 Oxygen–carbon dioxide diagram showing gas tensions. The lines represent the values of partial pressures of CO_2 (PCO_2) and O_2 (PO_2) that would result with addition of CO_2 to, and removal of O_2 from, air with initial composition I (normal atmospheric air at body temperature pressure saturated (BTPS)). If equal volumes of CO_2 and O_2 are exchanged, the resulting combinations of gas tensions are described by the line R = 1; if twice as much CO_2 is added as oxygen is removed, the gas tensions correspond to the line R = 2, etc.

and O_2 is removed from inspired room air (Fig. 2.9). If equal volumes are exchanged (i.e. the respiratory exchange ratio (R) is 1), the increase in PCO_2 is equal to the reduction in PO_2: the resulting values of PO_2 and PCO_2 then lie along a line starting at the inspired point (I in Fig. 2.9) and making an angle of $-45°$. If R is greater than 1, more CO_2 is added than O_2 is removed and the line is steeper. A fan of straight lines can therefore be drawn from point I, representing the values of PO_2 and PCO_2 for all possible values of R in the gas phase.

A similar approach can be taken with the various possible combinations of CO_2 removed from, and O_2 added to, the pulmonary arterial (mixed venous) blood (Fig. 2.10) – but here a problem arises, as the R lines are straight only if blood gas *contents* (concentrations) are plotted (Fig. 2.10a). If partial pressures of the gases are plotted, the non-linear dissociation curves for CO_2 and O_2 in blood result in alinear PCO_2–PO_2 relations for gas exchange in the blood phase (Fig. 2.10b). With certain assumptions, Figs 2.9 and 2.10b can now be superimposed in order to examine the possible combinations of PCO_2 and PO_2 that can occur within the lungs (Fig. 2.11). The main assumption is that in each individual lung 'unit' (alveolus and associated capillary) full equilibration of O_2 and CO_2 occurs, so that at the distal end of the capillary no gradient of either PO_2 or PCO_2

exists between alveolar gas and blood, i.e. there is no limitation of gas exchange by diffusion. The evidence suggests that this assumption is reasonable in most circumstances. The truism also applies that the number of oxygen molecules leaving the alveolar gas is the same as the number entering the blood (and vice versa for CO_2), i.e. in a given alveolus the value of R must be the same, whether calculated for gas or blood. But, of course, with the inevitable $\dot{V}_A/\dot{Q}$ mismatching present even in healthy lungs, the gas and blood R values, though identical in each individual lung unit, vary appreciably between units (see below.)

For every value of R there is one point of intersection in Fig. 2.11 that represents the PO_2 and PCO_2 that must obtain after equilibration in alveoli exchanging gas in the specified ratio. The line joining these points of intersection therefore represents all possible combinations of PO_2 and PCO_2 after equilibration in all the alveoli and pulmonary capillaries of lungs supplied with blood and gas with the compositions shown at $\bar{v}$ and I.[27]

2.3.2 'Ideal' alveolar air

The concept of 'ideal' alveolar air introduced by Riley and Cournand[28] utilizes the O_2–CO_2 relationship together with the respiratory exchange ratio for

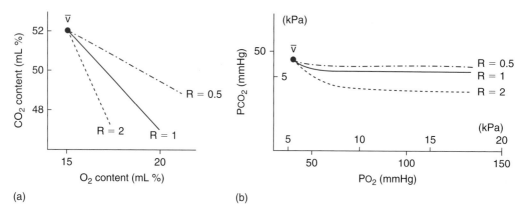

(a)   (b)

Figure 2.10 Oxygen–carbon dioxide diagrams showing (a) blood gas contents and (b) tensions. The lines represent the blood contents (concentrations) or partial pressures of CO_2 (Pco_2) and O_2 (Po_2) that would result with removal of CO_2 from, and addition of oxygen to, blood with initial composition $\bar{v}$ (corresponding to normal mixed venous (pulmonary arterial) blood at rest). If equal volumes of CO_2 and O_2 are exchanged, the resulting combinations of contents and tensions are described by the line R = 1; if twice as much CO_2 is removed as O_2 is added, the resulting values are described by the line R = 2, etc.

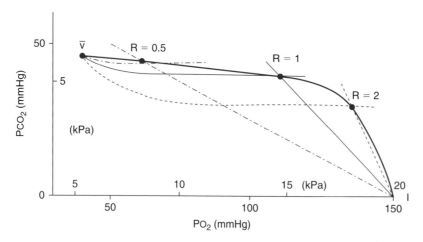

Figure 2.11 Superimposition of Figs 2.9 and 2.10b allows construction of the $\dot{V}_A/\dot{Q}$ line joining points where corresponding blood and gas R lines intersect. Since in an individual alveolus the local blood and gas R values are identical, this line describes all possible combinations of Pco_2 and Po_2 within lungs supplied with inspired air and mixed venous blood of compositions defined by I and $\bar{v}$ respectively. In an individual alveolus, the higher the R value, the higher the $\dot{V}_A/\dot{Q}$ ratio and the nearer the alveolar gas composition to inspired air, whereas a lower R implies a lower $\dot{V}_A/\dot{Q}$ ratio and closer proximity of gas tensions to those of mixed venous blood.

the lungs as a whole to identify the alveolar Po_2 and Pco_2 that would exist in all the alveoli of a given pair of lungs if there were no $\dot{V}_A/\dot{Q}$ mismatching. For example, if the overall R were 0.8, these gas tensions would be indicated uniquely by the intersection of the gas and blood lines for R = 0.8, since no other solution is possible (point i in Fig. 2.12). In this model the 'ideal' alveolar gas composition can thus be defined for any pair of lungs, given the overall R

value and the compositions of inspired air and mixed venous blood.

2.3.3 Alveolar air equation and Aa difference

In real life, even in healthy subjects, some degree of $\dot{V}_A/\dot{Q}$ mismatching is always present; in part, this results from the effects of gravity on ventilation and

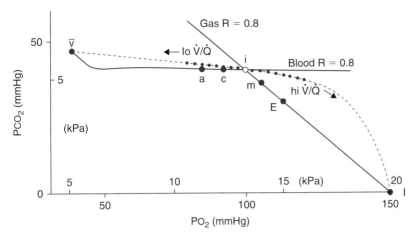

Figure 2.12 The 'ideal' alveolar gas tensions are defined by the point of intersection of the gas and blood R lines representing the overall respiratory exchange ratio for the lungs as a whole, typically 0.8. These intersect at point i on the $\dot{V}_A/\dot{Q}$ line (broken line), and the corresponding ideal P_{CO_2} and P_{O_2} represent values that would exist throughout the lungs exchanging gases with an R of 0.8 if ventilation and perfusion were perfectly matched and if the lungs were supplied with air and blood of compositions I and $\bar{v}$ respectively. The effect of $\dot{V}_A/\dot{Q}$ mismatching is to produce a range of combinations of P_{O_2} and P_{CO_2} in different lung units – but all can be represented as points on the $\dot{V}_A/\dot{Q}$ line. Each lung unit contributes to the mixed alveolar gas and mixed pulmonary capillary blood. The compositions of these are represented by points m and c on the respective gas and blood R lines. The gas expired at the mouth is further diluted by dead-space gas (with composition equivalent to inspired air) and is represented on the gas R line at point E. Similarly, the arterial blood gas tensions are affected by the admixture of a small anatomical shunt with the composition of mixed venous blood and are represented on the blood R line at point a.

perfusion individually (see Fig. 2.1). Since gravity has more effect on perfusion than on ventilation, the lung apices in the upright posture normally have a higher $\dot{V}_A/\dot{Q}$ and the bases a lower $\dot{V}_A/\dot{Q}$ than the overall average value.[1] In most lung diseases, the spread of $\dot{V}_A/\dot{Q}$ values is considerably greater and this usually reflects variations within, rather than between, lung regions. The effect of $\dot{V}_A/\dot{Q}$ inequalities is to produce variations in gas tensions between different alveoli. Intuitively it is obvious that alveoli with relatively more ventilation than perfusion will have a gas composition closer to inspired air, i.e. to the right of the ideal point on the O_2–CO_2 diagram (Fig. 2.12), whereas alveoli with relatively more perfusion than ventilation will have a composition nearer to mixed venous blood and to the left of the ideal point. But the gas compositions of all alveoli will still be on the same overall $\dot{V}_A/\dot{Q}$ line. A corollary of this analysis is that low $\dot{V}_A/\dot{Q}$ alveoli, which are nearer to the mixed venous point, also have R values lower than the overall value, whereas high $\dot{V}_A/\dot{Q}$ alveoli have higher-than-average R values.

The 'input' to the lungs is represented by the mixed venous (pulmonary arterial) blood and

inspired air; the 'output' comprises the pulmonary venous blood and expired air. Once blood draining all the pulmonary capillaries or gas expired from all the alveoli has mixed, their respective P_{O_2} and P_{CO_2} values will no longer be represented on the $\dot{V}_A/\dot{Q}$ line. The contribution of each lung unit to the pulmonary venous blood or to the expired gas is determined by the absolute amount of perfusion or ventilation that unit receives. The P_{O_2} and P_{CO_2} of the mixed blood and gas leaving the lungs are thus 'weighted' by perfusion and ventilation respectively. They can, however, be identified on the respective blood and gas R lines corresponding to the overall R value (Fig. 2.12); the effects of anatomical shunt and anatomical dead space are to move the points representing the composition of mixed arterial blood and mixed expired gas further along the same lines (Fig. 2.12).

This graphical analysis illustrates several points related to the effects of $\dot{V}_A/\dot{Q}$ mismatching. Because the blood R line for 0.8 has a very shallow slope at normal levels of P_{CO_2}, it would be anticipated that the effect of low $\dot{V}_A/\dot{Q}$ areas should be mainly to produce arterial hypoxaemia rather than hypercapnia.

Because of the problems of measuring mean alveolar gas tensions, the 'ideal' alveolar P_{CO_2} is often equated with the arterial P_{CO_2}; the justification for using this 'effective' alveolar P_{CO_2} is the shallow slope of the blood R line, as illustrated in Fig. 2.13. Clearly this approximation becomes less accurate with a greater spread of $\dot{V}_A/\dot{Q}$ ratios, when the shunt-like effect is greater – the clue to this is a markedly reduced arterial P_{O_2}. The effect of high $\dot{V}_A/\dot{Q}$ areas, on the other hand, is increasingly to separate the ideal alveolar P_{CO_2} from the mixed alveolar P_{CO_2} (Fig. 2.13).

With the alveolar P_{O_2}, the situation is different and clearly this cannot be approximated to the arterial value (Fig. 2.13). The P_AO_2 can, however, be calculated from the P_ACO_2 and the inspired P_{O_2} (P_IO_2) using the alveolar air equation, the simplified version of which is:[29]

$$P_AO_2 = P_IO_2 - \frac{P_ACO_2}{R} \qquad (2.4)$$

The 'effective' alveolar (i.e. arterial) P_{CO_2} is used to calculate an 'effective' alveolar P_{O_2}, which is very close to the 'ideal' value (Fig. 2.13). Typical values in a normal subject breathing air at sea level would be:

$$P_AO_2 = 150 - \frac{40}{0.8} = 100 \text{ mmHg}$$

or

$$P_AO_2 = 20 - \frac{5.3}{0.8} = 13.3 \text{ kPa}$$

(The P_{O_2} of inspired air (at body temperature pressure saturated, BTPS) at sea level is about 150 mmHg or 20 kpa.)

Using the measured arterial P_{O_2} and the alveolar air equation (Equation 2.4), the alveolar–arterial P_{O_2} difference (AaP_{O_2}) is calculated easily and is often used as a simple guide to the effects of 'venous

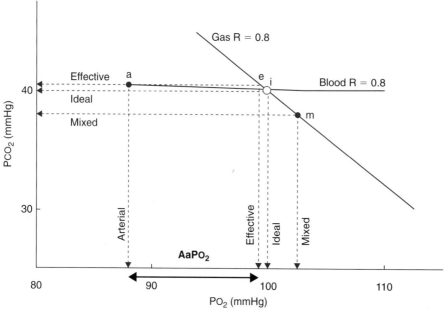

Figure 2.13 Various meanings of 'alveolar' gas tensions. The overall gas and blood R lines correspond to those illustrated in Fig. 2.12, with the 'ideal' alveolar P_{CO_2} and P_{O_2} defined by their point of intersection (i). Representative mixed alveolar gas tensions (m) are, in practice, not measurable. Since the blood R line is almost horizontal, the arterial P_{CO_2} (a) is close to the ideal and is used as the 'effective' (e) alveolar P_{CO_2}. The effective alveolar P_{O_2} can then be calculated using the alveolar air equation (see text) and is represented graphically by the P_{O_2} at point e, where a horizontal line through the arterial point intersects the gas R line. The effective alveolar tension of CO_2 (P_ACO_2) is thus a little higher and the effective alveolar tension of O_2 (P_AO_2) a little lower than the ideal values. The effect of low $\dot{V}_A/\dot{Q}$ alveoli is to widen the alveolar–arterial oxygen tension difference (AaP_{O_2}). As usually calculated, this represents the difference between effective P_AO_2 and Pa_{O_2} (heavy arrow).

admixture' (physiological shunt). In normal subjects breathing air it is usually less than 15 mmHg (2 kpa) (see below).

2.3.4 Three-compartment model of gas exchange

The CO_2–O_2 diagram has been of great value in understanding the mechanisms and consequences of ventilation/perfusion mismatching but is of no direct practical use. The concepts derived from this analysis are, however, used widely, notably in the 'three-compartment model' of Riley and Cournand.[28] In this analysis any pair of lungs can be considered as if it contained only three compartments (Fig. 2.14): (i) a population of 'ideal' alveoli in which the P_AO_2 and P_ACO_2 are the 'ideal' values as defined above; (ii) a population of alveoli with no perfusion, which therefore act as dead space; and (iii) a population of alveoli with no ventilation, which act as shunt. Note that the dead space compartment in this analysis includes not only alveoli that are totally unperfused but also a contribution from alveoli whose $\dot{V}_A/\dot{Q}$ is above average; similarly, the shunt includes not only alveoli that are totally unventilated but also a contribution from the lower-than-average $\dot{V}_A/\dot{Q}$ units (Fig. 2.15).

The effect of increased $\dot{V}_A/\dot{Q}$ mismatching in disease in the three-compartment model is to reduce the size of the alveolar compartment and to increase the size of the shunt and/or dead space compartments (usually both). This is illustrated diagrammatically for a normal and abnormal pair of lungs in Fig. 2.15. In this analysis, 'alveolar' ventilation occurs only in a single ideal compartment, since it is only here that air and blood meet and gas exchange can occur. The higher the ventilation of this compartment, the lower the ('ideal') alveolar PCO_2; as illustrated by Fig. 2.13, the 'ideal' and arterial PCO_2 are usually very close and therefore:

$$PaCO_2 \propto 1/\dot{V}_A \qquad (2.5)$$

hence the frequently made statement that 'a rise in arterial PCO_2 indicates a fall in alveolar ventilation' – but the 'alveolar ventilation' referred to is that of the 'ideal' compartment of the Riley–Cournand model and in that sense the statement is tautological.

The effect of high $\dot{V}_A/\dot{Q}$ alveoli is quantified by calculation of the physiological dead space, with appropriate values of expired and alveolar PCO_2 inserted in the Bohr equation (Equation 2.1). A graphical solution is illustrated in Fig. 2.16a; in the Riley and Cournand analysis, 'ideal' P_ACO_2 is usually estimated from arterial PCO_2, but if the PCO_2 of truly representative mixed alveolar gas could be sampled, then a different value would be obtained.

The direct corollary for quantitation of the effects of low $\dot{V}_A/\dot{Q}$ areas is the physiological shunt or venous admixture. The relevant equation is easily derived from the oxygen carried by the blood traversing the (ideal) alveolar and shunt compartments: the 'amount' of oxygen leaving the left ventricle each minute equals the total cardiac output ($\dot{Q}_t$) multiplied by the arterial oxygen content or concentration (CaO_2); in the three-compartment

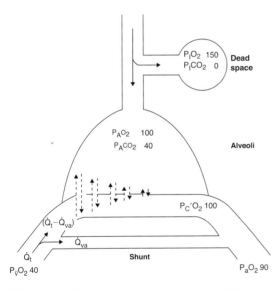

Figure 2.14 Three-compartment model comprising dead space, shunt and (ideal) alveoli. Gas tensions are shown in mmHg and the composition of dead-space gas is identical to that of inspired air. Broken arrows represent exchange of O_2 and CO_2 between alveolar gas and capillary blood; by the time red cells leave the pulmonary capillary, complete equilibration has occurred so that end-capillary PO_2, $Pc'O_2 = P_AO_2$. A proportion ($\dot{Q}_{va}$) of the total blood flow ($\dot{Q}_t$) bypasses functioning lung and effectively dilutes the oxygenated capillary blood with mixed venous blood.

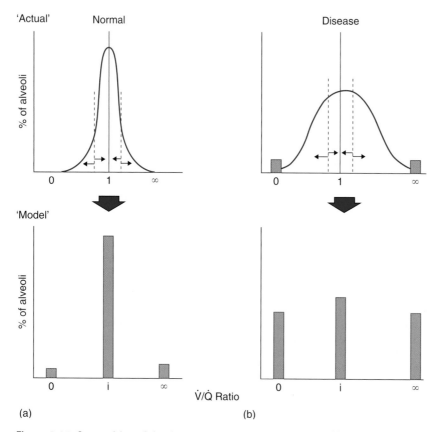

Figure 2.15 Composition of the three compartments in theoretical (a) normal and (b) diseased lungs. The upper diagrams are histograms of frequency of alveoli with various $\dot{V}_A/\dot{Q}$ ratios between zero (no ventilation) and infinity (no perfusion). In the normal lung the frequency distribution is narrow and centred on a mean $\dot{V}_A/\dot{Q}$ of about 1; in the diseased lung there are small numbers of units with $\dot{V}_A/\dot{Q}$ of 0 and infinity and the overall frequency distribution is much broader (in practice the distribution may be skewed or biphasic).[32] The three-compartment model (lower diagrams) describes the same lungs as if comprising only shunt, alveolar and dead-space compartments, with the $\dot{V}_A/\dot{Q}$ of the alveolar compartment determined by the intersection of blood and gas R lines on the CO_2-O_2 diagram. In effect, the model partitions the alveoli such that the shunt includes a contribution from those with lower-than-average $\dot{V}_A/\dot{Q}$ and the dead space a contribution from those with greater-than-average $\dot{V}_A/\dot{Q}$. In the diseased lung the wider dispersion of values leads to relatively larger dead space and shunt compartments and a smaller (ideal) alveolar compartment. As usually calculated, the 'physiological' dead space and 'physiological' shunt also encompass the anatomical dead space and shunt respectively.

model this is derived from two sources (Fig. 2.14) – blood that has come into equilibrium with alveolar gas, and blood that has bypassed ventilated alveoli. If the flow of blood through the latter (shunt or venous admixture) is $(\dot{Q}_{va})$, then the flow through the former is $(\dot{Q}_t - \dot{Q}_{va})$. The oxygen content of the shunted blood is the same as mixed venous $C\bar{v}o_2$; the relevant oxygen content of the blood draining the alveolar compartment is that which would be obtained by sampling at the distal end of the pulmonary capillaries $(Cc'o_2)$. Therefore:

$$Cao_2 \times \dot{Q}_t = (C\bar{v}o_2 \times \dot{Q}_{va}) + [Cc'o_2 \times (\dot{Q}_t - \dot{Q}_{va})]$$

or

$$\frac{\dot{Q}_{va}}{\dot{Q}_t} = \frac{Cc'o_2 - Cao_2}{Cc'o_2 - C\bar{v}o_2} \qquad (2.6)$$

Thus, to calculate the physiological shunt, three distinct measurements of blood oxygen content (concentration) are nseeded. Partial pressures of

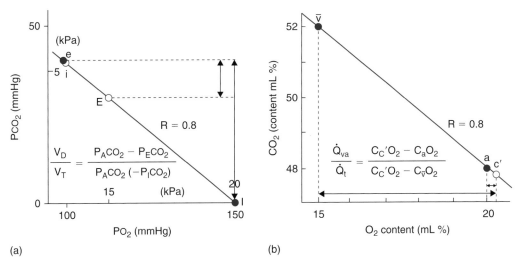

(a)   (b)

Figure 2.16 (a) Physiological dead space represented graphically in a normal subject on a CO_2–O_2 diagram. The alveolar and expired (E) gas tensions lie on the line relating PO_2 and PCO_2 in the gas phase for an overall R of 0.8. The value of P_ACO_2 used in the Bohr equation to derive dead space/tidal volume ratio (ratio of vertical arrows) is usually the effective (e) (i.e. arterial) PCO_2. The effect of high $\dot{V}_A/\dot{Q}$ units is to displace E towards the inspired point (I). (b) Physiological shunt fraction in (ratio of horizontal arrows) a normal subject represented graphically by plotting CO_2 and O_2 contents of blood for an overall R of 0.8; the effect of low $\dot{V}_A/\dot{Q}$ units is to displace the arterial point (a) further from the end capillary point (c′) and towards the mixed venous point ($\bar{v}$).

oxygen cannot be substituted directly in this equation because, unlike in a simple solution, the oxygen dissociation curve is grossly alinear and it is the contents rather than the tensions of oxygen in the contributing pulmonary capillaries that determine the composition of the mixed arterial blood. Usually, the mixed venous oxygen content is not available directly but, if a normal cardiac output and oxygen consumption ($\dot{V}O_2$) can be assumed, $C\bar{v}O_2$ can be estimated from the arterial value using the Fick relationship (Equation 2.2). We are left with the need to estimate the end-capillary oxygen content; this cannot be measured directly but it can be assumed that the end-capillary oxygen partial pressure is equal to the alveolar PO_2.

It may help to illustrate these relationships using average normal values of the variables. For example, if:

$$P_AO_2 = 100\,\text{mmHg}\ (13.3\,\text{kpa})$$

and

$$PaO_2 = 90\,\text{mmHg}\ (12.0\,\text{kpa})$$

then, since:

$$Pc'O_2 = P_AO_2;$$
$$Pc'O_2 = 100\,\text{mmHg}\ (13.3\,\text{kpa})$$

whence, from a standard dissociation curve:[30]

$$Sc'O_2 = 97.1\%$$

and

$$SaO_2 = 96.2\%$$

If the haemoglobin concentration is normal, fully saturated blood transports approximately 20 mL O_2 per 100 mL and therefore:

$$Cc'O_2 = 0.971 \times 20 = 19.42\,\text{mL}\ O_2/100\,\text{mL blood}$$

and

$$CaO_2 = 0.962 \times 20 = 19.24\,\text{mL}\ O_2/100\,\text{mL blood}$$

If the cardiac output and oxygen consumption are normal at 5 L min^{-1} and 250 mL min^{-1}

respectively, then from the Fick relationship (Equation 2.2):

$$C(a - \bar{v})o_2 = \frac{\dot{V}o_2}{\dot{Q}} = \frac{250}{5} = 50 \, mL \, L^{-1}$$

Or 5 mL O_2/100 mL blood
whence:

$$C\bar{v}o_2 = 19.24 - 5 = 14.24 \, mL \, o_2/100 \, mL \, blood$$

Therefore, applying the shunt equation (Equation 2.6):

$$\frac{\dot{Q}_{va}}{\dot{Q}_t} = \frac{Cc'o_2 - Cao_2}{Cc'o_2 - C\bar{v}o_2} = \frac{19.42 - 19.24}{19.42 - 14.24}$$
$$= 0.035$$

In other words, the lungs are functioning as if 3.5 per cent of the cardiac output were bypassing ventilated alveoli.

It is important to realize that both the Bohr (Equation 2.1) and shunt (Equation 2.6) equations describe general relations that can be applied to any actual or model lung that has alveoli in which gas exchange occurs together with a dead space and/or shunt. The volumes of the dead space or shunt, and whether they have real anatomical correlates or are only notional, depend simply on the values of alveolar gas tensions used in the equations (directly in the Bohr equations, and indirectly via the $Cc'o_2$ in the shunt equation). In the Riley–Cournand analysis, the relevant alveolar gas tensions are those in the hypothetical 'ideal' compartment.

2.3.5 'Alveolar' gas tensions

One question that we have so far skirted around is what exactly is alveolar air? It may be useful to summarize briefly the different senses in which the terms 'alveolar air', 'alveolar Po_2' and 'alveolar Pco_2' and 'alveolar ventilation' are used:

• In the classic Haldane–Priestley alveolar sample, the subject expires maximally into a long tube and an aliquot of the expired gas nearest the mouth is analysed. Undoubtedly this gas comes from alveoli, but it is probably not very representative as it is likely to arise from the more poorly ventilated alveoli, which tend to

empty latest in expiration. Consequently its gas tensions will be closer to mixed venous (higher Pco_2, lower Po_2) than the average.
• The end-tidal gas tensions are likely to be closer to the mean values, at least in normal subjects. By sampling at the end of a normal tidal breath, contamination by the anatomical dead space is avoided, but the expired Po_2 tends to fall and Pco_2 gradually tends to rise as the breath proceeds. The values obtained are therefore dependent on the size of the tidal volume. In disease, the slopes of the records of expired gas against time become much steeper; the end-tidal values are therefore more arbitrary and heavily weighted towards the better-ventilated alveoli.
• In anatomical terms, average alveolar gas tensions are easily defined but impossible to measure. Considerable inter- and intraregional differences in gas composition occur and the latter are markedly increased with the greater inequalities of ventilation/perfusion matching in disease. Even if gas from all alveoli could be mixed to produce representative mean tensions, these would still vary with time because of the tidal nature of ventilation and the pulsatile blood flow in the pulmonary capillaries.
• The ideal alveolar gas tensions, as described above, are an attempt to overcome the problems of sampling representative gas from real alveoli. They are usually closely related to:
• The effective alveolar gas tensions (Fig. 2.13) determined, in the case of P_Aco_2, directly from the arterial Pco_2 or, in the case of P_Ao_2, by calculation using the alveolar air equation (Equation 2.4).

If these several uses of the term 'alveolar' are borne in mind, it becomes easier to reconcile some apparent paradoxes; for example in one sense the alveolar (effective) and arterial Pco_2 are by definition the same, and yet in some clinical situations (e.g. suspected pulmonary embolism) the difference between alveolar (end-tidal) and arterial Pco_2 has been suggested as a useful clinical test. Again ventilation/perfusion mismatching classically produces hypoxaemia but not hypercapnia, since in the Riley–Cournand analysis CO_2 retention results from (ideal) alveolar hypoventilation (Equation 2.5) – yet if alveoli are defined in anatomical terms $\dot{V}_A/\dot{Q}$ mismatching in some conditions such as chronic obstructive pulmonary disease results in hypercapnia and can impair CO_2 output even more than oxygen uptake.[31] The classical analysis in terms of the three-compartment model ignores the fact that some alveoli inspire (from the dead space) previously expired air, a phenomenon that can increase appreciably in disease due to the types of inhomogeneity of ventilation described in Section 2.1.6.

2.3.6 Multiple inert gas elimination technique

More detailed analyses of $\dot{V}_A/\dot{Q}$ relationships in normal and diseased lungs have been developed by Wagner and colleagues using the multiple inert gas elimination technique (MIGET).[32] The ideal description of $\dot{V}_A/\dot{Q}$ relationships would be a profile in the form of a histogram (e.g. Fig. 2.15) and this is approached by MIGET (Fig. 2.17). The method involves the infusion of a solution of gases of different solubilities into the pulmonary artery and measurement of the concentrations of these gases in arterial blood and expired air. With a poorly soluble gas such as sulphur hexafluoride (SF_6), most is evolved into the alveolar air and little is retained in the blood. On the other hand more soluble gases tend to be retained in solution in the perfusing blood. The retention of any gas in a given lung unit is a function of the solubility of the gas and the $\dot{V}_A/\dot{Q}$ ratio of the particular unit. When a mixture of gases of different solubilities is infused in a steady state and the retention of each is measured it is possible to compute a distribution of $\dot{V}_A/\dot{Q}$ ratios that could give rise to the blood gas findings. A model of 50 compartments is used. The distribution produced may not be related uniquely to the retention–solubility characteristics recorded, but in general the simplest smooth distributions of $\dot{V}_A/\dot{Q}$ in relation to $\dot{V}_A$ or $\dot{Q}$ consistent with the data are recovered (Fig. 2.17). A later modification obviates the need for arterial blood sampling.[34] Wagner and colleagues have put this elegant technique to use in several clinical situations, and it has helped considerably in analysing the patterns and consequences of $\dot{V}_A/\dot{Q}$ mismatching in various diseases.[35] The 'multicompartment' model analysis offered by MIGET is clearly more realistic than the classical three compartments, but the more sophisticated analysis demands high-powered technology and is available in only a few centres.

2.4 REGIONAL LUNG FUNCTION

All of the tests discussed above evaluate the overall function of both lungs, with no attempt at spatial resolution, but in some clinical situations assessment of local function may be of value. Conventionally, this is obtained by use of radioactive isotopes with regional information obtained by external imaging. The classic studies of regional lung function utilized radioactively labelled

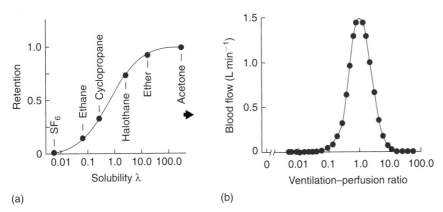

(a)

(b)

Figure 2.17 (a) Retention–solubility curve for arterial blood with six gases of varying solubility measured using the multiple inert gas elimination technique (MIGET). (b) The simplest smooth distribution of $\dot{V}_A/\dot{Q}$ ratios in relation to blood flow that can be derived from the retention–solubility information. Modified from ref 32 by kind permission of the American Thoracic Society.

oxygen and CO_2,[1,2] which is impracticable in most centres. The introduction of [133]xenon (^{133}Xe) made the techniques much more widely available.[36,37]

2.4.1 Radioisotopic measurements of regional ventilation

[133]Xenon is an inert, relatively insoluble gas with a long half-life. When a gas mixture containing a small concentration is breathed over several minutes, the isotope gradually accumulates until completely equilibrated with the gas in the lungs (as with the inert gas technique for measuring lung volume); a conventional scan or gamma camera image at the end of this period shows the count rates in different regions in proportion to the volume of ventilated lung. When the subject returns to breathing air, the xenon is washed out during tidal breathing and, by following the decay of radioactivity during the washout period, a direct index of regional ventilation per unit volume is obtained. The data can be analysed in a similar manner to the nitrogen washout used to assess overall ventilatory function, but the analysis is complicated by dissolved xenon recirculating from other tissues and by radiation from isotope that accumulates in the tissues of the chest wall.

Some information on regional ventilation can be obtained during the 'wash-in' of ^{133}Xe, but its long half-life means that the radioactivity recorded rapidly becomes more dependent on regional lung volume than on ventilation. This would not apply to a single inspiration, but a normal tidal breath does not allow accumulation of sufficient radioactivity for analysis. A full vital capacity inspiration is therefore usually employed, but its distribution may not necessarily reflect events during tidal breathing.

Most of the objections to the use of xenon for ventilation scanning are avoided by use of the short-lived isotope [81m]krypton ([81m]Kr).[38] This isotope has a much shorter half-life (11 s) than ^{133}Xe, so that progressive accumulation cannot occur and an equilibrium is reached between ventilation and radioactive decay. Images of tidal ventilation per unit volume can therefore be obtained directly, without the need to analyse washout curves or to take account of accumulation of the isotope outside the lungs. Although [81m]Kr itself is short-lived, immediate

access to a source is not essential as the parent isotope [81]rubidium has a half-life of 5 h. In practice, ^{133}Xe continues to be used for clinical purposes in many centres, but a major disadvantage is that views are obtainable in only one plane at a time.

Radioactively labelled fine aerosols offer an alternative to isotopic gases for studying the distribution of ventilation. One such is 'Technegas', an ultrafine dispersion of carbon aggregates labelled with radioactive technetium (^{99m}Tc). This allows multiple-view imaging and evaluation of central versus peripheral distribution of ventilation, in addition to the conventional topographic comparison.[39]

2.4.2 Radioisotopic measurements of regional perfusion

Even though its solubility is relatively low, radioactive xenon in solution can also be used to give information about regional perfusion. Counting over the lungs after an intravenous injection of ^{133}Xe detects its evolution into the perfused alveoli, which, because of the low solubility of the gas, is virtually complete after one circulation.[36] More commonly, however, regional perfusion is assessed after injection of microspheres labelled with [99m]Tc.[40] The particles become lodged temporarily in the pulmonary arterioles in proportion to the regional blood flow, but the proportion of vessels 'embolized' in this way is tiny. The optimal particle size is between $10\,\mu m$ and $50\,\mu m$; smaller particles pass through into the systemic circulation and those greater than $100\,\mu m$ in diameter obstruct undesirably large vessels. The technique gives clearer definition of local defects of perfusion than does dissolved xenon.

2.4.3 Clinical applications of regional function measurements

Assessment of ventilation and perfusion scans for clinical purposes is usually qualitative and based on pattern recognition. In healthy lungs regional distribution is broadly uniform, but the density of activity in two-dimensional images inevitably varies with the depth of lung at different levels (Fig. 2.18). The practised eye takes such variations into account. Localized defects are rare in healthy asymptomatic subjects, even including smokers.[41]

It may be possible to equate regions of the lung investigated by external scanning with particular

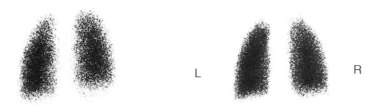

Figure 2.18 Posteroanterior ventilation (left) and perfusion (right) scans in a healthy subject showing normal distribution of isotopes.

lobes or segments, but more specific information is sometimes desired. This has been obtained by measurements during bronchoscopy with selective cannulation of the lobar or segmental bronchus. Differential spirometry and measurement of metabolic gas exchange in one or other lung were practised for many years but are little used now. The techniques, which are based on mass spectrometry, were originally established using a rigid broncho-scope[42] and later adapted for use with the fibre-optic bronchoscope.[23]

2.4.4 Modern imaging techniques

The recent revolution in imaging technology has resulted in several new approaches to evaluating regional ventilation and perfusion. To date most techniques have been used for research purposes, but clinical applications are likely to develop in the near future.

In its early days the applicability of computed tomography (CT) imaging in this field was limited by the time required to acquire sufficient data for reconstruction of lung 'slices'. The much faster modern equipment can be used in conjunction with isotopes such as xenon to give detailed regional information on ventilation, with iodi-nated contrast giving equivalent information on lung perfusion.[43,44] Magnetic resonance (MR) imaging is particularly good for evaluating regional perfusion[45,46] but can also be utilized for studying ventilation.[47] Position emission tomography (PET) after infusion of the nitrogen isotope $^{13}N_2$ has been used to study the effect of posture on topographical distribution of perfusion and ventilation in healthy subjects,[48] but its spatial resolution is less than that of CT and MR imaging.

Quantitative single photon-emission computed tomography (SPECT) has the capacity to produce detailed distributions of regional ventilation and perfusion, using, for example, inhaled Technegas (see above) and infused macroaggregates labelled with radioactive indium (^{113m}In) respectively.[49] This technique gives information on overall distribution similar to that obtained with MIGET (see Section 2.3.6). Although the overall severity of $\dot{V}_A/\dot{Q}$ disturbance may be underestimated by this method in comparison with MIGET, it has the advantage of producing detailed regional spatial distributions of ventilation and blood flow and potentially under more 'physiological' conditions than other imaging modalities.[49] SPECT ventilation studies have, for example, been used to demonstrate and measure airway closure and to visualize small, discrete areas of lung where this occurs.[50]

REFERENCES

1 West JB. Regional differences in gas exchange in the lung of erect man. *J Appl Physiol* 1962; **17**: 893–8.

2 West JB, Dollery CT. Distribution of blood flow and ventilation–perfusion ratio in the lung measured with radioactive CO_2. *J Appl Physiol* 1960; **15**: 405–10.

3 Connolly T, Bake L, Wood L, Milic Emili J. Regional distribution of a ^{133}Xe labelled gas volume inspired at constant flow rates. *Scand J Respir Dis* 1975; **56**: 150–59.

4 Hughes JMB, Glazier, JB, Maloney JE, West JB. Effect of lung volume on the distribution of pulmonary flow in man. *Respir Physiol* 1968; **4**: 58–72.

5 Agostoni E, D'Angelo E, Bonanni MV. The effect of the abdomen on the vertical gradient of pleural surface pressure. *Respir Physiol* 1970; **8**: 332–46.

6 Dosman J, Grassino A, Macklem PT, Engel LA. Factors influencing the oesophageal pressure gradient in upright man. *Physiologist* 1975; **18**: 194.

7 Albert RK, Hubmayr RD. The prone position elimi-nates compression of the lungs by the heart. *Am J Respir Crit Care Med* 2000; **161**: 1660–65.

8 Engel LA, Macklem PT. Gas mixing and distribution in the lung, in *Respiratory Physiology II* (ed. JG Widdicombe), University Park Press, London, 1977, pp. 37–82.

9 Cetti A, Moore AJ, Geddes DM. Collateral ventila-tion. *Thorax* 2006; **61**: 371–3.

10 Cournand A, Baldwin E, Darling RC, Richards DW. Studies on intrapulmonary mixture of gases: IV. Significance of pulmonary emptying rate and sim-plified open circuit measurement of residual air. *J Clin Invest* 1941; **20**: 681–9.

11 Fleming GM, Chester EH, Saniie J, Saidel GM. Ventilation inhomogeneity using multibreath nitrogen washout: comparison of moment ratios and other indexes. *Am Rev Respir Dis* 1980; **121**: 789–94.

12 Aurora P, Kozlowska W, Stocks J. Gas mixing effi-ciency from birth to adulthood measured by multi-ple-breath washout. *Respir Physiol Neurobiol* 2005; **148**: 125–39.

13 Comroe JH, Fowler WS. Lung function studies: VI. Detection of uneven alveolar ventilation during a single breath of oxygen. *Am J Med* 1951; **10**: 408–13.

14 Dollfuss, RE, Milic Emili J, Bates DV. Regional ven-tilation of the lung studied with boluses of xenon 133. *Respir Physiol* 1967; **2**: 234–46.

15 Teculescu, DB, Damel, MC, Costantino E, *et al.* Computerised single-breath nitrogen washout: pre-dicted values in a rural French community. *Lung* 1996; **174**: 43–55.

16 Fung YC, Sobin SS. Theory of sheet flow in lung alveoli. *J Appl Physiol* 1969; **26**: 472–88.

17 Hughes JMB. Pulmonary circulation and fluid balance, in *Respiratory Physiology II* (ed. JG Widdicombe), University Park Press, London, 1977, pp. 135–83.

18 Permutt S, Bromberger-Barnea B, Bane HN. Alveolar pressure, pulmonary venous pressure and the vascu-lar waterfall. *Med Thorac* 1962; **19**: 239–60.

19 Barnes, PJ, Liu SF. Regulation of pulmonary vascular tone. *Pharmacol Rev* 1995; **47**: 87–131.

20 Krogh A, Lindhard J. Measurements of the blood flow through the lungs of man. *Skand Arch Physiol* 1912; **27**: 100–125.

21 Cander L, Forster RE. Determination of pulmonary parenchymal tissue volume and pulmonary capillary blood flow in man. *J Appl Physiol* 1959; **14**: 541–51.

22 Sackner, MA, Greeneltch D, Heiman MS, *et al.* Diffusing capacity, membrane diffusing capacity, capillary blood volume, pulmonary tissue volume and cardiac output measured by a rebreathing tech-nique. *Am Rev Respir Dis* 1975; **111**: 157–65.

23 Williams SJ, Pierce RJ, Davies NJH, Denison DM. Methods of studying lobar and segmental function of the lung in man. *Br J Dis Chest* 1979; **73**: 97–112.

24 Lee G de J, DuBois AB. Pulmonary capillary blood flow in man. *J Clin Invest* 1955; **34**: 1380–90.

25 Haldane JS. *Respiration*. Yale University Press, New Haven, CT, 1922.

26 Rahn H. A concept of mean alveolar air and the ven-tilation–blood flow relationships during pulmonary gas exchange. *Am J Physiol* 1949; **158**: 21–30.

27 Rahn H, Fenn WO. *A Graphical Analysis of Respiratory Gas Exchange*, American Physiological Society, Washington, DC, 1955.

28 Riley RL, Cournand A. 'Ideal' alveolar air and the analysis of ventilation–perfusion relationships in the lungs. *J Appl Physiol* 1949; **1**: 825–47.

29 Campbell EJM. J Burns Amberson Lecture: the management of acute respiratory failure in chronic bronchitis and emphysema. *Am Rev Respir Dis* 1967; **96**: 626–39.

30 Severinghaus JW. Blood gas concentrations, in *Handbook of Physiology*, Section 3, *Respiration*, Vol. II. (eds WO Fenn and H Rahn), American Physiological Society, Baltimore, MD, 1965, pp. 1475–87.

31 West JB. Gas exchange when one lung region inspires from another. *J Appl Physiol* 1971; **30**: 479–87.

32 Wagner PD, Saltzman HA, West JB. Measurement of continuous distributions of ventilation–perfusion ratios: theory. *J Appl Physiol* 1974; **36**: 588–99.

33 West JB. Ventilation–perfusion relationships. *Am Rev Respir Dis* 1977; **116**: 919–43.

34 Wagner PD, Smith CM, Davies NJH, McEvoy RD, Gale GE. Estimation of ventilation–perfusion inequality by inert gas elimination without arterial sampling. *J Appl Physiol* 1985; **59**: 376–83.

35 Wagner PD, Rodriguez-Roisin R. Clinical advances in pulmonary gas exchange. *Am Rev Respir Dis* 1991; **143**: 883–8.

36 Ball WC, Stewart PB, Newsham LG, Bates DV. Regional pulmonary function studied with xenon 133. *J Clin Invest* 1962; **41**: 519–31.

37 Dollery CT, Hugh Jones P, Matthews CME. Use of radioactive xenon for studies of regional lung func-tion. *Br Med J* 1962; **2**: 1006–16.

38 Fazio F, Jones T. Assessment of regional ventilation by continuous inhalation of radioactive krypton-81m. *Br Med J* 1975; **3**: 673–6.

39 Amis TC, Crawford AB, Davison A, Engel LA. Distribution of inhaled 99mtechnetium labelled ultrafine carbon particle aerosol (Technegas) in human lungs. *Eur Respir J* 1990; **3**: 679–85.

40 Burdine JA, Sonnemaker RE, Ryder LA, Spjut HJ. Perfusion studies with technetium 99m human albumin microspheres. *Radiology* 1970; **95**: 101–7.

41 Fedullo PF, Kapitan K, Brewer NS, *et al.* Patterns of pulmonary perfusion scans in normal subjects: IV. The prevalence of abnormal scans in smokers 30 to 49 years of age. *Am Rev Respir Dis* 1989; **139**: 1155–7.

42 Hugh Jones P, West JB. Detection of bronchial and arterial obstruction by continuous gas analysis from individual lobes and segments of the lung. *Thorax* 1960; **15**: 154–64.

43 Simon BA. Regional ventilation and lung mechanics using X-ray CT. *Acad Radiol* 2005; **12**: 1414–22.

44 Hoffman EA, Chou D. Computed tomography studies of lung ventilation and perfusion. *Proc Am Thorac Soc* 2005; **2**: 492–8.

45 Fink C, Puderbach M, Bock M, *et al.* Regional lung perfusion: assessment with partially parallel three-dimensional MR imaging. *Radiology* 2004; **231**: 175–84.

46 Dehnert C, Risse F, Ley S, *et al.* Magnetic resonance imaging of uneven pulmonary perfusion in hypoxia in humans. *Am J Respir Crit Care Med* 2006; **174**: 1132–8.

47 Kauczor H, Hanke A, Beek EV. Assessment of lung ventilation by MR imaging: current status and future perspectives. *Eur Radiol* 2002; **12**: 1962–70.

48 Musch G, Layfield JDH, Harris RS, *et al.* Topographical distribution of pulmonary perfusion and ventilation, assessed by PET in supine and prone humans. *J Appl Physiol* 2002; **93**: 1841–51.

49 Petersson J, Sanchez-Crespo A, Rohdin M, *et al.* Physiological evaluation of a new quantitative SPECT method measuring regional ventilation and perfusion. *J Appl Physiol* 2004; **96**: 1127–36.

50 King, GG, Eberl S, Salome CM, Meikle SR, Woolcock AJ. Airway closure measured by a techne-gas bolus and SPECT. *Am J Respir Crit Care Med* 1997; **155**: 682–8.

3

Carbon Monoxide Diffusing Capacity (Transfer Factor)

The rate of diffusion of a gas through a membrane is proportional directly to the area and indirectly to the thickness of the membrane. The rate of diffusion also depends on the molecular weight of the gas and its solubility in the membrane. With oxygen, the rate of uptake across the alveolar–capillary membrane is determined not only by diffusion but also by perfusion, as haemoglobin rapidly becomes fully saturated with oxygen and further uptake then depends on replenishing the blood in the pulmonary capillaries. Uptake of carbon monoxide (CO), however, is little affected by the rate of blood flow and is much more dependent on diffusion. Originally, CO was introduced by Marie Krogh to assess the diffusing characteristics of the lung in an attempt to resolve a controversy.[1] In the early twentieth century there were two schools of thought among respiratory physiologists investigating gas exchange: Bohr and Haldane believed that uptake of oxygen could occur only by an active process of secretion from the alveoli into the blood, while August and Marie Krogh argued that the composition of alveolar gas and arterial blood were entirely compatible with passive diffusion between air and blood. The controversy was eventually resolved in favour of the latter view. Krogh used CO to assess pulmonary diffusion in order to avoid any dispute, since there was general agreement that CO was taken up by simple diffusion. This happy choice produced one of the simplest and most useful tests of respiratory function; although it was not applied generally until resurrected in the 1950s,[2] it is now in regular use in one form or another in every clinical lung function laboratory.

3.1 BREATH-HOLDING METHOD

With the method originally described by Krogh,[1] the subject inspires air containing a very low concentration of CO ($F_I CO$) (approximately 0.3%), holds the breath for a measured period and then breathes out, with an expired alveolar sample collected and its CO concentration measured. Krogh pointed out that the rate of uptake of a gas would be exponential, and she defined the permeability of the lungs (k) to CO as:

$$k = \frac{\log F_0 CO - \log F_t CO}{t \log e} = \frac{1}{t}\log e \frac{F_0 CO}{F_t CO} \quad (3.1)$$

where $F_0 CO$ is the initial alveolar gas concentration and $F_t CO$ is the gas concentration after breath-holding for t s. The value of k depends on the gas used – hence $k CO$ or $K CO$, the diffusion or transfer coefficient that has passed into general use. ($k CO$ and $K CO$ ($D_L CO/V_A$) as conventionally used differ because of volume measurement under either standard temperature pressure dry (STPD) or body temperature pressure saturated (BTPS) conditions.)

The initial CO concentration ($F_0 CO$) needed to apply Equation 3.1 is not that in the inspired test gas but the initial alveolar concentration after it has mixed with the air already in the lungs. This is obtained by including an inert tracer gas in the inspired mixture, most commonly helium.[2] It is assumed that the dilution of CO and helium in the lungs is similar but, whereas CO is also taken up by

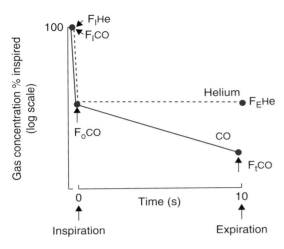

Figure 3.1 Diagrammatic representation of carbon monoxide (CO) and helium concentrations (log scale, as a percentage of the inspired concentration) against time during single-breath manoeuvre. Initially the two concentrations fall to a similar degree as the gases are diluted by air in the lungs. The helium concentration remains constant during breath-holding, while the CO concentration falls progressively. The rate of uptake of CO (Kco) is represented by the slope of the relation between [CO] and time.

the blood, helium is not (Fig. 3.1). Consequently, its concentration (F_EHe) in a subsequently expired sample can be taken as the alveolar concentration of helium after the test gas has mixed with the resident alveolar air. F_0CO is then calculated from the inspired (F_IHe) and expired helium concentrations:

$$F_0CO = \frac{F_EHe}{F_IHe} \times F_ICO \qquad (3.2)$$

The alveolar CO concentration at time t (usually 10 s in the standard test) is measured from an expired sample after flushing out the dead-space gas. The value of Kco calculated from Equation 3.1 represents the rate of uptake of CO per unit lung volume (usually per litre). The diffusing capacity (D_LCO) of the whole lung for CO is obtained by multiplying by the alveolar volume (V_A) at which the measurement was made:

$$D_LCO = Kco \times V_A \qquad (3.3)$$

The affinity of haemoglobin for CO is so high that the small amounts used in routine measurements of D_LCO do not give rise to any significant increase in CO tension (back pressure) in the blood.

Consequently, the driving pressure for CO can usually be equated with the alveolar pressure. However, smokers should be advised not to smoke on the day of the test as recent smoking can impair the uptake of CO due to the presence of carboxyhaemoglobin and the accompanying back pressure that reduces the effective driving pressure for the gas.

3.1.1 'Effective' alveolar volume

The single-breath measurement is usually performed at full inflation. In the method as originally standardized by Ogilvie et al., the alveolar volume used to calculate D_LCO was the total lung capacity measured in a separate manoeuvre by multiple-breath helium dilution (as described in Chapter 1, Section 1.3.4).[2] In a later modification, the single-breath estimate or 'effective' alveolar volume calculated from the dilution of the helium used in the test was proposed.[3] In normal subjects, the two resulting estimates of D_LCO are similar, but with maldistribution of ventilation in disease the single-breath estimate of V_A is less and the calculated D_LCO likewise. The convenience of all the measurements being available from a single manoeuvre has led most laboratories to adopt the single-breath estimate of 'effective' alveolar volume, but it is important to remember that D_LCO calculated in this way will be influenced by maldistribution of ventilation. The apparently better specificity of D_LCO measured using the multibreath volume estimate is offset in the very patients in whom large differences occur (severe airflow obstruction) by the poorly defined end point of the multibreath technique due to parts of the lung being ventilated very slowly. Kco is unaffected by these considerations and essentially assesses transfer of CO in the better-ventilated alveoli. If a multiple breath (or plethysmographic) estimate of V_A is used, the assumption that CO uptake in all alveoli would be equally good if they were ventilated evenly is unlikely to be valid.

3.1.2 Volume dependence of measurements

Conventionally, the measurement is made during breath-holding at full inflation as this exposes the maximum surface area available for gas exchange. If D_LCO is measured at a lower volume, its value is less.

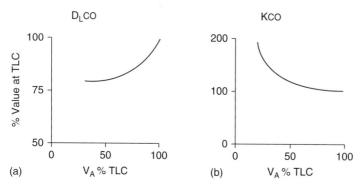

(a)   (b)

Figure 3.2 Theoretical variation of measurements of single-breath diffusing capacity (D_LCO) and rate of uptake of carbon monoxide (KCO) with the size of the breath inspired in a healthy subject. The volume of gas inspired determines the alveolar volume in which the test gas is distributed. As alveolar volume (V_A) falls, D_LCO also falls but proportionally less and the relationship is alinear. KCO is relatively volume-independent at high volumes but increases markedly at lower volumes.

Table 3.1 Pathological conditions that may reduce diffusing capacity (D_LCO)* and/or KCO

	↓ D_LCO	↓ KCO	Section
Chronic obstructive pulmonary disease	✓	✓	9.7
Emphysema	✓	✓	9.7, 9.13.1
Asthma	✓†	†	11.6
Pulmonary fibrosis	✓	✓	14.3.4
Sarcoidosis	✓	Mild or none	14.5.4
Pneumonectomy		†	14.2
Extrapulmonary restriction:			
Muscle weakness	✓	†	20.2.1.5
Skeletal deformity	✓	†	16.5, 16.6
Pleural disease	✓	†	16.4.2
Pulmonary vascular disease	✓	✓	15.1.3, 15.2.2
Pulmonary oedema	✓	✓	19.2.3
Mitral valve disease	✓	✓	19.3.1.2
Congenital R→L shunts	✓	✓	19.4.2
Anaemia	✓	✓	21.1.2
Renal failure	✓	✓	22.1.3
Hepatic cirrhosis	✓	✓	23.1.2
Collagen diseases, etc.:			
Rheumatoid arthritis	✓	Mild or none	25.2
Systemic sclerosis	✓	✓	25.3
Systemic lupus erythematosus	✓	✓	25.4

*Single-breath technique, using simultaneous alveolar volume (V_A).
†May be increased.

On the other hand, KCO increases at volumes below TLC (Fig. 3.2). This reflects the fact that the total volume of red blood cells (and therefore of haemoglobin binding sites) changes little with lung volume so that the uptake of CO per litre of ventilated lung is greater at lower volumes.[3,4] The volume dependence of the measurements has important clinical implications for the interpretation of results in pathological conditions where full expansion of the lungs is impeded (Tables 3.1 and 3.2).

3.1.3 Clinical uses of diffusing capacity

When tests of diffusion between alveolar gas and pulmonary capillary blood were introduced, it was thought that the greatest barrier to the transfer of

Table 3.2 Pathological conditions tending to increase diffusing capacity (D$_L$co)* and/or Kco

	↑ D$_L$co	↑ Kco	Section
Asthma	Sometimes ✓		11.6
Obesity	✓	✓	24.1.3
Pneumonectomy		✓	14.2
Extrapulmonary restriction:			
Muscle weakness		✓	20.2.1.5
Skeletal deformity		✓	16.5, 16.6
Pleural disease		✓	16.4.2
L→R shunts	✓	✓	19.4.1
Polycythaemia	✓	✓	21.2
Lung haemorrhage	✓†	✓†	22.1.5

*Single-breath technique using simultaneous alveolar volume (V$_A$).

†May be a rise against a background low value, e.g. in Goodpasture's syndrome.

gas was the alveolar–capillary membrane itself, but several other factors are also important. CO (or oxygen) has to traverse several layers of varying thickness between the alveoli and the red blood cells in the pulmonary capillaries. These include the alveolar epithelium, interstitium, endothelium, blood plasma, red cell membrane and red cell interior, after which it combines chemically with haemoglobin. This sequence explains both the strength and the weakness of the measurement of diffusing capacity in clinical practice as it can be impaired by many pathological processes. Consequently, it is a sensitive screening test for involvement of the lungs in various diseases, but its specificity is correspondingly poor (Table 3.1). The effects of anaemia and adjustment of the measurement to correct for it are discussed in Section 21.2.2. The various barriers to transfer of gas in effect represent a series of resistances. Evidence suggests that the major 'resistance' resides in the capillaries and red cells, so that the Kco, in particular, offers a useful functional index of the pulmonary microvasculature.[5]

In some conditions D$_L$co and, more commonly, Kco may be raised above the normal range (Table 3.2). In practice, the commonest causes of an increased overall D$_L$co are obesity and asthma,[6] while an increased Kco alone is commonly associated with conditions that impede full lung expansion from without (extrapulmonary restriction).

3.1.4 D$_m$ and V$_c$ components

The units of diffusing capacity demonstrate that the measurement is essentially a conductance, i.e. the reciprocal of resistance – the units of mL CO min^{-1} mmHg^{-1} (mmol min^{-1} kPa^{-1}) are analogous to those of airway conductance, 1 min^{-1} cmH$_2$O^{-1} (1 min^{-1} kPa^{-1}). When conductances are arranged in series, the overall conductance is obtained by adding reciprocals: the total diffusing capacity of the lungs (D$_L$) can therefore be expressed in terms of the diffusing capacity of the membrane (D$_m$) and a second component, which is dependent on the pulmonary capillary blood volume (V$_c$) and a constant term (θ) representing the specific gas uptake capacity per unit blood volume,[7] i.e.

$$\frac{1}{D_L} = \frac{1}{D_m} + \frac{1}{\theta V_c} \qquad (3.4)$$

As the only component in this equation that is dependent on diffusion is D$_m$, some authors prefer the term 'CO transfer factor' (T$_L$co) to describe the total 'diffusing capacity' (D$_L$co), but the latest international guidelines recommend the traditional term.[8]

Since CO and oxygen compete for the same binding sites on the haemoglobin molecule, the rate of uptake of CO is dependent on the prevailing Po$_2$. Use can be made of this to calculate the D$_m$ and V$_c$ components of Equation 3.4 by measuring D$_L$co at two or more levels of oxygenation (e.g. breathing room air and 100% oxygen).[7] The value of θ varies with Po$_2$ and can be obtained from standard tables. If the values of 1/D$_L$ measured at different levels of Po$_2$ are plotted against 1/θ, the slope of the linear relationship is 1/V$_c$, with 1/D$_m$ represented by the intercept on the ordinate (Fig. 3.3). Thus the alveolar membrane diffusing capacity and the volume of blood in the pulmonary capillaries can be estimated.

When measurements are made under hyperoxic conditions, the affinity of haemoglobin for CO is significantly reduced and a greater back pressure for CO results. This can be estimated by a simple rebreathing manoeuvre with the hyperoxic test gas and it needs to be deducted from the alveolar pressure to give the true driving pressure for CO.

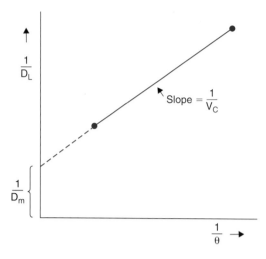

Figure 3.3 Derivation of membrane diffusing capacity and capillary blood volume. The reaction rate of carbon monoxide with oxyhaemoglobin (θ) is varied by making measurements of diffusing capacity ($D_L$co) at different levels of oxygenation of haemoglobin. $1/D_L$ is then plotted against $1/\theta$ (the latter obtained from standard tables) and, since $1/D_L = (1/V_c \times 1/\theta) + 1/D_m$ (Equation 3.4) (cf. $y = mx + c$), the slope of the relationship represents $1/V_c$ and the intercept on the y axis represents $1/D_m$.

D_m, diffusing capacity of pulmonary membrane; V_c, pulmonary capillary blood volume.

Although of considerable theoretical interest, measurements of D_m and V_c are disappointing in clinical practice. In principle they should give useful information that would aid analysis of the mechanisms of reduction of D_LCO in various clinical situations, but the answers are rarely clear-cut. One reason may be the inevitable errors associated with extrapolating a line based on only two points.

3.1.5 Practical issues

The precise details of the single-breath method for measuring D_LCO show several variations relating mainly to the F_IO_2 of the test gas and to calculation of the breath-hold time.[8,9] The F_IO_2 used can vary from 0.17 to 0.25; lower values are used to reduce the variation in uptake due to differences between inspired and expired oxygen, since the higher the alveolar PO_2 the ower the calculated D_LCO. In normal subjects it has been shown that D_LCO falls by 0.35 per cent per mmHg increase in alveolar PO_2.

Calculation of the precise breath-hold time normally includes proportions of the duration of the preceding inspiration and subsequent expiration, as some CO diffusion occurs during these periods as well as during the breath-hold itself. These practical details, equipment requirements and recommendations are discussed in detail elsewhere.[8,9]

Some breathless patients have difficulty holding the breath for the 10 s usually used. Reduction of the normally recommended breath-hold period from 10 s to 6 s produces no measurable change in normal subjects[10] but tends to underestimate D_LCO in patients with airway obstruction, probably because of impaired transport of CO from inspired gas through alveolar gas due to stratification and impaired equilibration.[11] Problems are also encountered with patients with a small vital capacity, e.g. less than 1 L, as adequate sampling of expired alveolar air requires flushing out of the dead space first. One or more of the alternative methods described below may help to circumvent these problems.

3.2 NON–BREATH-HOLDING METHODS

Several non-breath-holding techniques have been described, but experience with them is generally less than with the single-breath method.

3.2.1 Steady–state and rebreathing methods

The two classic steady-state methods are now largely of historical interest only. They differ only in the method of estimating the alveolar concentration of CO. With the method of Bates *et al.*,[12] this is obtained by sampling end-tidal gas, while that of Filley *et al.*[13] uses the concentration of carbon *dioxide* in expired air and alveolar gas (the latter obtained by assuming equality of alveolar and arterial PCO_2; see Chapter 2, Section 2.3). These values are inserted in the Bohr equation (Chapter 2, Equation 2.1) to calculate the physiological dead space/tidal volume ratio; then, using this value of V_D/V_T and the expired concentration of carbon monoxide, the Bohr equation is reapplied for CO to determine its alveolar concentration.

The steady-state techniques in general give lower values than the single-breath method, mainly because the measurements are made at a smaller alveolar volume. They are also more influenced by ventilation/perfusion inequalities and tend to be less reproducible. A rebreathing method has also been described for use both at rest and on exercise.[14]

3.2.2 Intrabreath method

In the more recent 'intrabreath' method, measurements of CO concentration are made at frequent intervals[15] or continuously[16,17] during a single exhalation. The technique, which requires rapidly responding analysers, is more suitable than the breath-holding method for measurements during exercise.[18] A similar concentration of CO to that in the test gas for the single-breath measurement is used, but the inert tracer gas used to derive lung volume is methane rather than helium. The subject takes a rapid full inhalation from residual volume and then exhales slowly at a fairly constant rate, determined by including a flow restrictor in the respiratory circuit. The values of $D_L CO$ obtained (at rest) inevitably differ somewhat from single-breath results as the measurement is not made at TLC. Normal reference values are being developed.[18]

REFERENCES

1 Krogh M. The diffusion of gases through the lungs of man. *J Physiol* 1915; **49**: 271–300.

2 Ogilvie CM, Forster RE, Blakemore WS, Morton JW. A standardised breath holding technique for the clinical measurement of the diffusing capacity of the lung for carbon monoxide. *J Clin Invest* 1957; **36**: 1–17.

3 McGrath MW, Thomson ML. The effect of age, body size and lung volume change on alveolar–capillary permeability and diffusing capacity in man. *J Physiol* 1959; **146**: 572–82.

4 Hughes JMB, Pride NB. In defence of the carbon monoxide transfer coefficient KCO (T_L/V_A). *Eur Respir J* 2001; **7**: 168–74.

5 Hughes JMB. The single breath transfer factor ($T_L CO$) and the transfer coefficient (KCO): a window on the pulmonary microcirculation. *Clin Physiol Funct Imaging* 2003; **23**: 63–71.

6 Saydain G, Beck KC, Decker PA, Cowl CT, Scanlon PD. Clinical significance of elevated diffusing capacity. *Chest* 2004; **125**: 446–52.

7 Roughton FJW, Forster RE. Relative importance of diffusion and chemical reaction rates in determining rate of exchange of gases in human lung, with special reference to true diffusing capacity of pulmonary membrane and volume of blood in the lung capillaries. *J Appl Physiol* 1957; **11**: 290–302.

8 MacIntyre N, Crapo RO, Viegi G, *et al.* Standardisation of the single breath determination of carbon monoxide uptake in the lung. *Eur Respir J* 2005; **26**: 720–35.

9 Quanjer PH. Standardised lung function testing. *Bull Eur Physiopathol Respir* 1983; **19** (suppl. 5): 39–44.

10 Neville E, Kendrick AH, Gibson GJ. A standardised method of estimating KCO on exercise. *Thorax* 1984; **39**: 823–7.

11 Graham BL, Mink JT, Cotton DJ. Effect of breath-hold time on $D_L CO$ (SB) in patients with airway obstruction. *J Appl Physiol* 1985; **58**: 1319–25.

12 Bates DV, Boucot NG, Dormer AE. The pulmonary diffusing capacity in normal subjects. *J Physiol* 1955; **129**: 237–52.

13 Filley GE, MacIntosh DJ, Wright GW. Carbon monoxide uptake and pulmonary diffusing capacity in normal subjects at rest and during exercise. *J Clin Invest* 1954; **33**: 530–39.

14 Hsia CCW, McBrayer DG, Ramanathan M. Reference values of diffusing capacity during exercise by a rebreathing technique. *Am J Respir Crit Care Med* 1995; **152**: 658–65.

15 Newth CJL, Cotton DJ, Nadel JA. Pulmonary diffusing capacity measured at multiple intervals during a single exhalation in man. *J Appl Physiol* 1977; **43**: 617–25.

16 Huang YC, Helms MJ, MacIntyre NR. Normal values for single exhalation diffusing capacity and pulmonary capillary blood flow in sitting, supine positions, and during mild exercise. *Chest* 1994; **105**: 501–8.

17 Wilson AF, Hearne J, Brenner M, *et al.* Measurement of transfer factor during constant exhalation. *Thorax* 1994; **49**: 1121–6.

18 Huang Y-CT, O'Brien SR, MacIntyre NR. Intrabreath diffusing capacity of the lung in healthy individuals at rest and during exercise. *Chest* 2002; **122**: 177–85.

4

Arterial Blood Gases and Acid–Base Balance

4.1 OXYGEN CARRIAGE BY THE BLOOD

When fully saturated, 1 g of haemoglobin combines with approximately 1.34 mL of oxygen, so that, with a normal haemoglobin concentration of 15 g per 100 mL of blood, the oxygen-carrying capacity of haemoglobin is 1.34×15, i.e. approximately 20 mL per 100 mL of blood. This greatly exceeds the volume of oxygen carried in solution, which, at a P_{O_2} of 100 mmHg, is only 0.3 mL per 100 mL of blood. Because of the shape of the haemoglobin–oxygen dissociation curve, haemoglobin is effectively fully saturated above a P_{O_2} of about 200 mmHg, but the amount of oxygen in solution continues to increase in direct proportion to the partial pressure.

The oxygen dissociation curve can be constructed by relating either oxygen content (concentration) or, more commonly, percentage saturation to P_{O_2} (Fig. 4.1). The two curves are almost interchangeable by adjusting the *y* axis, provided that the haemoglobin concentration is normal. Strictly, however, there is a small difference due to dissolved oxygen, which adds to oxygen concentration but not to saturation.

Normally, mixed venous blood at rest is about 75 per cent saturated (if the haemoglobin concentration is normal), but, because of the shape of the dissociation curve, this fall of 25 per cent below the arterial value is equivalent to a fall in P_{O_2} to less than half the arterial value, i.e. from approximately

90 mmHg (12 kPa) to 40 mmHg (5.3 kPa). Figure 4.1 also demonstrates the reserves of oxygen carriage bestowed by the shape of the dissociation curve, in that the arterial P_{O_2} can fall by an appreciable

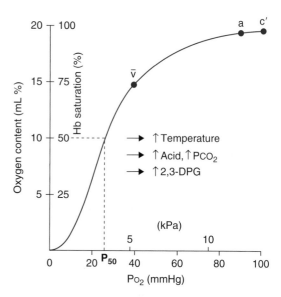

Figure 4.1 Haemoglobin–oxygen dissociation curve. The ordinate may be plotted in terms of either oxygen content (concentration) or percentage saturation. Approximate normal values for mixed venous $\bar{v}$, arterial (a) and end-pulmonary capillary blood (c′) are indicated. P_{50} represents the P_{O_2} when haemoglobin is 50 per cent saturated. The curve is shifted to the right with increases in temperature, acidity, P_{CO_2} (Bohr effect) or 2,3-diphosphoglycerate (DPG) concentration in the red cells.

extent from its normal value with only a modest reduction in the amount of oxygen transported. For clarity, Fig. 4.1 shows only a single dissociation curve but, at the level of the metabolizing tissues, oxygen delivery is facilitated by the shift to the right that occurs as CO_2 is taken up by the blood (Bohr effect): this implies that, for a given PO_2, oxygen carriage is less and therefore the blood releases more oxygen (Fig. 4.2). The position of the dissociation curve is also affected independently by pH, temperature and the concentration within the red cells of 2,3-diphosphoglycerate (2,3-DPG).

The shape of the oxygen dissociation curve has been described by various mathematical functions, but in practice the most frequently used index is the P_{50}, i.e. PO_2 at 50 per cent saturation. This can be measured in vitro after mixing equal volumes of fully saturated and fully desaturated blood that have been exposed to pure oxygen and to a vacuum respectively.[1] If equal volumes are mixed, the resulting blood is 50 per cent saturated and has a partial pressure (the P_{50}) of normally about 26 mmHg (3.5 kPa). Measurement of P_{50} is used to characterize various genetically determined abnormal haemoglobins that are associated with

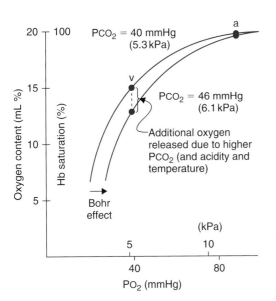

Figure 4.2 Haemoglobin–oxygen dissociation curve showing Bohr effect (shift to right), which occurs with higher P_{CO_2} in systemic capillaries in metabolizing tissues. For a given P_{O_2}, oxygen content and saturation are lower, which facilitates 'unloading' of oxygen from the blood to the tissues.

shifts of the dissociation curve to either right (increased P_{50}) or left (decreased P_{50}). Of course, an oxygen saturation in arterial blood as low as 50 per cent in vivo would be extreme and is rarely encountered, even in advanced disease. For this reason the 'P_{90}' has been proposed as a more clinically relevant landmark on the dissociation curve,[2] as values of SaO_2 around 90 per cent are quite commonly seen in clinical practice. Such a value is close to the 'knee' of the curve, but it depends greatly on pH – with a normal haemoglobin, values of pH between 7.26 and 7.56 would be associated with P_{90} ranging from approximately 48 mmHg to 67 mmHg.[2]

4.2 CARBON DIOXIDE CARRIAGE BY BLOOD

4.2.1 Modes of carbon dioxide carriage

The total amount of CO_2 carried by the blood (in millilitres per 100 mL) is appreciably greater than oxygen. About 5 per cent is in simple solution and a similar proportion is carried in chemical combination as carbamino compounds with proteins (including haemoglobin), but the great bulk (90%) is present as bicarbonate ions. Carbon dioxide entering red blood cells reacts with water under the influence of the enzyme carbonic anhydrase to form carbonic acid, most of which dissociates to hydrogen and bicarbonate ions:

$$CO_2 + H_2O \rightleftharpoons H_2CO_3 \rightleftharpoons H^+ + HCO_3^- \quad (4.1)$$

This deceptively simple reversible equilibrium underlies not only the carriage of CO_2 by the blood but also most of acid–base physiology.

4.2.2 Carbon dioxide dissociation curve

Normal arterial blood with a P_{CO_2} of 40 mmHg (5.3 kPa) carries approximately 48 mL CO_2 per 100 ml of blood, and resting mixed venous blood with a P_{CO_2} of 46 mmHg (6.1 kPa) carries about 52 ml CO_2 per 100 mL of blood (Fig. 4.3). The CO_2 content (concentration) difference between mixed venous and arterial blood is thus approximately 4 mL%, compared with a corresponding value for oxygen of 5 mL%. Each is determined by the cardiac output and by the rate of tissue metabolism, and the Fick equation can be applied to both:

$$\dot{Q} = \frac{\dot{V}O_2}{C(a - \bar{v})O_2} = \frac{\dot{V}CO_2}{C(\bar{v} - a)CO_2} \quad (4.2)$$

Whence, in an average normal subject at rest:

$$\frac{\dot{V}CO_2}{\dot{V}O_2} = R = \frac{C(\bar{v} - a)CO_2}{C(a - \bar{v})O_2} = \frac{4}{5} = 0.8 \quad (4.3)$$

where R is the respiratory exchange ratio (which at rest is approximately 0.8).

In the normal physiological range the CO_2 'dissociation curve' (i.e. relation of CO_2 concentration to PCO_2) is much steeper than the oxygen dissociation curve, since the corresponding differences in pressure between arterial and mixed venous blood are approximately 6 mmHg for CO_2 but 50 mmHg for oxygen. The CO_2 relationship is curvilinear, though less so than the oxygen curve. Consequently, if CO_2 retention occurs, then a given content difference (determined by tissue metabolism and cardiac output) implies an increasing difference in PCO_2 between mixed venous and arterial blood. The prevailing oxygen tension has an effect on the CO_2

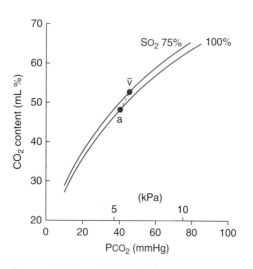

Figure 4.3 Carbon dioxide (CO_2) dissociation curve at levels of oxyhaemoglobin saturation (SO_2) corresponding approximately to normal arterial (100%) and mixed venous (75%) values. The relation is less curved than that for oxygen but its slope falls as PCO_2 increases. The dynamic 'physiological' relationship is indicated by the broken line between a and $\bar{v}$.

dissociation curve that is analogous to the Bohr effect of CO_2 on the oxygen dissociation curve. This is known as the Haldane (or Christiansen–Douglas–Haldane) effect and dictates that decreasing oxygenation shifts the curve to the left, i.e. at a given PCO_2 the volume of CO_2 carried increases (Fig. 4.3). As blood passes through metabolizing tissues, its affinity for oxygen consequently decreases, and its affinity for CO_2 increases, which makes sense in teleological terms. The reduction in oxygen saturation between arterial and venous blood is sufficient to produce a measurable shift of the CO_2 dissociation curve so that the effective relationship in vivo traverses two curves representing CO_2 dissociation at arterial and venous levels of oxygenation (Fig. 4.3).

4.3 BLOOD GAS MEASUREMENTS

4.3.1 Arterial blood gases

Modern automated blood gas analysers measure arterial PO_2, PCO_2 and pH directly using individual electrodes. The Astrup technique for interpolating $PaCO_2$ from pH measurements[3] was used in the era before directly recording $PaCO_2$ electrodes were available and is now largely of historic interest only, although some of the associated derived acid–base variables may still be calculated (see Section 4.5).

4.3.2 Capillary blood gases

An alternative to direct arterial blood sampling is use of 'arterialized' earlobe capillary sampling. With care this gives accurate estimation of arterial PCO_2 and pH, but PaO_2 is more vulnerable to error, particularly with values greater than about 80 mmHg (10.7 kPa).[4] At higher PaO_2 the arteriovenous PO_2 difference widens progressively because of the shape of the oxygen dissociation curve, and capillary PO_2 is then likely significantly to underestimate the arterial value.

4.3.3 Pulse oximetry

Monitoring of arterial oxygenation in clinical practice has been revolutionized in the past 25 years by the availability of simple, reliable pulse oximeters that estimate SaO_2 and can be used for continuous monitoring of patients, as well as during sleep and exercise studies and for convenient assessment of patients in the domiciliary setting. Modern oximeters emit and detect light at two wavelengths corresponding to oxygenated and deoxygenated haemoglobin. The estimate of SaO_2 obtained with a pulse oximeter is sometimes designated SpO_2 to distinguish it from directly measured arterial saturation. The probe is applied most commonly to the finger or earlobe and SpO_2 is measured by analysing only the pulsatile component of the absorbance in red and infrared light.[5] Carboxyhaemoglobin and methaemoglobin absorb light at the same wavelength so that the results become inaccurate in the presence of significant levels of either. Measurements can be falsely low in jaundiced patients and accuracy is also potentially compromised in deeply pigmented individuals.[6] In general the accuracy of pulse oximeters declines with values of SaO_2 below 75 per cent. Also, because of the shape of the oxygen dissociation curve, oximetry is much less sensitive to milder degrees of hypoxaemia than measurement of PaO_2.

4.3.4 Estimation of PcO_2 by rebreathing

A 'bloodless' technique for estimating mixed venous PcO_2 ($P\bar{v}CO_2$) during rebreathing was developed by Campbell and Howell but is little used nowadays. It is based on the principle that mixed venous blood is in equilibrium with a large 'pool' of CO_2 in the extracellular fluid, so that if a concentration of CO_2 close to $P\bar{v}CO_2$ is rebreathed from a small rubber anaesthetic bag it will rapidly reflect the PcO_2 of this pool. The measurement is made in two stages, starting with a 2-L bag containing pure oxygen. The first stage is simply a means of preparing a bag with a PcO_2 close to the mixed venous value; empirically this is usually achieved within 90 s. The subject then rests for a couple of minutes. In the second phase the prepared gas mixture is rapidly rebreathed for a few seconds to establish equilibrium with mixed venous blood. The PcO_2 of the mixture is then measured with a CO_2 gas analyser. Classically, at rest the $P\bar{v}CO_2$ is about 6 mmHg greater than $PaCO_2$, but with this technique the measurement made is the *oxygenated* mixed venous PcO_2, which is higher than the PcO_2 in the deoxygenated blood in the pulmonary arteries (Fig. 4.3). A more accurate estimate of arterial PcO_2 is given by multiplying the measured mixed venous value by 0.8.[7]

4.3.5 Transcutaneous PcO_2 monitoring

Self-evidently a pulse oximeter gives no information on PcO_2. Occasionally this presents clinical problems when monitoring patients with seriously compromised ventilation who are breathing oxygen, as relatively normal values of SaO_2 can induce a sense of false security if the possibility of a dangerous rise in $PaCO_2$ is not appreciated. Similarly simple and reliable non-invasive CO_2 monitoring would therefore be very valuable. Arterial PcO_2 can be estimated by use of a transcutaneous electrode to measure transcutaneous PcO_2 ($P_{tc}CO_2$). Hitherto, these instruments have sometimes been difficult to use, although they are applied more widely in neonates and infants, whose thinner skin improves accuracy. A recently introduced device applied, together with an oximeter sensor, to the ear gives reasonably accurate results and holds promise.[8] With improving technology, transcutaneous monitoring of PcO_2 seems likely to become more widely applied.

4.3.6 End tidal PcO_2 monitoring

Another approach to monitoring PcO_2, particularly popular in anaesthetic practice, is by capnography with measurement of end tidal CO_2 ($P_{ET}CO_2$). A CO_2 analyser is used to generate a continuous record of concentration at the mouth. The capnogram recorded during tidal expiration has a similar shape to that obtained during the single-breath nitrogen washout test (see Chapter 2, Section 2.1.9 and Fig. 2.5), except that the latter is recorded over a full vital capacity breath rather than the resting tidal volume. The end tidal PcO_2 (Fig. 4.4) is taken as an index of the arterial value, or at least as a guide to when an arterial sample should be taken.[9] Although of some value in subjects with healthy lungs, $P_{ET}CO_2$ is not an accurate predictor of $PaCO_2$ in patients with significant lung disease,[10] in whom ventilation/perfusion mismatching compromises interpretation of the alveolar 'plateau' (Fig. 4.4). Particularly in patients with airway obstruction, the expired 'plateau' becomes increasingly steep and poorly defined, such that the end tidal value is

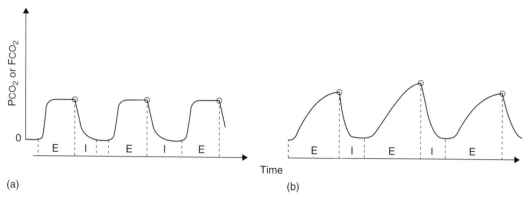

Figure 4.4 Schematic record of expired P_{CO_2} (or fractional concentration) during tidal breathing in **(a)** a healthy subject and **(b)** a patient with diffuse airway obstruction. E and I represent expiration and inspiration, respectively. In the healthy subject **(a)** expired P_{CO_2} is relatively constant once the anatomical dead space has emptied, while in the patient **(b)** P_{CO_2} rises progressively during expiration as less well ventilated alveoli (with higher P_{CO_2}) empty later. Consequently the end tidal value (o) is more arbitrary and variable.

somewhat arbitrary. A more important use of end tidal capnography in anaesthetic and intensive care practice is in monitoring expired CO_2 during endotracheal intubation to check that the tube is placed correctly in the airway rather than the oesophagus.

4.4 MECHANISMS OF HYPOXAEMIA

4.4.1 Hypoxia and cyanosis

At the level of the metabolizing tissues, the oxygen supply is dependent on both the oxygen content of the blood and the circulation – hence tissue hypoxia can develop even with a normal Pa_{O_2} if the circulation is sluggish. The classic clinical sign of oxygen lack is cyanosis, with central cyanosis reflecting impaired arterial oxygenation, and peripheral cyanosis resulting from either a low Pa_{O_2} or reduced peripheral perfusion. The presence of central cyanosis depends on the absolute concentration of deoxyhaemoglobin; it therefore becomes relatively more difficult to recognize in anaemic individuals, while it may be present in polycythaemia even with relatively normal Pa_{O_2}. The textbook teaching used to be that central cyanosis became detectable only when the arterial concentration of deoxyhaemoglobin increased to approximately 5 g/100 mL. With a normal haemoglobin concentration of 15 g/100 mL this would represent an Sa_{O_2} of only 67 per cent or a Pa_{O_2} of approximately 35 mmHg. In practice, central cyanosis is usually detectable with a much lower

Table 4.1 Mechanisms of hypoxaemia

Low inspired oxygen
Hypoventilation
Diffusion limitation
Anatomical R→L shunt
Ventilation/perfusion mismatching

concentration of deoxyhaemoglobin – of about 1.5 g/100 mL in arterial blood.[11] In fact, the 'textbook' view is based on an erroneous interpretation of a classic study by Lundsgaard and van Slyke,[12] as the level of 5 g/100 mL attributed to their work actually referred to the concentration of deoxyhaemoglobin in the tissue capillaries rather than in arterial blood.[13]

4.4.2 Pathophysiological mechanisms of hypoxaemia

The pathophysiological mechanisms that potentially can cause arterial hypoxaemia (i.e. reduced Pa_{O_2}) are listed in Table 4.1 and illustrated in Figs 4.5–4.8.

4.4.2.1 Reduced inspired P_{O_2}

At altitude the total barometric pressure is reduced, and consequently so is the inspired P_{O_2} ($P_I O_2$), even though the fractional concentration ($F_I O_2$) remains the same as at sea level. Therefore, the normal reference values for Pa_{O_2} need to be adjusted for people living at altitude.

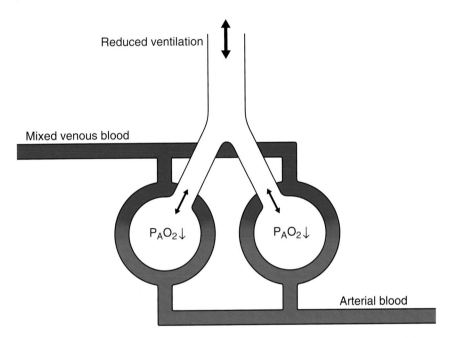

Figure 4.5 Causes of arterial hypoxaemia – hypoventilation: two-compartment model showing reduced, but evenly distributed, ventilation with normal blood flow. Alveolar P_{O_2} (P_AO_2) is less than normal; consequently blood draining each compartment is less well oxygenated than normal, resulting in low PaO_2.

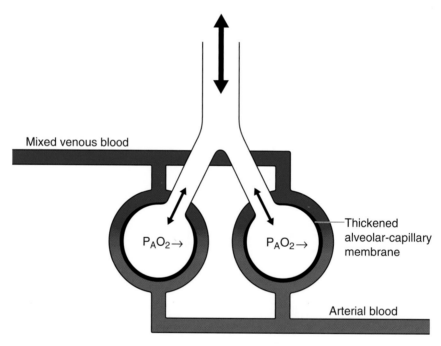

Figure 4.6 Causes of arterial hypoxaemia – limitation of oxygen diffusion: two compartment model showing normal and evenly distributed ventilation and perfusion, with consequently normal P_AO_2. Diffusion of oxygen is impaired due to thickening of the alveolar–capillary membrane, such that equilibration is incomplete by the time blood leaves each compartment.

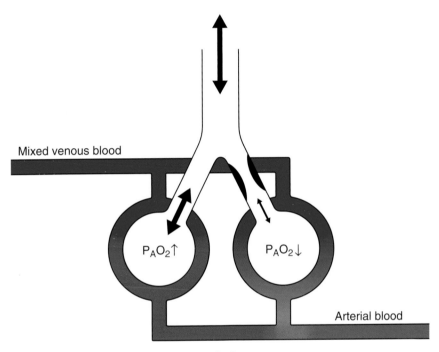

Figure 4.7 Causes of arterial hypoxaemia – $\dot{V}_A/\dot{Q}$ mismatching due to non-uniform distribution of ventilation but uniform distribution of perfusion: narrowing of airway to R compartment reduces its ventilation and $\dot{V}_A/\dot{Q}$ ratio with consequently a lower local P_AO_2. Relative overventilation and high $\dot{V}_A/\dot{Q}$ of L compartment with increased local P_AO_2 fails to compensate, so that mixing of blood from the two compartments results in low PaO_2 (see text for further amplification).

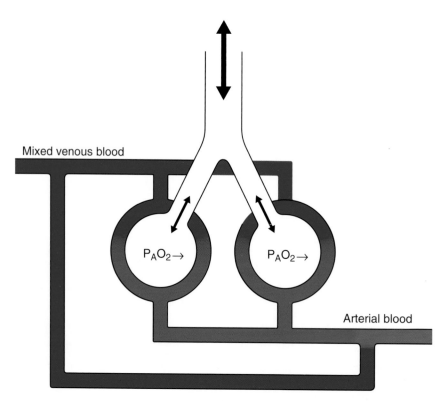

Figure 4.8 Causes of arterial hypoxaemia – right-to-left shunt: uniform distribution of ventilation and perfusion with normal oxygenation of blood in each compartment; arterial hypoxaemia results from shunted blood, which completely bypasses ventilated lung.

Altitude is a potential problem not only for people living and climbing there but also for air travellers. Although the cabin of a commercial aircraft is pressurized to avoid very low values of inspired Po_2 (P_IO_2), this is not equivalent to sea level. Usually the effective 'cabin altitude' is about 8000 feet (2500 m), which implies a reduction in P_IO_2 of approximately one-third. Although this presents no problems for people with good cardiopulmonary function, it may result in a dangerously low PaO_2 in patients who already have significant hypoxaemia at sea level. Various guidelines and protocols are available for use if such individuals wish to fly, e.g. the guideline produced by the British Thoracic Society, which recommends hypoxic challenge testing, in which blood gases are measured while breathing 15 per cent oxygen, for patients with more marked hypoxaemia at sea level.[14] An alternative approach is the use of an equation to predict the likely PaO_2 at altitude from sea-level measurements plus/minus some index of the severity of the underlying lung disease.[15] The recommendations can only be general, however, as the accuracy of prediction is only moderate and defining a 'safe' PaO_2 for an individual is largely speculative.

4.4.2.2 Hypoventilation

Hypoventilation implies a reduction in the total volume of air inspired and expired per minute (minute ventilation) (Fig. 4.5). In principle this causes a reduction in PaO_2 and an increase in $PaCO_2$. Such 'pure' hypoventilation is, however, quite uncommon, at least in the chronic stable situation. It occurs, for example, in patients with severe respiratory muscle weakness or severe skeletal abnormality, in which the respiratory muscles are unable either to generate a normal force or to apply it to expand the lungs. More common is acute or subacute hypoventilation, when breathing is depressed centrally, e.g. by sedative drugs.

The term 'alveolar hypoventilation', as usually used, is synonymous with hypercapnia. It implies a reduction in the *effective* ventilation but not necessarily in overall ventilation. In fact, in most situations associated with hypercapnia (e.g. in patients with chronic obstructive pulmonary disease, COPD), total ventilation is normal or even increased due to excessive dead space ventilation consequent on a restricted tidal volume and/or ventilation/perfusion mismatching (see Chapter 9, Section 9.6.3).

4.4.2.3 Impairment of gas diffusion

Hypoxaemia due to impaired diffusion of oxygen through the alveolar capillary membrane (Fig. 4.6) is uncommon. It is best exemplified by patients with interstitial fibrosis, particularly during exercise. On exercise the transit time for red blood cells through the pulmonary capillaries is reduced by the high blood flow. The reduced transit time combined with an increased resistance to diffusion may then prevent complete equilibration of alveolar and capillary Po_2.

4.4.2.4 Ventilation/perfusion mismatching and 'anatomical' shunt

Much the most common mechanism of hypoxaemia in clinical practice is mismatching of ventilation ($\dot{V}_A$) and perfusion ($\dot{Q}$) (Fig. 4.7), the underlying mechanisms of which are discussed in Chapter 2, Section 2.3.1. Quantitation in terms of detailed measurement of the distribution of $\dot{V}_A/\dot{Q}$ ratios is not feasible in routine clinical practice, but summary information on the severity of $\dot{V}_A/\dot{Q}$ mismatching can be deduced from the arterial blood gases. If the patient is in a reasonably steady state and if the inspired oxygen concentration is known, the alveolar air equation can be applied to estimate the 'ideal' alveolar Po_2, whence the alveolar–arterial gradient ($AaPo_2$) can be calculated and a semi-quantitative statement made about the presence or absence of a 'shunt-like' effect. If, in addition, expired air is collected, the Bohr equation can be applied to calculate the physiological dead space and thus to quantify the contribution of high $\dot{V}_A/\dot{Q}$ alveoli.

Unfortunately, the relation between the $AaPo_2$ and the percentage physiological shunt is non-linear (Fig. 4.9). Furthermore, since the shunt calculation is based on the oxygen content or saturation of blood, the shape of the oxygen dissociation curve implies that, for a given percentage venous admixture, the lower the P_AO_2, the narrower the $AaPo_2$ (Fig. 4.10). This accounts for the inverse correlation observed between $AaPo_2$ and $PaCO_2$,[16] since a rising $PaCO_2$ is inevitably associated with a falling P_AO_2, provided there is no change in inspired oxygen concentration. Conversely, at higher P_AO_2, the

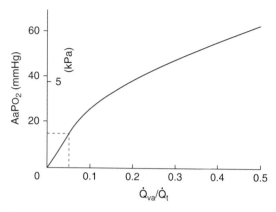

Figure 4.9 Relation between increasing physiological shunt ($\dot{Q}_{va}/\dot{Q}_t$) and alveolar–arterial tension difference (AaPo$_2$) at a constant $P_{A}O_2$ of 100 mmHg (13.3 kPa), with normal upper limits shown by broken lines.

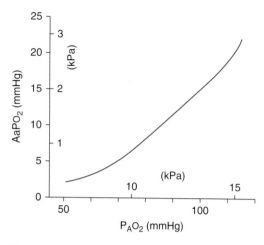

Figure 4.10 Relation between AaPo$_2$ and $P_{A}O_2$ with a constant physiological shunt of 0.05. With a reduction in $P_{A}O_2$ (e.g. in the presence of hypercapnia) the AaPo$_2$ narrows, and at higher $P_{A}O_2$ (hyperventilation or increased inspired oxygen) the AaPo$_2$ widens.

AaPO$_2$ widens, as is easily demonstrated during voluntary hyperventilation.

In clinical practice, the alveolar Po$_2$ is increased therapeutically by supplementing the inspired oxygen concentration when, for a given percentage physiological shunt (venous admixture), an increase in AaPo$_2$ would be expected (Fig. 4.9). But changing the composition of inspired air has an additional effect on the physiological shunt itself. This is best illustrated by the classic method of measuring Pao$_2$, and calculating the AaPo$_2$, after a few minutes breathing 100 per cent oxygen, in order to estimate the 'anatomical' shunt. The rationale is that the effects of any $\dot{V}_A/\dot{Q}$ mismatching can be eliminated by breathing pure oxygen since, given enough time, all the nitrogen will be washed out, even from the most poorly ventilated alveoli. The tendency of these alveoli with a low $\dot{V}_A/\dot{Q}$ ratio to lower the Po$_2$ of the arterial blood is therefore removed. The only 'shunt' remaining is then via channels that bypass the lungs or supply any alveoli that are totally unventilated (as shown in Fig. 4.8). The test is open to the objection that breathing 100 per cent O$_2$ will itself encourage alveolar collapse because of loss of the 'splinting' effect of poorly soluble nitrogen. In practice, however, it is a useful technique in the investigation of arterial hypoxaemia when this may be due to an abnormal right-to-left shunt through one or more structural channels. The usually quoted normal upper limit for the anatomical shunt measured in this way is 5 per cent of the cardiac output. In terms of the Pao$_2$, a value greater

than 550 mmHg (>73 kPa) is usually reached. Note that this is likely to represent an AaPo$_2$ in excess of 100 mmHg, emphasizing the dependence of AaPo$_2$ on alveolar Po$_2$. At such high levels of arterial Po$_2$, haemoglobin is fully saturated with oxygen. In effect, raising the Pao$_2$ to levels greater than 200–300 mmHg increases oxygen carriage by simple solution only. At these high values of Pao$_2$, increases in oxygen content and partial pressure become related linearly: as a rule of thumb, above a Pao$_2$ of 300 mmHg, each 20 mmHg of AaPo$_2$ represents an anatomical shunt of 1 per cent.

An alternative method of quantifying an 'anatomical' shunt is by intravenous injection of radio-labelled albumin particles large enough to lodge in the pulmonary microvasculature. With anatomical shunting a measurable proportion of the injected particles reaches the systemic circulation. This can be quantified using a gamma camera to count externally over organs with high blood flow such as the kidneys and brain. With large intrapulmonary shunts the results correlate well with the 100 per cent oxygen method.[17]

4.4.2.5 Indices of severity of hypoxaemia

If arterial hypoxaemia is due primarily to $\dot{V}_A/\dot{Q}$ mismatching, the percentage physiological shunt falls when pure oxygen is breathed (even though the $AaPO_2$ widens). To a lesser extent these opposing effects also come into play with any enrichment of the inspired oxygen, and the disappointing conclusion is that comparisons, not only of the $AaPO_2$, but also of the three-compartment analysis itself are difficult when the oxygen concentration the patient breathes changes. Of course, if sequential values of PaO_2 show a fall, the patient is clearly not improving – but if PaO_2 rises as the inspired PO_2 is increased, this could be caused either by the oxygen enrichment per se or by a true improvement with time in the efficiency of gas exchange, or both.

The uncertainty of assessing or predicting changes in arterial oxygenation when the inspired concentration is varied has prompted other approaches. One such is calculation of the ratio of arterial to alveolar PO_2 (a/A PO_2).[18] This is normally greater than 0.75 and changes little in normal subjects as F_IO_2 is increased, whereas the more traditional $AaPO_2$ difference increases. More commonly used, especially in patients with severe problems of oxygenation such as the acute respiratory distress syndrome (ARDS), is the ratio PaO_2/F_IO_2.[19] This provides a similar assessment of gas exchange and is directly available if the precise inspired oxygen concentration is known. In the context of the acute lung injury of ARDS, a value above 300 (PaO_2 in mmHg) is taken as insignificant while a value below 100 represents the most severe degree of hypoxaemia.[19]

4.5 ACID–BASE BALANCE

The carriage of CO_2 by the blood and its excretion by the lungs represents one of the two homeostatic mechanisms for regulating the acid–base status of the body. The lungs are able to adjust acid–base balance much more rapidly than the kidneys and, in effect, the lungs excrete about 100 times as much acid each day as do the kidneys.

4.5.1 Carbon dioxide–bicarbonate equilibrium

The subject of acid–base balance probably creates more confusion than any other area of clinical physiology. The aim of this account is to explain some simple principles and suggest pragmatic

guidelines. The three variables, hydrogen ion concentration (strictly hydrogen ion activity), bicarbonate ion concentration and carbonic acid concentration (and thus PCO_2) are inevitably linked by the carbonic acid association/dissociation equation (Equation 4.1), which bears restating:

$$CO_2 + H_2O \rightleftharpoons H_2CO_3 \rightleftharpoons H^+ + HCO_3^- \quad (4.1)$$

The dissociation constant of carbonic acid (K_A) is defined as for any reversible equilibrium as:

$$K_A = \frac{[H^+] \times [HCO_3^-]}{[H_2CO_3]}$$

but $[H_2CO_3]$ is related directly to the concentration of dissolved CO_2, which, in turn, is proportional to the solubility and partial pressure of CO_2. Therefore:

$$K_A = \frac{[H^+] \times [HCO_3^-]}{0.03\, PCO_2} \quad (PCO_2 \text{ in mmHg})$$

Taking logs:

$$\log K_A = \log[H^+] + \log \frac{[HCO_3^-]}{0.03\, PCO_2} \quad (4.2)$$

pH is the negative logarithm of the hydrogen ion concentration (activity) and pK_A is the negative logarithm of K_A, therefore:

$$pH = pK_A + \log \frac{[HCO_3^-]}{0.03\, PCO_2} \quad (4.3)$$

The value of pK_A has been found to be reasonably constant at 6.1 – hence the well-known Henderson–Hasselbalch equation:

$$pH = 6.1 + \log \frac{[HCO_3^-]}{0.03\, PCO_2(mmHg)} \quad (4.4)$$

or:

$$pH = 6.1 + \log \frac{[HCO_3^-]}{0.225\, PCO_2\,(kPa)}$$

For normal arterial blood $[HCO_3^-] \sim 24\,mM$ and $PCO_2 \sim 40\,mmHg$, therefore:

$$pH = 6.1 + \log \frac{24}{0.03 \times 40}$$
$$= 6.1 + 1.3 = 7.4$$

For many purposes (such as thinking rationally about the subject!), the 'negative logarithm to the base 10 of the hydrogen ion concentration' is a difficult concept to handle and the non-logarithmic form based on the equation derived by Henderson is easier to comprehend.[20] Since:

$$\frac{[H^+] \times [HCO_3^-]}{P_{CO_2}} = \text{a constant,}$$

$$[H^+] = \text{constant} \times \frac{P_{CO_2}}{[HCO_3^-]}$$

With P_{CO_2} in mmHg, $[HCO_3^-]$ in mM and $[H^+]$ in nM (10^{-9}M), then:[21]

$$[H^+] = 24 \times \frac{P_{CO_2}}{[HCO_3^-]} \qquad (4.5)$$

If P_{CO_2} is in kPa, the equivalent equation is:

$$[H^+] = 180 \times \frac{P_{CO_2}}{[HCO_3^-]}$$

For average normal arterial values:

$$[H^+] = 24 \times \frac{40}{24} = 40\,nM$$

i.e.

$$[H^+] = 40 \times 10^{-9} \text{ or } 4 \times 10^{-8}M^*$$

4.5.2 Primary acid–base disorders

Much of the confusion in understanding respiratory acid–base disturbances comes from muddling what are essentially chemical events (defined by Equation 4.1) with the physiological responses to those events. The immediate 'chemical' effects are clear from the reversible equilibrium. In a respiratory disturbance the primary change is in the CO_2 whereas in metabolic disturbance the primary change is in the $[H^+]$ or $[HCO_3^-]$:

- In *respiratory acidosis* the equilibrium in Equation 4.1 shifts immediately to the right so that the hydrogen ion concentration rises (pH falls) and the bicarbonate ion concentration also increases. This immediate rise in $[HCO_3^-]$ often causes surprise because 'acidosis' is mistakenly regarded as synonymous with a reduction in bicarbonate. In fact the vast majority of hydrogen ions produced are buffered by proteins so that the measured rise in $[HCO_3^-]$ is actually considerably greater than the concomitant rise in hydrogen ion concentration. The kidneys later compensate for the increase in acidity by retaining more bicarbonate. Although, in absolute terms, the increase in $[H^+]$ is small, organic systems generally tolerate acidity poorly and the hydrogen ion concentration is 'defended' vigorously. In general, in a typical patient with chronic, stable hypercapnia, about one-third of the increase in arterial $[HCO_3^-]$ will have occurred acutely in accordance with the above relationship and two-thirds by subsequent renal 'compensation'.
- In *respiratory alkalosis* the primary event is an increase in CO_2 excretion by overbreathing and therefore $[H^+]$ falls (pH rises), but most of the change is again buffered and $[HCO_3^-]$ falls. If this state is maintained for a matter of hours, fewer hydrogen ions but more bicarbonate ions are excreted by the kidneys and this tends to restore the $[H^+]$ towards normal.
- In *metabolic acidosis* $[H^+]$ rises (pH falls) and $[HCO_3^-]$ falls. The physiological response is rapid and any tendency for P_{CO_2} to rise is more than offset by the increased drive to breathe resulting from production of acid, so that the measured effect is a reduced Pa_{CO_2}.
- In metabolic alkalosis $[HCO_3^-]$ rises and $[H^+]$ falls (pH rises). The final result is rather variable as opposing influences are involved. Any increase in P_{CO_2} will tend to stimulate breathing but the lower acidity tends to inhibit it. The net effect is often the maintenance of Pa_{CO_2} in the normal range unless the alkalosis is severe[22] or unless CO_2 excretion is already compromised by poor lung function, in which case Pa_{CO_2} is more likely to increase.

---

*To convert $[H^+] = 4 \times 10^{-8}$ to pH, take the $\log_{10}$ and add a negative sign, i.e. $-(-8 + 0.6) = 7.4$.

Table 4.2 Commoner causes of primary acid–base disorders

Metabolic acidosis

Increased anion gap	Ketoacidosis (diabetic coma)
	Uraemia
	Lactic acidosis (tissue hypoxia)
	Poisoning, e.g. aspirin
Normal anion gap	Renal tubular acidosis
	Ureteric transplantation
	Severe diarrhoea
	Carbonic anhydrase inhibitors

Metabolic alkalosis

Severe vomiting	e.g. pyloric stenosis
Iatrogenic	Diuretics
	Corticosteroids
	Inappropriate bicarbonate infusion

Respiratory acidosis

Cerebral	Drugs (e.g. sedatives, hypnotics)
Raised intracranial pressure	(e.g. trauma, tumour, stroke)
	Primary alveolar hypoventilation
Spinal cord	Trauma
Motor neurons	Poliomyelitis
	Motor neuron disease
Peripheral nerves	e.g. Guillain–Barré syndrome
Motor end plate	Myasthenia gravis
	Relaxant drugs
Respiratory muscles	Dystrophies, myopathies
Thoracic cage	Trauma
	Scoliosis
	Thoracoplasty
Lung parenchyma	Severe pulmonary oedema ARDS, etc.
Airways	COPD
	Severe asthma
	Severe upper airway obstruction

Respiratory alkalosis

Intrapulmonary	Pulmonary fibrosis, infiltration
	Pneumonia
	Oedema
	Pulmonary embolism
	Acute asthma
Neurological	Central neurogenic hyperventilation
Psychological	Anxiety, psychogenic dyspnoea
Chemical	Hypoxaemia
	Aspirin poisoning
	Hepatic failure
Iatrogenic	Mechanical overventilation

ARDS, acute respiratory distress syndrome; COPD, chronic obstructive pulmonary disease.

Specific causes of each of these primary disturbances are listed in Table 4.2. Combined disturbances are common. It is sometimes helpful in elucidating the likely cause(s) of a metabolic acidosis to estimate the 'anion gap'.[23] This is obtained from measurements in venous blood and is based on the principle of electro-neutrality, i.e. the sum of all positive charges (cations) in a body fluid must equal the sum of all negative charges (anions). The main cations are sodium, potassium, calcium and magnesium, and the main anions are chloride, bicarbonate, proteins, sulphate, phosphate and the anions of organic acids. The anion gap estimates any anions not measured and traditionally it is simplified to the most abundant in blood, i.e. $[Na^+] - ([Cl^-] + [HCO_3^-])$. When calculated in this way it has a normal value of between $5 \times 10^{-3}\,M$ and $14 \times 10^{-3}\,M$. A metabolic acidosis with increased anion gap results from excess of either endogenous organic acids (lactic acidosis, ketoacidosis or renal failure) or exogenous acids (e.g. resulting from ingestion of alcohols or salicylic acid).

4.5.3 Graphical analysis of acid–base balance

Once two of the three variables P_{CO_2}, $[HCO_3^-]$ and pH (or $[H^+]$) are measured, the third can be calculated. The relation between any pair can be used graphically to examine acid–base status, and the third variable then appears as a series of isopleths on the graph. Each of the three possible modes of display has its devotees: the relation between log P_{CO_2} and pH may be the most familiar as it is the basis of the Siggaard–Andersen nomogram,[3] while the plot of $[HCO_3^-]$ versus pH has been used extensively by Davenport.[24] The non-logarithmic versions are more approachable, and the most widely used are the relations between $[H^+]$ and P_{CO_2},[25,26] and between $[HCO_3^-]$ and P_{CO_2} (Fig. 4.11).[21,25,27] The latter is in effect the CO_2 dissociation curve in different guise.

Either relation illustrates respiratory acid–base disturbances well. The $[H^+]$ versus P_{CO_2} plot eloquently demonstrates a metabolic acidosis, while the $[HCO_3^-]$ versus P_{CO_2} relationship does greater justice to metabolic alkalosis.

For interpretation of clinical acid–base data, it is desirable to relate the measured values to the

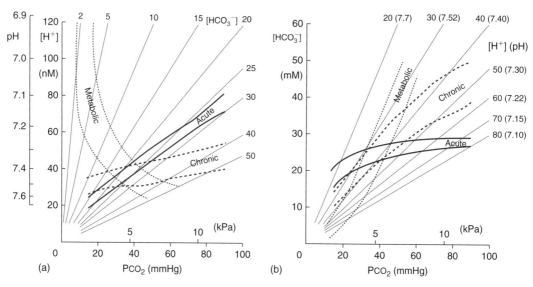

Figure 4.11 Two non-logarithmic ways of looking at acid–base disturbances. **(a)** Relates hydrogen ion activity, [H⁺], to Pco₂ with isopleths of constant [HCO₃⁻]. **(b)** Relates [HCO₃⁻] to Pco₂ with isopleths of constant [H⁺] (pH). The bands indicate the approximate ranges likely with uncomplicated acid–base disturbances; solid lines represent the 95 per cent 'significance bands' for acute respiratory acidosis[25] and acute respiratory alkalosis;[28] broken lines show similar ranges for chronic respiratory acidosis[29] and chronic respiratory alkalosis.[30] Data in metabolic acidosis and alkalosis (dotted lines) represent the combined ranges of two studies.[31,32]

expected quantitative relations among the three variables Pco₂, [HCO₃⁻] and [H⁺] (or pH) for the different types of acid–base disturbance. Over the years sufficient data have been accumulated for this to be done with some confidence, and Fig. 4.11 shows the likely relationships in single, uncomplicated disturbances. Only the data in acute respiratory acidosis[25] and alkalosis,[28] however, are based on the study of normal humans; those in chronic respiratory disturbances,[29,30] and in metabolic acidosis[31,32] and alkalosis,[31] have been obtained from carefully selected patients in an apparently steady state in whom complicating factors were as far as possible excluded.

To illustrate the use of these relations a theoretical example is shown in Fig. 4.12. Starting with normal values (1) the subject first develops an acute respiratory acidosis (2); the Paco₂ is held at a constant level while renal retention of bicarbonate occurs and [H⁺] falls to the value appropriate for a chronic 'compensated' respiratory acidosis (3). A further acute rise in Paco₂ then supervenes (4). Note that the rise from 3 to 4 parallels the 'acute' relationship and the subject finishes at point 4 between the 'acute' and 'chronic' bands

with an 'acute-on-chronic' respiratory acidosis. This type of analysis shows that a given single set of data should always be interpreted in the light of previous values and the clinical situation. When opposing influences are involved, an apparently simple, uncomplicated disturbance may conceal a combination of two or more different acid–base abnormalities. For complete interpretation of values at a point on any acid–base diagram it is necessary to know not only where the subject has ended up but also how he or she got there.

The difference in units between [H⁺] and [HCO₃⁻] conceals the very narrow range of acidity over which the organism functions – with the acute rise from points 1 and 2 in Fig. 4.12 [HCO₃⁻] rises by 2.2 mM (2.2×10^{-3} M) and [H⁺] by 15 nM (15×10^{-9} M) – in other words 99.999993 per cent of the hydrogen ions are immediately buffered. Two-thirds of the remainder are eventually negated by renal compensation.

4.5.4 Other acid–base indices

The relation between pH and log Pco₂ is used in the Astrup method for estimating arterial Pco₂.[3] The

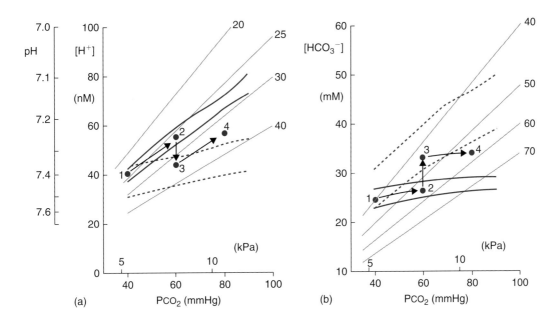

Figure 4.12 Example of use of non-logarithmic acid–base diagrams in respiratory acidosis. Bands for acute and chronic respiratory acidosis as in Fig. 4.11. Starting with normal values (1), the hypothetical subject develops an acute respiratory acidosis (2), renal retention of bicarbonate occurs (3) and then a further acute rise in Pco_2 occurs (4). The actual values at each stage are:

	Pco_2 (mmHg)	[H⁺] (nM)	pH	[HCO₃⁻] (mM)
1	40	40	7.4	24.0
2	60	55	7.26	26.2
3	60	44	7.36	32.7
4	80	57	7.24	33.7

measurement actually made is pH, but by also measuring pH in vitro at different known values of Pco_2 the pH of the blood is interpolated on the graph and a presumptive $Paco_2$ read off. The technique is subject to the fundamental error that the relations of pH and log Pco_2 in blood in vitro and in vivo differ because of the influence of the remainder of the extracellular fluid in the intact organism.

Some of the indices of acid–base status are relics of this now obsolete approach, but they still have their advocates. The derived indices, which include standard bicarbonate, base excess and deficit, and total buffer base, often hinder understanding of respiratory acid–base disturbances. They are used mainly to distinguish and quantify the 'respiratory' and 'metabolic' components of a given disturbance. It should,

however, be noted that 'metabolic' in this context includes renal compensation for a primary respiratory disorder. In a respiratory acidosis or alkalosis, therefore, such indices distinguish the 'acute' from the 'chronic'. The situation is usually clearer if the actual rather than the standard bicarbonate is used, with a 'metabolic' acidosis or alkalosis more usefully defined as a primary disturbance resulting from an excess or deficit of hydrogen ions. In practice, in an uncomplicated 'acute-on-chronic' respiratory acidosis the reduction in pH below its normal value is a useful guide to the magnitude of the acute change.[33]

Hitherto, the most frequently available index of CO_2 carriage and acid–base status has been the venous 'bicarbonate', although many biochemistry laboratories no longer include it as part of the routine electrolyte profile. The measurement usually made is the 'total CO_2 content', of which only 90 per cent is actually bicarbonate ions. Although often overlooked, it can be very useful as a rough check on the validity of blood gas measurements as large discrepancies may suggest technical errors or an unrepresentative arterial sample. A raised venous 'bicarbonate' can also be a clue to unsuspected respiratory failure or may suggest that CO_2 retention is 'chronic' (i.e. present for at least a day or two) in patients presenting for the first time.

4.5.5 The 'strong ion' approach to analysing acid–base balance

Inevitably, the analysis presented above is oversimplified. A more comprehensive approach based on the principles of physical chemistry was proposed by Stewart[34] and subsequently developed by others.[35,36] This focuses on the factors that independently determine $[H^+]$, reducing the emphasis on $[HCO_3^-]$, which in this analysis is a dependent rather than independent variable. According to the 'strong ion' analysis, the independent variables controlling acid–base balance are three: the P_{CO_2}, the 'strong ion difference' (SID) and the total weak acid concentration (a weak acid is one that is partly dissociated rather than completely ionized). The SID is the difference between the charge of the strong (completely dissociated) cations and anions in plasma: in effect this boils down to $[Na^+] + [K^+] - [Cl^-]$. A higher value of SID reduces acidity (higher pH). The weak acids in blood are predominantly proteins, particularly albumin, with a small contribution from inorganic phosphate.

This analysis defines six rather than four primary acid–base disorders. Respiratory disturbances remain as before, but metabolic acidosis and alkalosis can each be either of two types, resulting from increases or decreases in SID or in total weak acid concentration. Metabolic acidosis results from either decreasing SID or increasing [weak acid], while increasing SID or decreasing [weak acid] produces alkalosis.

In practice, this approach is of most value in understanding complex metabolic disturbances, as are commonly seen in patients receiving intensive care. In particular, the analysis highlights the important role of albumin concentration. Albumin is a weak acid and therefore a reduction

in its concentration has an alkalinizing effect. Consequently, a metabolic acidosis resulting from a reduction in SID may be underestimated or concealed in patients with hypoalbuminaemia.[37] Again, it is well recognized that infusion of large volumes of normal saline can result in an acidosis: in terms of the strong ion theory this is readily explicable as due to a reduction in plasma SID as plasma $[Cl^-]$ increases proportionally to a greater extent than $[Na^+]$.[38] An important determinant of SID is renal function, in particular via the regulatory effect of the kidneys on plasma chloride concentration. Thus, with 'renal compensation' for a respiratory acidosis, the strong ion approach emphasizes the increase in SID consequent on increased excretion of chloride ions, rather than the traditional explanation in terms of retention of bicarbonate.[39]

REFERENCES

1 Edwards MJ, Martin RJ. Mixing technique for the oxygen–haemoglobin equilibrium and Bohr effect. *J Appl Physiol* 1966; **21**: 1898–902.
2 Rebuck AS, Chapman KR. The P_{90} as a clinically relevant landmark on the oxyhaemoglobin dissociation curve. *Am Rev Respir Dis* 1988; **137**: 962–3.
3 Astrup P, Jorgensen K, Siggaard-Andersen O, Engel, K. The acid–base metabolism: a new approach. *Lancet* 1960; **1**: 1035–9.
4 Hughes JMB. Blood gas estimations from arterialised capillary blood versus arterial puncture: are they different? *Eur Respir J* 1996; **9**: 184–5.
5 Tremper KK. Pulse oximetry. *Chest* 1989; **95**: 713–14.
6 Ries AL, Prewitt LM, Johnson JJ. Skin colour and ear oximetry. *Chest* 1989; **96**: 287–90.
7 McEvoy JDS, Jones NL, Campbell EJM. Mixed venous and arterial PCO_2. *Br Med J* 1974; **4**: 687–90.
8 Parker SM, Gibson GJ. Evaluation of a transcutaneous carbon dioxide monitor ('TOSCA') in adult patients in routine respiratory practice. *Respir Med* 2007; **101**: 261–4.
9 Saura P, Blanch L, Lucangelo U, *et al.* Use of capnography to detect hypercapnic episodes during weaning from mechanical ventilation. *Intensive Care Med* 1996; **22**: 374–81.
10 Morley TF, Giaimo J, Maroszan E, *et al.* Use of capnography for assessment of the adequacy of alveolar ventilation during weaning from mechanical ventilation. *Am Rev Respir Dis* 1993; **148**: 339–44.

11 Goss GA, Hayes JA, Burdon JGW. Deoxyhaemoglobin concentrations in the detection of central cyanosis. *Thorax* 1988; **43**: 212–13.

12 Lundsgaard C, van Slyke DD. Cyanosis. *Medicine* 1923; **2**: 1–76.

13 Martin L, Khalil H. How much reduced haemoglobin is necessary to generate central cyanosis? *Chest* 1990; **97**: 182–5.

14 British Thoracic Society. Managing passengers with respiratory disease planning air travel: British Thoracic Society recommendation. *Thorax* 2002; **57**: 289–304.

15 Dillard TA, Berg BW, Ragagopal KR, Dooley JM, Mehm WJ. Hypoxaemia during air travel in patients with chronic obstructive pulmonary disease. *Ann Intern Med* 1989; **111**: 326–7.

16 Gray BA, Blalock JM. Interpretation of the alveolar–arterial oxygen differences in patients with hypercapnia. *Am Rev Respir Dis* 1991; **142**: 4–8.

17 Whyte MKB, Peters AM, Hughes JMB, *et al.* Quantification of right to left shunt at rest and during exercise in patients with pulmonary arteriovenous malformations. *Thorax* 1992; **47**: 790–96.

18 Gilbert R, Keighley JF. The arterial/alveolar oxygen tension ratio: an index of gas exchange applicable to varying inspired oxygen concentrations. *Am Rev Respir Dis* 1974; **109**: 142–5.

19 Murray JF, Matthay MA, Luce JM, Flick MR. An expanded definition of the adult respiratory distress syndrome. *Am Rev Respir Dis* 1988; **138**: 720–23.

20 Henderson LJ. The theory of neutrality regulation in the animal organism. *Am J Physiol* 1908; **21**: 427–48.

21 Campbell EJM. RIpH. *Lancet* 1962; **1**: 681–3.

22 Javaheri S, Kazemi H. Metabolic alkalosis and hypoventilation in humans. *Am Rev Respir Dis* 1987; **136**: 1011–15.

23 Gabow PA, Kaehny WD, Fennessey PV, *et al.* Diagnostic importance of an increased serum anion gap. *N Engl J Med* 1980; **303**: 854–8.

24 Davenport HW. *ABC of Acid–Base Chemistry*, 6th edn, University of Chicago Press, Chicago, IL, 1974.

25 Brackett NC, Cohen JJ, Schwartz WB. Carbon dioxide titration curve of normal man. *N Engl J Med* 1965; **272**: 6–12.

26 Flenley DC. Another non-logarithmic acid–base diagram? *Lancet* 1971; **1**, 961–5.

27 Cohen JJ, Schwarz WB. Evaluation of acid–base equilibrium in pulmonary insufficiency. *Am J Med* 1966; **41**: 163–7.

28 Arbus GS, Hebert JA, Levesque PR, *et al.* Characterisation and applications of the 'significance band' for acute respiratory alkalosis. *N Engl J Med* 1969; **280**: 117–23.

29 Brackett NC, Wingo CF, Muren O, Solano JT. Acid–base response to chronic hypercapnia in man. *N Engl J Med* 1969; **280**: 124–30.

30 Grimbert R, Raynaert M, Perret C. Acid–base response to chronic hypocapnia in man. *Bull Eur Physiopath Respir* 1977; **13**: 659–67.

31 Bone JM, Cowie J, Lambie AT, Robson JS. The relationship between arterial P_{CO_2} and hydrogen ion concentration in chronic metabolic acidosis and alkalosis. *Clin Sci* 1974; **46**: 113–23.

32 Verdon F, van Melle G, Perret C. Respiratory response to acute metabolic acidosis. *Bull Eur Physiopath Respir* 1981; **17**: 223–35.

33 Jeffrey AA, Warren PM, Flenley DC. Acute hypercapnic respiratory failure in patients with chronic obstructive lung disease: risk factors and use of guidelines for management. *Thorax* 1992; **47**: 34–40.

34 Stewart PA. Modern quantitative acid–base chemistry. *Can J Physiol Pharmacol* 1983; **61**: 1444–61.

35 Fencl V, Leith DE. Stewart's quantitative acid–base chemistry: applications in biology and medicine. *Respir Physiol* 1993; **91**: 1–16.

36 Jones NL. A quantitative physicochemical approach to acid–base physiology. *Clin Biochem* 1990; **23**: 189–95.

37 Fencl V, Jabor A, Kasda A, Figge A. Diagnosis of metabolic acid–base disturbances in critically ill patients. *Am J Respir Crit Care Med* 2000; **148**: 339–44.

38 Constable PD. Hyperchloraemic acidosis: the classic example of strong ion acidosis. *Anest Analg* 2003; **96**: 919–22.

39 Alfaro V, Torras R, Ibanez J, Palacios L 1996. A physical-chemical analysis of the acid–base response to chronic obstructive pulmonary disease. *Can J Physiol Pharmacol* 2003; **74**: 1229–35.

5

Tests of Ventilatory Control

In health, ventilation is very closely adjusted to metabolic demands and the ventilatory control system has to compensate rapidly for changes such as the increased metabolism of exercise or a reduction in inspired oxygen partial pressure (e.g. at altitude). Ventilatory control is modified in many conditions and it can also be influenced by several drugs. The 'metabolic' or reflex system of respiratory control includes receptors that respond to mechanical or chemical stimuli; a central controller with an inherent rhythmicity and output, which are modulated by sensory information; a neural pathway comprising afferent nerves, the brainstem, spinal cord, and intercostal and phrenic nerves; and an effector 'organ', the respiratory muscles. The efficiency of the respiratory muscles in adjusting ventilation to meet metabolic requirements is in turn dependent on the mechanical and gas-exchanging properties of the lungs.

The 'respiratory centres' in the brainstem are inaccessible and therefore much of our knowledge of central respiratory control has been inferred from studies in animals. The extent to which these are relevant to respiratory control in intact humans is sometimes open to doubt. Conventional clinical measurements usually assess the integrity of the whole respiratory control pathway including receptors, neural connections and end-organ response; consequently abnormalities of the control of ventilation may be difficult to localize. In recent years, traditional tests of ventilatory responsiveness to carbon dioxide and hypoxia have been supplemented by newer techniques offering considerable insight into the control pathways in humans and

the various regions of the central nervous system involved. These techniques include use of cortical evoked sensory potentials,[1] transcranial magnetic stimulation,[2] and dynamic imaging of the brain by positron emission tomography[3] and magnetic resonance.[4] Studies, initially done in healthy subjects, are gradually being extended to patients with various diseases, with increasing understanding of the complexities involved, but so far none has become a generally applicable clinical test. As with other aspects of neurological function, a consequence of these studies is the realization that the respiratory control mechanisms exhibit much greater 'plasticity' than appreciated hitherto – i.e. the capacity to develop persistent changes of morphology or function (or both) depending on previous experience.[5] Such adaptations of the respiratory control systems in disease might be considered analogous with, for example, compensatory adjustments of ventilation/perfusion matching or the development of hyperinflation, which in terms of gas exchange and lung mechanics, respectively, can reduce the functional impact of disease.

5.1 NEURAL CONTROL MECHANISMS

Both mechano- and chemoreceptors send information to the brainstem respiratory neurons, providing a negative feedback system that adjusts breathing in response to changing conditions. Receptors that respond to mechanical stimuli are located in several sites, including the airways (stretch and irritant receptors), adjacent to the alveoli (J-receptors) and the chest wall (tendon organs and muscle spindles). The pattern of breathing adopted by patients with abnormal respiratory mechanics is determined by information sensed by these receptors and transmitted via afferent nerves, in particular the vagus nerve but also the glossopharyngeal, phrenic and intercostal nerves. The effects of varying afferent information on breathing pattern can be simulated using artificial resistive or elastic loads, but in practice no direct clinical tests of the neural afferents regulating ventilation are available. The only situation where stimulation of such receptors is open to clinical study is in the investigation of the cough reflex by assessing the tussive response to inhalation of irritant agents such as citric acid.[6]

Various respiratory centres – e.g. inspiratory, expiratory, apneustic, pneumotaxic – have been described in animals, usually by observing the pattern of breathing as the brainstem is stimulated or sectioned at various levels. In recent years, most attention has been focused on a group of neurons in the ventrolateral medulla, known as the pre-Bötzinger complex. These appear to have a critical role as the rhythm generator or 'pacemaker' for regular tidal breathing, although other groups of neurons may also be involved.[7]

In humans, information on the control pathways has been synthesized from various 'natural experiments' in which isolated pathological lesions in specific sites have been correlated with particular abnormalities of breathing. Some of these are discussed in Chapter 20, Section 20.1.1 in relation to the effects of neurological diseases. From these and other studies, Plum inferred two separate pathways of ventilatory control (Fig. 5.1).[8] The 'metabolic', unconscious or automatic pathway of motor control originates from the rhythm generator in the brainstem and its descending efferent connections to the spinal motor neurons via bulbospinal pathways in the ventrolateral spinal cord. A second, 'behavioural', motor pathway controls breathing during voluntary acts, including speech, breath-holding and voluntary deep breathing (and therefore during performance of most conventional respiratory function tests). This motor pathway originates in the cerebral

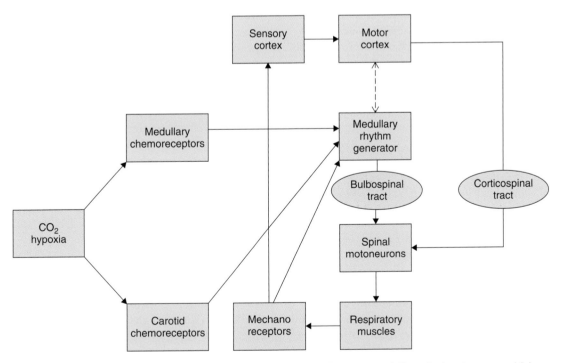

Figure 5.1 Simplified schematic representation of pathways of ventilatory control. The spinal motoneurons driving the respiratory muscles are controlled by both the automatic (metabolic) pathway originating in the medulla and the voluntary (behavioural) pathway originating in the cerebral cortex.

cortex, traverses the reticular formation and descends via the corticospinal tracts in the dorsolateral columns of the spinal cord. The behavioural and metabolic spinal motor pathways are thus distinct; whether they connect above the spinal motor neurons is uncertain.[9] Their separate locations have important implications for neurosurgeons involved in spinal cord surgery, and interruption of each produces very different effects. For example, during slow-wave (deep) sleep (SWS), ventilation is dependent primarily on the metabolic control system; breathing during SWS may be grossly disturbed if this pathway is damaged, even though during wakefulness behavioural control may compensate sufficiently to maintain adequate ventilation. Alternatively, if metabolic control is intact but the behavioural pathway is interrupted, the subject has a monotonously regular breathing pattern, which he or she is unable to modify ('locked-in syndrome' – see Chapter 20, Section 20.1.3).

Tests of the chemical control of breathing (see below) are often assumed to assess medullary function, i.e. 'metabolic' control, but by the very nature of the unnatural breathing manoeuvres and apparatus imposed on the subjects, it is likely that important behavioural influences are introduced. For the optimal study of automatic or metabolic control, behavioural influences need to be kept to a minimum; this may be best achieved by measurements of resting tidal ventilation without a mouthpiece, especially during SWS[10] (see Chapter 6, Section 6.2.2).

5.2 CHEMICAL CONTROL OF BREATHING

Ventilation is exquisitely sensitive to increasing P_{CO_2} and rather less so to decreasing P_{O_2}. Carbon dioxide produces its effect mainly by increasing the acidity of the cerebrospinal fluid (CSF), which stimulates chemoreceptors in the brainstem. There is probably also a direct stimulant effect of CO_2 itself.[11] Chemosensitive neurons are found in many areas in the brainstem, and the relative importance of surface and deeper receptor cells remains in doubt.[12] The peripheral chemoreceptors are also stimulated by CO_2, accounting for about one-third of the ventilatory response.[13]

The stimulant effect of hypoxaemia is mediated mainly by the chemoreceptors in the carotid and aortic bodies and their afferent neural connections. The ventilatory response to hypoxia is, however, complex as it depends on the pattern, intensity and time course of exposure.[14] The initial stimulant effect is followed by a reduced response, which, with sustained hypoxia over several days, blends with longer-term acclimatization. In the latter situation hypocapnia resulting from the initial hyperventilation has a counter-effect, but some acclimatization to hypoxia occurs even under isocapnic conditions.

5.2.1 Ventilatory response to carbon dioxide

The traditional method of testing the integrity of the ventilatory response to CO_2 is by measuring ventilation as the subject breathes an increased CO_2 concentration. This can be achieved in a steady state while breathing gas mixtures containing different concentrations of CO_2,[15] or, more commonly in clinical practice, the continually increasing ventilation is measured while the subject rebreathes a gas mixture containing CO_2.[16]

To assess the effects of CO_2 alone, it is important to prevent hypoxia, which, via the peripheral chemoreceptors, has a synergistic effect. With the rebreathing technique this is achieved by starting with a hyperoxic mixture, e.g. 5 per cent CO_2 and 95 per cent O_2. Ventilation is conveniently measured by enclosing the rebreathing bag in a rigid box or bottle, with a port to which a one-way valve and pneumotachograph/integrator or gas meter are attached. Carbon dioxide is sampled continuously at the mouth and the end tidal P_{CO_2} is usually used as an index of the stimulus. Ventilation and P_{CO_2} are then plotted every quarter- or half-minute. The relationship is usually rectilinear (Fig. 5.2) and is classically described in terms of its slope (S) and the intercept on the P_{CO_2} axis (B), which have been equated with the 'sensitivity' and 'threshold' of the control system respectively. Under normal conditions the rebreathing and steady-state techniques give similar slopes but the rebreathing response is shifted to the right, i.e. the intercept is higher, by 6–8 mmHg.[16,17] The difference is attributed to the delay in transit of CO_2 from the alveolar air to the central chemoreceptors in the brain.

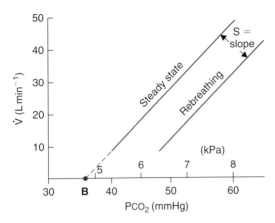

Figure 5.2 Schematic ventilatory responses to carbon dioxide (CO_2) measured by steady-state and rebreathing techniques. Classically the response is described in terms of its slope (S) and intercept at zero ventilation on the PCO_2 axis (B). In normal subjects the two techniques produce similar slopes but the rebreathing response has a higher intercept.

In healthy subjects the ventilatory response to CO_2 can be altered by inducing changes in acid–base status. A metabolic acidosis shifts the response line to the left, i.e. ventilation for a give PCO_2 is increased,[18] whereas respiratory acidosis[19] or metabolic alkalosis[20] has the converse effect, i.e. ventilation for a given PCO_2 is less than normal. With the steady-state CO_2 response the difference is due mainly to a shift in the intercept value, but there may also be a slightly greater slope in metabolic acidosis[17] and a reduction in slope in metabolic alkalosis, especially if the resting $PaCO_2$ is elevated.[20] With the rebreathing CO_2 response, metabolic acidosis and alkalosis can produce changes in both slope[17] and intercept.[21]

In clinical practice, when hypercapnia accompanies a reduced ventilatory response to CO_2, it may be impossible to determine which is cause and which effect. It could reasonably be argued that a low central sensitivity to CO_2 predisposes to CO_2 retention. On the other hand, since:

$$[H^+] = 24 \frac{PCO_2}{[HCO_3{}^-]} \qquad (5.1)$$

a given rise in PCO_2 will result in a smaller rise in $[H^+]$ if the $[HCO_3{}^-]$ is already high. Since local $[H^+]$ is the main stimulus to the medullary chemoreceptors, a smaller rise in ventilation would

be expected. Consequently, the slope of the ventilatory response to CO_2 varies inversely with the arterial bicarbonate concentration,[22] so that some reduction is virtually inevitable in patients with chronic hypercapnia. In addition, many patients with hypercapnia have disordered respiratory mechanics, which will impair the ventilatory response to stimulation even further. The main clinical role of measuring the ventilatory response to CO_2 is in recognition of abnormal ventilatory control insufficient to cause a persistent rise in resting $PaCO_2$ in patients with relatively normal mechanical respiratory function.

5.2.2 Ventilatory response to hypoxia

In general, the short-term ventilatory responses to hypercapnia and hypoxia are multiplicative. This synergism can be utilized to assess the response to hypoxia by comparing the steady-state responses of ventilation to CO_2 at widely differing values of alveolar PO_2, such as 200 mmHg and 40 mmHg.[23] More commonly the inspired PO_2 is lowered gradually by the addition of nitrogen[24] or by rebreathing;[25] in both techniques P_ACO_2 is monitored continuously and maintained constant. In healthy subjects the stimulus can be represented by the alveolar (end tidal) PO_2, but in patients (especially those with airway obstruction) this is a poor guide to the arterial PO_2 and continuous monitoring of arterial oxygen saturation by oximetry is preferable.

The ventilatory response to PO_2 under isocapnic conditions has the form of a rectangular hyperbola (Fig. 5.3a). Weil et al. described it by the relationship:[24]

$$\dot{V}_E = \dot{V}_{EO} + \frac{A}{P_AO_2 - 32} \qquad (5.2)$$

where $\dot{V}_{EO}$ is the asymptote of ventilation at infinite PO_2 and the parameter A is a shape factor used to characterize the magnitude of the ventilatory response; the larger the value of A, the greater the response. Alternatively, ventilation can be plotted against the reciprocal of P_AO_2 to approximate a straight line. The relation between ventilation and P_AO_2 resembles the mirror image of the oxygen dissociation curve with inflection points at similar values of PO_2, so that plotting $\dot{V}_E$ against oxygen saturation instead of PO_2 gives a linear relationship

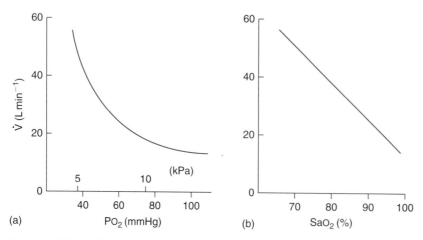

Figure 5.3 (a) Ventilatory response to Pao$_2$ showing hyperbolic shape. (b) If ventilation is plotted against arterial oxygen saturation, the relation approximates a straight line.

(Fig. 5.3b). This is convenient in practice as measurements of Sao$_2$ are available directly from an oximeter.[25] The linear relationship is a consequence of the shape of the relationship between oxygen consumption and oxygen delivery at the receptor site. The actual stimulus to the chemoreceptors is Po$_2$ rather than oxygen content or saturation.[14]

The rebreathing ventilatory response to progressive hypoxia is sufficiently reproducible for use as a clinical test.[26] It has, for example, been used to demonstrate the relatively specific action of the respiratory stimulant drug almitrine on the peripheral chemoreceptors.[27]

An alternative approach for assessing function of the peripheral chemoreceptors is to examine the transient response of ventilation to changes in inspired Po$_2$. This can be done by measuring the reduction of ventilation that occurs after removal of any resting hypoxic stimulus by the subject taking a few breaths of oxygen,[28] or by measuring the increase of ventilation after a single vital capacity[23] or a few tidal breaths[29] of an anoxic mixture. In each case a transient change in ventilation is seen within two or three breaths, with the short latency implying an effect via the peripheral chemoreceptors. Transient responses to hypoxaemia correlate with steady-state or rebreathing responses in most subjects, but occasionally their use reveals individuals in whom a disproportionately large transient response indicates a high hypoxic sensitivity that is obscured by a central depressant effect of hypoxia.[23,26] Such tests are poorly standardized

for clinical purposes, and in patients with airway obstruction and hyperinflation the results are inevitably affected by poor alveolar gas mixing.

5.3 OTHER WAYS OF EVALUATING RESPIRATORY CENTRE OUTPUT

For assessing the chemical control of ventilation in normal subjects, the minute ventilation is a reasonably reliable index of the output from the respiratory centres, but in disease it has serious disadvantages. If the effector system (chest wall, lungs or airways) is deranged, its efficiency is reduced and a given stimulus emanating from the central rhythm generator is likely to evoke a subnormal response in terms of ventilation.[30] Alternatively, a normal ventilatory response in such circumstances is likely to imply a respiratory centre output that is greater than normal. It is therefore sometimes desirable to measure the response at a more proximal point in the effector pathway (Fig. 5.4). Electrical activity in the phrenic nerves has been used in animals but is impracticable as a quantitative index in humans; the diaphragmatic electromyelogram (EMG) is used in research[31] but is not generally available as a clinical test. The work of breathing, calculated from measurements of oxygen consumption[32] or from pressure–volume studies,[33] has been used productively in detailed analysis of mechanical disorders but it is inconvenient and tedious. More frequently used is measurement of

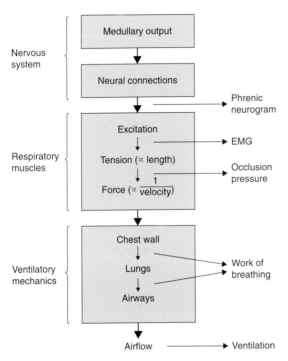

Figure 5.4 Indices of respiratory drive obtained at different levels in the effector pathway. Each index is potentially affected by abnormalities at any of the preceding levels. Ventilation, which is the most convenient measurement, is the least specific.

EMG, electromyelogram.

the pressure developed isometrically at the start of inspiration.[34–36] The principle is that mouth (i.e. alveolar) pressure during a transient occlusion at the start of inspiration gives an index of respiratory 'drive' that might be expected to be independent of lung and airway mechanics. In theory, it should not matter whether the airways are narrow or the lungs are stiff, as no air flows during this short period of occlusion. The index used most commonly is the mouth occlusion pressure ($P_{0.1}$) developed 0.1 s after the onset of inspiration.[34] This period of occlusion is sufficiently short for it to be over before the subject can sense or react to it. The measurement can be made during either tidal or stimulated breathing. In general, in the face of adverse respiratory mechanics a greater pressure, reflected as an increased $P_{0.1}$, is required to maintain normal ventilation. On average, values of $P_{0.1}$ at rest are greater than normal in patients with either increased airway resistance or reduced pulmonary compliance, but there is considerable overlap with healthy

subjects.[35] However, reduced $P_{0.1}$ responses to CO_2 are seen not only with impaired central respiratory drive but also in some subjects with airway obstruction and pulmonary hyperinflation (see Chapter 9, Section 9.9) or with chronic weakness of the respiratory muscles (see Chapter 20, Section 20.2.1.6). In the acute situation of patients receiving assisted ventilation, abnormally high $P_{0.1}$ values have been shown to predict failure to wean, as such a finding implies a high mechanical load.[37]

$P_{0.1}$ can also be measured during stimulation with CO_2 or hypoxia by measurement at intervals during a conventional rebreathing procedure; instead of ventilation, $P_{0.1}$ is plotted against the stimulus. Originally it was suggested that the relation of $P_{0.1}$ to P_ACO_2 during rebreathing was best described by a logarithmic function,[34] but other authors found a linear plot adequate.[38] In principle (Fig. 5.5) this technique should help to distinguish a reduction in the ventilatory response to CO_2 due to abnormal peripheral mechanics (where $P_{0.1}$ versus PCO_2 would be normal) from a low ventilatory response due to central insensitivity to CO_2 (where $P_{0.1}$ versus PCO_2 would be reduced). However, in patients with airway obstruction similar reservations apply as with measurements at rest. First, due to delayed equilibration of pressures, $P_{0.1}$ measured at the mouth does not accurately reflect pressure within the lungs in patients with severe airway narrowing.[39] Second, inspiratory muscle efficiency is impaired by severe hyperinflation so that $P_{0.1}$ as an index of 'neuromuscular drive' should ideally be interpreted in relation to the capacity of the inspiratory muscles at an equivalent absolute lung volume.[40] Third, if, as commonly occurs in airway obstruction, the end expiratory volume increases further (dynamic hyperinflation) during rebreathing, this is likely also to influence the $P_{0.1}$, as the pressure recorded then reflects a combination of active inspiratory muscle contraction and passive recoil of the respiratory system (see Chapter 9, Section 9.9).

Because of these difficulties of interpretation and because of a desire to assess respiratory control at its most 'physiological' and with least interference from behavioural influences, the emphasis has shifted away from stimulation by hypercapnia and hypoxaemia to a more detailed analysis of resting breathing. Milic Emili pointed out that ventilation can be analysed not only in terms of its classical

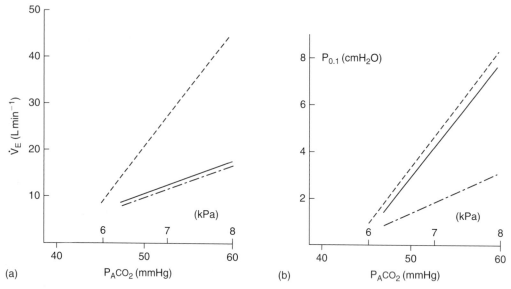

Figure 5.5 Theoretical use of mouth occlusion pressure to distinguish reduced ventilatory responses to carbon dioxide (CO_2) caused by abnormal lung mechanics (solid line) and impaired central drive (dashed/dotted line). (a) If ventilation is plotted against CO_2 these are indistinguishable and in both cases the response is reduced below the normal (dashed line). (b). If $P_{0.1}$ is plotted against $P_A CO_2$ the subject with abnormal pulmonary mechanics shows a normal response, but if central drive is impaired the $P_{0.1}$ is reduced.

components, tidal volume (V_T) and breathing frequency (f), but also in relation to the duration of inspiration (T_I) and the mean inspiratory flow (V_T/T_I):[41]

$$\dot{V} = V_T \times f = \frac{V_T}{T_I} \times \frac{T_I}{T_{TOT}} \times 60 \, \text{L min}^{-1}$$

$$(5.3)$$

where T_{TOT} is the average duration of each breath ($60/f$ s.). The variable T_I/T_{TOT}, i.e. the proportion of each breath spent on inspiration, is termed the 'inspiratory duty ratio' and the terms V_T/T_I and T_I/T_{TOT} have been interpreted as 'drive' and 'timing' components of ventilation, which to some extent are controlled independently. It should, however, be noted that the 'drive' indicated by V_T/T_I is still dependent also on pulmonary mechanics.

REFERENCES

1 Zifko UA, Young BG, Remtulla H, Bolton CF. Somatosensory evoked potentials of the phrenic nerve. *Muscle Nerve* 1995; **18**: 1487–9.

2 Similowski T, Straus C, Coic L, Derenne JP. Facilitation-independent response of the diaphragm to cortical magnetic stimulation in conscious man. *Am J Respir Crit Care Med* 1996; **154**: 1771–7.

3 Corfield DR, Fink GR, Ramsay SC, *et al.* Evidence for limbic system activation during CO_2-stimulated breathing in man. *J Physiol* 1995; **488**: 77–84.

4 Evans KC, Shea SA, Saykin AJ. Functional MRI localisation of central nervous system regions associated with volitional inspiration in humans. *J Physiol* 1999; **520**: 383–92.

5 Mitchell GS, Johnson SM. Neuroplasticity in respiratory motor control. *J Appl Physiol* 2003; **94**: 358–74.

6 Fuller RW, Jackson DW. Physiology and treatment of cough. *Thorax* 1990; **45**: 425–30.

7 Feldman JL, Del Negro CA. Looking for inspiration: new perspectives on respiratory rhythm. *Nat Rev Neurosci* 2006; **7**: 232–42.

8 Plum F. Neurological integration of behavioural and metabolic control of breathing, in *Breathing: Hering–Breuer Centenary Symposium* (ed. R. Porter), Churchill, London, 1970, pp. 159–81.

9 Guz A. Brain, breathing and breathlessness. *Respir Physiol* 1997; **109**: 197–204.

10 Phillipson EA, Bowes G. Control of breathing during sleep, in *Handbook of Physiology: The Respiratory System* (eds Cherniack NS and Widdicombe JG), American Physiological Society, Bethesda, MD, 1986, pp. 649–89.

11 Millhorn DE, Eldridge FL. Role of ventrolateral medulla in regulation of respiratory and cardiovascular systems. *J Appl Physiol* 1986; **61**: 1249–63.

12 Remmers JE. A century of control of breathing. *Am J Respir Crit Care Med* 2005; **172**: 6–11.

13 Bellville JW, Whipp BJ, Kaufman RD. Central and peripheral chemoreflex loop gain in normal and carotid body-resected subjects. *J Appl Physiol* 1979; **46**: 843–53.

14 Powell FL, Milsom WK, Mitchell GS. Time domains of the hypoxic ventilatory response. *Respir Physiol* 1998; **112**: 123–34.

15 Cunningham DJC, Cormack RS, O'Riordan JLH, *et al*. An arrangement for studying the respiratory effects in man of various factors. *Q J Exp Physiol* 1975; **42**: 294–303.

16 Read DJC. A clinical method for assessing the ventilatory response to CO_2. *Australas Ann Med* 1976; **16**: 20–32.

17 Linton RAF, Poole-Wilson PA, Davies RJ, Cameron IR. A comparison of the ventilatory response to carbon dioxide by steady-state and rebreathing methods during metabolic acidosis and alkalosis. *Clin Sci* 1973; **45**: 239–49.

18 Cunningham DJC, Shaw DG, Lahiri S, Lloyd BB. The effect of maintained ammonium chloride acidosis on the relation between pulmonary ventilation and alveolar oxygen and carbon dioxide in man. *Q J Exp Physiol* 1961; **46**: 323–34.

19 Falchuk KH, Lamb TW, Tenney SM. Ventilatory response to hypoxia and CO_2 following CO_2 exposure and $NaHCO_3$ ingestion. *J Appl Physiol* 1996; **21**: 393–8.

20 Goldring RM, Cannon PJ, Heinemann HO, Fishman AP. Respiratory adjustment to chronic metabolic alkalosis in man. *J Clin Invest* 1968; **47**: 188–202.

21 Oren A, Whipp BJ, Wasserman K. Effects of chronic acid–base changes on the rebreathing hypercapnic ventilatory response in man. *Respiration* 1991; **58**: 181–5.

22 Heinemann HO, Goldring RM. Bicarbonate and the regulation of ventilation. *Am J Med* 1974; **57**: 361–70.

23 Kronenberg R, Hamilton RN, Gabel R, *et al*. Comparison of three methods for quantitating respiratory response to hypoxia in man. *Respir Physiol* 1972; **16**: 109–25.

24 Weil JV, Byrne-Quinn E, Sodal IE, *et al*. Hypoxic ventilatory drive in normal man. *J Clin Invest* 1970; **49**: 1061–72.

25 Rebuck AS, Campbell EJM. A clinical method for assessing the ventilatory response to hypoxia. *Am Rev Respir Dis* 1974; **109**: 345–50.

26 Shaw RA, Schonfeld SA, Whitcomb ME. Progressive and transient hypoxic ventilatory drive tests in healthy subjects. *Am Rev Respir Dis* 1982; **126**: 37–40.

27 Stradling JR, Barnes P, Pride NB. The effects of almitrine on the ventilatory response to hypoxia and hypercapnia in normal subjects. *Clin Sci* 1982; **63**: 401–4.

28 Dejours A. Control of respiration by arterial chemoreceptors. *Ann NY Acad Sci* 1963; **109**: 682–95.

29 Edelman NH, Epstein PE, Lahiri S, *et al*. Ventilatory response to transient hypoxia and hypercapnia in man. *Respir Physiol* 1973; **17**: 302–14.

30 Cherniack RM, Snidal DP. The effect of obstruction to breathing on the ventilatory response to CO_2. *J Clin Invest* 1956; **35**: 1286–90.

31 Luo YM, Hart N, Mustafa N, *et al*. Effect of diaphragm fatigue on neural respiratory drive. *J Appl Physiol* 2001; **90**: 1691–9.

32 Brodovsky D, Macdonell JA, Cherniack RM. The respiratory response to carbon dioxide in health and in emphysema. *J Clin Invest* 1960; **39**: 724–9.

33 Milic Emili J, Tyler JM. Relation between work output of respiratory muscles and end tidal CO_2 tension. *J Appl Physiol* 1963; **18**: 497–504.

34 Whitelaw WA, Derenne J-P, Milic Emili J. Occlusion pressure as a measure of respiratory centre output in conscious man. *Respir Physiol* 1975; **23**: 181–99.

35 Scott GC, Burki NK. The relationship of resting ventilation to mouth occlusion pressure: an index of resting respiratory function. *Chest* 1990; **98**: 900–906.

36 Whitelaw WA, Derenne J-P. Airway occlusion pressure. *J Appl Physiol* 1993; **74**: 1475–83.

37 Herrara M, Blasco J, Venegas J, *et al*. Mouth occlusion pressure ($P_{0.1}$) in acute respiratory failure. *Int Care Med* 1985; **11**: 134–9.

38 Cherniack NS, Lederer DH, Altose MD. Occlusion pressure as a technique in evaluating respiratory control. *Chest* 1978; **70** (suppl.): 137–41.

39 Marazzini L, Cavestri R, Gori D, *et al*. Difference between mouth and oesophageal occlusion pressure during CO_2 rebreathing in chronic obstructive pulmonary disease. *Am Rev Respir Dis* 1978; **118**: 1027–33.

40 Gribbin HR, Gardiner IT, Heinz GJ, *et al*. The role of impaired inspiratory muscle function in limiting the ventilatory response to CO_2 in chronic airflow obstruction. *Clin Sci* 1983; **64**: 487–95.

41 Milic Emili J. Recent advances in clinical assessment of control of breathing. *Lung* 1982; **160**: 1–17.

6

Respiratory Measurements During Sleep

Measurements of respiratory function during sleep have increased dramatically in the past 25 years, the main driver being the belated recognition of the obstructive sleep apnoea syndrome as a major health problem. Over the same period advances in technology have encouraged wide availability of appropriate equipment, in particular simple and reliable oximeters to measure oxygen saturation and more refined methods for measuring flow and volume changes. Several compact portable recording systems for continuous monitoring overnight are now available. Unlike the situation in the conscious subject, during sleep meaningful direct measurements of resting ventilation and breathing pattern are readily made.

Traditionally, sleep studies were performed in hospital and involved the recording of numerous signals, including several channels of electroencephalography (EEG), electro-oculography (EOG) and electromyography (EMG). For many, detailed polysomnography (PSG) under supervision overnight in hospital remains the gold standard for investigation of possible sleep apnoea,[1] but the practicalities of cost and access for the large number of patients requiring investigation have driven the development of limited recording systems (sometimes known as respiratory polysomnography) that omit neurophysiological recording signals. These are increasingly used for domiciliary recording, which, in practice, is sufficient in the majority of patients with suspected sleep apnoea. More detailed investigation using traditional polysomnography is required for some patients, particularly those with comorbidity such as chronic airway disease or neuromuscular disease, as well as for the recognition and investigation of other sleep disorders that may enter the differential diagnosis.

6.1 NORMAL SLEEP STRUCTURE

A major advance in understanding sleep was the recognition of its considerable neurophysiological heterogeneity. Electrophysiological recordings led to the classification of sleep in various stages that depend on the dominant electrical rhythms detected. The universally used system developed by Rechtschaffen and Kales separates sleep into rapid eye movement (REM) and non-REM sleep.[2] In REM sleep the EOG identifies characteristic jerky eye movements, the EEG shows low-amplitude, mixed-frequency waves, and EMG recordings from peripheral muscles show intermittent suppression of activity. Non-REM sleep is divided into four stages of increasing depth, again characterized by signals of particular frequencies on the EEG (Table 6.1). Stages I and II are sometimes considered together as light sleep, and stages III and IV as deep or slow-wave sleep (SWS) because of the increasing dominance of low-frequency, high-amplitude waves. Classically, sleep is staged in 'epochs' of 30 s, with the dominant wave-forms in each epoch dictating the classification, but inevitably the distinction is sometimes somewhat arbitrary.

Table 6.1 Electrophysiological classification of sleep stages

Stage	EEG	EOG	EMG
Relaxed wakefulness	Alpha rhythm, 8–13 Hz	Variable, voluntary, blinking	Variable, high tonic activity
Non-REM sleep			
I	Mixed frequency, low amplitude	Rolling movements	Decreasing tonic activity
II	As I, plus high-amplitude K complexes and sleep spindles	Fewer movements	Decreasing tonic activity
III	High amplitude, low frequency, delta waves <50%	Picks up EEG	Little activity
IV	Delta waves >50%	Picks up EEG	Little activity
REM sleep	Mixed frequency, low amplitude	Jerky movements in phasic REM	Low tonic activity, phasic twitches

EEG, electroencephalography; EMG, electromyography; EOG, electro-oculography; REM, rapid eye movement.

REM sleep itself shows two distinct patterns, with the rapid eye movements clustered in brief periods ('phasic REM') interspersed with relative quiescence of eye movements ('tonic REM'). The characteristic REM-related suppression of muscle activity, which includes suppression of most respiratory muscles, occurs in phasic REM (see below).

In normal adults, sleep starts with gradually deepening non-REM sleep and periods of SWS tend to occur mostly in the earlier part of the night. The first period of REM sleep appears typically after 1–2 h, with subsequent REM epochs approximately every 90 min. Each period of REM sleep lasts for 15–30 min, with the duration tending to lengthen later in the night.

6.2   BREATHING DURING SLEEP

Overall, sleep is accompanied by a modest reduction in ventilation[3,4] and a small increase in $PaCO_2$ of between 2 mmHg and 8 mmHg.[4,5] There is a similar fall in average PaO_2, which corresponds to a reduction in oxygen saturation of about 2 per cent.[6] There is also an overall reduction in metabolism, with falls in oxygen consumption and CO_2 production of about 10 per cent compared with the resting awake state.[7] Clearly, however, in view of the rise in $PaCO_2$, the reduction in ventilation is proportionally greater than the reduction in CO_2 production, highlighting the important differences between respiratory control awake and asleep (see below). There is a small reduction in functional residual capacity (FRC)[8] and an important increase in the resistance of the

supraglottic airway associated with less tone in the muscles that support it.[9,10] The sleep-related fall in ventilation and rise in $PaCO_2$ occur independently of the increase in upper airway resistance, as they are seen also in subjects breathing via a tracheal stoma, which bypasses the area of narrowing.[11] The pattern of tidal breathing shows some variation, with waxing and waning ('periodic breathing'), particularly at the onset of sleep. This pattern, which results from instability of respiratory control, is exaggerated by hypoxia and consequently is particularly apparent at altitude.

6.2.1   Control of breathing during sleep

During wakefulness, breathing is modulated by various afferent signals from chemoreceptors and mechanoreceptors and is also influenced by the activity of the brain above the medulla (see Chapter 5, Section 5.1). During sleep, supramedullary influences are reduced or absent and the main afferent input is from the chemoreceptors, with the ventilatory output determined by the associated reflex mechanisms. Respiratory control then depends on a negative feedback system, with any changes in ventilation resulting in a signal (changes in blood gases and acidity in the vicinity of the chemoreceptors) that tends to correct that change and restore stability. Overall, the conventional ventilatory responses to both CO_2 and hypoxia are reduced in sleep compared with in the awake state.[12]

Importantly, during sleep the influence of alertness, or the 'wakefulness drive', which exerts a stabilizing influence, is lost and consequently any

Table 6.2 Factors potentially destabilizing breathing during sleep in different situations

	Normal subjects – sea level	Normal subjects – altitude	Cardiac failure
Hypoventilation/higher $PaCO_2$ (↑ 'plant gain')	+		
Loss of wakefulness drive	+	+	+
Self-perpetuation (underdamping)	+	+	+
Hypoxia		+	±
↑ ventilatory response to CO_2 (↑ 'controller gain')		+	+
Prolonged circulation time			+
Metabolic alkalosis			±

+, relevant; ± sometimes relevant.

perturbations of the controlling loop lead more readily to unstable breathing.[13] Breathing is further destabilized if the afferent information changes rapidly or if there is a delay in registering and responding to the stimulus (Table 6.2).[12] If this happens the control system tends to overcompensate or 'overshoot', resulting in periodic breathing with hyperpnoea alternating with hypopnoea or apnoea.

The sequence of events can be modelled by examining the relationships between alveolar ventilation and $PaCO_2$. Since these are inversely proportional to each other (see Chapter 2, Section 2.3.4), their relationship for a given CO_2 output is represented by a hyperbola (the 'isometabolic line'), as illustrated in Fig. 6.1. If ventilation is determined by the responsiveness of the respiratory chemoreceptors to $PaCO_2$, then the prevailing value ('set point') is set by the intersection of the ventilatory response and isometabolic lines (point 1 in Fig. 6.1). If $PaCO_2$ were to be transiently reduced (e.g. by assisted ventilation), ventilation would diminish, as determined by the ventilatory response line, until, in principle, a $PaCO_2$ would be reached at which apnoea occurred (the apnoeic threshold). This hypocapnia-induced apnoea threshold is, however, highly dependent on the sleep–wake state, being very sensitive and reproducible in non-REM sleep but more variable in REM sleep and often absent in wakefulness.[14] The absence of a detectable apnoea threshold when awake is due the 'wakefulness drive', which helps to maintain the stability of breathing; it is depicted in Fig. 6.1 by the horizontal line, which defines the consequent minimum awake ventilation.[15] When an individual falls asleep, responsiveness to CO_2 is diminished and the ventilatory response line shifts to the right, with the potential apnoeic threshold now revealed by loss of the wakefulness drive. Ignoring any change in CO_2

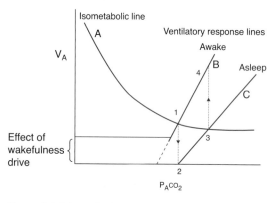

Figure 6.1 Schematic diagram of factors influencing ventilation awake and at sleep onset. For a given carbon dioxide (CO_2) output, the relation of ventilation (shown here as alveolar ventilation, V_A) to PCO_2 is hyperbolic (isometabolic line A). The awake ventilatory response line (B) intersects line A at the 'set point' (1), which determines the prevailing PCO_2. The horizontal extension of line B represents the 'wakefulness drive' that prevents ventilation falling to zero when the subject is awake (i.e. there is no apnoeic threshold awake). With sleep onset the ventilatory response line moves to the right (line C) and the wakefulness drive is lost, exposing an apnoeic threshold; potentially the subject then becomes apnoeic (point 2) until CO_2 accumulates sufficiently to establish a new stable set point (3). If the subject then awakens, the higher PCO_2 stimulates increased ventilation until PCO_2 falls to point 1. Repeated arousal will tend to perpetuate the ventilatory instability. Modified from ref.15.

output, the set point then moves to the right, at a higher $PaCO_2$ and lower V_A than when awake (point 3 in Fig. 6.1). At the higher $PaCO_2$ the hyperbolic isometabolic line decrees that a given change in ventilation will produce a bigger change in $PaCO_2$, i.e. the responsiveness of the arterial blood gases to changes in ventilation is greater. In control system theory this phenomenon is known as an increase in 'plant gain',

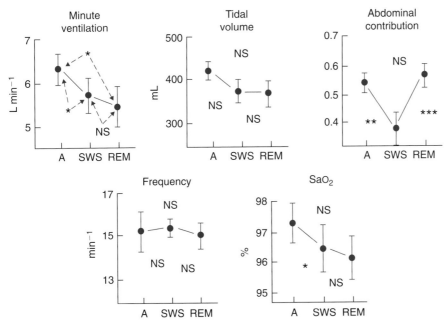

Figure 6.2 Effect of sleep state on ventilation and its subdivisions and on arterial oxygen saturation in six normal subjects. Values are mean ± SEM. Redrawn from: Stradling JR *et al.* Changes in ventilation and its components in normal subjects during sleep. *Thorax* 1985; **40**: 364–70, with permission from the BMJ Publishing Group.

*$P<0.05$; **$P<0.01$; ***$P<0.001$.
A, awake; NS, not significant; REM, rapid-eye-movement sleep; SWS, slow-wave sleep.

while the converse – i.e. the effect of blood gases on ventilation – is known as 'controller gain'. Both contribute to the overall 'loop gain' of the control system.[16] On falling asleep, therefore, an individual may experience brief apnoea (point 2 in Fig. 6.1) until sufficient CO_2 accumulates to move him or her to the new set point (point 3 in Fig. 6.1). However, if, as commonly occurs in the early stages of sleep, the individual transiently arouses, the drive to breathe would immediately increase again, resulting in increased ventilation (point 4 in Fig. 6.1). In this way the stage is set for periodic breathing to develop at the onset of sleep. The tendency is increased by high ventilatory responsiveness to CO_2, as occurs under hypoxic conditions (e.g. at altitude), and also by prolongation of the circulation time, as occurs in cardiac failure, which lengthens the period between changes in blood gases and their detection by the chemoreceptors. In the latter two situations periodic breathing may persist through the night, itself disrupting sleep with frequent arousals, which then perpetuate the instability. Recurrent arousals may result from either apnoea-related hypoxia or the subsequent ventilatory overshoot. The factors that

potentially can destabilize breathing during sleep are listed in Table 6.2.

6.2.2 Breathing in non-REM sleep

Once sleep is established, and particularly in SWS, ventilation is typically regular but overall is reduced by about 15 per cent compared with the awake state (Fig. 6.2).[4] The reduction is due mainly to a smaller tidal volume with little overall change in breathing frequency. During SWS the pattern of ventilation shows an increase in the relative contribution of ribcage expansion and corresponding decrease in abdominal displacement compared with in the awake state.[4,17] Electromyographic studies in a small number of normal subjects have shown relatively greater activation of the intercostal muscles, but there is also an increase in diaphragmatic activity in some individuals.[17] This greater activation occurs in the face of the overall reduction in ventilation and is probably a response to the increased resistance of the upper airway during sleep. The latter occurs irrespective of posture and is confined to the supraglottic segment of the airway, the resistance of which approximately doubles while that of the remainder of the airway remains fairly constant.[9,10] The higher resistance during sleep is due to an overall decline in the tonic activity of the muscles such as genioglossus that support the upper airway, and there is a corresponding reduction in upper airway dimensions. Another contributory factor may be loss of caudal traction[18] accompanying the reduction in FRC that occurs with sleep onset.[8]

6.2.3 Breathing in REM sleep

The most characteristic feature of breathing during REM sleep is its variability, which probably accounts for the apparently discrepant results of various studies in the literature. Overall, most data suggest lower ventilation than in the awake state.[15] Compared with non-REM sleep, some studies show similar average ventilation, while others suggest a further reduction. Ventilation is most markedly reduced and the pattern of breathing is most irregular in phasic REM sleep. The pattern of activation of the inspiratory muscles, and consequently the distribution of volume change between ribcage and abdomen, is very different in REM sleep compared with non-REM sleep, with a much greater relative displacement of the abdomen,[3,17] a pattern seen most markedly during the final epoch of REM sleep towards the end of the night.[19] It results from inhibition and hypotonia of all muscles apart from the diaphragm. In this respect the non-diaphragmatic muscles during REM sleep behave similarly to postural muscles. The upper airway dilator muscles become similarly hypotonic and the consequent increase in airway compliance contributes to the greater frequency of apnoeas during REM sleep. Even though the electrical activity of the diaphragm may increase, the resulting transdiaphragmatic pressure is less due to impaired efficiency of diaphragmatic contraction in the absence of support from the other inspiratory muscles.[20]

Patients with compromised ventilation from whatever cause are particularly vulnerable during phasic REM sleep when they depend almost exclusively on activation of the diaphragm. This produces a characteristic oximetry pattern of REM-related hypoventilation, which is seen, for example, in patients with severe chronic airway disease, respiratory muscle weakness and skeletal deformities such as scoliosis (Fig. 6.3). The periods of desaturation are typically concentrated in three or four periods during the night corresponding to the epochs of REM sleep. The magnitude of reduction in SaO_2 depends on the baseline (awake) level, as the shape of the oxygen dissociation curve dictates a greater fall for a given reduction of ventilation if the initial level is already low.[24] The level of oxygenation during the REM epochs is not constant, with a typical pattern of reductions for 10–20 s associated with phasic periods of REM sleep and some recovery during the intervening periods of tonic REM (Fig. 6.3).

6.2.4 Sleep–disordered breathing and arousal

Ventilatory stimulation at the point of arousal results in transient hyperventilation mediated by a reflex effect.[25] The arousal response is essentially a defence mechanism that ensures maintenance or re-initiation of ventilation. Both mechanical and chemical stimuli may have a role in provoking arousal. In healthy subjects woken from non-REM sleep by various stimuli, including added resistance, hypoxia and hypercapnia, the magnitude of the inspiratory effort in an individual at the point of arousal is similar irrespective of the nature of the stimulus,[26] suggesting that the effort itself is the final common pathway in the afferent sequence.

6.3 RESPIRATORY MEASUREMENTS DURING SLEEP

Several physiological measurements can be made during sleep, either singly or, more commonly, in various combinations. The choice depends on various factors, including the nature of the problem under investigation, the context in which it is being investigated and the facilities available. The more commonly recorded are discussed individually below. Details of recording the electrophysiological signals of the electroencephalogram (EEG), electro-oculogram (EOG) and electromyogram (EMG) are beyond the scope of this account.

6.3.1 Respiratory effort

Effort can be measured directly by continuous monitoring of the oesophageal pressure using either an oesophageal balloon or a catheter-mounted miniature transducer. This is the most reliable

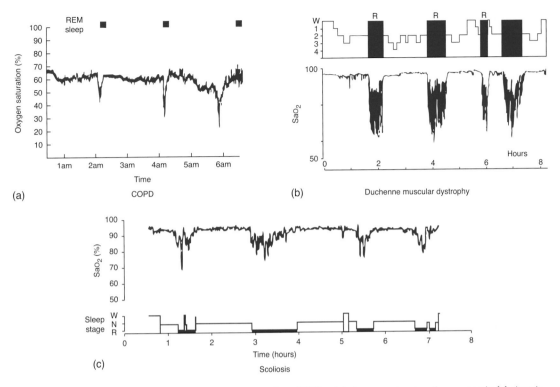

Figure 6.3 Characteristic pattern of rapid-eye-movement sleep (REM)-related oxygen desaturation as seen in (a) chronic obstructive pulmonary disease (COPD), (b) respiratory muscle weakness (Duchenne muscular dystrophy) and (c) severe scoliosis. The periods of marked reduction in oxygen saturation (Sao_2) relate to epochs of REM sleep (solid blocks); note that the pattern of desaturation is not constant, with dips that correspond to phasic REM sleep. (a) and (b) redrawn from refs 21 and 22, with permission from the American Thoracic Society. (c) redrawn from: Sawicka EH, Branthwaite MA. Respiration during sleep in Kyphoscoliosis. *Thorax* 1987; **42**: 801–8, with permission from the BMJ Publishing Group.

method for confident distinction between central and obstructive apnoeas, but its invasive nature precludes its widespread use. Oesophageal pressure monitoring can be particularly helpful in patients with respiratory muscle weakness or in very obese patients in whom chest wall displacement may be greatly diminished and respiratory events difficult to classify using external sensors. Pressure measurements can also detect periods of increased upper airway resistance during sleep, even in the absence of detectable changes in ventilation or oxygenation.[27] Multiple pressure measurement at several levels in the pharynx and oesophagus may be helpful in identifying the site(s) of airway narrowing.[28]

6.3.2   Chest wall motion

Movements of the ribcage, abdomen or both can be recorded by various devices, including magnetometers[29] and, more commonly, a respiratory inductance

plethysmograph (RIP).[30,31] Use of such devices to measure ventilation is discussed in Chapter 1, Section 1.4. Reasonably accurate measurements are possible after appropriate calibration, provided that the subject stays in the same posture,[31] but the results are compromised by changes in posture and usually are regarded only as semi-quantitative.[30] Another important role of monitoring chest wall movements is to detect paradoxical motion of the ribcage and abdomen, which is a key diagnostic criterion of obstructive, as opposed to central, apnoeas and hypopnoeas. With accurate calibration, the summed RIP signal during an obstructive apnoea would be zero but, in practice, recognition of an out-of-phase pattern together with other features such as intermittent snoring usually suffices for the recognition of an obstructive event. Sometimes, however, external sensors are insufficiently sensitive to detect the respiratory effort during an obstructive apnoea, which may then be classified incorrectly

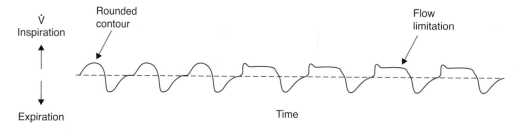

Figure 6.4 Schematic pattern of inspiratory flow illustrating development of flow limitation with plateaux of flow.

as 'central'.[32] Occasionally, in undoubted obstructive apnoea, the RIP signal suggests qualitatively normal movement of the ribcage and abdomen. This has been attributed to changes in the shape of the ribcage or abdomen without changing volume, due to alterations in the vertical (craniocaudal) dimension related to flexion and extension of the spine.[20] Poor sensitivity of external monitoring devices can be particularly problematic in subjects with severe obesity.

6.3.3 Airflow

The most definitive method for measuring airflow is use of a pneumotachograph incorporated into a tight-fitting facemask, a technique that represents the reference standard, particularly for detailed research.[33] In clinical practice, however, semi-quantitative methods are more commonly used. Thermistors or thermocouples positioned on the upper lip adjacent to the nostrils and mouth detect changes in temperature related to inspiratory and expiratory flow. However, the relation between the resulting signal and airflow is very alinear and their use can underestimate the frequency of abnormal respiratory events, particularly hypopnoeas.[34] Increasingly, temperature-sensitive devices are being replaced by measurement of nasal pressure via small nasal 'prongs' (similar to those used for oxygen delivery). These generally measure flow more accurately,[35] although nasal obstruction leading to less nasal breathing and more mouth breathing occasionally causes underestimation.[36] In practice, this appears to matter little for clinical purposes, and comparison with pneumotachography shows that accurate assessment of obstructive sleep apnoea is possible even in patients who complain of nasal obstruction.[37] An additional advantage of nasal pressure measurement is that it allows detailed

examination of the contour of the inspiratory airflow signal in order to identify the characteristic appearance of airflow limitation (Fig. 6.4).[38] Periods of flow limitation (usually associated with snoring) may themselves be sufficient to disrupt sleep, even in the absence of apnoea or hypopnoea, and may contribute to the symptomatology of patients with sleep-breathing disturbance associated with upper airway narrowing. Recognition of inspiratory flow limitation is also used by auto-adjusting continuous positive airway pressure (CPAP) machines to optimize the pressure required by increasing it until sufficient to overcome the flow limitation.

6.3.4 Respiratory impedance

Forced oscillation via a nasal mask has been used to assess the upper airway during sleep and to detect episodes of increased impedance associated with apnoeas and hypopnoeas as well as for monitoring the effectiveness of CPAP treatment in overcoming these.[39,40] Experience to date is limited, but the method appears promising and the application of forced oscillation has been shown not to modify upper airway muscle tone or to disrupt sleep itself.[41]

6.3.5 Oximetry

Pulse oximeters are used universally in overnight sleep recordings, either as a single sensor or in combination with other measurements. It is important to ensure that the sampling rate of the oximeter is adequate for detecting the dips in oxygenation that follow transient apnoeas and hypopnoeas. With several instruments, the averaging time of measurement can be modified over a range that may extend from 3 s to more than 20 s. The shorter the averaging time, the more accurate the result, and increasing beyond 10 s can seriously underestimate the magnitude of desaturation.[42] Reducing the sampling frequency improves the memory capacity of the instrument but at the cost of lower sensitivity.

Either an ear probe or finger probe can be used, with the former sometimes recommended because of the more rapid response,[43] but in practice the latter suffices for most purposes. The data recorded can be analysed in various ways, including a cumulative plot of SaO_2 against time[44] or a histogram displaying the relative time at different values of SaO_2.[45] The latter gives a time-weighted average SaO_2, but this is relatively insensitive to transient dips as the most revealing section is the 'tail' of the distribution representing the time spent at lower values. The latter is quantified in terms of the proportion of time with SaO_2 less than particular values, e.g. 90 per cent, 80 per cent. Alternatively, a nadir value can be quoted but, by definition, this represents only one instant during the night and is therefore intrinsically more variable.

6.3.6 Measurement of PCO_2

PCO_2 during sleep can be monitored by end tidal sampling or by using a transcutaneous PCO_2 electrode. The disadvantages of end tidal PCO_2 measurement in general are discussed in Chapter 4, Section 4.3.6 and its use to estimate arterial PCO_2 during sleep is of doubtful value.[46] Transcutaneous PCO_2 measurements are sometimes made during sleep, particularly in paediatric practice, but they are used less often in adults in whom hitherto they have been less reliable. Also, during conventional polysomnography, the slow response time of a PCO_2 electrode seriously compromises its value, although it can be useful in subjects with suspected sleep-related hypoventilation. Improving technology is likely to encourage more widespread use of transcutaneous PCO_2 monitoring in the future (see Chapter 4, Section 4.3.5).

6.3.7 Audiovisual recording

Recording of snoring is incorporated in many sleep study systems, usually using a small microphone attached over the trachea. This is a useful adjunct to other signals for distinguishing central and obstructive respiratory events. Video recording allows identification of sleeping posture that may have a major influence of sleep-breathing

abnormalities. Alternatively, posture can be assessed using small sensors attached to the skin.

6.3.8 Pulse transit time analysis

The pulse transit time (PTT) represents the time for transmission of the arterial pressure wave from the aortic valve to the periphery and is recorded by detecting the peripheral pulse shock wave. The velocity of the wave depends on the stiffness of the arterial walls and is related inversely to the blood pressure. Consequently, as blood pressure rises, PTT shortens. It therefore increases with the normal inspiratory fall in blood pressure and decreases during the increases in blood pressure that accompany arousal.[47] Using oesophageal pressure as the reference, PTT has been shown to have good sensitivity and specificity for distinguishing central and obstructive events.[48]

6.4 DEFINITIONS

6.4.1 Apnoeas, hypopnoeas and apnoea hypopnoea index

A period of apnoea is defined arbitrarily as cessation of airflow for at least 10 s. Following the original description by Gastaut et al., apnoeas are classified as 'central' if both airflow and chest wall movement cease, 'obstructive' if out-of-phase chest wall movement continues with no flow at the nose or mouth, and 'mixed' if an initially central pattern develops into an obstructive pattern as effort increases (Fig. 6.5).[49] Originally a sleep apnoea syndrome was diagnosed if there were at least 30 apnoeas occurring in both non-REM sleep and REM sleep during a 7-h nocturnal period.[50] However, it was subsequently recognized that many older healthy people have a frequency of apnoeas exceeding this limit. In addition, it became clear that the obstructive sleep apnoea syndrome can be seen with frequent periods of hypopnoea without complete apnoea.[51] Consequently, sleep studies are often reported in terms of the apnoea/hypopnoea index (AHI), i.e. the number of apnoeas plus hypopnoeas per hour of sleep. If sleep time is not recorded accurately, the index is reported per hour of study.

Unfortunately, the definition of a hypopnoea varies with the technology used to measure it.

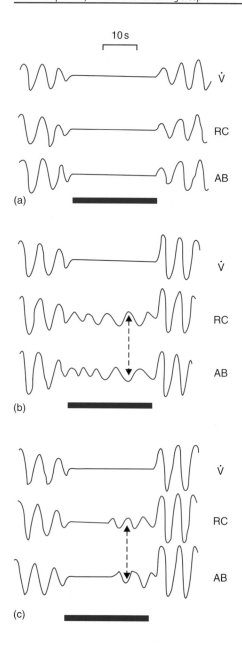

Figure 6.5 Schematic diagram of three patterns of sleep apnoea. Each panel shows airflow at the mouth (V̇, inspiration upward) and anteroposterior diameters of ribcage (RC) and abdomen (AB). (a) Central apnoea with cessation of chest wall movement. (b) Obstructive apnoea with continued chest wall movement and RC and AB moving out of phase with each other (<–––>). (c) Mixed apnoea in which movements and flow cease together but movement restarts before flow.

According to the definition proposed by the American Academy of Sleep Medicine, a hypopnoea is either (i) a decrease of more than 50 per cent from baseline in the amplitude of a valid measurement of breathing during sleep; or (ii) a clear amplitude reduction of a validated measurement of breathing during sleep that does not reach the above criterion but that is associated with either an oxygen desaturation greater than 3 per cent or an arousal.[33]

6.4.2 Other events and indices

An additional type of sleep-breathing event is sometimes reported, a respiratory effort-related arousal (RERA), which is a sequence of breaths with increasing effort leading to arousal but which fails to meet the criteria for apnoea or hypopnoea. Strictly, this requires recording of oesophageal pressure to identify progressively increasing efforts, with an abrupt reduction in effort associated with the arousal.

The term 'respiratory disturbance index' (RDI) is sometimes used interchangeably with the apnoea/hypopnoea index, but its use is not consistent in the literature. Some authors use RDI instead of AHI when measurements are obtained with simplified recording systems (i.e. without neurophysiological signals), in which case the denominator is hours of study rather than hours of sleep,[52] whereas others define RDI as the sum of apnoeas and hypopnoeas plus RERAs divided by the total sleep time.[53]

An alternative index, used particularly when oxygen saturation alone is recorded, is the ODI (or 'dip rate'). This is usually defined as the number of transient dips in SaO_2 of 4 per cent or more per hour. The ODI is usually used when sleep time is not recorded, so the denominator is hours of study. In patients with the obstructive sleep apnoea syndrome, the ODI is generally rather less than AHI.

6.4.3 Effect of definitions on diagnosis

Not surprisingly, the numerical values of the indices calculated from sleep studies vary with the precise definitions used, and this can affect the assessment of severity of sleep apnoea syndromes.[54] This is most obvious with the difference in the denominator when AHI is measured per hour of study or per hour of sleep as, clearly, the former can underestimate the latter. Inconsistencies also affect the numerator, which varies depending on whether a reduction in flow or volume displacement is used to recognize hypopnoea, as well as on the requirement for, and magnitude of, any associated desaturation. In a large community study, it was shown that the median RDI could vary by as much as tenfold, depending on the precise definitions of apnoea and hypopnoea used.[54] Similarly, in a sleep clinic population investigated by polysomnography, the prevalence of disease estimated using different thresholds of AHI varied considerably, depending on the definitions used.[55]

6.4.4 Central apnoea and hypoventilation syndromes

A central sleep apnoea syndrome is recognized by the presence of five or more central apnoeas plus hypopnoeas per hour of sleep.[33] Central apnoeas may be associated with Cheyne–Stokes breathing in which there is characteristic cyclical fluctuation, with periods of central apnoea and hypopnoea alternating with hyperpnoea in a gradual waxing and waning fashion (see Chapter 19, Section 19.2.4). Conventionally, hypoventilation during sleep is distinguished from hypopnoea by its longer duration and the consequent rise in $PaCO_2$. Unlike individuals with sleep apnoea syndromes, who generally have normal arterial blood gases when awake, patients with the obesity hypoventilation syndrome (formerly known as the Pickwickian syndrome) have daytime hypercapnia and hypoxaemia that worsen during sleep (see Chapter 24, Section 24.2).

6.5 SLEEP INVESTIGATION SYSTEMS

The range of equipment available for investigations during sleep ranges from comprehensive polysomnography with 12–16 signals at one extreme to oximetry alone at the other, with several devices that incorporate varying combinations of signals in between. The American Sleep Disorders Association classifies sleep investigation systems into four types (Table 6.3).[1]

6.5.1 In-hospital polysomnography

Type I systems represent detailed polysomnography, including neurophysiological recordings, performed under supervision in hospital. This is regarded as the

Table 6.3 Classification of sleep study systems*

Type 1	Standard (attended) polysomnography
Type 2	Comprehensive (portable) polysomnography
Type 3	Modified portable systems ('respiratory polysomnography')
Type 4	Single or dual-signal systems (oximetry ± 1 other signal)

*Based on recommendations of American Sleep Disorders Association.

reference standard and in the USA is recommended as the investigation of choice for most patients.[1]

6.5.2 Domiciliary polysomnography

Type 2 systems, or 'comprehensive portable polysomnography', record essentially the same signals as type 1 systems, but the recording device is smaller so that recordings can be made in the domiciliary setting. Appreciable time and care need to be taken in setting up such systems, and loss of one or more signals overnight occurs in up to a third of patients,[56] although others have reported better success. Perhaps surprisingly, when domiciliary polysomnography was compared with measurements in a sleep laboratory, most subjects preferred the latter.[57]

6.5.3 Limited sleep study systems ('respiratory polysomnography')

Type 3 monitoring systems omit neurophysiological recording and incorporate four to six channels, which include oxygen saturation and various combinations of chest wall movement, airflow, body position and sound monitoring. Several different systems are now available, designed for use in the home and validated to varying degrees by comparison with in-hospital polysomnography. Clinical demand, limitation of resources and the realization that most patients undergoing investigation for the obstructive sleep apnoea syndrome do not require full polysomnography have encouraged most sleep services to expand their capacity using these systems.

Although the systems differ in detail, some generalizations can be made about their use. Self-evidently, they do not aim to measure the stage or even the duration of sleep. Consequently, various sleep-related indices (such as AHI) are expressed in relation to the study time rather than sleep time.

A further general point is that the automated algorithms employed in various limited sleep study systems are often unreliable, and studies need to be checked manually.[58,59] The sensitivity and specificity of these devices for diagnosing the obstructive sleep apnoea syndrome have been reported in several studies. Comparisons using limited study systems, both in hospital[58-60] and in the subject's home,[61-63] with the 'gold standard' of polysomnography have generally been reassuring. The failure rate for studies at home is reported to be as low as 10 per cent,[62] but other authors have found the need for subsequent more detailed investigation in a greater proportion.[64] False negative results occur, particularly in subjects with only mild or moderate sleep apnoea.[60] Clearly, the values of sensitivity and specificity calculated in different comparative studies depend on the criteria and thresholds used for diagnosis.

More productive than crude estimation of sensitivity and specificity is comparison of the pre-test probability with the outcome of the study. This approach allows more meaningful assessment of the value of the investigation for ruling in or ruling out the condition in question. It also highlights the important point that a 'negative' result needs to be interpreted in the light of the clinical likelihood (pre-test probability) of the condition. If this is high, then a 'negative' result should prompt further, more detailed investigation, whereas if it is low, a negative investigation helps to confirm the absence of the condition.[65]

6.5.4 Nocturnal oximetry

Type 4 monitors either are oximeters alone or record oximetry together with one other channel, usually nasal pressure[65-67] or snoring.[68,69] Figures reported for the sensitivity and specificity of oximetry alone for diagnosing patients with obstructive sleep apnoea syndrome vary considerably between different studies and depend critically on the populations studied. Some authors find very limited value,[66,70-72] whereas others have reported acceptable accuracy particularly in carefully selected patients.[73,74] In one study, oximetry was actually inferior to clinical assessment.[71] By contrast, in another study in which the end point was taken as compliance with effective treatment, oximetry alone proved to be as effective as polysomnography in predicting the outcome.[74]

REFERENCES

1 Flemons WW, Littner MR, Rowley JA, et al. Home diagnosis of sleep apnoea: a systematic review of the literature. Chest 2003; **124**: 1543–79.

2 Rechtschaffen A, Kales A (eds). A Manual of Standardized Terminology, Techniques and Scoring System for Sleep Stages in Human Subjects. Brain Information Service, UCLA, Los Angeles, CA, 1968.

3 Stradling JR, Chadwick GA, Frew AJ. Changes in ventilation and its components in normal subjects during sleep. Thorax 1985; **40**: 364–70.

4 Bulow K. Respiration and wakefulness in man. Acta Physiol Scand 1963; **59** (suppl. 209).

5 Dempsey JA, Smith CA, Przybylowski T, et al. The ventilatory responsiveness to CO_2 below eupnoea as a determinant of ventilatory stability in sleep. J Physiol 2004; **560**: 1–11.

6 Gries RE, Brooks LJ. Normal oxyhaemoglobin saturation during sleep. How low does it go? Chest 1996; **110**: 1489–92.

7 White DP, Zwillich CW. Metabolic rate and breathing during sleep. J Appl Physiol 1985; **59**: 384–91.

8 Ballard RD, Irvin CG, Martin RJ, et al. Influence of sleep on lung volumes in asthmatics and normals. J Appl Physiol 1990; **68**: 2034–41.

9 Hudgel DW, Martin RJ, Johnson B, Hill P. Mechanics of the respiratory system and breathing pattern during sleep in normal humans. J Appl Physiol 1984; **56**: 133–7.

10 Wiegand DA, Latz B, Zwillich CW, Wiegand L. Upper airway resistance and geniohyoid muscle activity in normal men during wakefulness and sleep. J Appl Physiol 1990; **69**: 1252–61.

11 Morrell MJ, Harty HR, Adams L, Guz A. Breathing during wakefulness and NREM sleep in humans without an upper airway. J Appl Physiol 1996; **81**: 274–81.

12 Douglas NJ. Control of breathing during sleep. Clin Sci 1984; **67**: 465–71.

13 Khoo MC, Gottschalk A, Pack AI. Sleep-induced periodic breathing and apnoea: a theoretical study. J Appl Physiol 1991; **70**: 2014–24.

14 Dempsey JA. Crossing the apnoeic threshold: causes and consequences. Exp Physiol 2004; **90**: 13–24.

15 Stradling JR. Obstructive sleep apnoea and related syndromes, in Respiratory Medicine, 3rd edn (eds Gibson GJ, Geddes DM, Costabel U, Sterk PJ and Corrin B), Saunders, London, 2003, pp. 1068–101.

16 Cherniak NS, Longobardo GS. Mathematical models of periodic breathing and their usefulness in understanding cardiovascular and respiratory disorders. Exp Physiol 2006; **91**: 295–305.

17 Tabachnik E, Muller NL, Bryan AC, Levison H. Changes in ventilation and chest wall mechanics during sleep in normal adolescents. *J Appl Physiol* 1981; **51**: 557–64.

18 Van der Graafe WB. Thoracic influence on upper airway patency. *J Appl Physiol* 1998; **65**: 2124–31.

19 Tusiewicz K, Moldofsky H, Bryan AC and Bryan MH (1977) Mechanics of the rib cage and diaphragm during sleep. J. Appl. Physiol. 43, 600-2

20 Lopes JM, Tabachnik E, Muller NL, Levison H, Bryan AC. Total airway resistance and respiratory muscle activity during sleep. *J Appl Physiol* 1983; **54**: 773–7.

21 Douglas NJ, Flenley DC. Breathing during sleep in patients with obstructive lung disease. *Am Rev Respir Dis* 1990; **141**: 1055–70.

22 Smith PEM, Calverley PMA, Edwards RHT. Hypoxaemia during sleep in Duchenne muscular dystrophy. *Am Rev Respir Dis* 1988; **137**: 884–8.

23 Sawicka EH, Branthwaite MA. Respiration during sleep in kyphoscoliosis. *Thorax* 1987; **42**: 801–8.

24 Stradling JR, Lane DJ. Nocturnal hypoxaemia in chronic obstructive pulmonary disease. *Clin Sci* 1983; **64**: 213–22.

25 Trinder J, Ivens C, Kleiman J, Klevelaan D, White DP. The cardiorespiratory activation response at an arousal from sleep is independent of the level of CO_2. *J Sleep Res* 2006; **15**: 174–82.

26 Gleeson K, Zwillich CW, White DP. The influence of increasing ventilatory effort on arousal from sleep. *Am Rev Respir Dis* 1990; **142**: 295–300.

27 Virkkula P, Silvola J, Maasilta P, Malmberg H, Salmi T. Esophageal pressure monitoring in detection of sleep-disordered breathing. *Laryngoscope* 2002; **112**: 1264–70.

28 Reda M, Gibson GJ, Wilson JA. Pharyngoesophageal pressure monitoring in sleep apnea syndrome. *Otolaryngol Head Neck Surg* 2001; **125**: 324–31.

29 Sharp JT, Druz WS, Foster JR, Wicks MS, Chokroverty S. Use of the respiratory magneto-meter in diagnosis and classification of sleep apnea. *Chest* 1980; **77**: 350–53.

30 Whyte KF, Gugger M, Gould GA, *et al.* Accuracy of respiratory inductive plethysmograph in measuring tidal volume during sleep. *J Appl Physiol* 1991; **71**: 1866–71.

31 Cantineau JP, Escourrou P, Sartene R, Gaultier C, Goldman M. Accuracy of respiratory inductive plethysmography during wakefulness and sleep in patients with obstructive sleep apnoea. *Chest* 1992; **102**: 1145–51.

32 Staats BA, Bonekat HW, Harris CD, Offord KP. Chest wall motion in sleep apnea. *Am Rev Respir Dis* 1984; **130**: 59–63.

33 American Academy of Sleep Medicine. Sleep-related breathing disorders in adults: recommendations for syndrome definition and measurement techniques in clinical research. *Sleep* 1999; **22**: 667–89.

34 Farré R, Montserrat JM, Rotger M, Ballester E, Navajas D. Accuracy of thermistors and thermo-couples as flow-measuring devices for detecting hypopnoeas. *Eur Respir J* 1998; **11**: 179–82.

35 Heitman SJ. Atkar RS, Hajduk EA, Wanner RA, Flemons WW. Validation of nasal pressure for the identification of apneas/hypopnoeas during sleep. *Am J Respir Crit Care Med* 2002; **166**: 386–91.

36 Sériers F, Marc I. Nasal pressure recording in the diagnosis of sleep apnoea hypopnoea syndrome. *Thorax* 1999; **54**: 506–10.

37 Thurnheer R, Xie X, Bloch KE. Accuracy of nasal cannula pressure recordings for assessment of ventilation during sleep. *Am J Respir Crit Care Med* 2001; **164**: 1914–19.

38 Hosselet JJ, Norman RG, Ayappa I, Rapoport DM. Detection of flow limitation with a nasal cannula/pressure transducer system. *Am J Respir Crit Care Med* 1998; **157**: 1461–7.

39 Badia JR, Farré R, Montserrat JM, *et al.* Forced oscillation technique for the evaluation of severe sleep apnoea/hypopnoea syndrome: a pilot study. *Eur Respir J* 1998; **11**: 1128–34.

40 Steltner H, Staats R, Timmer J, *et al.* Diagnosis of sleep apnea by automatic analysis of nasal pressure and forced oscillation impedance. *Am J Respir Crit Care Med* 2002; **165**: 940–44.

41 Badia JR, Farré R, Rigau R, *et al.* Forced oscillation measurements do not affect upper airway muscle tone or sleep in clinical studies. *Eur Respir J* 2001; **18**: 335–9.

42 Farré R, Montserrat JM, Ballester E, *et al.* Importance of the pulse oximeter averaging time when measuring oxygen desaturation in sleep apnea. *Sleep* 1998; **21**: 386–90.

43 American Thoracic Society. Indications and standards for cardiopulmonary sleep studies. *Am Rev Respir Dis* 1989; **139**: 559–68.

44 Slutsky AS, Strohl KP. Quantification of oxygen saturation during episodic hypoxaemia. *Am Rev Respir Dis* 1980; **121**; 893–5.

45 Meanock CI, Guyatt AR, Cumming G. The assessment of nocturnal oxygen saturation. *Clin Sci* 1983; **65**: 507–13.

46 Sanders MH, Kern NB, Costantino JP, *et al.* Accuracy of end tidal and transcutaneous PCO_2 monitoring during sleep. *Chest* 1994; **106**: 472–83.

47 Pitson DJ, Sandell A, van den Hout R, Stradling JR. Use of pulse transit time as a measure of inspiratory

effort in patients with obstructive sleep apnoea. *Eur Respir J* 1995; **8**: 1669–74.

48 Argod J, Pepin JL, Levy P. Differentiating obstructive and central sleep respiratory events through pulse transit time. *Am J Respir Clin Care Med* 1998; **158**: 1778–83.

49 Gastaut H, Tassinari CA, Duron B. Polygraphic study of the episodic diurnal and nocturnal (hypnic and respiratory) manifestations of the Pickwick syndrome. *Brain Res* 1966; **1**: 167–86.

50 Guilleminault C, Tilkian A, Dement WC. The sleep apnoea syndrome. *Annu Rev Med* 1976; **27**: 465–84.

51 Gould GA, Whyte KF, Rhind GB, *et al.* The sleep hypopnoea syndrome. *Am Rev Respir Dis* 1988; **137**: 895–8.

52 Li CK, Flemons WW. State of home sleep studies. *Clin Chest Med* 2003; **24**: 283–95.

53 Lee-Chiong TL. Monitoring respiration during sleep. *Clin Chest Med* 2003; **24**: 297–306.

54 Redline S, Kapur VK, Sanders MH, *et al.* Effects of varying approaches for identifying respiratory disturbances on sleep apnea assessment. *Am J Respir Crit Care Med* 2000; **161**: 369–74.

55 Manser RL, Rochford P, Pierce RJ, Byrnes GB, Campbell DA. Impact of different criteria for defining hypopneas in the apnea-hypopnea index. *Chest* 2001; **120**: 909–14.

56 Portier F, Portmann A, Czernichow P, *et al.* Evaluation of home versus laboratory polysomnography in the diagnosis of sleep apnea syndrome. *Am J Respir Crit Care Med* 2000; **162**: 814–18.

57 Fry JM, DiPhillipo MA, Curran K, Goldberg R, Baran AS. Full polysomnography in the home. *Sleep* 1998; **21**: 635–42.

58 Esnaola S, Duran J, Infante-Rivard C, Rubio R, Fernandez A. Diagnostic accuracy of a portable recording device (MESAM IV) in suspected obstructive sleep apnoea. *Eur Respir J* 1996; **9**: 2597–605.

59 Zucconi M, Ferini-Strambi L, Castronovo V, Oldani A, Smirne S. An unattended device for sleep-related breathing disorders: validation study in suspected obstructive sleep apnoea syndrome. *Eur Respir J* 1996; **9**: 1251–6.

60 Verse T, Pirsig W, Junge-Hulsing B, Kroker B. Validation of the POLY-MESAM seven-channel ambulatory recording unit. *Chest* 2000; **117**: 1613–18.

61 Redline S, Tosteson T, Boucher MA, Millman RP. Measurement of sleep-related breathing disturbances in epidemiologic studies: assessment of the validity and reproducibility of a portable monitoring device. *Chest* 1991; **100**: 1281–6.

62 Parra O, Garcia-Esclasans N, Montserrat JM, *et al.* Should patients with sleep apnoea/hypopnoea syndrome be diagnosed and managed on the basis of home sleep studies? *Eur Respir J* 1997; **10**: 1720–24.

63 Ballester E, Solans M, Vila X, *et al.* Evaluation of a portable respiratory recording device for detecting apnoeas and hypopnoeas in subjects from a general population. *Eur Respir J* 2000; **16**: 123–7.

64 Whittle AT, Finch SP, Mortimore IL, MacKay TW, Douglas NJ. Use of home sleep studies for diagnosis of the sleep apnoea/hypopnoea syndrome. *Thorax* 1997; **52**: 1068–73.

65 Mayer P, Meurice JC, Philip-Joet F, *et al.* Simultaneous laboratory-based comparison of ResMed Autoset with polysomnography in the diagnosis of sleep apnoea/hypopnoea syndrome. *Eur Respir J* 1998; **12**: 770–75.

66 Kiely JL, Delahunty C, Matthews S, McNicholas WT. Comparison of a limited computerised diagnostic system (Res Care Autoset) with polysomnography in the diagnosis of obstructive sleep apnoea syndrome. *Eur Respir J* 1996; **9**: 2360–64.

67 Gugger M. Comparison of ResMed AutoSet (version 3.03) with polysomnography in the diagnosis of the sleep apnoea/hypopnoea syndrome. *Eur Respir J* 1997; **10**: 587–91.

68 White JES, Smithson AJ, Close PR, *et al.* The use of sound recording and oxygen saturation in screening snorers for obstructive sleep apnoea. *Clin Otolaryngol* 1994; **19**: 218–21.

69 Issa FG, Morrison D, Hadjuk E, *et al.* Digital monitoring of sleep-disordered breathing using snoring sound and arterial oxygen saturation. *Am Rev Respir Dis* 1993; **148**: 1023–9.

70 Douglas NJ, Thomas S, Jan MA. Clinical value of polysomnography. *Lancet* 1992; **339**: 347–50.

71 Gyulay S, Olson LG, Hensley MJ, *et al.* A comparison of clinical assessment and home oximetry in the diagnosis of obstructive sleep apnea. *Am Rev Respir Dis* 1993; **147**: 50–53.

72 Epstein LJ, Doriac GR. Cost effectiveness analysis of nocturnal oximetry as a method of screening for sleep apnea-hypopnea syndrome. *Chest* 1998; **113**: 97–103.

73 Vazques JC, Tsai WH, Flemons WW, *et al.* Automated analysis of digital oximetry in the diagnosis of obstructive sleep apnea. *Thorax* 2000; **55**: 302–7.

74 Whitelaw WA, Brant RF, Flemons WW. Clinical usefulness of home oximetry compared with polysomnography for assessment of sleep apnea. *Am J Respir Crit Care Med* 2005; **171**: 188–93.

7

Exercise Tests

The performance of exercise requires an increase in the metabolism of the relevant muscles, which results in generation of adenosine triphosphate (ATP). Concomitantly, the transport of oxygen to, and carbon dioxide from, the muscles increases. The efficiency of this process depends on the integration of several factors, with the respiratory muscles, lungs, chest wall, pulmonary circulation, heart, systemic circulation, blood and exercising muscles all contributing. Defects at various points, either singly or in combination, can impair efficiency and limit the exercise ability of an individual.

Exercise tests vary considerably in their complexity and in the number and type of measurements made. At the simplest level walking along a corridor with the patient might be regarded as part of the clinical examination, while at the other extreme, arterial cannulation and making multiple measurements breath by breath during exercise allow detailed assessment of pulmonary gas exchange. The type of test chosen depends on the information required. A clinical exercise test can be helpful in various situations (Table 7.1). In principle it has the advantage of allowing assessment of the patient and his or her performance at the time he or she is most likely to experience symptoms. This can often be revealing in relation to the symptom of breathlessness, which to some patients means excessive ventilation and to others difficulty in breathing because of adverse pulmonary mechanics; occasionally it may even reflect the symptoms associated with myocardial ischaemia. Formal quantitation of exercise performance allows more objective estimation of disability than the clinical history alone, since the patient's interpretation will be coloured by his or her own expectations and previous level of regular activity. An exercise test can provide useful information on the likely factors limiting exercise, in particular on whether the limitation is due primarily to respiratory or circulatory problems. In the early stages of some diseases, exercise tests reveal abnormalities, such as reduced arterial oxygenation, that are well compensated at rest, while in the particular context of asthma a simple exercise test may be diagnostic (see Chapter 11, Section 11.9.2). Other common indications are listed in Table 7.1. More comprehensive accounts of exercise physiology and exercise tests as practised by respiratory (rather than cardiac) laboratories are available elsewhere.[1–4]

Table 7.1 **Common indications for exercise testing**

Assessment of unexplained breathlessness
Identification of factors limiting exercise intolerance
Objective measurement of exercise capacity
Monitoring natural history of disease and/or effects of therapy
Estimation of prognosis (e.g. chronic cardiac failure)
Preoperative evaluation (e.g. before lung resection, volume-reduction surgery, transplantation)
Tailoring of training/rehabilitation programmes
Recognizing oxygen desaturation/evaluating benefit of ambulatory oxygen
Diagnosing exercise-induced asthma

7.1 PHYSIOLOGICAL RESPONSES TO EXERCISE

7.1.1 Metabolic responses

In a trained athlete the oxygen consumption ($\dot{V}O_2$) during maximal exercise may be as much as 20 times that at rest.[5] In healthy individuals muscle metabolism during moderate exercise follows mainly aerobic pathways, but at high levels of exercise the delivery of oxygen to the muscles becomes critical and anaerobic metabolism with production of lactic acid is increasingly important.

The respiratory quotient (RQ) of tissues metabolizing aerobically varies from 0.7 (for fat alone) to 1.0 (for glycogen); the average value tends to be higher in exercising muscles than in muscles at rest (approximately 0.9 compared with a mean resting value of 0.8). During light and moderate exercise the demand of exercising muscles for oxygen is satisfied by a combination of increased oxygen supply (i.e. increased blood flow) and an increase in the 'extraction ratio', i.e. the proportion of the oxygen delivered by arterial blood that is extracted by the metabolizing tissues. At rest the extraction ratio is approximately 0.25–0.35, but it can increase to as much as 0.8 at maximum exercise in fit subjects.[6] As work rate increases, however, the amount of oxygen that can be extracted becomes insufficient for energy requirements and additional energy is then supplied by anaerobic metabolism. This produces carbon dioxide (CO_2) without consuming oxygen and therefore causes the RQ to rise disproportionately.

It is important to note that the respiratory exchange ratio (R) measured at the mouth is not necessarily the same as the tissue RQ: the difference is obvious in the 'unsteady' state, where the rates of adaptation to changes of metabolism, circulation and ventilation may differ. But, even in an apparently steady state, although the oxygen uptake measured at the mouth is close to the tissue consumption, this is not necessarily true for CO_2 production, since the stores of CO_2 in the body are very much larger than those of oxygen. Consequently, the values of R and RQ may deviate as the CO_2 output seen at the mouth is the net result of metabolic production and entry into, or exit from, the body stores.[7]

7.1.1.1 The 'anaerobic threshold'

It has been suggested that the onset of anaerobic metabolism is recognizable as a threshold at which the consequent increase in blood lactate concentration is accompanied by disproportionate increases in CO_2 production and ventilation, with the drive to ventilation increasing markedly because of the associated metabolic acidosis. The 'anaerobic threshold' (AT) is defined in terms of the threshold level of $\dot{V}O_2$ at which the specified changes are detected. Its value is reduced in some clinical situations in which oxygen supply is likely to be compromised, but its literal use is a considerable oversimplification.[1,8] It has been shown, for example, that muscles can release lactate even in the face of an apparently adequate oxygen supply; metabolizing muscles can even use lactate as a substrate, as also can other tissues. Anaerobic metabolism does not 'switch on' abruptly; rather, the production of lactate by, and its removal from, exercising muscles are continuous processes. It is also noteworthy that the disproportionate rise in ventilation often used as a guide to the AT can be seen during progressive exercise by subjects with myophosphorylase deficiency (McArdle's syndrome), a condition in which no lactate is generated; in these individuals the excessive ventilation leads to a fall in [H^+] (rise in pH), i.e. a respiratory alkalosis rather than the characteristic metabolic acidosis that accompanies lactate production.[9]

Greater amounts of lactate are produced during periods of relative tissue hypoxia; this occurs, for example, with impaired cardiac output or when breathing air with a reduced PO_2 (e.g. at altitude). During progressive exercise the blood concentration of lactate depends on a balance between its production and removal, so that, rather than a discrete threshold, there is a progressive and exponential rise in concentration over a period as the rate of production starts to exceed the capacity of the body to remove it.[8] There is a consequent disproportionate increase in ventilation accompanying the associated metabolic acidosis, although the apparent 'thresholds' for ventilation and blood lactate concentration do not necessarily coincide.[8] It is therefore recommended that the AT should not be interpreted literally but rather should be regarded as a pragmatic descriptive term[2] used to

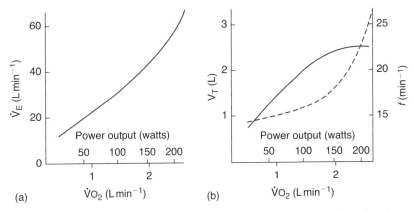

(a)

(b)

Figure 7.1 (a) Schematic pattern of ventilation during progressive exercise related to oxygen consumption and power output (workload) in a normal subject. The relation is linear up to approximately 50 per cent of $\dot{V}O_2$max, after which ventilation increases disproportionately. (b) Tidal volume (solid line) and breathing frequency (broken line) during progressive exercise as in (a). At lower workloads the increasing ventilation is due mainly to increases in tidal volume with little change in frequency; tidal volume reaches a maximum at about 50–60 per cent of vital capacity and the subsequent rise in ventilation is due to increasing frequency alone.

recognize a disproportionate increase in ventilation and the effects of this on gas exchange during progressive exercise. As such, the concept has proven useful in evaluating the response of an individual to exercise and in assessing the likely factors contributing to exercise limitation. The methods for measurement of AT are discussed below.

7.1.2 Ventilatory adaptations to exercise

7.1.2.1 Ventilatory mechanics during exercise

The stimuli to increase breathing on exercise are several, including both chemical (CO_2, acidity) and neurogenic factors. In normal subjects the relation between ventilation and work performed (Fig. 7.1a) is linear up to about 50–60 per cent of maximum $\dot{V}O_2$. Above this level ventilation increases disproportionately. Carbon dioxide output ($\dot{V}CO_2$) also rises disproportionately to $\dot{V}O_2$, with the result that $\dot{V}_E$ remains related closely to $\dot{V}CO_2$ except at high workloads (Fig. 7.2).

The increase in ventilation at low and moderate workloads is achieved mainly by increasing tidal volume, with initially a relatively small contribution from breathing frequency (Fig. 7.1b). Usually, maximum tidal volume is reached at a value of 50–60

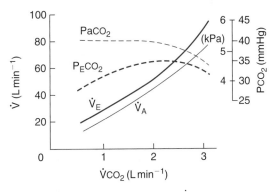

Figure 7.2 Schematic pattern of total ($\dot{V}_E$) and alveolar ($\dot{V}_A$) ventilation during exercise related to carbon dioxide (CO_2) output. In mild and moderate exercise, alveolar ventilation is closely regulated to CO_2 output, with the result that arterial $P{CO_2}$ remains constant. Although the volume of the physiological dead space increases, this is outweighed by the rise in tidal volume so that V_D/V_T falls and consequently expired $P{CO_2}$ ($P_E{CO_2}$) rises and is closer to $P_a{CO_2}$ than at rest. With heavy exercise $\dot{V}_A$ (and therefore $\dot{V}_E$) increases disproportionately and both $P_a{CO_2}$ and $P_E{CO_2}$ fall. Redrawn from ref. 1.

per cent of the VC; above this, further increases in ventilation result from increasing breathing frequency alone. This relation of maximum tidal volume to VC holds also in disease, with the ratio between the two being largely independent of the specific disease concerned.[10]

The constraint on further increases in tidal volume is mainly mechanical and is a consequence of the curvilinear pressure–volume relation of the lungs and the progressive fall in lung compliance as the end inspired volume rises. Detailed study of the static pressure–volume curve of the lungs in normal subjects on exercise shows that, compared with rest, there is some reduction in the compliance over a given volume range, probably due to stiffening of the lungs by the greater volume of blood in the pulmonary capillaries.[11] The reduced compliance is accompanied by a minor reduction in TLC and a more definite fall in VC with an increase in RV. The latter may be due either to inability to complete a true full expiration during exercise or to the more congested pulmonary capillaries supporting the alveolar walls and thus inhibiting full deflation.

The increased tidal flows of exercise approach the maximum available, especially towards the end of expiration (Fig. 7.3). The tendency for limitation of expiratory flow to occur (i.e. exercise flow reaching maximum, as defined by the maximum expiratory flow–volume (MEFV) curve) is greater in older healthy subjects in whom it can be seen at moderate levels of exercise.[12] This age-related difference is attributable to the loss of elastic recoil of the lungs and consequently lower maximum expiratory flow with age. In an individual, maximum expiratory flows are slightly greater during exercise than at rest, due to slight bronchodilatation.[12]

In younger subjects the exercise-related increase in tidal volume is accommodated by an increase in end inspiratory lung volume (EILV) and a reduction in end expiratory lung volume (EELV). The latter may aid the inspiratory muscles by increasing their fibre length and reducing the radius of curvature of the diaphragm compared to resting FRC, thus 'priming' them for subsequent inspiration. In older healthy subjects the EELV shows a fall during moderate exercise but increases again (to close to resting FRC) in more severe exercise,[13] presumably as a result of the greater tendency to expiratory flow limitation at lower lung volumes. With increasing age expiratory flow limitation is demonstrable over an increasing proportion of the exercise tidal volume, but whether these constraints limit exercise capacity in elderly people is uncertain.[13]

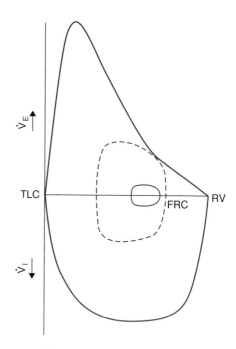

Figure 7.3 Schematic diagram of tidal flow–volume relations at rest (thin solid line) and on heavy exercise (broken line) compared with maximum flow–volume curves (thick solid line) in a young healthy subject. Expiratory flow approaches maximum at end expiration on heavy exercise.

The normal maximum exercise ventilation is approximately 70 per cent of the sprint maximum voluntary ventilation (MVV) measured over 15 s, but it is closer to the sustained isocapnic MVV measured over 4 min. Maximal exercise and maximal voluntary ventilation are sometimes compared in an individual in order to analyse the factors likely to be limiting ventilation, but this is of dubious validity as the breathing strategies differ considerably. During voluntary hyperventilation normal subjects tend to increase rather than decrease their EELV, and much greater expiratory effort is expended, with consequently much more muscular work performed for a given ventilation than when breathing naturally during exercise. In practice, the ventilatory 'reserve' at maximal exercise is more appropriately calculated by comparing exercise ventilation with a maximum predicted from the resting FEV_1, by multiplying by 35 (see below).[2]

7.1.2.2 Alveolar and dead space ventilation

The appropriateness of the ventilatory response to the metabolic demand of exercise can be assessed by measuring either the mixed expired P_{CO_2} (P_ECO_2) or alveolar P_{CO_2} (P_ACO_2). The former is related to the overall ventilation ($\dot{V}_E$):

$$P_ECO_2 \propto \frac{\dot{V}CO_2}{\dot{V}_E} \qquad (7.1)$$

while P_ACO_2 is related to alveolar ventilation ($\dot{V}_A$):

$$P_ACO_2 \propto \frac{\dot{V}CO_2}{\dot{V}_A} \qquad (7.2)$$

P_ACO_2 in this context is usually used in the sense of the 'ideal' alveolar P_{CO_2} of the Riley and Cournand three-compartment model (see Chapter 2, Section 2.3.4), with $\dot{V}_A$ representing the ventilation of the 'ideal' alveolar compartment; hence, P_ACO_2 can be approximated to arterial P_{CO_2}. During low and moderate levels of exercise, $PaCO_2$ remains fairly constant, implying that alveolar ventilation is normally closely adjusted to CO_2 output (Fig. 7.2). At high levels of exercise $PaCO_2$ falls. On the other hand, P_ECO_2 rises at low or moderate levels of exercise. In conjunction with a stable $PaCO_2$ this indicates that overall ventilation increases relatively less than alveolar ventilation – i.e. ventilation of the dead space makes a proportionally smaller contribution during exercise. This can be quantified using the Bohr equation (see Equation 2.1 in Chapter 2) to calculate the V_D/V_T ratio, which falls on exercise. Although, in absolute terms, the physiological dead space increases a little, this is more than outweighed by the rise in tidal volume, leading to a lower V_D/V_T ratio and therefore an overall improvement in the efficiency of distribution of the tidal volume compared with rest.[14]

In patients it is sometimes useful to analyse the ventilation in this way, in terms of its alveolar and dead-space components. The keys to this analysis are the values of P_{CO_2} – if P_ECO_2 is below normal for the level of exercise, the total ventilation must be excessive (Equation 7.1). End tidal P_{CO_2} ($P_{ET}CO_2$) is sometimes used as a surrogate for arterial (or alveolar) P_{CO_2} in order to separate alveolar

and dead space hyperventilation, but considerable caution is needed. As discussed in Chapter 4, Section 4.3.6, end tidal values can seriously underestimate $PaCO_2$ (or P_ACO_2) in patients with airway disease. Moreover, in healthy subjects during exercise, the converse may apply, with $P_{ET}CO_2$ exceeding $PaCO_2$.[15] If $P_{ET}CO_2$ is low but $PaCO_2$ is normal, dead space ventilation and the V_D/V_T ratio are high. Note, however, that a normal overall ventilation (normal P_ECO_2) could conceal the combination of low alveolar ventilation ($PaCO_2$ high) and high dead space ventilation.

The ratios of ventilation to oxygen consumption ($\dot{V}_E/\dot{V}O_2$) or CO_2 production ($\dot{V}_E/\dot{V}CO_2$) are known as the ventilatory equivalents for oxygen and CO_2 respectively. In light to moderate exercise, both fall compared with resting values due to the relative fall in dead space ventilation. In more severe exercise, with the increasing ventilatory drive associated with metabolic acidosis, $\dot{V}_E/\dot{V}O_2$ rises again. This usually occurs before any increase in $\dot{V}_E/\dot{V}CO_2$ (see below and Fig. 7.5f, p. 127) as ventilation is independent of oxygen consumption but closely linked to CO_2 output. Use is made of the different profiles of these two indices in one of the methods for calculating the anaerobic threshold (see p. 127).

7.1.3 Circulatory responses

In health, cardiac output increases progressively on exercise in relation to $\dot{V}O_2$ but the relationship is slightly curvilinear, with a lower rate of increase at higher workloads.[16] During mild exercise, both increasing stroke volume and heart rate contribute. The stroke volume, however, approaches a maximum at a relatively low level of exercise, and subsequent increases in cardiac output depend on increasing heart rate (Fig. 7.4). The increase in stroke volume is due partly to an increase in venous return and partly to a greater ejection fraction with a smaller end diastolic volume. The relation between heart rate and $\dot{V}O_2$ is steeper in women than in men because of the lower average lean body mass in women.[17]

The supply of oxygen to the tissues increases relatively more than the cardiac output because they extract a greater proportion of oxygen from the arterial blood. The systemic blood pressure increases on exercise but to a lesser extent than the cardiac output, implying a reduction in peripheral vascular

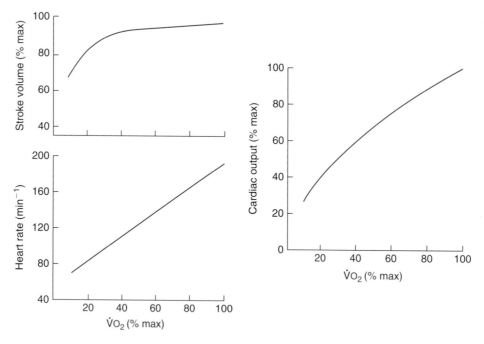

Figure 7.4 Schematic pattern of normal cardiac response to exercise, based on data of Astrand *et al.*[16] In mild exercise, both heart rate and stroke volume increase, but the latter approaches its maximum at relatively low workloads; subsequent increases in cardiac output result from the greater heart rate only.

resistance. The 'oxygen pulse', defined as the $\dot{V}_{O_2}$ divided by the heart rate, represents the volume of oxygen extracted by the metabolizing tissues per beat; this is sometimes used as an indirect estimate of stroke volume, but it is also affected by the arteriovenous oxygen content difference. An increased slope of the relationship between heart rate and $\dot{V}_{O_2}$ usually implies a small stroke volume. This pattern is seen in patients with cardiac disease but also in many other conditions, including deconditioning in otherwise healthy subjects. Maximum heart rate declines with age and is commonly predicted using one of two simple equations – either $220 -$ age in years or $210 -$ (age in years $\times 0.65$). Both give similar values for subjects under the age of 40 years, but the latter tends to be more accurate in older healthy individuals.[2]

7.1.4 Ventilation/perfusion matching on exercise

7.1.4.1 Effects of exercise intensity

The overall matching of ventilation to perfusion normally improves on moderate exercise, as implied by the lower V_D/V_T ratio. This improvement is also apparent if the contribution of lung units with low $\dot{V}_A/\dot{Q}$ ratios is quantified as the proportion of venous admixture or physiological shunt $(\dot{Q}_{va}/\dot{Q}_t)$; normally this falls on moderate exercise.[14] The alveolar arterial oxygen tension difference (AaP_{O_2}) remains constant or falls slightly at low or moderate workloads, but at higher loads the AaP_{O_2} often widens. The increase is due to the higher P_AO_2 and in very heavy exercise a fall in PaO_2 may also occur.[18] P_AO_2 rises for two reasons – because of an increase in alveolar ventilation disproportionate to $\dot{V}_{CO_2}$ and also because of an increase in R (since $P_AO_2 = P_IO_2 - P_ACO_2/R$ – Equation 2.4 in Chapter 2). In either case AaP_{O_2} widens without necessarily implying a deterioration in pulmonary gas exchange (see Chapter 4, Section 4.4.2.4). When very fit young individuals exercise heavily PaO_2 can fall by as much as 30 mmHg (4 kPa) and SaO_2 by up to 15 per cent.[18] The reduction in SaO_2 reflects not only the fall in PaO_2 but also a pH- and temperature-dependent shift of the haemoglobin–oxygen dissociation curve to the right, resulting in a lower SaO_2 for a given PaO_2. Ventilation/perfusion mismatching is the main cause of hypoxaemia on heavy exercise. Although, on very heavy exercise, $\dot{V}_A/\dot{Q}$ matching tends to deteriorate, its effects are countered to some extent by an overall increase in $\dot{V}_A/\dot{Q}$ ratio (i.e. the increase in alveolar ventilation is relatively greater than the increase in pulmonary blood flow). Other factors also come into consideration on heavy exercise. At levels close to maximum, diffusion limitation may contribute because of the very rapid transit of red blood cells through the pulmonary capillaries. The effects of both $\dot{V}_A/\dot{Q}$ mismatching and diffusion limitation are amplified further by the lower mixed venous (pulmonary arterial) PO_2 consequent on the greater extraction of oxygen from the blood by the metabolizing muscles. Finally, opening of small intrapulmonary right-to-left anatomical shunts may be an additional factor. Although such shunts are not necessarily detectable by conventional gas exchange techniques, they have been demonstrated by bubble contrast echocardiography in healthy young subjects exercising maximally and shown to correlate with $AaPO_2$.[19]

An increase in the diffusing capacity for carbon monoxide on exercise is demonstrable using both the breath-holding and intrabreath methods.[20] This results from a combination of more even distribution of ventilation and the higher volume and flow of blood in the pulmonary capillaries.

7.1.4.2 Effects of muscles used on gas exchange

Most of the foregoing and most conventional testing relate to exercise performed predominantly with the legs. Occasionally, however, arm exercise is used in individuals with problems of mobility or in training and rehabilitation of patients with respiratory limitation. Comparison of upper and lower limb exercise shows that symptom-limited maximum $\dot{V}O_2$, ventilation and heart rate are all less when the arms are used.[21] Comparison of peak arm and leg exercise at an equivalent $\dot{V}O_2$ also shows differences, with higher ventilation and $\dot{V}CO_2$, higher P_AO_2 and PaO_2 and narrower $AaPO_2$ with the former. In part these findings represent relative hyperventilation with arm exercise, probably due to the demonstrably greater lactate production, which in turn results from the smaller exercising muscle bulk.[21]

7.1.5 Limiting factors and fitness

In health the limit to increasing exercise is set by cardiovascular and peripheral muscle function rather than by ventilatory function. The maximum heart rate predicted from the subject's age (see p. 124) is approached by a normal subject at the breaking point of exercise. In contrast, comparison of the maximum ventilation attained on exercise with what can be achieved voluntarily shows that normal subjects reach only between one-half and three-quarters of their ventilatory capacity at the breaking point of exercise, i.e. normally there is an appreciable 'ventilatory reserve'.

In patients with airway obstruction, the maximum voluntary ventilation predicted by multiplying FEV_1 by 35 considerably underestimates the maximum that can be achieved on exercise, which, in this population, is given more realistically by:

$$\text{Maximum exercise } \dot{V}_E = (FEV_1 \times 18.9) + 19.7$$

$$(7.3)$$

(or, for ease of memory,[1] $(FEV_1 \times 20) + 20$).

In disease the limit(s) to exercise are frequently multifactorial and often depend on the sensations perceived in addition to likely physiological limits. In cardiac disease the stroke volume is most often the limiting factor (provided that angina does not lead to premature termination of exercise), but deconditioning and impaired peripheral muscle function may be contributory. In lung disease, pulmonary mechanics, hypoxaemia due to abnormal gas exchange, and weakness of the respiratory muscles may all be important, with peripheral muscle deconditioning and impaired cardiovascular fitness also sometimes contributing. In practice it can be very difficult to distinguish general deconditioning (unfitness) associated with a sedentary lifestyle from early or mild cardiac disease.[22]

The concept of 'fitness' is easy to understand but more difficult to define precisely. With training, normal subjects achieve more exercise as a result of a combination of factors. A larger stroke volume and ejection fraction, improved muscle blood flow, increased muscle bulk and cellular metabolic adaptations may all contribute. In physiological studies, the degree of fitness is quantified by measuring the maximum oxygen uptake at exhausting exercise. This is often not feasible in clinical studies and the $\dot{V}O_2$max used to define maximum performance is more correctly termed the peak $\dot{V}O_2$ or 'symptom limited $\dot{V}O_2$max'.

7.2 PROGRESSIVE EXERCISE TESTS

7.2.1 Methodology

Most static tests of lung function can be performed by a technician or clinical physiologist, but formal exercise testing usually requires the presence of a physician. Although fatalities are very rare, cardiac dysrhythmias are not infrequent in middle-aged patients and occasionally require intervention. It is important that the patient be allowed to terminate the test if he or she develops distressing symptoms. Continuous monitoring of the electrocardiogram (ECG) should be the rule for patients with suspected cardiac disease and for all over the age of 40 years.

Detailed cardiopulmonary exercise tests require either a bicycle ergometer or a treadmill. Each has its advantages: use of a bicycle is less prone to movement artefacts, and exercise is easier to standardize as the external work rate is more readily quantified, but it is less familiar to many middle-aged patients and it puts relatively more strain on the leg muscles. A treadmill allows more natural exercise but is less convenient for use with a mouthpiece and noseclip and sometimes more difficult for the patient to stop if distressing symptoms develop.

Progressive exercise tests are usually performed using standard increments of power output, e.g. 10 W, 15 W or 25 W, with periods of 1–3 min at each level. Alternatively a 'ramp' protocol can be used in which the work rate is increased continuously but very gradually. This can result in a higher peak work rate but the overall physiological responses to the two types of incremental test are similar.[2,23] The measurements usually made are heart rate, ventilation, oxygen uptake, CO_2 production and oxygen saturation. Values can be averaged over the last 15–30 s of each period or recorded on a breath-by-breath basis, provided that rapidly responding gas analysers are used. It is important to note that oximeters can over- or underestimate SaO_2 in normal subjects on heavy exercise, possibly related to local perfusion, and

similar errors may be relevant to patients, particularly those in whom there is any circulatory limitation.[24] Although the conditions of progressive exercise testing are strictly non-steady-state, reproducible results are usually obtained and appropriate reference values are available.[25–28] It may be useful for the subject to record the severity of breathlessness at the end of each increment using one of the methods described in Section 7.5.2.

The subject is encouraged to continue exercising until symptoms become very uncomfortable or until instructed to stop by the operator (e.g. if certain ECG changes are observed). In most cases patients discontinue exercise because of breathlessness or discomfort in the legs (or both). If the subject feels faint or develops chest pain suggestive of ischaemia, the test should be terminated.

7.2.2 Evaluation of results

The results are assessed in terms of (i) the maximal values achieved (particularly peak $\dot{V}O_2$, ventilation and heart rate) and (ii) their interrelations during submaximal exercise. Strictly, maximum oxygen uptake requires demonstration that a plateau has been reached, but in practice the peak exercise $\dot{V}O_2$ ('symptom-limited $\dot{V}O_2$max) is taken as equivalent. Its value depends on body size and declines with age. Sometimes $\dot{V}O_2$max is 'normalized' by expressing it in terms of body size or weight ($\dot{V}O_2$/kg), but this does not 'normalize' fully as smaller individuals have higher weight-corrected values and obese individuals have lower values.[2]

Submaximal values of the various physiological measurements can be evaluated in many different ways, most commonly by plotting them against the simultaneous $\dot{V}O_2$ as an indication of the 'metabolic load'. The externally measured work rate (in watts) can be used as an alternative, but the relation between $\dot{V}O_2$ and workload varies between individuals, due particularly to variations in body weight. Obesity adds to the 'cost' of exercise such that the relationship between $\dot{V}O_2$ and work rate is displaced upwards in obese people, i.e. to a higher $\dot{V}O_2$ for a given work rate, although the slope of the graph is not affected.

A large number of different displays can be generated from a single progressive exercise test. The comprehensive example in Fig. 7.5 is taken from

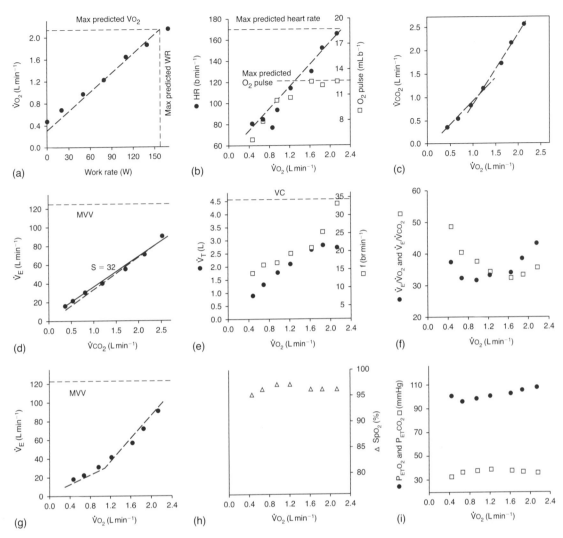

Figure 7.5 Various measurements obtained during progressive exercise to symptom-limited maximum in a healthy elderly individual. Points represent average values during 1 min at each workload. See text for explanation. Redrawn from ref. 2, with permission from the American Thoracic Society.

a recent guideline produced by the American Thoracic Society and the American College of Chest Physicians – but many other combinations of measurements can be examined instead of, or in addition to, the nine illustrated. In this example, Fig. 7.5a illustrates the relation of $\dot{V}O_2$ to work rate and all bar one of the other plots relate various measurements to $\dot{V}O_2$. Figure 7.5b shows the heart rate and oxygen pulse with superimposed an indication of the average predicted maxima for the individual concerned. Figure 7.5c shows the curvilinear (or biphasic) relation between $\dot{V}CO_2$ and

$\dot{V}O_2$ with linear regressions plotted through the data points of the two phases. The point of intersection represents one estimate of the AT ('V slope' method[29]). Figure 7.5d shows the more nearly rectilinear relation of ventilation to $\dot{V}CO_2$ (cf. Fig. 7.2). The plot of tidal volume and breathing frequency (7.5e) shows the tendency for a maximum V_T to develop (cf. Fig. 7.1b). In Fig. 7.5f ventilatory equivalents for both oxygen and CO_2 are plotted; the $\dot{V}O_2$ at the nadir $\dot{V}_E/\dot{V}O_2$ gives an alternative estimate of AT (ventilatory equivalents method[30]). Figure 7.5g–i illustrates respectively

Table 7.2 Typical patterns of functional abnormality during progressive exercise in various conditions

	Peak values			Submaximal values				
	Vo_2max	Ventilatory reserve[†]	HR_{max}	$\dot{V}_E$*	HR*	AT	V_D/V_T	Pao_2/Sao_2[‡]
COPD	↓	0 or ↓	↓	↑ or →	↑	→(↓)	↑	→ or ↓
ILD	↓	↓		↑	↑	→(↓)	↑	↓
CHF	↓	↓ or →	→(↓ if severe)	↑	↑	↓	↑	→
PVD	↓	→	→	↑	↑	↓	↑	↓
Unfitness	↓	→	→	↑(→)	↑	↓(→)	→	→
Psychogenic breathlessness	↓	↑ or →	↓	↑	↑ or →	→	→	→

*In relation to Vo_2.

[†]Maximum voluntary ventilation (MVV) (predicted from forced expiratory volume in 1 s, FEV_1) minus maximum exercise ventilation.

↓, lower than predicted (bracketed arrows indicate less common pattern).

↑, higher than predicted (bracketed arrows indicate less common pattern).

→, similar to predicted (bracketed arrows indicate less common pattern).

[‡]Compared with resting values.

AT, anaerobic threshold; CHF, congestive heart failure; COPD, chronic obstructive pulmonary disease; HR, heart rate; ILD, interstitial lung disease; Pao_2, arterial oxygen tension; PVD, pulmonary vascular disease; Sao_2, oxygen saturation; V_D/V_T, dead space/tidal volume ratio; $\dot{V}_E$, maximum expiratory flow.

ventilation (with 'MVV' predicted from FEV_1), oxygen saturation and end tidal gas tensions.

7.2.3　Patterns of abnormality in disease

The approach to evaluating the response to exercise depends on the reason for performing the test. Some of the common indications are listed in Table 7.1. One of the commonest is as an aid to the differential diagnosis of breathlessness. In this situation the approach is one of pattern recognition, as certain characteristic patterns are associated with the commoner pathological causes of breathlessness (Table 7.2). However, the distinctions are often fuzzy and most types of abnormality are seen in more than one type of disease. It is important to make use of collateral information, such as the results of imaging and cardiological investigations, as well as resting lung function measurements.

7.3　'STEADY-STATE' EXERCISE TESTS

Historically, 'steady-state' exercise testing was employed when detailed analysis of gas exchange on exercise was desired, as the relatively slow responses of earlier gas analysers demanded stable signals. Modern rapidly responding analysers largely obviate the need for this as they allow valid assessment of rapidly changing signals (e.g. breath by breath) during progressive exercise. High-intensity, constant-load exercise still has advantages over progressive

exercise tests in certain contexts. In particular, it has been shown to be of value as a sensitive method for repeat studies following various interventions – e.g. in monitoring the effects of drugs,[31] rehabilitation or lung-volume-reduction surgery. Steady-state testing is also the appropriate method for analysing ventilatory mechanics during exercise, in particular with use of measurements of inspiratory capacity and comparisons of tidal and maximum flow to detect the evolution of expiratory flow limitation and dynamic hyperinflation.[32] A steady-state test is usually preceded by a progressive exercise test to determine the individual's capacity, and a work rate of 50–70 per cent of the maximum achieved is then employed. For detailed gas exchange analysis the subject needs to exercise for about 6 min before a reasonably steady state is achieved. Alternatively, when assessing therapeutic interventions, the duration of exercise at the same workload pre- and post- may be used, often in combination with assessment of breathlessness (see Section 7.5).

7.4　WALK TESTS

7.4.1　Self-paced walk tests

Walking with the patient up and down a hospital corridor while monitoring oxygen saturation may be sufficient to determine whether significant desaturation occurs, particularly in more disabled people. Stair-climbing is a traditional method for assessing the fitness of patients for thoracic surgery[33] and has some prognostic significance.[34] In recent years, measurement of the maximum distance walked in a fixed period has become a popular way of assessing performance in individuals with moderate or severe respiratory disability. Initially the 12-min walking distance was proposed,[35] but subsequently shorter distances have been employed,[36] with most now using the 6-min walk test (6 MWT).[37] The patient is instructed simply to walk as quickly as he or she can for the prescribed period over a previously marked distance on the level (usually a hospital corridor). The patient is allowed to stop at his or her own discretion because of symptoms, but the time of any rest is included in the period of the test. The 6 MWT has the advantages over progressive exercise testing using a cycle or treadmill that equipment requirements are minimal and that little technical expertise is needed. Also, a self-paced walk test relates more closely to the normal activities of daily living than do maximal tests. The results do, however, correlate moderately well with measurements of $\dot{V}O_2max$.[38] One or two practice tests are advised as the distance walked tends to increase with experience,[39] and encouragement during the test should be standardized.[40] Indications for 6 MWT include evaluating the effects of therapeutic interventions, quantifying functional status, predicting morbidity pre-surgery and determining the optimal time for lung transplantation. In relation to therapeutic interventions, it has been estimated that the minimal clinically significant difference in distance walked between two tests is 54 m and, in general, a difference greater than 70 m is required for confident recognition of improvement.[41] The distance walked by healthy subjects varies with age, height, weight and sex, and appropriate reference equations are available.[42,43]

7.4.2 Shuttle walk tests

In the incremental shuttle walk test,[44] the subject walks at up to 12 increasing speeds along a 10-m distance, with the speed increasing each minute and controlled by audio signals. The test is terminated when the subject becomes too breathless to maintain the required speed or fails to complete a shuttle in the time allowed. The test is therefore closer than the 6 MWT to a symptom-limited test

on a cycle ergometer and the results correlate well with $\dot{V}O_2max$.[45] An endurance shuttle walk test, analogous to steady-state exercise using a bicycle ergometer, has also been developed;[46] its performance relates well to the outcome of rehabilitation in patients with chronic obstructive pulmonary disease (COPD).

7.5 ASSESSMENT OF BREATHLESSNESS

7.5.1 Physiological background

Breathlessness is the predominant symptom of patients with abnormal respiratory function. In general, patients complain of breathlessness because ventilation is either excessive or difficult.[47] In the latter case the difficulty may reflect an abnormal 'load' (high resistance, low compliance) or impaired capacity (e.g. muscle weakness or hyperinflation impairing the mechanical advantage of the respiratory muscles) or both. Some authorities distinguish 'dyspnoea' from 'breathlessness', but in effect the terms are interchangeable when used to describe the symptom as opposed to the breathlessness experienced by normal subjects during exercise.

The sensation described as 'breathlessness' varies considerably in quality between individuals. The sensation appreciated by a patient with asthma, for instance, is very different from that perceived by individuals with pulmonary fibrosis, cardiac failure or respiratory muscle weakness. These differences have been analysed both in model situations in healthy subjects[48] and in patients with different conditions[49] by presenting them with a number of phrases describing the nature of the sensation experienced and asking them to choose those terms that most closely resemble that sensation. When the responses are subjected to cluster analysis, recognizable patterns emerge that correspond broadly to the different ventilatory stimuli used (in model situations) or to the type of disease and corresponding mechanical abnormality present. For example, patients with reduced pulmonary compliance identify terms related to rapid breathing, while patients with airway obstruction choose the terms that identify wheeziness or distress.[50] With such a complexity of sensations and terminology, it is perhaps surprising that precise and reasonably reproducible measurements of 'breathlessness' can be obtained, but presumably this results from consistency of the sensation within individuals.

Although breathlessness can arise from many causes, it appears to depend ultimately on the perception of respiratory effort and the psychological reaction to that effort. Attempts to define a unique neurological pathway have been unsuccessful, but there is clear evidence that afferent information from the respiratory muscles is a necessary component. In general, the level of breathlessness depends on the appropriateness of the proprioceptive information received in relation to awareness of the motor output driving ventilation.

Detailed analysis in patients with various cardiorespiratory diseases shows that the severity of breathlessness can be related to several aspects of mechanical performance of the respiratory system.[51,52] The variables that have been shown to affect severity include: (i) inspiratory pleural pressure as a proportion of $P_I$max – an index of the force of inspiratory contraction in relation to the capacity of the inspiratory muscles; (ii) peak inspiratory flow – an index of the velocity of shortening of the inspiratory muscles; (iii) tidal volume divided by vital capacity – an index of the degree of contraction of the muscles; (iv) breathing frequency, i.e. number of contractions per minute; and (v) T_I/T_{TOT} – the 'duty cycle', which indicates the proportion of each breath during which the inspiratory muscles contract. The independent relations between breathlessness and each of these variables describe in mathematical terms how the intensity of effort required to produce a given level of ventilation increases in various circumstances: when resistance increases or compliance decreases, when the muscles are weak, when their velocity of contraction increases or when their capacity is impaired due to shortening (e.g. when the lungs are hyperinflated).

Afferent information from extraneous sources is also relevant to the intensity of the sensation, as exemplified by the demonstration in normal subjects in whom breathlessness was induced by either CO_2 or resistance breathing that blowing cold air on the cheeks reduces the sensation without affecting ventilation.[53] This finding corresponds to the well-known clinical benefit of airflow over the face of patients with severe respiratory distress.

Table 7.3 Modified Borg scale[55,56]

0	Nothing at all (just noticeable)
0.5	Very, very slight
1	Very slight
2	Slight
3	Moderate
4	Somewhat severe
5	Severe
6	
7	Very severe
8	
9	Very, very severe (almost maximal)
10	Maximal

7.5.2 Methods of measurement of breathlessness

The Medical Research Council (MRC) scale describes breathlessness in relation to the activities of everyday life. Although relatively crude, the MRC grades correlate with performance in a shuttle walk test.[54] When breathlessness is assessed during clinical exercise testing, one of two simple semi-quantitative methods is usually applied. In the Borg scale of perceived exertion,[55,56] the subject is presented with a non-linear numerical scale corresponding to adjectives describing the severity of the relevant symptom (Table 7.3). This represents a 'category scale' from which the subject is asked to choose the description closest to severity of the symptom. With the alternative visual analogue scale (VAS),[57] the subject is presented with a straight line of 10- or 20-cm length with descriptions only at either end, usually 'not at all breathless' and 'extremely breathless'. The upper limit may be related to an individually set maximum such as that recognized during a standard period of heavy exercise or the end of a CO_2 rebreathing manoeuvre.[57] More commonly, the maximum point is not 'anchored' in this way but is left for the individual to interpret in relation to his or her subjective experience. Other exercise-related symptoms such as leg discomfort can be assessed similarly.

Borg or VAS measurements are most commonly obtained at intervals during progressive exercise, but they can also be measured during steady-state exercise. Measurements may be influenced by the type of exercise undertaken. During steady-state exercise, ventilatory measurements are more or

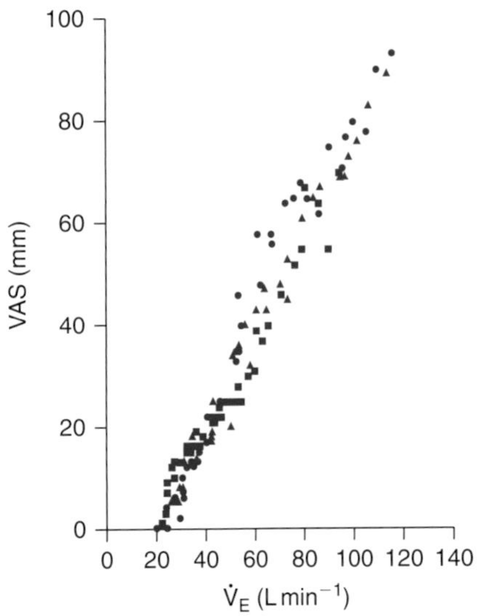

Figure 7.6 Relation of visual analogue scale (VAS) score for breathlessness to ventilation during progressive exercise in a normal subject. Three separate exercise tests are shown (■, ▲, ●). Note the threshold level of ventilation below which no breathlessness is scored and the consistent linear relation above this threshold.

less stable after 4 min but the severity of breathlessness at a given level of exercise continues to rise after this period, independent of ventilation.[58] This finding suggests that the sensation reported may be influenced by other factors such as fatigue during prolonged exercise testing.

The methods of measuring 'breathlessness' are applicable equally to the 'normal' breathlessness experienced by healthy subjects during exercise and to the symptomatic breathlessness of patients with cardiorespiratory disease. If the level of breathlessness (VAS) is plotted against ventilation during progressive exercise, normal subjects exhibit a threshold level of ventilation below which no breathlessness is scored. Once the threshold is exceeded the relation of VAS to ventilation is approximately linear (Fig. 7.6). Within an individual the relation of breathlessness to ventilation is usually tightly coupled, but they can be dissociated artificially, e.g. by having the subject breathe through a resistance, when the degree of breathlessness increases for a given ventilation.[57]

Variation between healthy individuals in the level of breathlessness resulting from a given stimulus or a given level of ventilation is large. There is a weak relation between the intensity of breathlessness and overall level of fitness,[59] but there appears to be no relation between magnitude of the breathlessness response to ventilation and the ventilatory response to chemical stimuli.[59]

The choice between VAS and Borg assessments is an individual one. The results are closely related, both in normal subjects and in patients with airway disease.[60,61] Studies of reproducibility of each technique have shown a tendency for reduced responses to ventilation on repeat testing in the short term,[60,62] emphasizing the need for a control group or placebo when studying the effects of any interventions. Over longer periods, reproducibility using the Borg method in healthy subjects is good,[63] though some authors have reported that reproducibility of VAS measurements is better.[64]

REFERENCES

1 Jones NL. *Clinical Exercise Testing*, 3rd edn, W.B. Saunders, London, 1987.
2 American Thoracic Society/American College of Chest Physicians. ATS/ACCP statement on cardiopulmonary exercise testing. *Am J Respir Crit Care Med* 2003; **167**: 211–77.
3 Wasserman K, Hansen JE, Sue D, Stringer D, Whipp BJ. *Principles of Exercise Testing and Interpretation*, 4th edn, Lippincott, Williams & Wilkins, Philadelphia, PA, 2005.
4 Palange P, Ward SA, Carlsen, K-H, *et al.* Recommendations on the use of clinical exercise testing in clinical practice. *Eur Respir J* 2007; **29**: 185–209.
5 Johnson BD, Saupe KW, Dempsey JA. Mechanical constraints on exercise hyperpnoea in endurance athletes. *J Appl Physiol* 1992; **73**:874–86.
6 Dantzker DR, Foreman B, Gutierrez G. Oxygen supply and utilization relationships: a reevaluation. *Am Rev Respir Dis* 1991; **143**: 675–9.
7 Clode M, Campbell EJM. The relationship between gas exchange and changes in blood lactate concentration during exercise. *Clin Sci* 1969; **37**: 263–72.
8 Myers J, Ashley E. Dangerous curves: a perspective on exercise, lactate and the anaerobic threshold. *Chest* 1997; **111**: 787–95.
9 Hagberg JM, Coyle EF, Carroll JE, *et al.* Exercise hyperventilation in patients with McArdle's disease. *J Appl Physiol* 1982; **52**: 991–4.
10 Gowda K, Zintel T, McFarland C, Orchard R, Gallagher CG. Diagnostic value of maximum exercise tidal volume. *Chest* 1990; **98**: 1351–4.

11 Stubbing DG, Pengelly LD, Morse JLC, Jones NL. Pulmonary mechanics during exercise in normal males. *J Appl Physiol* 1980; **49**: 506–10.

12 Johnson BD, Badr MS, Dempsey JA. Impact of the aging pulmonary system on the response to exercise. *Clin Chest Med* 1994; **15**:229–46.

13 DeLorey DS, Babb TG. Progressive mechanical ventilatory constraints with aging. *Am J Respir Crit Care Med* 1999; **160**: 169–77.

14 Jones NL, McHardy GJR, Nalmark A, *et al.* Physiological dead space and alveolar arterial gas pressure differences during exercise. *Clin Sci* 1966; **31**: 19–29.

15 Lewis DA, Sietsema KE, Casaburi R, Sue DY. Inaccuracy of non-invasive estimates of V_D/V_T in clinical exercise testing. *Chest* 1994; **106**: 1476–80.

16 Astrand P-O, Cuddy TE, Saltin B, Stenberg J. Cardiac output during submaximal and maximal work. *J Appl Physiol* 1964; **19**: 268–74.

17 Cotes JE, Berry G, Burkinshaw L, *et al.* Cardiac frequency during submaximal exercise in young adults; relation to lean body mass, total body potassium and amount of leg muscle. *Q J Exp Physiol* 1973; **58**: 239–50.

18 Dempsey JA, Wagner PD. Exercise-induced arterial hypoxaemia. *J Appl Physiol* 1999; **87**: 1997–2006.

19 Strickland MK, Welsh RC, Haykowsky MJ, *et al.* Intrapulmonary shunt and pulmonary gas exchange during exercise in humans. *J Physiol* 2004; **561**: 321–9.

20 Huang Y-CT, O'Brien SR, MacIntyre NR. Intrabreath diffusing capacity of the lung in healthy individuals at rest and during exercise. *Chest* 2002; **122**: 177–85.

21 Martin TW, Zeballos RJ, Weisman IM. Gas exchange during maximal upper extremity exercise. *Chest* 1991; **99**: 420–25.

22 Martinez FJ, Stanopoulos I, Acero R, *et al.* Graded comprehensive cardiopulmonary exercise testing in the evaluation of dyspnoea unexplained by routine evaluation. *Chest* 1994; **105**: 168–74.

23 Revill SM, Beck KE, Morgan MD. Comparison of the peak exercise response measured by the ramp and 1-min step cycle exercise protocols in patients with exertional dyspnea. *Chest* 2002; **121**: 1099–105.

24 Hansen JE, Casaburi R. Validity of ear oximetry in clinical exercise testing. *Chest* 1987; **91**: 333–7.

25 Jones NL, Makrides L, Hitchcock C, Chypchar T, McCartney N. Normal standards for an incremental progressive cycle ergometer test. *Am Rev Respir Dis* 1985; **131**: 700–708.

26 Blackie SR, Fairbarn MS, McElvaney NG, *et al.* Normal values and ranges for ventilation and breathing pattern at maximal exercise. *Chest* 1991; **100**: 136–42.

27 Hansen JE, Sue DY, Wasserman K. Predicted values for clinical exercise testing. *Am Rev Respir Dis* 1984; **129**: 549–55.

28 Neder JA, Nery LE, Peres C, Whipp BJ. Reference values for dynamic responses to incremental cycle ergometry in males and females aged 20 to 80. *Am J Respir Crit Care Med* 2001; **164**: 1481–6.

29 Sue DY, Wasserman K, Moricca RB, Casaburi R. Metabolic acidosis during exercise in patients with chronic obstructive pulmonary disease: use of the V-slope method for anaerobic threshold determination. *Chest* 1988; **94**: 931–8.

30 Belman MJ, Epstein LJ, Doornbos D, *et al.* Non-invasive determinations of the anaerobic threshold: reliability and validity in patients with COPD. *Chest* 1992; **102**: 1028–34.

31 Oga T, Nishimura K, Tsukino M, *et al.* The effects of oxitropium bromide on exercise performance in patients with chronic obstructive pulmonary disease: a comparison of three different exercise tests. *Am J Respir Crit Care Med* 2000; **161**: 1897–901.

32 O'Donnell DE, Revill SM, Webb KA. Dynamic hyperinflation and exercise intolerance in chronic obstructive pulmonary disease. *Am J Respir Crit Care Med* 2001; **164**: 770–77.

33 Bolton JWR, Weisman DS, Haynes JL, *et al.* Stair climbing as an indicator of pulmonary function. *Chest* 1987; **92**: 783–8.

34 Olsen G, Bolton JWR, Weisman DS, Hornung CA. Stair climbing as an exercise test to predict the post-operative complications of lung resection: two years' experience. *Chest* 1991; **99**: 587–90.

35 McGavin CR, Gupta SP, McHardy GJR. Twelve-minute walking test for assessing disability in chronic bronchitis. *Br Med J* 1976; **1**: 822–3.

36 Butland RJA, Pang J, Gross ER, Woodcock AA, Geddes DM. Two, six and 12 minute walking tests in respiratory disease. *Br Med J* 1982; **284**: 1607.

37 American Thoracic Society. ATS statement: guidelines for the six-minute walk test. *Am J Crit Care Med* 2002; **166**: 111–17.

38 Solway S, Brooks D, Lacasse Y, Thomas S. A qualitative systematic overview of the measurement properties of functional walk tests used in the cardiorespiratory domain. *Chest* 2001; **119**: 256–70.

39 Knox AJ, Morrison JFJ, Muers MF. Reproducibility of walking test results in chronic obstructive airways disease. *Thorax* 1988; **43**: 388–92.

40 Guyatt GH, Pugsley SO, Sullivan MJ, *et al.* Effect of encouragement on walking test performance. *Thorax* 1984; **39**: 818–22.

41 Redelmeier DA, Bayoumi AM, Goldstein RS, Guyatt GH. Interpreting small differences in

functional status: the six minute walk test in chronic lung disease patients. *Am J Respir Crit Care Med* 1997; **155**: 1278–82.

42 Enright PL, Sherrill DL. Reference equations for the six-minute walk in healthy adults. *Am J Respir Crit Care Med* 2000; **158**: 1384–7.

43 Enright PL, McBurnie MA, Bittner V, *et al*. The 6-minute walk test: a quick measure of functional status in elderly adults. *Chest* 2003; **123**: 387–98.

44 Singh SJ, Morgan MD, Scott S, Walters C, Hardman AE. Development of a shuttle walking test of disability in patients with chronic airways obstruction. *Thorax* 1992; **47**: 1019–24.

45 Singh SJ, Morgan MD, Hardman AE, Rowe C, Bardsley PA. Comparison of oxygen uptake during a conventional treadmill test and the shuttle walking test in chronic airflow limitation. *Eur Respir J* 1994; 7: 2016–20.

46 Revill SM, Morgan MD, Singh SJ, Williams J, Hardman AE. The endurance shuttle walk: a new field test for the assessment of endurance capacity in chronic obstructive pulmonary disease. *Thorax* 1999; **54**: 213–22.

47 Campbell EJM, Howell JBL. The sensation of breathlessness. *Br Med Bull* 1963; **19**: 36–40.

48 Simon PM, Schwartzstein RM, Weiss JW, *et al*. Distinguishable sensations of breathlessness induced in normal volunteers. *Am Rev Respir Dis* 1989; **140**: 1021–7.

49 Simon PM, Schwartzstein RM, Weiss JW, *et al*. Distinguishable types of dyspnea in patients with shortness of breath. *Am Rev Respir Dis* 1990; **142**: 1009–14.

50 Elliott MW, Adams L, Cockcroft A, *et al*. The language of breathlessness: use of verbal descriptors by patients with cardiopulmonary disease. *Am Rev Respir Dis* 1991; **144**: 826–32.

51 Leblanc P, Bowie DM, Summers E, Jones NL, Killian KJ. Breathlessness and exercise in patients with cardiorespiratory disease. *Am Rev Respir Dis* 1986; **133**: 21–5.

52 Mahler DA, Faryniarz K, Lentine T, *et al*. Measurement of breathlessness during exercise in asthmatics: predictor variables, reliability and responsiveness. *Am Rev Respir Dis* 1991; **144**: 39–44.

53 Schwartzstein RW, Lahive K, Pope A, Weinberger SE, Weiss JW. Cold facial stimulation reduces breathlessness induced in normal subjects. *Am Rev Respir Dis* 1987; **136**: 58–61.

54 Bestall JC, Paul EA, Garrod R, *et al*. Usefulness of the Medical Research Council (MRC) dyspnoea scale as a measure of disability in patients with chronic obstructive pulmonary disease. *Thorax* 1999; **54**: 581–6.

55 Borg G. Psychophysical bases of perceived exertion. *Med Sci Sports Exerc* 1982; **14**: 377–81.

56 Mahler DA, Rosiello RA, Harver A, *et al*. Comparison of clinical dyspnoea ratings and psychophysical measurements of respiratory sensation in obstructive airway disease. *Am Rev Respir Dis* 1987; **135**: 1229–33.

57 Stark RD, Gambles SA, Lewis JQ. Methods to assess breathlessness in healthy subjects. *Clin Sci* 1981; **61**: 429–39.

58 O'Neill PA, Stark RD, Allen SC, Stretton TB. The relationship between breathlessness and ventilation during steady-state exercise. *Clin Respir Physiol* 1986; **22**: 247–50.

59 Adams L, Chronos N, Lane R, Guz A. The measurement of breathlessness induced in normal subjects: individual differences. *Clin Sci* 1986; **70**: 131–40.

60 Wilson RC, Jones PW. A comparison of the visual analogue scale and modified Borg scale for the measurement of dyspnoea during exercise. *Clin Sci* 1989; **76**: 277–82.

61 Muza SR, Silverman MT, Gilmore GC, Hellerstein HK, Kelsen SG. Comparison of scales used to quantitate the sense of effort to breathe in patients with chronic obstructive pulmonary disease. *Am Rev Respir Dis* 1990; **141**: 909–13.

62 Belman MJ, Brooks LR, Ross DJ, Mohsenifar Z. Variability of breathlessness measurement in patients with chronic obstructive pulmonary disease. *Chest* 1991; **99**: 566–71.

63 Wilson RC, Jones PW. Long term reproducibility of Borg scale estimated of breathlessness during exercise. *Clin Sci* 1991; **80**: 309–12.

64 Grant S, Aitchison T, Henderson E, *et al*. A comparison of the reproducibility and the sensitivity to change of visual analogue scales, Borg scales, and Likert scales in normal subjects during submaximal exercise. *Chest* 1999; **116**: 1208–17.

8

Normal Variation

Variations in lung function between and within individuals result from several factors, many of which may need to be taken into account in the interpretation of clinical data. For the commonly performed tests, a number of equations based on large populations of healthy individuals are available, from which an average predicted or reference value can be calculated. For most tests, the reference equations incorporate factors for sex, age and body size (usually represented by height); account may, however, also need to be taken of ethnic variation, body weight, the posture of the subject or the time of day when the test was performed. Summarized here are some of the more important causes of variation between and within normal subjects as a background against which changes in disease need to be viewed.

8.1 EFFECTS OF BODY AND LUNG SIZE

8.1.1 Effects on lung volumes

Large individuals generally have large lungs, with the total lung capacity varying as much as three-fold in the healthy adult population. The effect of size is due mainly to differences in the total number of alveoli, and the consequent variation is reflected in all the subdivisions of lung volume, including the FEV_1. Stature is the most appropriate

and convenient index of body size to use for predicting most lung volumes. Bodyweight or body mass index (BMI) has little effect independent of height in individuals in the normal and mildly overweight range. Exceptions are the effect of weight on FRC and expiratory reserve volume (ERV), which, because of the important influence of the abdomen on the position of the diaphragm, are smaller in overweight individuals. Over the BMI range $20–30\,kg\,m^{-2}$, FRC falls by about 25 per cent and ERV by about one-half.[1] Use of BMI in reference equations, however, takes no account of the relative contributions of fat and muscle or of the distribution of body fat. The greater the proportion of fat,[2] and, particularly, of abdominal fat,[3] the more effect overweight has on the usual spirometric lung volumes (FEV_1, VC). The effects of frank obesity (BMI $>30\,kg\,m^{-2}$) are described in Chapter 24, Section 24.1.

The effect of variations in lung size is seen also in measurements, such as the single-breath carbon monoxide diffusing capacity (D_LCO), that are directly dependent on lung volume. KCO (D_LCO per litre alveolar volume), however, is independent of size. As would be expected, variation in body size also affects oxygen consumption and carbon dioxide (CO_2) output, but other effects may be less obvious, e.g. the variation between healthy subjects in measurements of pulmonary compliance[4] and the ventilatory responses to CO_2[5] and hypoxia[6] can all be reduced by scaling for body or lung size.

8.1.2 Effects on airway function

The effect of body size on airway function is less clear-cut. Since the airways and alveoli have different embryological origins, some disproportion might be expected. This effect is seen, for example, with the FEV_1/VC ratio, which tends to be slightly lower in very tall healthy individuals with large lung volumes. Over a large range of heights airway and lung size correlate weakly with each other, but within narrower ranges of body size there can be considerable variation in their relative function. It might be expected that the large normal variation in maximum expiratory flows at a particular volume (e.g. 50% VC) would be reduced by dividing by the absolute lung volume in order to correct for variations in lung size. In practice, however, this has little effect in reducing the variance in adults,[7] although between children of widely different sizes the expectation is borne out.[8] In adult subjects of similar size, relationships have been shown between both $\dot{V}_E$max at high lung volumes and FEV_1 and tracheal dimensions assessed radiographically,[9] but incorporation of large airway size in the prediction of $\dot{V}_E$max has only a minor effect.[10]

8.1.3 Size corrections

It is important to distinguish volume correction used to take account of variation in body size *between* individuals from correction for measurements made at different lung volumes *within* an individual. For example, calculation of specific airway conductance allows both of these, but use of specific compliance is valid only for comparison between subjects because, whereas airway conductance increases with lung volume in both senses, compliance is greater in larger lungs but in an individual it decreases as lung volume increases.

In clinical lung function testing, size correction of measurements of volume or flow can be applied in two ways, with very different implications. For example, the common convention of expressing lung volumes as percentages of the predicted values aims to take account of variations in body size; in effect it brings together midgets and giants without concealing any changes in lung function induced by disease. Instead of litres or litres per second, the units are 'per cent predicted TLC (VC)' or 'predicted TLCs (VCs) per second'. It

should be noted, however, that, if a group of individuals with a particular disease is being compared with a group of healthy subjects, the results from the latter should also be expressed in relation to the predicted TLC for each, a point that is sometimes glossed over by 'forcing' every normal subject to have a 'predicted' value of 100 per cent.

Where a measurement is itself dependent on the lung volume at which it is made (e.g. maximum flow or lung recoil pressure), it can also be related to volume as a percentage of the measured TLC (or VC). This mode of expression as 'per cent actual TLC (VC)' is a relative scale – a means of assessing whether changes in the given variable are proportionally less or more than the changes in lung volume. This is rarely an appropriate means of assessing abnormalities in disease and it requires theoretical justification before it is applied. One situation where it may be valid is after pneumonectomy, where clearly the predicted TLC for two lungs is no longer relevant.

8.2 EFFECTS OF GENDER

Many of the normal sex differences in respiratory function result from differences in body size but, even after taking account of size, important differences are seen with some tests. After adolescence the VC and TLC of boys exceed those of girls of similar height, with most of the difference attributable to differences in proportions of the body frame.[11] For a given stature men have larger lungs than women, due to a greater complement of alveoli: differences in airway size are less marked and consequently the FEV_1/VC ratio tends to be slightly less in men.[12] Maximum respiratory pressures are greater in men than in women,[13] and this also explains the greater maximum lung recoil pressure in men.[14] Variation in pulmonary compliance parallels the differences in volume,[4] as does the CO diffusing capacity, but K_{CO} is similar in the two sexes.[15] Breathing and oxygenation during sleep in men and women of normal build are similar.[16]

8.3 GENETIC INFLUENCES

After correction for stature, marked differences in lung function are seen between races, with subjects of European origin generally having values of VC and TLC up to 10–15 per cent larger than non-European people. Small lung volumes are seen particularly in south Indians, sub-Saharan Africans and Australian aborigines people.[17] As with the effect of gender, it appears that differences in body frame and proportions are important in determining the total complement of alveoli, as size-independent indices of lung distensibility suggest no ethnic differences.[18]

Genetic influences on lung function have also been demonstrated by twin[19] and family studies.[20,21] FEV_1 and VC are more concordant between monozygotic than dizygotic twins,[19] but this may be determined largely by closer body height.[22] Ventilatory responses to both hypoxia and CO_2 appear to have a particularly strong genetic component.[23] Recent interest has focused on polymorphisms of specific genes that may relate to functional measurements and the rate at which these decline with age.[24]

8.4 ENVIRONMENTAL INFLUENCES

8.4.1 Intrauterine and early childhood events

Several studies have shown that low birth weight is associated with lower size-corrected FEV_1 and/or VC in later childhood and adult life,[25,26] suggesting that suboptimal lung development may be due to fetal undernutrition. One study has also reported lower D_LCO and exercise capacity at age 19 years in individuals born prematurely (<32 weeks' gestation) or with low birth weight (<1500 g).[27] However, an adverse effect of low birth weight has not been a universal finding, with some cohorts showing either no effect on later spirometric volumes[28] or a small effect that is no longer statistically significant after taking account of confounding socioeconomic factors.[29]

Neonatal lung disease or pneumonia in infants under the age of 2 years is associated more consistently with reductions in FEV_1 and VC in adult life.[26,28,30] In one large study of middle-aged subjects, average differences of 0.39 L and 0.6 L respectively were found between those with and without a history of infantile pneumonia.[28]

8.4.2 Altitude

The most obvious effects of altitude on respiratory function tests relate to reduction in inspired PO_2. Even at modest altitude this results in a lower PaO_2 and a need to adjust the normal range and consequently, also, the criteria for institution of oxygen therapy in patients with lung disease.[31] Concomitantly, the arterial PCO_2 is reduced as ventilation is stimulated by hypoxaemia. After ascent to altitude, breathing during non-rapid eye movement (REM) sleep shows more marked periodicity (resembling Cheyne–Stokes breathing), which is abolished by increasing the inspired PO_2 (see Chapter 6, Section 6.2.1).

High-altitude natives show several noteworthy differences from their compatriots born at sea level. Compensatory changes in oxygen-carrying capacity of the blood occur with the development of polycythaemia and a change in the P_{50}. Altitude natives also tend to have larger lung volumes than those born at sea level; this may be the result of hypoxia stimulating lung growth in early childhood, as has been demonstrated in experimental animals. A higher CO diffusing capacity is attributed to greater blood flow to the lung apices associated with higher pulmonary arterial pressure.[32] Chronic hypoxaemia has important effects on ventilatory drive: high-altitude natives have blunted responses to hypoxia,[33] and long-term residence at altitude by low-level natives appears to produce similar effects.[34]

Atmospheric air at altitude has a lower density than at sea level, resulting in an increase in maximum expiratory flow, especially at high lung volumes. Consequently, peak expiratory flow (PEF) is increased but the conventional peak flow meter underestimates PEF in this situation and a correction has to be applied if the true value is required.[35] FEV_1 and VC are not affected significantly by altitudes up to 2300 m.[36]

8.4.3 Diet and nutrition

Several epidemiological studies have shown that better spirometric function is associated with higher intake or blood levels of certain vitamins and minerals, although cause and effect cannot necessarily be inferred from the mainly cross-sectional studies reported to date. The most consistent apparently beneficial effects are seen with high intakes of fruit (particularly apples[37]), vitamins C and E[37,38] and β-carotene[39] and higher circulating levels of vitamin E.[40]

8.4.4 Atmospheric pollution

It is likely that exposure to atmospheric pollutants has important effects on respiratory function, but studies in this area are confounded by difficulties in accurate retrospective quantitation of both short- and long-term exposure to potentially noxious inhaled gases and particulates. Short-term exposure to ozone is known to produce an acute decline in spirometric indices,[41] and a preliminary study of university students in California suggested that estimated higher lifetime exposure to environmental ozone was associated with mildly impaired airway function.[42] A longitudinal study of New York firemen, in whom spirometric measurements were available before and after the collapse of the World Trade Center in 2001, showed a clear (average 0.37 L) reduction in FEV_1 during the year after exposure to the dust, with a dose–response effect as assessed by the intensity of exposure at the time of the disaster.[43]

Indoor atmospheric pollution is also relevant in some communities, particularly in countries where biomass is used as cooking fuel. This is associated with a high concentration of respirable particulates in the air, e.g. PM10 – particles with a diameter of 10 μm or less. In one study of non-smoking women in Mexico, FEV_1 and FEV_1/VC were lower in those using biomass-burning stoves than in those who cooked with gas, and FEV_1 was lower in those with higher domestic concentrations of PM10.[44]

8.4.5 Passive smoking

Maternal smoking is associated with lower FEV_1 and maximal expiratory flows in children and young adults.[45,46] The effect is probably due to exposure in utero as well as during childhood.[47,48] Similar effects have been shown in non-smoking adults regularly exposed to passive smoking either at home or in the workplace.[49]

8.4.6 Tobacco smoking

With active smoking we enter the grey area between normality and disease. Smoking is, however, so prevalent that a note needs to be made here of its 'normal' effects on lung function. Smoking-related airway disease is considered more fully in Chapter 9.

Even a single cigarette produces a measurable increase in the airway resistance of a normal subject, and this can persist for up to an hour.[50] Asymptomatic smokers as a group have lower FEV_1, VC, FEV_1/VC, maximum expiratory flows and CO diffusing capacity than non-smokers.[51,52] The effect on D_LCO is related partly to the higher carboxyhaemoglobin content of blood in smokers (account can be taken of this by estimating the 'back pressure' of CO by rebreathing from a bag), but there is an additional effect, probably due to a lower volume of blood in the pulmonary capillaries of smokers.[53] The difference between smokers and non-smokers is exaggerated if the measurement is made in the supine posture, when smokers may fail to demonstrate the expected rise in D_LCO and KCO.[54]

Much interest has centred on the relation between smoking and bronchial hyperresponsiveness (BHR) to non-specific stimuli such as histamine and methacholine. Bronchial responsiveness is distributed as a continuous variable in the community,[55] but, on average, apparently healthy smokers have greater responsiveness than non-smokers.[56] The level of BHR is related to both the amount smoked previously (pack-years) and the current consumption.[57] Although BHR has been demonstrated in smokers with normal spirometric function[58] or only subtle evidence of small airway dysfunction,[59] overall there is a strong relation with FEV_1,[56,58] even after excluding subjects outwith the usually accepted 'normal' range.[59] Confident attribution of cause and effect is, however, not yet possible as a relation between bronchial responsiveness and airway calibre would be expected for geometric reasons, as outlined in Chapter 1, Section 1.6.3.8. Conversely, it has been argued that the level of responsiveness may influence the harmful effects of smoking and hence determine the level of airway function.[59] The latter hypothesis is supported by the finding that the age-related decline in FEV_1 in smokers varies with the level of bronchial responsiveness.[60] In one longitudinal study, continued smoking was associated with increasing BHR over and above the effect of declining baseline function.[61] A correlate of BHR is greater spontaneous diurnal variation of indices of airway function such as PEF; such an increase has been shown in smokers compared with non-smokers.[62]

Cessation of smoking is associated most notably with an increase in $D_L CO$ and KCO, which occurs within a week of quitting.[63,64] In older individuals no change in mechanical function is likely but a small increase in FEV_1 is demonstrable in young adults.[65]

8.5 GROWTH AND AGEING

8.5.1 Effects of lung growth

Lung volumes and maximum expiratory flows increase progressively during childhood and generally correlate well with stature. If the specific (i.e. volume-corrected) compliance of the lungs is related to stature, however, there appears to be a slight decline with growth,[66] implying a change in the elasticity of the lungs. The nature of this is not clear, but the relatively lower lung recoil in young children may have important implications for the maintenance of airway patency; e.g. their lower lung recoil pressure correlates with the relatively larger closing volumes in young children.[67]

As a result of their different embryological origins, development of the larger airways is in advance of alveolar development; the lungs of a term infant at birth contain a full complement of relatively mature airways but alveolar multiplication continues during childhood until about 10–12 years of age.[68] The more mature airways may be the cause of the relatively high specific airway conductance found shortly after birth. During later childhood the relationship of airway conductance to lung volume is similar to that of adults.[69] If maximum expiratory flow is expressed as 'TLCs per second' there is no change with growth.[8]

The FEV_1/VC ratio tends to be greater in children than adults, often approaching 100 per cent. Because of its dependence on lung size, the CO diffusing capacity increases with stature, but KCO is higher in smaller children and falls with age.[70]

Up to puberty, lung volumes increase steadily, approximately in proportion to height, but around puberty there is a marked increase in all indices, especially in boys (Fig. 8.1).[71,72] However, the pubertal growth spurt in lung function lags a few months behind the spurt of height,[73] and function continues to increase after somatic growth has ceased,[74] reaching peak values around the ages of 18–20 years in

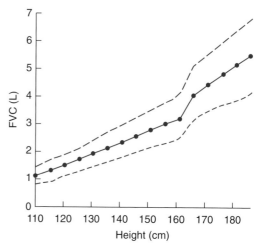

Figure 8.1 Mean (±2 SD) effect of growth on forced vital capacity (FVC) in boys aged 4–19 years in relation to height, showing disproportionate increase corresponding to the time of puberty. Redrawn from: Rosenthal M *et al.* Lung function in white children aged 4–19 years: I. Spirometry. *Thorax* 1993; 48: 794–802, with permission from the BMJ Publishing Group.

females and a little later in men. The pattern varies between individuals, however, so that those in the age range 18–25 years represent a heterogeneous group comprising some whose lungs are still growing, some who have reached a plateau and some whose function has already started to decline.[73]

8.5.2 Effects of ageing

From the early twenties there is a gradual decline in most indices. Most studies have, however, been cross-sectional comparisons of cohorts of healthy subjects. The present lung function of a 70-year-old may well have been influenced by factors of, for example, environment and nutrition, which will not apply over the next 50 years to an individual who is now 20 years old, and so extrapolation of these data to sequential changes in an individual is unlikely to be valid. Longitudinal data suggest that, although FEV_1 shows an accelerating decline with age, the magnitude of this decline is less, and its apparent age of onset is later, than would be suggested by cross-sectional analyses.[75]

8.5.2.1 Lung and airway mechanics

The lungs share the general ageing changes of connective tissue elsewhere in the body – just as the

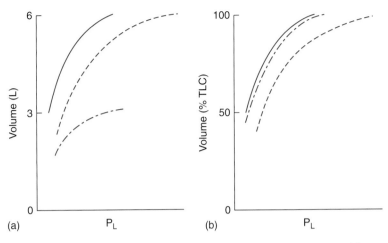

Figure 8.2 Schematic changes in static pressure–volume curve of lungs with growth and ageing. Lung recoil pressure (P_L) is plotted against volume (a) in absolute terms, and (b) as a percentage of total lung capacity (TLC) for a normal young adult (dashed line), an elderly adult (unbroken line) and a child (dashed/dotted line). In the child the compliance of the lungs is lower approximately in proportion to lung volume (a), but at any given percentage of TLC, P_L is less than in the young adult (b). With ageing in adult life the main change is a reduction in recoil pressure, but there is also a slight increase in compliance in the tidal range.

turgor of the skin is lost in elderly people, so also elastic recoil of the lungs diminishes. In consequence the pressure–volume curve is shifted to lower values of recoil pressure at all lung volumes (Fig. 8.2).[14] There is also an increase in the slope of the relationship, i.e. pulmonary compliance, but this is minor. Such an increase in lung distensibility might be expected to increase lung volumes (see Fig. 1.7e in Chapter 1) – but most series show no change in TLC with age, possibly due to the countering effect of a fall in muscle strength with the two opposing influences cancelling out. The passive elastic properties of the chest wall also change with age in the direction of decreasing compliance.[76] Although TLC changes little, if at all, with age, its subdivisions change markedly, with a decline in VC balanced by an increase in RV (Fig. 8.3). FRC also increases, both in absolute terms and as a proportion of TLC.

Respiratory resistance measured by forced oscillation falls a little in elderly people,[77] and specific airway conductance measured plethysmographically remains remarkably constant with age.[78] FEV_1, the FEV_1/VC ratio and maximum flows, especially at low lung volumes, decline progressively. Consequently, the contour of the maximum flow–volume curve alters and it develops a greater

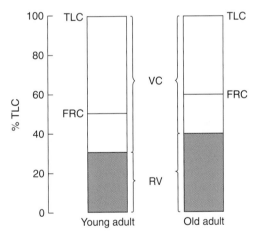

Figure 8.3 Changes in the subdivisions of lung volume with ageing. Total lung capacity (TLC) shows little or no change, but residual volume (RV) increases at the expense of vital capacity (VC). Functional residual capacity (FRC) also rises with age as a consequence of the reduced lung recoil pressure.

convexity to the volume axis (Fig. 8.4), with an appearance that qualitatively is similar to that seen with diffuse airway obstruction (see Chapter 9, Section 9.2.3.2). These appearances result from loss of recoil of both the lungs and the airways themselves, with the result that they are more easily

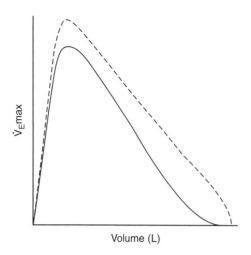

Figure 8.4 Schematic change in the contour of the maximum expiratory flow–volume curve with ageing. In the normal young subject (dashed line) the descending part of the curve is approximately straight or shows a slight concavity to the volume axis. By comparison, the curve for the elderly subject (unbroken line) shows a slightly lower peak, a smaller vital capacity (VC) and a convexity to the volume axis. The abrupt reduction in maximum expiratory flow ($\dot{V}_E$max) as residual volume (RV) is approached in the young subject implies that factors other than airway narrowing determine the point at which maximal expiration is terminated (see text for further discussion).

compressible and therefore narrow relatively more during forced expiration. Their unstressed dimensions, however, are not reduced and may actually be slightly greater than in young subjects; this explains the unchanged airway conductance in relation to volume, despite the loss of airway support consequent on the lower lung recoil pressure. The increasing residual volume with age is a reflection of the same alterations in mechanical properties of the airways, with greater narrowing and closure of airways as effort is applied to expire below FRC. Whereas in younger healthy subjects RV is reached when the increasing outward recoil of the chest wall balances the expiratory effort, in older individuals dynamic airway narrowing prevents further deflation, and the shape of the terminal part of the maximum expiratory flow–volume (MEFV) curve differs as a result (Fig. 8.4).[79] The age-related reduction of maximum expiratory flow, particularly at lower lung volumes, implies that tidal expiratory flow may become maximal,

even at rest, with consequent flow limitation during tidal breathing. Using the negative expiratory pressure technique, this phenomenon has been shown to occur in a large proportion of healthy elderly subjects, in whom it may contribute to dyspnoea, even in the absence of overt cardiopulmonary disease.[80]

The level of bronchial responsiveness to methacholine increases with age in proportion to the reduction in FEV_1.[81]

8.5.2.2 Ventilation, perfusion and gas exchange

The changes in mechanical function with ageing are accompanied by less even ventilation. The slope of phase III of the single breath test increases with age;[82] phase IV (closing volume), which may not even be present in some young subjects, is detected earlier in expiration, so that the ratio CV/VC rises progressively.[83] The overall efficiency of gas exchange declines with a gradually falling arterial PO_2 and widening $AaPO_2$.[84,85] The lower PaO_2 is attributable to greater mismatching of ventilation and perfusion, with no evidence of increased shunting with normal ageing.[86] The contribution of lung units with high $\dot{V}_A/\dot{Q}$ ratios also increases with age, such that the physiological dead space rises and represents an increasing proportion of the tidal volume.[84]

The CO diffusing capacity falls with age for several reasons, including the reduced efficiency of ventilation, which produces a lower effective alveolar volume, a reduction in the ratio of alveolar surface area to volume,[87] and a reduction in pulmonary capillary blood volume.[88] The effect of gas distribution is removed by calculation of the K_{CO}, but the other factors result in a fall in this also.[15]

8.5.2.3 Ventilatory control and exercise

The ventilatory responses to both hypoxia and hypercapnia are less in elderly people compared with young people.[89] Exercise capacity declines with ageing[90] because of a combination of reduced muscle strength, deconditioning and fitness generally. The maximum heart rate and cardiac output fall with age and the ventilatory response to exercise is greater in older subjects.[91]

8.6 POSTURE

Most tests of respiratory function are performed with the subject standing or sitting upright and differences between the two are trivial.[92] Measurements at the bedside are usually made with the patient semi-recumbent, where the postural influence is intermediate between upright and supine. Postural differences in routine measurements are all related directly or indirectly to gravity. During tidal breathing in the supine posture, abdominal motion makes the greater contribution to chest wall expansion, whereas in the upright posture, ribcage movement is dominant.[93] The effect of posture on static lung volumes is greatest for FRC and ERV, which are appreciably less when the subject is supine because gravity no longer acts to keep the diaphragm and abdominal contents out of the thorax. Changes in other subdivisions of lung volume are much less, but there is a small fall in VC (usually less than 15%) in the supine posture. In part, this results from displacement of air by greater pooling of blood in the chest. The magnitude of this postural change in VC decreases with age.[94]

In the supine posture, the gravitational forces that influence the distribution of ventilation and blood flow act along the anteroposterior axis. Regional distribution of blood flow is more uniform, which probably accounts for the smaller physiological dead space when lying down.[95] More even distribution of ventilation might also be expected in the supine position, but, particularly in older subjects the effect is complicated by the lower FRC and consequent greater likelihood of airway narrowing and closure during tidal breathing. In younger individuals the $AaPo_2$ is less and the Pao_2 usually slightly higher in the supine position,[96] whereas in older healthy subjects the reverse may occur, with an increased $AaPo_2$ and a lower Pao_2 supine compared with upright.[97] The arterial Pco_2 tends to be slightly higher supine,[96] but the ventilatory response to CO_2 is apparently independent of posture.[98] Ventilation/perfusion matching is further improved in the prone posture, in which the distorting effect of the anteriorly positioned heart is avoided (see Chapter 13, Section 13.5).

The CO diffusing capacity and Kco are both higher in the supine posture because of the increased volume of blood in the pulmonary capillaries. As with VC, the postural differences become less marked with age,[99] possibly because of more even perfusion in the upright posture associated with a higher pulmonary artery pressure in elderly people.[100]

8.7 DIURNAL VARIATION

Diurnal variation in lung function in the awake subject is seen most clearly in asthma, but smaller changes occur in non-asthmatic subjects. The changes are attributable to circadian variation in airway size. The lowest values of FEV_1, VC and PEF occur during the night, a pattern that persists even if the subject has not slept.[101] Daytime measurements show increases between 9 a.m. and noon, followed by a decline later in the day.[102] The average variation in forced expiratory measurements is between 3 per cent and 5 per cent and is greater in younger adults and smokers.[102] This diurnal variation needs to be considered in longitudinal studies, if careful assessments of drug responses are required or if the effects of exposure to potentially hazardous agents at work are being studied. TLC remains constant, but RV falls in the morning as VC rises.[102] Variation in D_Lco is apparently out of phase with airway function as measurements are highest in the early morning with a small but progressive fall during the day. This reduction may be due to the combined effects of increasing carboxyhaemoglobin concentration secondary to multiple testing and a small decline in haemoglobin concentration during the day.[103]

8.8 CHANGES DURING THE MENSTRUAL CYCLE AND PREGNANCY

8.8.1 Effects of the menstrual cycle

The well-known effect of the menstrual cycle on severity of asthma in some women prompted study of changes in non-asthmatic individuals, but no effect either on resting airway function or on bronchial responsiveness to methacholine is demonstrable.[104] Similarly, there appears to be no significant effect of the menstrual cycle on CO uptake.[105] However, there are changes in ventilation, with the higher concentration of circulating progesterone in the luteal phase of the cycle causing ventilatory stimulation with increases at rest,[106] on exercise[107] and during CO_2 rebreathing.[108]

8.8.2 Effects of pregnancy

Pregnancy affects tests of respiratory function in several ways, most obviously via the direct mechanical consequences of the enlarging uterus; other relevant factors include the increased cardiac output and blood volume and the greater ventilatory drive resulting from circulating progesterone.

The effects on lung mechanics become most apparent in the third trimester. The most notable is a fall in FRC; RV also falls and VC often shows a small rise so that TLC is usually unchanged.[109,110] Maximum respiratory pressures are unaffected,[111] except during labour (see below). Maximum flows and FEV_1, however, are not measurably increased.[109]

Oxygen consumption increases with pregnancy, but the increase in ventilation is disproportionately high both at rest and on exercise.[112,113] Hyperventilation is an early feature,[111] which undoubtedly contributes to the breathlessness noted by many women from an early stage of pregnancy. $PaCO_2$ is consequently reduced and falls progressively with advancing pregnancy,[114] pregnant women showing a chronic respiratory alkalosis with a persistently low $[HCO_3^-]$ and $[H^+]$ (the average arterial pH during pregnancy is 7.47).[114] PaO_2 typically shows a small rise and the $AaPO_2$ may also increase due to the relatively larger increase in alveolar PO_2 consequent on the hyperventilation. PaO_2 supine is lower than upright values in late pregnancy.[115]

The maximum aerobic capacity $\dot{V}O_2$max is increased in pregnancy, but maximum CO_2 output is slightly reduced, implying a reduced respiratory exchange ratio at maximum exercise.[113] Since resting $\dot{V}O_2$ is increased, the available increase in $\dot{V}O_2$ between rest and exercise is less than normal. A rise in D_LCO might be expected to accompany the hypervolaemia of pregnancy; the few available data surprisingly show either no change[116] or a slight fall,[109] but in the latter study the effect of the fall in haemoglobin concentration was not taken into account.

Hypoxaemia during sleep might be expected in view of the marked reduction in FRC, especially in late pregnancy. One study of women at 36 weeks of an uncomplicated pregnancy, however, showed normal nocturnal oxygenation.[117] Also, comparison of the apnoea/hypopnoea index during late pregnancy and postpartum shows a lower value in the former.[115,117] Subjects predisposed to obstructive sleep apnoea, on the other hand, may show a deterioration during pregnancy.[118] Although central stimulation of activity of the respiratory muscles by circulating progesterone may contribute to the preservation of oxygenation during sleep in late pregnancy, this occurs despite a tendency for the pharyngeal airway to narrow, particularly in the third trimester.[119] Snoring is common in pregnancy, implying some instability of the upper airway, and is particularly common in women with pre-eclampsia in whom upper airway dimensions are smaller still,[120] possibly due to the associated fluid retention causing oedema of the airway. The snoring, particularly in pre-eclampsia, is accompanied by demonstrable inspiratory flow limitation, though usually without oxygen desaturation.[121]

During labour, forceful diaphragmatic contraction contributes to the marked increases in abdominal pressure, potentially setting up the conditions for the development of diaphragmatic fatigue. In one study of six patients a reduction in $P_I$max during labour was demonstrated, together with a progressive decline in the ratio of high to low frequency components of the diaphragmatic electromyogram (EMG), a pattern consistent with fatigue.[122]

8.9 NORMAL OR ABNORMAL?

The ideal reference data against which to assess the lung function of a patient would be his or her premorbid function, but, except in short-term challenge tests, such information is not usually available. For the more common tests, prediction equations based on large series of healthy subjects are used. Most equations incorporate terms for age, sex and height, and sometimes ethnic origin; an indication of the residual deviation around the mean values is also usually quoted. The usefulness of such reference equations depends critically on the size and comparability of the reference population. Most laboratories in the UK use those recommended previously by the European Community and the European Respiratory Society (ERS).[123,124] The working party that produced these recommendations developed a series of 'summary equations' based on the pooled data from several reports. This philosophy has been questioned on statistical grounds, and the summary equations were not formally re-endorsed in the joint ERS/American Thoracic Society (ATS) guidelines on standardizing lung function testing.[125] Nonetheless, the equations published originally in 1983 have generally been found acceptable and appropriate.[123]

The view in North America is different, with the ATS recommending that each laboratory should choose equations from the literature that best suit a group of healthy subjects studied in that laboratory.[126] In the USA, the large National Health and Nutrition Examination Survey (NHANES) has generated reference equations based on data from several thousands of individuals, incorporating ethnicity as well as other relevant variables.[127] No Europe-wide equivalent is available yet, but equations have been derived from populations of healthy subjects in many countries.[17,125] Clearly, whether 'summary' or individual equations are used, it is important to check that they predict values close to those measured in healthy subjects in the same laboratory.

Extrapolation of reference equations beyond the limits of variation of the population studied is potentially unwise, but it does appear that extrapolation to the extremes of stature encountered in otherwise healthy subjects produces valid results.[128] Caution should, however, be exercised in applying historical reference equations in view of the likely effects of environmental factors on different cohorts of subjects .[129] Reductions over time in potentially adverse influences, such as childhood infections, imply that equations derived cross-sectionally are likely progressively to underestimate functional indices as time passes.[75]

The level at which the result of an individual test should be considered 'abnormal' is inevitably somewhat arbitrary. Historically, values outside the range 80–120 per cent of mean predicted were often regarded as abnormal, but this takes no account of the extent of variation of different tests in the reference population. More appropriately, the actual deviation of a result from the mean reference value should be related to the standard deviation (SD) of the results of the test in the healthy population. The number of SDs by which a result differs from the mean predicted for that individual is the 'standardized residual' or 'z score'. Thus, provided the population is normally distributed, a result 1 SD less than predicted has a z of -1.

Defining the limits of 'normality' involves a trade-off between the sensitivity and specificity of the test in question. If the limits are set very wide, the test gains specificity in that an abnormal ('positive') result has a very high likelihood of being truly abnormal (i.e. there would be few 'false positives'), but it loses sensitivity as fewer 'true positives' are identified. On the other hand, if the 'normal' limits are set too narrow, the converse applies, with greater sensitivity but poor specificity. In practice, in clinical lung function testing, the limits of normality are often set between z scores of -1.65 and $+1.65$. With a normal distribution the intervening range then encompasses 90 per cent of the healthy population, i.e. one in ten healthy individuals would have results lying outside this range, with 5 per cent below and 5 per cent above these limits (Fig. 8.5). The case for using these limits is strengthened by the knowledge that for most tests (though not all, e.g. TLC, D_LCO) the likely abnormality is in one predictable direction, e.g. reduced, rather than increased, FEV_1. Thus, assuming a normal distribution of values in the healthy population, a result that is more than 1.65 SD below the mean predicted (i.e. $z < -1.65$) would be seen in only 5 per cent of the healthy population.

The alternative method of expressing results as a percentage of the mean predicted value is still preferred by many as it gives a better 'feel' for the severity of an abnormality. It is, for example, used widely in assessment of chronic obstructive pulmonary disease (COPD), where FEV_1 per cent predicted is the criterion that defines the different grades of severity (see Chapter 9, Section 9.1). This approach is often assumed to take account of variation in body size, but this is not necessarily the case.[130] Also, comparison of per cent predicted values between subjects of different ages is potentially misleading, and comparisons between the results of different tests in a given individual in order to define the site of an abnormality (e.g. 'large' versus 'small' airways) is not valid as the normal ranges of different tests vary considerably. In summary, there are advantages in using both z scores and per cent predicted, but the above

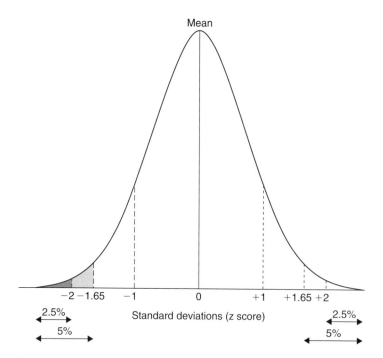

Figure 8.5 Normal distribution showing proportions of the healthy population encompassed by different 'normal' ranges. A z score between -2 and $+2$ includes the test results of 95 per cent of the normal population, with 2.5 per cent above and 2.5 per cent below these limits. If the 'normal' range is defined in terms of z scores between approximately -1.65 and $+1.65$, 5 per cent of the population will have values above and 5 per cent below these limits.

caveats with respect to the latter need to be borne in mind.

REFERENCES

1 Jones RL, Nzekwu M-MU. The effects of body mass index on lung volumes. *Chest* 2006; **130**: 827–33.
2 Lazarus R, Gore CJ, Booth M, Owen N. Effects of body composition and fat distribution on ventilatory function in adults. *Am J Clin Nutri* 1998; **68**: 35–41.
3 Ochs-Balcom HM, Grant BJB, Muti P, *et al.* Pulmonary function and abdominal adiposity in the general population. *Chest* 2006; **129**: 853–62.
4 Yernault JC, Baran D, Englert M. Effect of growth and ageing on the static mechanical lung properties. *Bull Eur Physiopath Respir* 1977; **13**: 777–88.
5 Rebuck AS, Rigg JRA, Kangalee M, Pengelley LD. Control of tidal volume during rebreathing. *J Appl Physiol* 1974; **37**: 475–8.
6 Hirshman CA, McCullough RE, Weil JV. Normal values for hypoxic and hypercapnic ventilatory drives in man. *J Appl Physiol* 1975; **38**: 1095–8.
7 Green M, Mead J, Turner JM. Variability of maximum expiratory flow–volume curves. *J Appl Physiol* 1974; **37**: 67–74.
8 Zapletal A, Motoyama EK, van de Woestijne KP, *et al.* Maximum expiratory flow–volume curves and airway conductance in children and adolescents. *J Appl Physiol* 1969; **26**: 308–16.
9 Osmanliev D, Bowley N, Hunter DM, Pride NB. Relation between tracheal size and forced expiratory volume in one second in young men. *Am Rev Respir Dis* 1982; **126**: 179–82.
10 Collins DV, Cutillo AG, Armstrong JD, *et al.* Large airway size, lung size and maximal expiratory flow in healthy non smokers. *Am Rev Respir Dis* 1986; **134**: 951–5.
11 Jacobs DR, Nelson ET, Dontas AS, *et al.* Are race and sex differences in lung function explained by frame size? *Am Rev Respir Dis* 1992 **146**: 644–9.
12 Schwartz J, Katz SA, Fegley RW, Tockman MS. Sex and race differences in the development of lung function. *Am Rev Respir Dis* 1988; **138**: 1415–21.
13 Wilson SH, Cooke NT, Edwards RHT, Spiro SG. Predicted normal values for maximal respiratory

pressures in Caucasian adults and children. *Thorax* 1984; **39**: 535–8.

14 Gibson GJ, Pride NB, O'Cain C, Quagliato R. Sex and age differences in pulmonary mechanics in normal non-smoking subjects. *J Appl Physiol* 1976; **41**: 20–25.

15 Bradley J, Bye C, Hayden SP, Hughes DTD. Normal values of transfer factor and transfer coefficient in healthy males and females. *Respiration* 1979; **38**: 221–6.

16 Catterall JR, Calverley PMA, Shapiro CM, Flenley DC, Douglas NJ. Breathing and oxygenation during sleep are similar in normal men and normal women. *Am Rev Respir Dis* 1985; **132**: 86–8.

17 Cotes JE, Chinn DJ, Miller MR. *Lung Function*, 6th edn, Blackwell, Oxford, 2006.

18 Donnelly PM, Yang T-S, Peat JK, Woolcock AJ. What factors explain racial differences in lung volumes. *Eur Respir J* 1991; **4**: 829–38.

19 Redline S, Tishler PV, Lewitter FI, *et al.* Assessment of genetic and nongenetic influences on pulmonary function: a twin study. *Am Rev Respir Dis* 1987; **135**: 217–22.

20 Cotch MF, Beaty TH, Cohen BH. Path analysis of familial resemblance of pulmonary function and cigarette smoking. *Am Rev Respir Dis* 1990; **142**: 1337–43.

21 Coultas DB, Hanis CL, Howard CA, Skipper BJ, Samet JM. Heritability of ventilatory function in smoking and non smoking New Mexico Hispanics. *Am Rev Respir Dis* 1991; **144**: 770–75.

22 Ghio AJ, Crapo RO, Elliott CG, *et al.* Heritability estimates of pulmonary function. *Chest* 1989; **96**: 743–6.

23 Kawakami Y, Yamamoto H, Yoshikawa T, Shida A. Chemical and behavioural control of breathing in adult twins. *Am Rev Respir Dis* 1984; **129**: 703–7.

24 Van Diemen CC, Postma DS, Vonk JM, *et al.* A disintegrin and metalloprotease 33 polymorphisms and lung function decline in the general population. *Am J Respir Crit Care Med* 2005; **172**: 329–33.

25 Canoy D, Pekkanen J, Elliott P, *et al.* Early growth and adult respiratory function in men and women followed from the fetal period to adulthood. *Thorax* 2007; **62**: 396–402.

26 Tennant PWG, Gibson GJ, Pearce MS. Lifecourse predictors of adult respiratory function: results from the Newcastle Thousand Families Study. *Thorax* 2008; **63**: 823–30.

27 Vrijlandt EJ, Gerritsen J, Boezen HM, Grevink RG, Duiverman EJ. Lung function and exercise capacity in young adults born prematurely. *Am J Respir Crit Care Med* 2006; **173**: 890–96.

28 Shaheen SO, Sterne JAC, Tucker JS, Florey C du V. Birth weight, childhood lower respiratory tract infection and adult lung function. *Thorax* 1998; **53**: 549–53.

29 Lima R da C, Victora CG, Menezes AMB, Barros FC. Respiratory function in adolescence in relation to low birth weight, preterm delivery, and intrauterine growth restriction. *Chest* 2005; **128**: 2400–407.

30 Shaheen SO, Barker DJP, Sheill AW, *et al.* The relationship between pneumonia in early childhood and impaired lung function in late adult life. *Am J Respir Crit Care Med* 1994; **149**: 616–19.

31 Perez-Padilla R, Torre-Bouscoulet L, Muino A, *et al.* Prevalence of oxygen desaturation and use of oxygen at home in adults at sea level and at moderate altitude. *Eur Respir J* 2006; **27**: 594–9.

32 DeGraff AC, Grover RF, Johnson RL, *et al.* Diffusing capacity of the lung in Caucasians native to 3100 m. *J Appl Physiol* 1970; **29**: 71–6.

33 Severinghaus JW, Bainton CR, Carcelen A. Respiratory insensitivity to hypoxia in chronically hypoxic man. *Respir Physiol* 1966; **1**: 308–34.

34 Weil JV, Byrne-Quinn E, Sodal IE, *et al.* Acquired attenuation of chemo-receptor function in chronically hypoxic man at high altitude. *J Clin Invest* 1971; **50**: 186–95.

35 Thomas PS, Harding RM, Milledge JS. Peak expiratory flow at altitude. *Thorax* 1990; **45**: 620–21.

36 Vaughan TR, Weber RW, Tipton WR, Nelson HS. Comparison of PEFR and FEV_1 in patients with varying degrees of airway obstruction; effect of modest altitude. *Chest* 1989; **95**: 558–62.

37 Butland BK, Fehily AM, Elwood PC. Diet, lung function, and lung function decline in a cohort of 2512 middle aged men. *Thorax* 2000; **55**: 102–8.

38 Tujague JB, Bastaki M, Holland N, Balmes JR, Tager IB. Antioxidant intake, GSTM1 polymorphism and pulmonary function in healthy young adults. *Eur Respir J* 2006; **27**: 282–8.

39 Guenegou A, Leynaert B, Pin I, *et al.* Serum carotenoids, vitamins A and E, and 8 year lung function decline in a general population. *Thorax* 2006; **61**: 320–26.

40 Black PN, Scragg R. Relationship between serum 25–hydroxyvitamin D and pulmonary function in the third national health and nutrition examination survey. *Chest* 2005; **128**: 3792–8.

41 Kinney PL, Ware JH, Spengler JD, *et al.* Short term pulmonary function change in association with ozone levels. *Am Rev Respir Dis* 1989; **139**: 56–61.

42 Kunzli N, Lurmann F, Segal M, *et al.* Association between lifetime ambient ozone exposure and pulmonary function in college freshmen: results of a pilot study. *Environ Res* 1997; **72**: 8–23.

43 Banauch GI, Hall C, Weiden M, *et al.* Pulmonary function after exposure to the World Trade Center

collapse in the New York City Fire Department. *Am J Respir Crit Care Med* 2006; **174**: 312–19.

44 Regalado J, Perez-Padilla R, Sansores R, *et al.* The effect of biomass burning on respiratory symptoms and lung function in rural Mexican women. *Am J Respir Crit Care Med* 2006; **174**: 901–5.

45 Rona RJ, Chinn S. Lung function, respiratory illness and passive smoking in British primary school children. *Thorax* 1993; **48**: 533–6.

46 O'Connor GT, Weiss ST, Tager IB, Speizer FE. The effect of passive smoking on pulmonary function and non specific bronchial responsiveness in a population-based sample of children and young adults. *Am Rev Respir Dis* 1987; **135**: 800–804.

47 Moshammer H, Hoek G, Luttmann-Gibson H, *et al.* Parental smoking and lung function in children: an international study. *Am J Respir Crit Care Med* 2006; **173**: 1255–63.

48 Corbo GM, Agabiti N, Forastiere F, *et al.* Lung function in children and adolescents with occasional exposure to environmental tobacco smoke. *Am J Respir Crit Care Med* 1996; **154**: 695–700.

49 Mazjesi M-R, Kazemi H, Johnson DC. Effects of passive smoking on the pulmonary function of adults. *Thorax* 1990; **45**: 27–31.

50 Nadel JA, Comroe JH. Acute effects of inhalation of cigarette smoke on airway conductance. *J Appl Physiol* 1960; **16**: 713–16.

51 Krumholz RA, Chevalier RB, Ross JC. Cardiopulmonary function in young smokers. *Ann Intern Med* 1964; **60**: 603–10.

52 Higgins MW, Enright PL, Kronmal RA, *et al.* Smoking and lung function in elderly men and women: the Cardiovascular Health Study. *J Am Med Assoc* 1993; **269**: 2741–8.

53 Sansores RH, Paré P, Abbound RT. Acute effect of cigarette smoking on the carbon monoxide diffusing capacity of the lung. *Am Rev Respir Dis* 1992; **146**: 951–8.

54 Hyland RH, Krastins IRB, Aspin N, *et al.* Effect of body position on carbon monoxide diffusing capacity in asymptomatic smokers and non-smokers. *Am Rev Respir Dis* 1978; **117**: 1045–53.

55 Rijcken B, Schouten JP, Weiss ST, *et al.* The distribution of bronchial responsiveness to histamine in symptomatic and in asymptomatic subjects: a population-based analysis of various indices of responsiveness. *Am Rev Respir Dis* 1989; **140**: 615–23.

56 Rijcken B, Schouten JP, Mensinga TT, *et al.* Factors associated with bronchial responsiveness to histamine in a population sample of adults. *Am Rev Respir Dis* 1993; **147**: 1447–53.

57 Cerveri I, Bruschi C, Zoia M, *et al.* Smoking habit and bronchial reactivity in normal subjects: a

58 Britton J, Pavord I, Richards K, *et al.* Factors influencing the occurrence of airway hypersensitivity in the general population: the importance of atopy and airway calibre. *Eur Respir J* 1994; **7**: 881–7.

59 Rijcken B, Schouten JP, Weiss ST, Speizer FE, van der Lende R. The relationship between airway responsiveness to histamine and pulmonary function level in a random population sample. *Am Rev Respir Dis* 1988; **137**: 826–32.

60 Frew AJ, Kennedy SM, Chan-Yeung M. Methacholine responsiveness, smoking and atopy as risk factors for accelerated FEV_1 decline in male working populations. *Am Rev Respir Dis* 1992; **146**: 878–83.

61 Chinn S, Jarvis D, Luczynska CM, *et al.* An increase in bronchial responsiveness is associated with continuing or restarting smoking. *Am J Respir Crit Care Med* 2005; **172**: 956–61.

62 Higgins BG, Britton JR, Chinn S, *et al.* Factors affecting peak expiratory flow variability and bronchial reactivity in a random population sample. *Thorax* 1993; **48**: 899–906.

63 Knudson RJ, Kaltenborn WT, Burrows B. The effects of cigarette smoking and smoking cessation on the carbon monoxide diffusing capacity of the lung in asymptomatic subjects. *Am Rev Respir Dis* 1989; **140**: 645–51.

64 Sansores RH, Paré P, Abboud RT. Effect of smoking cessation on pulmonary carbon monoxide diffusing capacity and capillary blood volume. *Am Rev Respir Dis* 1992; **146**: 959–64.

65 Sherrill DL, Holberg CJ, Enright PL, Lebowitz MD, Burrows B. Longitudinal analysis of the effects of smoking onset and cessation on pulmonary function. *Am J Respir Crit Care Med* 1994; **148**: 591–7.

66 Zapletal A, Paul T, Samanek M. Pulmonary elasticity in children and adolescents. *J Appl Physiol* 1976; **40**: 953–61.

67 Mansell A, Bryan C, Levison H. Airway closure in children. *J Appl Physiol* 1972; **33**: 711–14.

68 Janssens JP, Pache JC, Nicod LP. Physiological changes in respiratory function associated with ageing. *Eur Respir J* 1999; **13**: 197–205.

69 Polgar G, Weng TR. The functional development of the respiratory system. *Am Rev Respir Dis* 1979; **120**: 625–95.

70 O'Brodovich HM, Mellins RB, Mansell AL. Effects of growth on the diffusion constant for carbon monoxide. *Am Rev Respir Dis* 1982; **125**: 670–73.

71 Rosenthal M, Bain SH, Cramer D, *et al.* Lung function in white children aged 4–19 years: I. Spirometry. *Thorax* 1993; **48**: 794–802.

72 Rosenthal M, Cramer D, Bain SH, *et al.* Lung function in white children aged 4–19 years: II. Single breath analysis and plethysmography. *Thorax* 1993; **48**: 803–8.

73 Wang X, Dockery DW, Wypij D, *et al.* Pulmonary function growth velocity in children 6 to 18 years of age. *Am Rev Respir Dis* 1993; **148**: 1502–8.

74 Sherrill DL, Camilli A, Lebowitz MD. On the temporal relationships between lung function and somatic growth. *Am Rev Respir Dis* 1989; **140**: 638–44.

75 Burrows B, Lebowitz MD, Camilli AE, Knudson RJ. Longitudinal changes in force expiratory volume in one second in adults: methodologic considerations and findings in healthy non-smokers. *Am Rev Respir Dis* 1986; **133**: 974–80.

76 Mittman C, Edelman NH, Norris AH, Shock NW. Relationship between chest wall and pulmonary compliance and age. *J Appl Physiol* 1965; **20**: 1211–16.

77 Guo YF, Herrmann F, Michel J-P, Janssens J-P. Normal values for respiratory resistance using forced oscillation in subjects >65 years old. *Eur Respir J* 2005; **26**: 602–8.

78 Pelzer AM, Thomson ML. Effect of age, sex, stature and smoking habits on human airway conductance. *J Appl Physiol* 1966; **21**: 469–76.

79 Leith DE, Mead J. Mechanism determining residual volume of the lungs in normal subjects. *J Appl Physiol* 1967; **23**: 221–7.

80 de Bisschop C, Marty ML, Tessier JF, *et al.* Expiratory flow limitation and obstruction in the elderly. *Eur Respir J* 2005; **26**: 594–601.

81 Sparrow D, O'Connor GT, Rosner B, Segal MR, Weiss ST. The influence of age and level of pulmonary function on non-specific airway responsiveness: the normative aging study. *Am Rev Respir Dis* 1991; **143**: 978–82.

82 Buist AS, Ross BB. Quantitative analysis of the alveolar plateau in the diagnosis of early airway obstruction. *Am Rev Respir Dis* 1973; **108**: 1078–87.

83 Buist AS, Ross BB. Predicted values for closing volumes using a modified single breath nitrogen test. *Am Rev Respir Dis* 1973; **107**: 744–52.

84 Mellemgaard K. The alveolar–arterial oxygen difference. *Acta Physiol Scand* 1966; **67**: 10–20.

85 Sorbini CA, Grassi V, Solinas E, Muiesan G. Arterial oxygen tension in relation to age in healthy subjects. *Respiration* 1968; **25**: 3–13.

86 Cardus J, Burgos F, Diaz O, *et al.* Increase in pulmonary ventilation–perfusion inequality with age in healthy individuals. *Am J Respir Crit Care Med* 1997; **156**: 648–53.

87 Gillooly M, Lamb D. Airspace size in lungs of lifelong non-smokers. *Thorax* 1993; **48**: 39–43.

88 Guenard H, Marthan R. Pulmonary gas exchange in elderly subjects. *Eur Respir J* 1996; **9**: 2573–7.

89 Kronenberg RS, Drage CW. Attenuation of the ventilatory and heart rate responses to hypoxia and hypercapnia with aging in normal men. *J Clin Invest* 1973; **52**: 1812–19.

90 Jones NL, Summers E, Killian KJ. Influence of age and stature on exercise capacity during incremental cycle ergometry in men and women. *Am Rev Respir Dis* 1989; **140**: 1373–80.

91 Poulin MJ, Cunningham DA, Peterson DH, *et al.* Ventilatory response to exercise in men and women 55 to 86 years of age. *Am J Respir Crit Care Med* 1994; **149**: 408–15.

92 Townsend MC. Spirometric forced expiratory volumes measured in the standing versus the sitting posture. *Am Rev Respir Dis* 1984; **130**: 123–4.

93 Sharp JT, Goldberg NB, Druz WS, Danon J. Relative contributions of rib cage and abdomen to breathing in normal subjects. *J Appl Physiol* 1975; **39**: 608–18.

94 Michels A, Decoster K, Derde L, Vleurinck C, van de Woestijne KP. Influence of posture on lung volumes and impedance of respiratory system in healthy smokers and non-smokers. *J Appl Physiol* 1991; **71**: 294–9.

95 Riley RL, Permutt S, Said S, *et al.* Effect of posture on pulmonary dead space in man. *J Appl Physiol* 1959; **14**: 339–44.

96 Bjurstedt H, Hesser CM, Liljestrand G, *et al.* Effects of posture on alveolar arterial CO_2 and O_2 differences and on alveolar dead space in man. *Acta Physiol Scand* 1962; **54**: 65–82.

97 Ward RJ, Tolas AG, Benveniste RJ, *et al.* Effect of posture on normal arterial blood gas tensions in the aged. *Geriatrics* 1966; **21**: 139–43.

98 Rigg JRA, Rebuck AS, Campbell EJM. Effect of posture on the ventilatory response to CO_2. *J Appl Physiol* 1974; **37**: 487–90.

99 Chang SC, Chang HI, Liu SY, Shiao GM, Perng RP. Effects of body position and age on membrane diffusing capacity and pulmonary capillary blood volume. *Chest* 1992; **102**: 139–42.

100 Stam H, Kreuzer FJA, Verspille A. Effect of lung volume and positional changes on pulmonary diffusing capacity and its components. *J Appl Physiol* 1991; **71**: 1477–88.

101 Spengler CM, Shea SA. Endogenous circadian rhythm of pulmonary function in healthy humans. *Am J Respir Crit Care Med* 2000; **162**: 1038–46.

102 Borsboom GJ, van Pelt W, van Houwelingen HC, *et al.* Diurnal variation in lung function in subgroups from two Dutch populations: consequences for

longitudinal analysis. *Am J Respir Crit Care Med* 1999; **159**: 1163–71.

103 Frey TM, Crapo RO, Jensen RL, Elliott CG. Diurnal variation of the diffusing capacity of the lung: is it real? *Am Rev Respir Dis* 1987; **136**: 1381–4.

104 Pauli BD, Reid RL, Munt PW, Wigle RD, Forkert L. Influence of the menstrual cycle on airway function in asthmatic and normal subjects. *Am Rev Respir Dis* 1989; **140**: 358–62.

105 Bacon CJ, Prior JC, Abboud RT, Oldham AR, McKenzie DC. Changes in pulmonary transfer factor with menstrual cycle phase. *Respir Physiol Neurobiol* 2005; **146**: 195–203.

106 England SJ, Farhi LE. Fluctuations in alveolar carbon dioxide and in base excess during the menstrual cycle. *Respir Physiol* 1976; **26**: 157–61.

107 Schoene RB, Robertson HT, Pierson DJ, Peterson AP. Respiratory drives and exercise in menstrual cycles of athletic and non-athletic women. *J Appl Physiol* 1981; **50**: 1300–305.

108 Dutton K, Blanksby BA, Morton AR. CO_2 sensitivity changes during the menstrual cycle. *J Appl Physiol* 1989; **67**: 517–22.

109 Gazioglu K, Kaltreider NL, Rosen M, Yu PN. Pulmonary function during pregnancy in normal women and in patients with cardiopulmonary disease. *Thorax* 1970; **25**: 445–50.

110 Nørregaard O, Schultz P, Østergaard A, Dahl R. Lung function and postural changes during pregnancy. *Respir Med* 1989; **83**: 467–70.

111 Contreras G, Gutierrez M, Beroiza T, *et al.* Ventilatory drive and respiratory muscle function in pregnancy. *Am Rev Respir Dis* 1991; **144**: 837–41.

112 Knuttgen HG, Emerson K. Physiological response to pregnancy at rest and during exercise. *J Appl Physiol* 1974; **36**: 549–53.

113 Lotgering FK, van Doorn MB, Struijk PC, Pool J, Wallenburg HCS. Maximal aerobic exercise in pregnant women: heart rate, O_2 consumption, CO_2 production and ventilation. *J Appl Physiol* 1991; **70**: 1016–23.

114 Lucius H, Gahlenbeck H, Kleine H-O, *et al.* Respiratory functions, buffer system and electrolyte concentrations of blood during human pregnancy. *Respir Physiol* 1970; **9**: 311–17.

115 Prodromakis E, Trakada G, Tsapanos V, Spriopoulos K. Arterial oxygen tension during sleep in the third trimester of pregnancy. *Acta Obstet Gynecol Scand* 2004; **83**: 159–64.

116 McAuliffe F, Kametas N, Rafferty GF, Greenough A, Nicolaides K. Pulmonary diffusing capacity in pregnancy at sea level and at high altitude. *Respir Physiol Neurobiol* 2003; **134**: 85–92.

117 Brownell LG, West P, Kryger MH. Breathing during sleep in normal pregnant women. *Am Rev Respir Dis* 1986; **133**: 38–41.

118 Edwards N, Blyton DM, Hennessy A, Sullivan CE. Severity of sleep-disordered breathing improves following parturition. *Sleep* 2005; **28**: 737–41.

119 Izci B, Vennelle M, Liston WA, *et al.* Sleep-disordered breathing and upper airway size in pregnancy and post-partum. *Eur Respir J* 2006; **27**: 321–7.

120 Izci B, Riha RL, Martin SE, *et al.* The upper airway in pregnancy and pre-eclampsia. *Am J Respir Crit Care Med* 2003; **167**: 137–40.

121 Connolly G, Razak AR, Hayanga A, *et al.* Inspiratory flow limitation during sleep in pre-eclampsia: comparison with normal pregnant and non-pregnant women. *Eur Respir J* 2001; **18**: 672–6.

122 Nava S, Zanotti E, Ambosino N, *et al.* Evidence of acute diaphragmatic fatigue in a 'natural' condition: the diaphragm during labour. *Am Rev Respir Dis* 1992; **146**: 1226–30.

123 Quanjer PH. Standardized lung function testing. *Clin Respir Physiol* 1983; **19** (suppl. 5).

124 Quanjer PH. Standardized lung function testing. *Eur Respir J* 1993; **6** (suppl. 16).

125 Pelligrino R, Viegi G, Brusasco V, *et al.* Interpretative strategies for lung function tests. *Eur Respir J* 2005; **26**: 948–68.

126 American Thoracic Society. Lung function testing: selection of reference values and interpretative strategies. *Am Rev Respir Dis* 1991; **144**: 1202–18.

127 Hankinson JL, Odencratz JR, Fedan KB. Spirometric reference values from a sample of the general U.S. population. *Am J Respir Crit Care Med* 1999; **159**: 179–87.

128 Aitken ML, Schoene RB, Franklin J, Pierson DJ. Pulmonary function in subjects at the extremes of stature. *Am Rev Respir Dis* 1985; **131**: 166–8.

129 Van Pelt W, Borsboom GJJM, Rijcken B, *et al.* Discrepancies between longitudinal and cross-sectional change in ventilatory function in 12 years of follow-up. *Am Rev Respir Dis* 1994; **149**: 1218–26.

130 Miller MR, Pincock AC. Predicted values: how should we use them? *Thorax* 1988; **43**: 265–7.

PART B

FUNCTION IN RESPIRATORY DISEASE

Chronic Obstructive Pulmonary Disease and Obliterative Bronchiolitis

9.1 TERMINOLOGY AND DEFINITIONS

The terminology of chronic airway disease is confused and confusing. 'Chronic obstructive pulmonary disease' (COPD) has become the most widely used diagnostic term for describing individuals with chronic airway obstruction that is largely irreversible. Other terms, which in effect are synonymous, include chronic obstructive lung (airway) disease, chronic airway (airflow) obstruction (limitation) and the traditional British 'chronic bronchitis and emphysema'. The functional features particular to asthma (variable airway obstruction) are considered in Chapter 11. It should be noted, however, that both asthma and smoking-induced COPD are sufficiently common to occur together quite frequently. To complicate matters further, many patients with asthma have a degree of persistent airway narrowing and some, despite little apparent spontaneous variability of airway function, show a marked improvement after treatment with corticosteroids, such that they are then diagnosed as asthmatic.

The term 'airflow obstruction' is sometimes preferred to 'airway obstruction' as it admits narrowing due to loss of support from the surrounding alveoli (as in emphysema), without necessarily any anatomical changes in the airways themselves. The severity of airflow obstruction that results from loss of lung recoil alone is, however, debatable[1,2] and panacinar emphysema can sometimes be present without significant airflow limitation.[3,4] Within the broad spectrum of patients with COPD, subgroups with predominantly 'bronchial' or 'emphysematous' types of airway narrowing are recognizable,[5] but the majority of patients occupy the middle ground with features of both (see Section 9.13.1).

The presence of airway obstruction is usually recognized by a reduction in the ratio of FEV_1 to VC or FVC. In view of the normal age-related decline of FEV_1/(F)VC, the ratio should be compared to appropriate predicted values (as with any other index), rather than using an arbitrary value to separate airway narrowing from normality. The common convention of using 75 per cent or 70 per cent as such a cut-off level is potentially misleading,

Table 9.1 Classification of severity of chronic obstructive pulmonary disease (COPD) in terms of forced expiratory volume (FEV) per cent predicted

	Mild	Moderate	Severe	Very severe
*[+]GOLD (7)	>80	30–80	<30	
*[+]NICE/BTS (8)	50–80	30–49	<30	
*[+]ERS/ATS (9)	>80	50–80	30–50	<30

*With $FEV_1/FVC \leq 0.7$.
[+]Severity of 'airflow obstruction'.
[+]Post-bronchodilator.
FVC, forced vital capacity.

particularly in elderly people, in whom it can considerably overestimate the frequency of COPD in otherwise healthy individuals.[6] On the other hand, a value of FEV_1/VC of 70 per cent in a young adult would definitely be abnormal.

The severity of airway obstruction in COPD is usually assessed by expressing the FEV_1 as a percentage of the mean predicted value. Categorization of severity in this way is, however, arbitrary and the limits and definitions vary between different guidelines (Table 9.1).[7–9]

9.2 AIRWAY MECHANICS

9.2.1 Mechanisms of airway narrowing

The characteristic functional features of patients with diffuse intrathoracic airway narrowing are increased resistance to airflow during quiet breathing and a reduction in maximum flow at all lung volumes, particularly on expiration.[1] In patients with chronic bronchitis, mucous hypersecretion and mucous gland hypertrophy are characteristic histological findings, but these are most marked in the larger, more central airways, whereas the obstruction to airflow is determined mainly by the calibre of more peripheral airways.[10,11]

Dayman in 1951 distinguished the two main mechanisms that contribute to airflow obstruction – intrinsic narrowing and loss of airway support.[12] More recent detailed measurements using computed tomography (CT)[13] have confirmed that the FEV_1 in COPD is related to both the magnitude of airway wall thickening and the severity of emphysema. The recoil pressure of the lungs is an important determinant of bronchial calibre and accounts for the normal decrease in airway resistance (i.e. increasing calibre) when measurements are made at progressively higher lung volumes (see Fig. 1.27 in Chapter 1). The intrapulmonary airways can be regarded as surrounded by a series of supporting struts, the alveolar walls. Since the airways themselves are elastic, reduction in the number or effectiveness of these attachments in emphysema reduces airway calibre and impairs function.[14] The centricacinar type of emphysema, which is related closely to cigarette smoking, is particularly relevant to airway narrowing.[15]

'Intrinsic' narrowing of the airways results from thickening of their walls with inflammatory changes and consequent bronchiolar and peribronchiolar fibrosis ('remodelling'). The presence of excess mucous exudate in the small airways may also contribute.[16] Similar factors influence airway calibre during inspiration and expiration, but during the latter the additional role of dynamic compression comes into play. Measurements in expiration (especially forced expiration) are therefore the most abnormal, but maximum inspiratory flow and inspiratory airway resistance are unlikely to be normal in individuals with symptomatic airway disease.[17]

9.2.2 Sites of airway narrowing in chronic obstructive pulmonary disease

Measurements of airway resistance in vivo in patients with diffuse airway disease have confirmed earlier autopsy data, showing that the main site of the increase is in the smaller conducting airways of less than 2 mm diameter.[10,11] These airways are found between the fourth and fourteenth generations of the tracheobronchial tree.[11] This has been called the 'silent zone' of the lungs,[18] as the large increase in overall cross-sectional area of this more distal part of the bronchial tree implies that extensive disease can develop here before conventional tests of airway function are demonstrably abnormal (see Chapter 1, Section 1.6.3). As disease progresses, however, tests such as FEV_1 become abnormal and recent three-dimensional CT imaging has confirmed that FEV_1 relates more closely to the dimensions of the distal small airways than to the larger proximal airways.[19] The main sites of expiratory dynamic airway compression, however, are in more proximal airways, although further towards the alveoli than in healthy subjects.

9.2.3 Forced expiration and inspiration

The effect of the narrowed small airways during forceful expiration is to produce rapid attenuation of the driving alveolar pressure, such that equal pressure points develop more peripherally than normal.[20] The elastic properties of the airway walls themselves may also be altered, rendering them more susceptible to dynamic compression.[2] The net result is that expiratory flow limitation occurs more readily than normal. This is best illustrated by comparison of the isovolume pressure–flow (IVPF) curve with that of a normal subject at the same proportion of the vital capacity (Fig. 9.1). As well as a reduction in airway conductance (increase in resistance) during quiet breathing (represented by the gradient of the IVPF curve as it passes the origin), maximum expiratory flow at any lung volume (% VC) is reduced, and so also is the 'minimum effective pressure', i.e. the lowest driving pressure required to generate this maximum flow. In normal subjects, maximum expiratory flow is entirely effort-dependent in the upper quarter or so of the VC (see Fig. 1.32 in Chapter 1); in patients with chronic airflow obstruction, the more peripheral location of the equal pressure points and the greater compressibility of the airways conspire to reduce the dependence on effort, with the result that minimum effective pressures can be demonstrated at relatively higher volumes than in normal subjects. Less dependence on effort adds to the value and reproducibility of measurements such as the FEV_1 in patients with diffuse airway obstruction. Even peak expiratory flow (PEF), which is sometimes suspect because in healthy subjects it is entirely dependent on effort, may be less so in patients with airflow obstruction. (Both measurements are of course dependent on effort in the sense that they demand a preceding full inspiration and a modicum of expiratory push.)

In subjects with chronic airflow obstruction of varying severity, PEF and FEV_1 are correlated (Fig. 9.2),[21] but they are not interchangeable, as with more severe narrowing PEF (% predicted) is often better preserved than FEV_1 (% predicted), i.e. PEF may underestimate the severity of airway narrowing. With less severe obstruction the converse is true, with PEF potentially underestimating FEV_1.[22] The

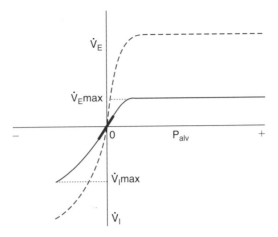

Figure 9.1 Isovolume pressure–flow (IVPF) curve at 50 per cent vital capacity (VC) for a normal subject (broken line, redrawn from Fig. 1.30 (see Chapter 1) and a patient with severe airflow obstruction (unbroken line). The slope of the IVPF curve close to the origin (thickened portion) represents airway conductance and is markedly reduced. Maximum expiratory flow ($\dot{V}_E$ max) is relatively more affected than maximum inspiratory flow ($\dot{V}_I$ max). The alveolar pressure (P_{alv}) necessary to produce $\dot{V}_E$ max is less than normal, i.e. expiratory flow is less effort-dependent than in the normal subject.

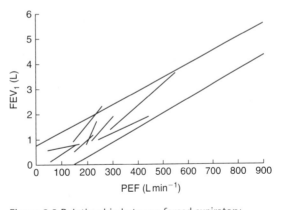

Figure 9.2 Relationship between forced expiratory volume in 1 s (FEV_1) and peak expiratory flow (PEF) in patients with airway obstruction of varying severity. The equation of the overall relationship was FEV_1 (L) = 0.00589 × PEF (L min^{-1}) − 0.065, and the band shows 95 per cent confidence limits. The thin lines show individual relationships in eight patients studied sequentially during recovery from exacerbations. Redrawn from: Kelly CA, Gibson GJ. Relation between FEV_1 and peak expiratory flow in patients with chronic airflow obstruction. *Thorax* 1988; **43**: 335–6, with permission from the BMJ Publishing Group.

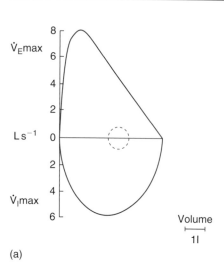

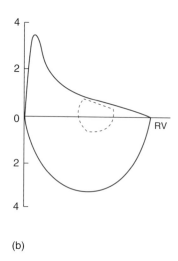

(a)   (b)

Figure 9.3 Schematic maximum flow–volume curves in (a) a normal subject and (b) a patient with severe airway obstruction (FEV$_1$/VC = 1.2/3.5). In the patient maximum expiratory flow ($\dot{V}_E$ max) is more affected than maximum inspiratory flow ($\dot{V}_I$ max) and the expiratory curve shows a characteristic convexity towards the volume axis. Also shown (broken lines) are flow–volume relations during a resting tidal breath; in the normal subject, considerable reserves of flow are available but the patient achieves maximum flow during tidal expiration. (Volumes recorded as change in thoracic volume, with subjects seated within a variable volume body plethysmograph.)

FEV$_1$, forced expiratory volume in 1 s; RV, residual volume; VC, vital capacity.

ratio FEV$_1$/VC is relatively sensitive to mild disease, but in patients with established disease it is a poor guide to the severity of airway obstruction,[23] which in general is better assessed in terms of FEV$_1$ expressed as either a percentage of the predicted value or a z score (see Chapter 8, Section 8.9).

9.2.3.1 'Negative effort dependence'

In some patients the paradoxical effect of a diminishing FEV$_1$ with greater effort is seen. This 'negative effort dependence' is essentially a consequence of Boyle's law (pressure × volume is constant). The rapid generation of a very positive alveolar pressure at the beginning of forced expiration compresses intrathoracic gas, to a degree predicted by Boyle's law. For example, if a maximum expiratory pressure of 100 cmH$_2$O (10 kPa) (one-tenth of an atmosphere) were applied in square-wave fashion, then thoracic gas volume (TGV) would be reduced by 10 per cent. This would have a relatively small effect on the volume expired by a normal subject but much more of an effect in a patient with airway obstruction, as the absolute volume reduction may represent a large proportion of the VC. Since maximum expiratory flow is critically dependent on lung volume, more vigorous efforts producing greater compression result in lower flow and lower FEV$_1$, as less volume is expired in the first second. Such an effect is demonstrable, though minor, in healthy subjects[24] but is much greater in patients with airway obstruction, particularly those with a large residual volume.

9.2.3.2 Maximum flow–volume curves

The maximum expiratory flow–volume (MEFV) curve in generalized intrathoracic airway narrowing shows a characteristic appearance with reduced flows at all volumes, but particularly in the latter part of the vital capacity, so that the contour of the curve becomes markedly convex to the volume axis (Figs 9.3 and 9.4). Qualitatively, the shape of the curve resembles that of older healthy subjects and, in effect, the appearances are an exaggeration of the normal ageing change, emphasizing the need to relate the appearances to those expected for the age of the individual.

If, as is usually the case, the volume expired is displayed against maximum flow, the curve typically shows a sharper peak than if flow is related to change in thoracic volume (as recorded with the

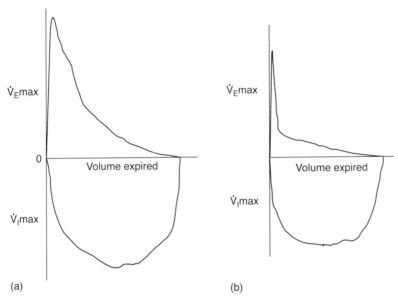

Figure 9.4 Maximum flow–volume curves in (a) a subject with moderately severe chronic obstructive pulmonary disease (COPD) and (b) more severe disease showing the so-called 'airway collapse' pattern (*x* axis represents volume expired), with a sharp initial peak followed by rapid decline in flow to very low levels for the remainder of the forced expiration. Pattern (b) is not specific for emphysema.

FFN: $\dot{V}_E$ max, maximum expiratory flow; $\dot{V}_I$ max, maximum inspiratory flow.

subject enclosed in a variable volume plethysmograph) (see Fig. 1.34 in Chapter 1). The difference reflects the effects of compression of thoracic gas by the expiratory effort; this is visualized when change in TGV is displayed but not by volume expired. The volume expired during the short time that peak flow is generated is determined mainly by the volume of the conducting airways (anatomical dead space), but during the same period thoracic volume diminishes much more because of the gas compression. As the effort is released towards the end of the manoeuvre, the relation between maximum expiratory flow and TGV is influenced by opposing effects of rarefaction of thoracic gas and continuing expiration. The total volume change (body temperature pressure saturated, BTPS) from beginning to end of the manoeuvre is, of course, identical.*

Particular patterns of the MEFV curve are sometimes identified in patients with COPD, in particular the so-called 'airway collapse' pattern, with a very sharp peak followed by a marked decrease (Fig. 9.4). Although sometimes equated with the

presence of emphysema and loss of support to the airway due to the reduced elastic recoil of the lungs, this appearance is not specific for that condition, as it can also be seen (and may be reversible) in asthma. This appearance is related more closely to the overall severity of airway narrowing.[25]

The maximum inspiratory flow–volume (MIFV) curve usually has a normal overall shape but, for the reasons discussed above, there is a reduction in V_I max at all volumes.[17] The diagnostic value of the appearances of MEFV and MIFV curves in patients with localized proximal airway narrowing are discussed in Chapter 12, Section 12.1.2.

9.2.4 Tidal breathing and expiratory flow limitation

Comparison of the flows developed during tidal breathing with the maxima during forceful efforts gives a visual impression of the available reserves of, and constraints upon, tidal breathing (Fig. 9.3) and in particular the greater reserves of inspiratory than

---

* It should be noted that, for convenience, flow–volume curves are often obtained with a subject seated in a body plethysmograph with the door open and using the pneumotachograph attached to the mouthpiece. In this situation the signal recorded is the volume expired. Change in TGV can be recorded only by using a variable volume plethysmograph with the door closed.

expiratory flow. Frequently, flow during tidal expiration coincides with, or even appears to exceed, the maximum at that volume; this phenomenon is seen regularly in patients with values of FEV_1 of 1 L or less. Recordings of tidal volume against time in such patients also show the characteristic expiratory slowing.[26] In mechanical terms the most economical pattern of tidal breathing is determined by the combination of pulmonary compliance and airway resistance; e.g. patients with pulmonary fibrosis and 'stiff' lungs breathe most economically with a relatively small tidal volume and rapid frequency (see Chapter 14, Section 14.3.1). On the other hand, patients with COPD, who usually have a high compliance and high airway resistance, might be expected to breathe more economically with large tidal volumes and slow breathing frequency. However, as is apparent from Fig. 9.3, increasing the tidal volume by prolonging expiration below FRC will reap very little reward because the flows that can be achieved are so low. Extending the tidal volume upwards within the restricted range available by increasing the end expiratory and end inspiratory volumes certainly allows higher flows, but these are achieved at the expense of greater work against elastic forces at the higher operating lung volume. The other option for increasing ventilation when demands require (as during exercise) is, of course, to increase the frequency of breathing. In practice, therefore, patients with chronic airflow obstruction, like those with pulmonary fibrosis, tend to breathe with a rapid frequency and relatively small tidal volume. Because of the poor efficiency of gas exchange, their overall ventilation needs to be greater than normal unless the arterial P_{CO_2} is allowed to rise. Although the greater resistance to airflow is encountered in expiration, all the work has to be done during inspiration and it is therefore not surprising that many patients find greater discomfort breathing in than out.

The phenomenon of expiratory flow limitation during tidal breathing was first appreciated by comparing tidal and maximal flows,[27] as illustrated in Fig. 9.3. The concept implies that tidal expiratory flow at a particular volume (whether at rest or on exercise) has reached a limit and cannot be increased by greater effort. Although an elegant way of illustrating the problem, comparing tidal and maximal flow in this way is open to several objections. These arise partly because the flow–volume

curves are usually superimposed with reference to volume expired (assuming that full inflation – TLC – is a fixed reference point); this ignores the effect of gas compression during forceful expiration, which, as discussed above, is particularly marked in patients with a large RV, such that 'isovolume' in terms of the volume expired below TLC is likely to be very different from 'iso TGV', and it is the latter that determines lung recoil pressure and therefore airway calibre. Other problems arise because of the very different volume and time histories of tidal and maximum expiration. Stretching the lungs by a full inspiration, the duration of the inspiration and the time the breath is held before expiration can all alter lung recoil and thus airway calibre.[28] Thus, even at 'iso TGV', mechanical conditions within the lungs differ during maximal and tidal expiration.

An alternative method for identifying flow limitation is the more recently introduced negative expiratory pressure technique, in which a modest suction pressure is applied at the mouthpiece during tidal expiration. It is assumed that any increase in flow (apart from a brief transient due to emptying the upper airway) implies the absence of flow limitation (Fig. 1.38 in Chapter 1).[29,30] The extent of flow limitation can vary with posture; it contributes to breathlessness on exercise,[31] and it may be an important determinant of orthopnoea.[32] Overall the prevalence of expiratory flow limitation in patients with COPD is high and, although there is a correlation with the reduction in FEV_1, this is not close.[29,30]

In patients with expiratory flow limitation due to COPD, the expectation on applying negative pressure at the mouth is that flow will not increase, but in some situations expiratory flow may actually decrease. This occurs particularly in patients with a very compliant upper airway, such as those with the obstructive sleep apnoea syndrome, and the coexistence of the two conditions may cause problems of interpretation.[33] Another approach to identifying flow limitation in COPD is by using forced oscillation, which may be more sensitive than the negative expiratory pressure method.[34]

9.2.5 Measurements of airway resistance

Tests of forced expiration are the most commonly used in routine clinical assessment of patients with airway narrowing. They have the advantages of good reproducibility, ease of performance and simple equipment. Measurement of airway resistance is favoured by some laboratories. This can be obtained either by plethysmography (panting or tidal breathing) or by the forced oscillation method (see Chapter 1, Section 1.6.4). Correlation between these two methods is good,[35] although correlations between tidal and forced manoeuvres are generally poorer.[35,36] None of these techniques is particularly sensitive to early disease (see Section 9.12.2). Although in normal subjects airway resistance is dominated by the central airway, which is the narrowest part of the bronchial tree, once the resistance of the more peripheral airways rises sufficiently this will no longer apply. Consequently, patients with symptomatic airway disease have clearly abnormal values of both resistance and forced expiratory measurements.

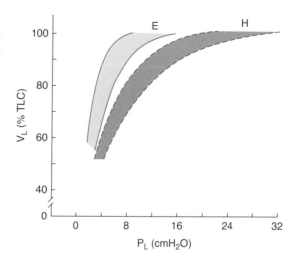

Figure 9.5 Range of static expiratory pressure–volume (PV) curves in 25 patients with emphysema (E) compared with healthy subjects (H) with volume expressed as per cent actual total lung capacity (TLC). Even in relation to relative lung volume, lung recoil pressure is greatly diminished and compliance is increased. Redrawn with permission from ref. 39.

P_L, lung recoil pressure; V_L, lung volume.

9.3 LUNG DISTENSIBILITY AND LUNG VOLUMES

9.3.1 Static pressure–volume curve of the lungs

The abnormalities of lung distensibility in COPD are in effect an exaggeration of the normal changes with age – but unlike normal ageing, the total lung capacity is usually considerably increased in COPD. The most abnormal pressure–volume (PV) curves are seen in patients with severe emphysema. This is most evident if the PV curve is plotted with lung volume expressed as per cent predicted TLC, but even in relation to actual TLC pulmonary compliance is increased and lung recoil pressures are reduced (Fig. 9.5).[2,37] Correspondingly, the parameter K of a monoexponential function fitted to the static PV curve (see Chapter 1, Section 1.2.2) is increased.[38,39] Correlations of K with the severity of emphysema assessed pathologically[40] or by CT scanning[41] have been reported, but some individuals with severe emphysema have apparently normal K values.[42] K is in effect an index of the size of the ventilated airspaces and it reflects the severity of microscopic emphysema. In some individuals with severe disease, progressive closure during expiration of airways subtending emphysematous lung modifies the shape of the PV curve, thereby reducing the value of K.[42] Destruction of alveolar architecture and increased

lung distensibility are not necessarily cause and effect, as in mild disease the reduction in elastic recoil and consequent increase in lung volume may be out of proportion to the severity of emphysema.[43]

Loss of lung recoil pressure and increases in compliance are sometimes regarded as specific for emphysema, but some abnormality of lung distensibility is seen in almost all patients with chronic airflow obstruction. In the early days of oesophageal pressure measurements it was thought that pulmonary compliance was less than normal in emphysema, but this erroneous conclusion was drawn from measurement of dynamic compliance, which, because of grossly uneven ventilation, is markedly reduced compared with the static value.

9.3.2 Static lung volumes

It is unusual in COPD not to find some increase in TLC if measured plethysmographically.[44] Measurements by gas dilution are likely to underestimate TLC in individuals with airway obstruction (see Chapter 1, Section 1.3.4) and can be misleading. On the other hand, plethysmography can sometimes overestimate lung volumes in subjects with airway disease, due to exaggerated phase differences between mouth and alveolar pressure during panting against a shutter (see Fig. 1.18 in Chapter 1). In practice, provided that the panting frequency is restricted to around 1 Hz, the effect is small, averaging only about 0.3 L.[45]

The increased lung distensibility in COPD might be expected also to increase the vital capacity, and a supernormal value is seen occasionally in early emphysema. However, any increase in VC at its upper limit is rapidly overtaken by the rising residual volume that 'prunes' the lower part of the VC, so that in most patients with established airway obstruction the VC is less than normal and it declines as the severity of airway narrowing increases. The FVC is usually even more reduced and considerably underestimates the true VC in many patients with airway narrowing.[46]

The characteristic increase in RV in COPD results mainly from progressive closure or virtual closure of airways during expiration. This occurs at larger volumes than normal because of both loss of lung recoil and 'intrinsic' narrowing of the airways. Towards the end of full expiration, flow continues at a very slow rate until terminated abruptly by the start of inspiration. The limit to further expiration is probably set by the uncomfortable sensation of prolonged forceful expiration through the few narrowed airways that are still patent. The RV increases relatively more than the TLC, so that the RV/TLC ratio is greater than normal. The magnitude of increases in RV and RV/TLC depends on the severity of airway narrowing, with general correlations between each and FEV_1.[44]

9.3.3 Lung hyperinflation

To the radiologist, hyperinflation of the lungs implies an increased TLC, as this is the volume at which chest radiographs are conventionally taken. In the functional and clinical context, however, hyperinflation implies an increased volume over the normal tidal breathing range, and in particular an increase in FRC. The term FRC is usually used synonymously with end expiratory lung volume (EELV).[47] In healthy subjects at rest, FRC coincides with the relaxation volume (V_r), at which outward elastic recoil of the chest wall exactly balances the inward recoil of the lungs and all the respiratory muscles are at rest (see Chapter 1, Section 1.1.1). In COPD the reduction in lung recoil alters this balance such that the relaxation volume increases (Fig. 9.6). In addition to this 'static hyperinflation', however, dynamic factors elevate FRC above V_r even at

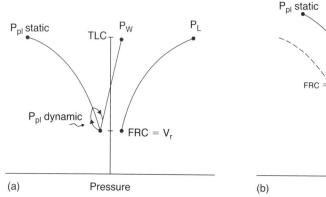
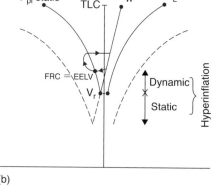

(a)   Pressure   (b)

Figure 9.6 Static and dynamic hyperinflation in chronic obstructive pulmonary disease (COPD) illustrated by schematic pressure–volume relationships. (a) Normal functional residual capacity (FRC), equal to the 'relaxation volume' (V_r), which is determined by the balance between lung recoil (P_L) inwards and chest wall recoil (P_W) outwards. Pleural pressure (P_{pl}) during breath-holding (P_{pl} static) is the mirror image of P_L and defines the pressure needed to maintain lung inflation at a particular volume; P_{pl} dynamic describes pleural pressure during a tidal breath, with the area of the tidal loop determined by the airway resistance. (b) Analogous relations in a patient with COPD and hyperinflation (broken lines repeat (a) for comparison). Chest wall recoil is assumed to be unchanged, but the loss of lung recoil increases the relaxation volume (static hyperinflation). Additional dynamic hyperinflation occurs because expiratory flow limitation causes premature termination of tidal expiration before V_r is reached and consequently end expiratory lung volume (EELV = FRC) is greater than V_r. The dynamic hyperinflation is likely to increase further with the greater ventilatory demands of exercise.

rest and, characteristically, FRC increases even further on exercise. By contrast, in healthy subjects FRC on exercise often falls below V_r due to increasing expiratory (abdominal) muscle contraction (see Chapter 7, Section 7.1.2.1).

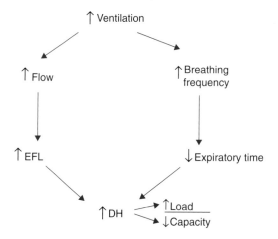

Figure 9.7 Progressive dynamic hyperinflation: potential contributory factors and consequences.

DH, dynamic hyperinflation; EFL, expiratory flow limitation.

Dynamic hyperinflation, both at rest and during exercise, occurs when inspiration begins before the 'natural' end of expiration is reached, i.e. before passive recoil of lungs and chest wall are balanced at V_r. The inspiratory muscles begin to contract and the next inspiration is initiated before expiratory flow ceases. Even at rest this phenomenon contributes significantly to the elevated FRC (Fig. 9.6).[48,49] Dynamic hyperinflation is dependent on both expiratory flow and expiratory time (Fig. 9.7).[49] When ventilation increases, the time available for expiration falls, encouraging its premature termination. Dynamic hyperinflation tends to be more severe in patients with more severe airway obstruction. It increases not only during exercise[50] but also during acute exacerbations of COPD.[51]

Since TLC does not change significantly during exercise, increasing hyperinflation can be monitored by measuring inspiratory capacity (IC),[52] which falls as tidal breathing occurs over a higher 'operating lung volume' range (Fig. 9.8).[50] The greater ventilatory demand of exercise in the face of a limited IC implies that increased ventilation may

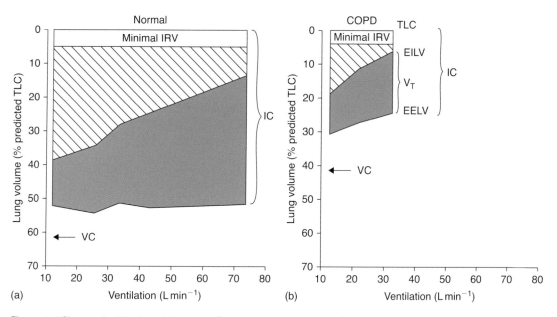

Figure 9.8 Changes in tidal breathing range ('operational lung volumes') as ventilation increases during exercise in (a) normal subjects and (b) patients with advanced chronic obstructive pulmonary disease (COPD). In the patients, the tidal range is severely constrained because of both the progressively increasing end expiratory lung volume (EELV = FRC, i.e. increasing dynamic hyperinflation) and end inspiratory lung volume (EILV), which approaches total lung capacity (TLC), leaving only a minimal inspiratory reserve volume (IRV). Redrawn from ref. 50, with permission from the American Thoracic Society.

FRC, functional residual capacity; IC, inspiratory capacity; VC, vital capacity; V_T, tidal volume.

be achievable only by a faster breathing frequency. This further decreases expiratory time (Fig. 9.7) and a vicious cycle of progressive dynamic hyperinflation may result.[49]

Although included here under the heading of lung volumes, dynamic hyperinflation and its effects on IC are, of course, a direct consequence of airway narrowing due to expiratory flow limitation (see Section 9.2.4). The breathing strategy is a response to the need for increased ventilation, but the consequent 'cost' borne by the respiratory muscles is a major contributor to breathlessness on exertion.

9.4 RESPIRATORY MUSCLE FUNCTION

The importance of respiratory muscle function in COPD has been recognized increasingly in recent years. The respiratory muscles are required to work against an increased load, while their capacity is potentially impaired by geometric, metabolic and nutritional factors. Respiratory muscle function is relevant to exercise performance, breathlessness, ventilatory control and the development of respiratory failure. The overall impression is that respiratory muscle function is better preserved than might be expected, considering the constraints under which the muscles operate.

9.4.1 Statics – respiratory muscle strength

In general, the position of full inflation is determined by a balance between recoil of the respiratory system and the strength of the inspiratory muscles (see Fig. 1.7a in Chapter 1). An increase in TLC of the magnitude sometimes seen in COPD (which may be as much as 150% of the predicted value) necessarily implies an alteration in the mechanical advantage of the inspiratory muscles, as the force needed to distend the lungs and chest wall is generated at thoracic volumes well above their normal working range. The interpretation of measurements of maximum respiratory pressures depends on whether they are considered in relation to the absolute volume (i.e. % predicted TLC) or relative volume (% actual TLC). At FRC or RV, maximum inspiratory pressure ($P_I$max) is less negative and transdiaphragmatic pressure (P_{di}max) is less than values found in normal subjects.[53] On the other

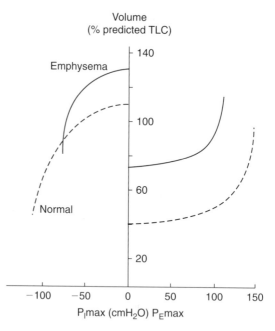

Figure 9.9 Average values of maximum static inspiratory alveolar pressure ($P_I$max) and maximum static expiratory alveolar pressure ($P_E$max) in groups of normal subjects (broken lines) and patients with emphysema (solid lines) plotted between residual volume (RV) and total lung capacity (TLC). Based on data of Decramer et al.[55]

hand, if maximum inspiratory pressures are related to absolute rather than relative lung volumes, they appear normal or even 'supernormal' (Fig. 9.9).[54] Measurements of P_{di}max during forceful voluntary inspiratory efforts[53] or phrenic nerve stimulation[56] have shown that diaphragmatic function is remarkably well preserved when account is taken of the hyperinflation.

These observations imply that the respiratory muscles, and particularly the diaphragm, are capable of adapting to hyperinflation by an alteration in the length–tension characteristics of the muscle. Various changes in diaphragmatic function contribute to this adaptation to the extra load imposed by increased airway resistance and hyperinflation. These include an alteration in the fibre composition of the muscle, with a greater proportion of fatigue-resistant type I muscle fibres,[57,58] a higher concentration of mitochondria and oxidative capacity,[58,59] and shortening of the muscle sarcomeres.[59] Despite its theoretical importance, it appears that reduction in diaphragmatic curvature has less effect on diaphragmatic function than reduction in muscle length.

The expiratory muscles are not at a similar mechanical disadvantage in the presence of an increased thoracic volume. Rochester and Braun therefore argued that maximum static expiratory alveolar pressure (P_Emax) could be used as an index of respiratory muscle strength when analysing the respective contributions of weakness and mechanical disadvantage to the impairment of P_Imax found in many patients.[60] Using this argument in a group of patients with COPD, Rochester and Braun found that the value of P_Emax (i.e. severity of weakness) explained 46 per cent and diaphragmatic length explained 35 per cent of the variance in P_Imax. They concluded, therefore, that impairment of static inspiratory muscle function in COPD was due to a combination of mechanical disadvantage and general muscle weakness. Recent evidence suggests that expiratory muscle function is rather better preserved than limb muscle function in COPD, possibly because of deconditioning in more disabled individuals.[61]

Generalized muscle weakness in COPD may be due to various nutritional and metabolic factors associated with inadequate intake, increased energy expenditure, blood gas disturbances and electrolyte deficiencies. Several studies have examined the effect of dietary supplementation on respiratory muscle function in malnourished patients with COPD. Some uncontrolled studies reported benefit, but controlled studies show no improvement in lung function or exercise capacity.[62]

Various controlled and uncontrolled studies have also examined the beneficial effects of specific training of the respiratory muscles. In general, training of muscles is task-specific, i.e. the benefits are seen in the task trained but not necessarily in other activities. Thus, it is possible to improve respiratory muscle strength by appropriate training but without necessarily providing any benefit to exercise performance. A meta-analysis of controlled studies of respiratory muscle training in COPD showed that training by either resistive breathing or isocapnic hyperventilation increased strength or endurance, but there was no improvement in exercise capacity.[63] A further recent controlled study, however, showed overall improvements in the sensations of breathlessness and fatigue following training.[64]

9.4.2 Dynamics – effects on tidal breathing

Hyperinflation of the thorax and consequent flattening of the diaphragm is associated with a change in the normal pattern of activation of the respiratory muscles with relatively greater activity of the inspiratory intercostals and accessory muscles and consequently relatively more displacement of the rib cage and less of the abdomen.[65] The normal inspiratory positive swing of abdominal pressure during tidal breathing is attenuated and in advanced disease the net change may become negative. The tidal swing in pleural pressure is inevitably increased because of the abnormally high airway resistance and also the reduced lung compliance associated with breathing at high volumes (see Fig. 9.6).

Early studies suggested that tidal expiration in COPD is essentially passive, but later work using intramuscular needle electrodes showed phasic expiratory electromyographic (EMG) activity in the deepest layer of abdominal muscles (transversus abdominis) in subjects with more severe airway narrowing.[66] There is generally less post-inspiratory 'braking' by persisting inspiratory muscle contraction than occurs in normal subjects.[67] With dynamic hyperinflation the inspiratory muscles begin to contract, and the next inspiration is initiated, before expiratory airflow ceases. This adds to the burden on the inspiratory muscles because there is a greater elastic load associated with tidal breathing over a higher volume range where lung compliance is less and the inspiratory muscles have to overcome an extra pressure (intrinsic positive end expiratory pressure, $PEEP_i$) before lung inflation can commence. This was first recognized in acutely ill patients during mechanical ventilation, where it is easily identifiable as a positive pressure if the airway is occluded at end expiration. The same phenomenon is present to a lesser extent in stable patients with COPD as a consequence of dynamic hyperinflation.[68]

The main inspiratory action of the diaphragm during tidal breathing, as in healthy subjects, is like a piston moving caudally.[69] The flattening of the diaphragm accommodates some of the increase in lung volume in COPD, but the larger part depends on expansion of the ribcage.[70,71] It was previously assumed that, over the tidal breathing range, the zone of apposition of the diaphragm to the parietal pleura lining the inner surface of the ribcage was diminished,[69] but direct measurement by ultrasonography suggests that this is not necessarily so.[71]

9.4.3 Respiratory muscle fatigue in chronic obstructive pulmonary disease

Patients with COPD have a limited force reserve and consequently increased potential to develop respiratory muscle fatigue.[72] This has been demonstrated in experimental studies using the various indices described in Chapter 1, Section 1.5.4.2, but the relevance of the results to normal breathing is unclear. Voluntary hyperventilation sufficient to reduce $PaCO_2$ by 10 mmHg has been shown to be associated with a change in the EMG high/low ratio compatible with the development of fatigue,[73] and patients with COPD develop slowed relaxation of the inspiratory muscles after exercise.[74] On the other hand, transdiaphragmatic pressure in response to cervical magnetic stimulation shows no decline following strenuous exercise,[75] suggesting that overt fatigue of the diaphragm is unlikely to be clinically significant. As discussed above, one important adaptation to the increased mechanical load in COPD is to breathe with a small tidal volume. Because of the irreducible dead space this breathing pattern predisposes to the development of hypercapnia, but it may also represent a mechanism that obviates the development of muscle fatigue.

9.5 BRONCHIAL RESPONSIVENESS

9.5.1 Effects of bronchodilators

Since bronchodilators have a measurable effect on the normal airway, it is unlikely that completely 'irreversible' airway obstruction exists. The most appropriate way of assessing the response to a bronchodilator response is somewhat contentious. Improvements in FEV_1 in COPD are characteristically small and on average less than seen in asthma, albeit with considerable overlap,[76] as the distribution of responses in the population of individuals with chronic airway obstruction is unimodal rather than bimodal (Fig. 9.10).[77] Consequently, using bronchodilator responsiveness to identify 'reversibility' of airway obstruction is inevitably arbitrary. Those who advocate such a distinction usually require both a percentage increase (e.g. 12%) and a minimum absolute increase (e.g. 200 mL) in FEV_1 to identify a 'significant' response.[78] With short-acting β-agonists there is a clear dose–response relationship and larger doses also produce a more prolonged effect.[79] Because of the small increases in FEV_1, other indices are sometimes advocated. Of simpler measurements, the increase in (relaxed) VC often exceeds that in FEV_1. (Sometimes the proportional increase in VC is greater than that in FEV_1 so that the ratio FEV_1/VC actually declines, despite clear evidence of improvement, emphasizing that this

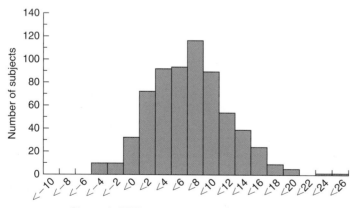

Change in FEV_1 % predicted after both bronchodilators

Figure 9.10 Unimodal distribution of change in forced expiratory volume in 1 s (FEV_1) (in absolute terms with volume expressed as % predicted) after bronchodilators (salbutamol + ipratropium) in 660 patients with chronic obstructive pulmonary disease (COPD). Redrawn from: Calverley PMA *et al.* Bronchodilator reversibility testing in chronic obstructive pulmonary disease. *Thorax* 2003; **58:** 659–64, with permission from the BMJ Publishing Group.

ratio is a poor guide to severity in established airway obstruction.)

Most recent interest has focused on the effects of bronchodilators on hyperinflation. Bronchodilators reduce FRC and increase IC both at rest[80] and on exercise, and several studies have shown that less hyperinflation is associated with less breathlessness and improved exercise capacity.[80–83] Exercise performance is often included in controlled trials of bronchodilators, with endurance (exercise time) during a constant work rate submaximal test used as a primary outcome measurement.[82,83] An endurance shuttle walk offers a simpler alternative.[84]

In everyday clinical assessment, however, the increase in FEV_1 remains the most commonly used index of bronchodilator response; in practice, its main value is in identifying unusually large responses (e.g. >0.4 L) in patients with chronic airway disease, which should alert the observer to the likelihood of asthma.

9.5.2 Effects of corticosteroids

The optimal method of assessing response to corticosteroids is an equally vexed question, as conventional respiratory function tests are of little value in predicting useful responses.[85] A meta-analysis of studies addressing the frequency of response to oral steroids in patients with stable chronic airway obstruction (excluding previously diagnosed asthma) showed that the proportion with an increase in FEV_1 greater than 20 per cent after a course of oral steroids was approximately 10 per cent greater than after placebo.[86] Whether such 'responders' are subsequently labelled 'asthmatic' is a semantic point, but in such a common clinical situation this frequency of response implies large numbers of patients.

Studies of treatment with inhaled steroids aimed at evaluating their effects on long-term decline of FEV_1 have consistently shown a modest increase over the first 3 months of treatment, even though the rate of decline thereafter is usually unaffected.[87,88] The short- to medium-term effect is assumed to be due to a reduction in inflammation in the airways. The general recommendation to use inhaled steroids routinely in the treatment of patients with COPD and more severe airway obstruction[7–9] is based on data related to the number of exacerbations rather than on evidence of improvement in respiratory function.

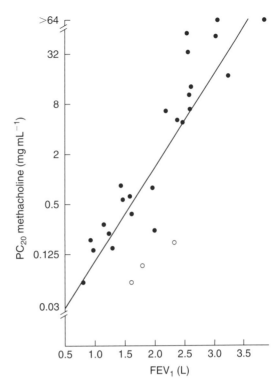

Figure 9.11 Relation between forced expiratory volume in 1 s (FEV_1) and bronchial responsiveness to methacholine (PC_{20} mg mL^{-1}) in patients with chronic obstructive pulmonary disease (COPD). Redrawn from: Ramsdale EH *et al*. Methacholine bronchial responsiveness in chronic bronchitis: relationship to airflow obstruction and cold air responsiveness. *Thorax* 1984; **39**: 912–18, with permission from the BMJ Publishing Group.

9.5.3 Effects of bronchoconstrictors

Patients with COPD generally show less responsiveness to bronchoconstrictor stimuli than do those with asthma, but often the apparent response is greater than that seen in the healthy population. The proportion of patients with COPD who show bronchial hyperresponsiveness (BHR) in various studies has varied from 45 per cent to 70 per cent.[89] In addition to the magnitude of the response, there are other important differences between bronchial reactivity in the two patient populations. A characteristic feature of asthma is marked sensitivity to chemical and other stimuli even when airway function is effectively normal. In COPD, however, there is a clearer relationship between sensitivity to histamine or methacholine and pre-challenge ventilatory function (Fig. 9.11).[90,91] Second, the range of stimuli producing responses in

COPD is more limited than in asthma, with responses seen more consistently to direct chemical stimuli than to indirect challenges such as exercise, hyperventilation and hypertonic saline, which in asthma produce their effects by release of mediators.[92] A plateau response to challenge (as is seen in healthy subjects) can be demonstrated in some, though not all, patients with COPD.[93]

The relation between BHR and pre-challenge airway function in COPD (unlike asthma) emphasizes the important role of airway dimensions in determining the response (see Chapter 1, Section 1.6.8.3). Detailed structure–function comparison has shown that BHR, as assessed by measurements of PC_{20} (see Chapter 1, Section 1.6.8.2), is related inversely to airway wall thickness;[91] the same study and another in patients with emphysema due to α_1-antitrypsin (AAT) deficiency[94] also highlighted a relation to loss of lung elasticity. The presence of emphysema may in addition underlie the loss of the normal bronchodilating effect of deep inspiration following methacholine challenge.[95] Epidemiological studies have shown that BHR in COPD predicts accelerated decline of FEV_1[96,97] and perhaps the development of COPD in initially asymptomatic individuals.[97]

Another manifestation of increased bronchial responsiveness is abnormal diurnal variation of ventilatory function, most often assessed in terms of spontaneous lability of PEF. Greater than normal variation is seen in many patients with COPD, and this correlates with sensitivity to methacholine challenge.[98] Another important clinical aspect of BHR is the response to therapeutic doses of β-blocking drugs. The adverse effect of these drugs in asthma has occasioned appropriate caution in their use in non-asthmatic patients with COPD. Bronchoconstriction is demonstrable in COPD following administration of non-selective agents such as propranolol,[99] but cardioselective agents such as metoprolol are generally considered safe, with no deterioration in FEV_1 or loss of the bronchodilator response to selective β_2-agonists,[100,101] although metoprolol has been shown to increase non-specific bronchial responsiveness, with a modest fall in PC_{20}.[101] The bigger concern is that, occasionally, β-blockers 'unmask' asthma by causing bronchoconstriction in previously undiagnosed individuals with chronic airway obstruction.

9.6 PULMONARY GAS EXCHANGE AND OXYGEN TRANSPORT

9.6.1 Distribution of ventilation

The distribution of ventilation is uneven at an early stage in the development of airflow obstruction. This is readily demonstrable using the single-breath nitrogen test (Fig. 9.12). The 'plateau' shows a rising concentration as the more poorly

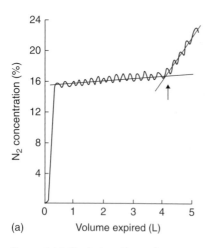
(a)

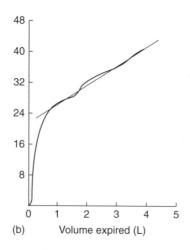
(b)

Figure 9.12 Single-breath test for uneven ventilation in (a) a normal subject and (b) a patient with severe airflow obstruction. In the normal subject, phase III shows only a slight slope and a clear closing volume is identifiable (arrow). In the patient, the slope of phase III is much steeper, cardiogenic oscillations are less marked and no phase IV can be identified.

ventilated alveoli empty later in expiration. The same effect can be shown with the multiple-breath nitrogen technique, where the time and ventilation required to wash out the nitrogen while breathing pure oxygen are increased. The uneven ventilation results from both patchy distribution of disease in the small airways and emphysema.[102]

Collateral ventilation – i.e. the ventilation of alveolar structures through passages or channels that bypass the normal airways[103] – is particularly common in emphysema. In healthy lungs the resistance of potential collateral channels is much greater than that of normal airways, but the reverse may be true in COPD.[104] Collateral ventilation can even occur between lobes, particularly in patients with homogeneous rather than heterogeneous distribution of emphysema.[105]

9.6.2 Distribution of pulmonary blood flow

Compensatory adjustments of pulmonary blood flow occur on a regional basis so that radioisotope scans in patients with airway obstruction often show gross irregularities of ventilation and perfusion but usually apparently fairly good regional matching of the two (Fig. 9.13). The local reduction in blood flow is caused by active vasoconstriction of pulmonary arterioles in areas of severe hypoxia.

Compensatory vasoconstriction on a regional basis is, however, only a crude means of matching ventilation and perfusion and considerable mismatching remains within lung regions, leading to a large physiological dead space and increased physiological shunt.

The mechanism regulating hypoxic vasoconstriction probably contributes to the development of pulmonary hypertension in advanced airway obstruction. Increasing the oxygen concentration of inspired air in such patients leads both acutely and over the longer term to reductions in pulmonary artery pressure by reversal of hypoxic vasoconstriction. Usually, clinical evidence of pulmonary hypertension is present only in severe airflow obstruction, but an abnormal rise in pulmonary artery pressure on exercise may occur in patients with milder disease.[106] In those with cor pulmonale and clinical evidence of right heart failure, the cardiac output is usually normal or greater than normal.[106]

9.6.3 Ventilation/perfusion mismatching

The main mechanism impairing the efficiency of pulmonary gas exchange in COPD is ventilation/perfusion mismatching. Arterial hypoxaemia is the rule, with or without hypercapnia. The contribution of lung units with low $\dot{V}_A/\dot{Q}$ ratios can be assessed by

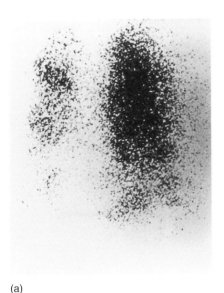
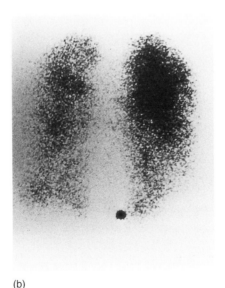

(a)   (b)

Figure 9.13 Ventilation (a) and perfusion (b) scans in a patient with chronic obstructive pulmonary disease (COPD), showing patchy, but apparently fairly well-matched, regional distribution of isotope.

calculation of the alveolar–arterial P_{O_2} difference (AaP_{O_2}) or, if a normal cardiac output is assumed, by calculation of the percentage physiological shunt as described in Chapter 2, Section 2.3.4. The contribution of high $\dot{V}_A/\dot{Q}$ lung units can be quantified by simultaneous collection of expired gas and arterial blood and application of the Bohr equation to calculate the dead space/tidal volume (V_D/V_T) ratio (see Equation 2.1 in Chapter 2); this is virtually always increased but in practice is rarely measured.

According to the classical three-compartment analysis of gas exchange, the presence of a raised Pa_{CO_2} indicates alveolar hypoventilation, i.e. underventilation of the 'ideal' alveoli. With severe $\dot{V}_A/\dot{Q}$ mismatching this 'compartment' becomes progressively smaller (see Chapter 2, Section 2.3.4). However, in reality, CO_2 retention results from $\dot{V}_A/\dot{Q}$ mismatching,[107,108] despite the classical teaching that any tendency for P_{CO_2} to rise can normally be countered by increasing total ventilation. In effect, some alveoli inspire the expired air of others, either in series (as in centrilobular emphysema) or via collateral pathways, and this has serious consequences for the elimination of CO_2, which may even exceed the effects on oxygen uptake.[108]

The multiple inert gas elimination technique (MIGET) allows detailed analysis of the mechanisms and effects of $\dot{V}_A/\dot{Q}$ mismatching in COPD. Wagner *et al.* studied 23 patients and found that the distribution of both ventilation and perfusion was usually bimodal (Fig. 9.14).[109] Most patients had a population of lung units with approximately normal ventilation and perfusion and a second population with either predominantly high $\dot{V}_A/\dot{Q}$ ratios (little perfusion) or predominantly low $\dot{V}_A/\dot{Q}$ ratios (little ventilation); a few patients showed both high and low patterns. Of those who showed clinical, radiographic and functional features of the predominantly 'emphysematous' type of airflow obstruction, the great majority had an abnormal population of high $\dot{V}_A/\dot{Q}$ units. In terms of the three-compartment model, this is equivalent to a large physiological dead space, with resting blood gases well preserved, but at the cost of excessive ventilation. By contrast, in patients with predominantly 'bronchial' features, the patterns of gas exchange were less clear-cut. Such patients usually have more severe hypoxaemia, and therefore an abnormal population of low $\dot{V}_A/\dot{Q}$ units might be expected; this is indeed seen in some patients (Fig. 9.14), but in others the hypoxaemia and venous admixture effect result from an overall reduction in mean $\dot{V}_A/\dot{Q}$ ratio, without any identifiable subgroup of low $\dot{V}_A/\dot{Q}$ lung units.

In a subsequent study of mild COPD, the results of the MIGET technique were compared with morphological data on lungs subsequently resected surgically.[110] Increased dispersion of both perfusion and ventilation were confirmed, and both, as well as the AaP_{O_2}, could be correlated with the severity of emphysema. A relationship was also found between the dispersion of ventilation and evidence of inflammatory changes in small airways. Breathing 100 per cent O_2 increased the dispersion of perfusion, worsening $\dot{V}_A/\dot{Q}$ mismatching overall,

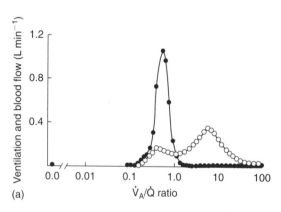
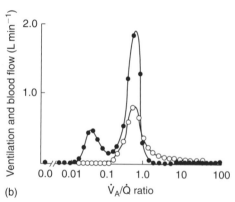

Figure 9.14 Distribution of ventilation/perfusion ($\dot{V}_A/\dot{Q}$) ratios determined by the multiple inert gas elimination technique (MIGET) in two patients with chronic obstructive pulmonary disease (COPD). **(a)** Bimodal distribution of ventilation (o), producing a large proportion of lung units with high $\dot{V}_A/\dot{Q}$ ratio (large physiological dead space) in a patient with predominant emphysema. **(b)** Bimodal distribution of perfusion (●) with increased population of lung units with low $\dot{V}_A/\dot{Q}$ ratios (large physiological shunt) in a patient with predominant bronchial disease. Redrawn from ref. 109 with permission from the American Society for Clinical Investigation.

presumably due to release of hypoxic vasoconstriction. Nevertheless PaO$_2$ increased to an average value of 481 mmHg, which, according to the traditional use of this test, implies only a mildly increased 'anatomical' shunt. In terms of the three-compartment model analysis, the deleterious effects of 100 per cent oxygen on $\dot{V}_A/\dot{Q}$ matching are seen also as an apparent increase in physiological dead space,[111] as better ventilated lung alveoli are 'deprived' of their perfusion in favour of less well-ventilated alveoli.

9.6.4 Determinants of arterial carbon dioxide tension

(See Table 9.2.)

In patients with chronic airflow obstruction there is a general inverse relationship between the FEV$_1$ and the resting PCO$_2$, best described by a hyperbolic

Table 9.2 Factors potentially contributing to hypercapnia in chronic obstructive pulmonary disease (COPD)

Severity of airway narrowing
Inspiratory muscle weakness/dysfunction
Small tidal volume, high V$_D$/V$_T$
Obesity
Excess alcohol consumption
Low innate ventilatory responsiveness
Uncontrolled oxygen treatment
Metabolic alkalosis
Sedatives, hypnotics, strong analgesics

V$_D$/V$_T$, dead space/tidal volume ratio.

function (Fig. 9.15a).[112] A proportion of patients, usually of the 'bronchial' type (see Section 9.13.1), have a resting value of PCO$_2$ well above the average predicted from their FEV$_1$. This may reflect an innately low premorbid ventilatory response to CO$_2$, but various other factors may also contribute, including inspiratory muscle dysfunction (Fig. 9.15b).[60] Several studies have emphasized the importance of the size of the tidal volume in determining whether or not CO$_2$ retention occurs.[113,114] Since the essential determinant of the arterial PCO$_2$ is not the overall ventilation, but the effective alveolar ventilation (see Equation 2.5 in Chapter 2), the pattern of breathing with rapid frequency and relatively small tidal volume adopted by patients with chronic airway obstruction (see Section 9.2.4) may have serious consequences for gas exchange if the mechanical benefits of a relatively small tidal volume are offset by a high V$_D$/V$_T$ ratio. Patients with COPD and hypercapnia can be distinguished most clearly from their fellows with normal PaCO$_2$ by a small tidal volume and more rapid frequency. Such a pattern is adopted by those with the highest mechanical load to breathing and the weakest inspiratory muscles or, more particularly, by those with the most adverse ratio of load to capacity. In a large study Bégin and Grassino showed that PaCO$_2$ correlated with V$_D$/V$_T$, FEV$_1$ or pulmonary resistance (R$_L$) (each an index of the mechanical 'load') and with the ratios R$_L$/P$_{max}$ or mean inspiratory pressure (again an index of load) to P$_I$max

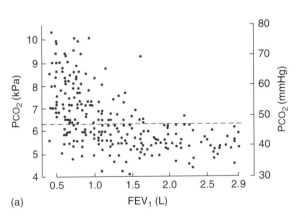

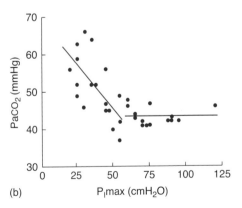

(a)   (b)

Figure 9.15 Factors that determine arterial PCO$_2$ levels in chronic obstructive pulmonary disease (COPD): both the forced expiratory volume in 1 s (FEV$_1$) (a) and maximum inspiratory pressure (P$_I$max) (b) relate inversely to PCO$_2$, but both are usually markedly impaired before hypercapnia develops (conversion: 1 kpa = 7.5 mmHg). (a) redrawn from: Lane DJ et al. Relation between airways obstruction and CO$_2$ tension in chronic obstructive airways disease. *Br Med J* 1968; **3**: 707–9, with permission from the BMJ Publishing Group. (b) redrawn from ref. 60, with permission from the American Thoracic Society.

(capacity).[113] $PaCO_2$ was also related to bodyweight, an association that accords with clinical experience of 'blue bloaters'. Although adoption of such a breathing pattern may avoid overloading the inspiratory muscles, reducing the risk of consequent fatigue and irreversible ventilatory failure, this is achieved at the cost of hypercapnia. A further factor that may be relevant is the function of the upper (pharyngeal) airway, as one study showed an association between hypercapnia in COPD and habitual snoring, possibly related to excess alcohol consumption.[115]

9.6.5 Tissue oxygen supply

Oxygen supply to the tissues depends not only on the arterial PO_2 but also on the haemoglobin concentration, acid–base status, red cell 2,3-diphosphoglycerate (2,3-DPG) and local blood flow. An increased red cell mass commonly accompanies arterial hypoxaemia in patients with COPD. Comparison is made with the effects of hypoxia on normal subjects at altitude but, in patients with COPD and hypoxaemia, the magnitude of the response sometimes appears to be exaggerated,[116] although direct comparison may not be valid, as single values of PaO_2 or SaO_2 may be unrepresentative. A further complicating factor in smokers is the presence of a significant level of carboxyhaemoglobin. This both reduces the oxygen-carrying capacity of haemoglobin and alters the position of the haemoglobin–oxygen dissociation curve and may affect the severity of secondary polycythaemia.[116] The apparently beneficial 'adaptation' of polycythaemia increasing blood oxygen content in hypoxaemic COPD may be outweighed by an increase in viscosity of the blood, and venesection may improve exercise capacity.[117]

9.7 CARBON MONOXIDE DIFFUSING CAPACITY

There is no good evidence that the transfer of oxygen and CO_2 across the alveolar capillary membrane in COPD is limited by incomplete diffusion. The diffusing capacity for CO (D_LCO) is, however, reduced in virtually all patients with symptomatic disease and particularly in the presence of severe emphysema. The D_LCO is reduced in part because of maldistribution of ventilation and also because emphysema reduces the overall alveolar surface area. The reduction in KCO seen in most patients largely reflects the latter. Many studies have shown a clear inverse relationship between KCO and the extent of emphysema found at autopsy,[5] in surgically resected lungs[118] and by CT scanning.[119] In generally, if the KCO is well preserved, severe generalized emphysema is effectively excluded. This probably represents the single most useful application of the measurement in clinical practice; the demonstration of a low KCO in a patient with airway obstruction usually implies a degree of alveolar destruction, whereas a normal or high value suggests asthma and should be an encouragement to pursue treatment more vigorously. As might be expected, the pulmonary capillary blood volume (V_c) is reduced in emphysema; it correlates inversely with severity but is no better a discriminant for emphysema than the simpler single breath D_LCO.[120]

9.8 RESPIRATORY FUNCTION DURING SLEEP

Worsening of pulmonary gas exchange during sleep is common in patients with COPD, especially in those whose blood gases are most abnormal by day. Hypoxaemia is particularly severe during rapid-eye-movement (REM) sleep,[121] when SaO_2 can fall to alarming levels. Increases in $PaCO_2$ are much less marked. Because of the considerable differences in the body 'stores' of oxygen and CO_2, transient deterioration in gas exchange results in much larger changes in PaO_2 and oxygen saturation than in $PaCO_2$. The main cause of the deterioration is hypoventilation,[122] related to the reduced ventilatory drive during sleep. On average, in patients with daytime hypercapnia, an overall increase in $PaCO_2$ of about 5 mmHg occurs from evening to early morning, with bigger increases in those with the highest daytime values.[123]

During REM sleep there is marked inhibition of the intercostal, scalene and sternomastoid muscles, with preservation of diaphragmatic activity, resulting in reduced expansion of the ribcage. Inhibition occurs during periods of rapid eye movements (phasic REM sleep) rather than continuously during REM sleep, so that the pattern of REM-related desaturation is of transient falls in SaO_2 interspersed by partial recovery (see Fig. 6.3 in Chapter 6).[122]

Overall, the strongest predictor of nocturnal oxygenation in COPD is the daytime level, with the relationship determined largely by the shape of the haemoglobin–oxygen dissociation curve.[124] In one study it was shown that nocturnal desaturation more than 4 per cent below the baseline awake level is very unlikely to occur if daytime SaO_2 is 95 per cent or greater but is virtually inevitable with daytime SaO_2 of 93 per cent or less.[125] In patients with mild daytime hypoxaemia and a narrow range of daytime PaO_2 (56–70 mmHg), two studies have shown an additional independent predictive effect of $PaCO_2$, with higher daytime $PaCO_2$ being associated with more severe nocturnal desaturation.[126,127]

The clinical value of sleep studies in patients with COPD has been a matter of debate. The issue is relevant because of the need to recognize patients whose prognosis is improved by long-term oxygen treatment (LTOT). The benefits of LTOT are well established in patients with daytime hypoxaemia,[128,129] but there is no good evidence that sleep measurements add to the prognostic information in terms of survival or the development of pulmonary hypertension.[126,130] For this reason, overnight measurements are not generally recommended as routine in patients with COPD. Detailed sleep assessment is, however, clearly indicated if the clinical features suggest the possibility of coexistent obstructive sleep apnoea syndrome.

9.9 TESTS OF VENTILATORY CONTROL

The relative roles of central and peripheral factors in ventilatory control and the genesis of hypercapnia in patients with COPD have been debated for many years. Recently the pendulum has swung towards peripheral mechanisms, due to better understanding of the constraints imposed by disordered lung mechanics and the associated impairment of inspiratory muscle function in the face of pulmonary hyperinflation.

The problems of interpreting an abnormal ventilatory response in the presence of disordered peripheral respiratory mechanics are discussed in Chapter 5, Section 5.3. In most patients with significant chronic airflow obstruction, the ventilatory response to CO_2 is impaired, as would be expected with the increased load due to airway narrowing. Attempts to assess more directly the output of the respiratory

centres by measuring diaphragmatic EMG,[131] work of breathing[132] and mouth occlusion pressure during CO_2 stimulation[133] have sometimes shown a proportion of patients with airflow obstruction (usually with chronic hypercapnia) in whom the reduction of ventilatory response appeared out of proportion to the disordered mechanics and in whom central insensitivity to CO_2 was therefore inferred. However, even an abnormally low occlusion pressure may not necessarily signify a central mechanism, for several reasons: first, the associated hyperinflation is likely to reduce the mechanical advantage of, and therefore the pressure generated by, the inspiratory muscles;[134] second, pressure measured at the mouth may not accurately reflect intrathoracic pressure in the presence of severe airway narrowing;[135] and third, if the end expiratory volume (FRC) is above the neutral relaxation volume of the lungs and thorax (dynamic hyperinflation), $P_{0.1}$ at the mouth will underestimate the output of the inspiratory muscles, since some of their energy is used to maintain the increased volume.[68] These considerations imply that $P_{0.1}$ will tend to underestimate the true central respiratory drive in COPD. The findings that the $P_{0.1}$ response to rebreathing CO_2 may be normal, and that even in hypercapnic patients resting values of $P_{0.1}$ are usually increased,[136] therefore imply that neural drive to breathe is actually increased rather than decreased and that alternative explanations for hypercapnia need to be sought.

A further problem with interpretation of responses to rebreathing in patients with hypercapnia relates to the stimulus measured; usually this is end tidal PCO_2, which in a rebreathing circuit is assumed to reflect arterial PCO_2. However, the ultimate stimulus to the central chemoreceptors is increasing hydrogen ion concentration and, in the presence of chronic hypercapnia, a given change in $PaCO_2$ will generate a smaller increase in $[H^+]$ (see Chapter 5, Section 5.2.1). Consequently, change in PCO_2 overestimates the relevant stimulus. Therefore, even leaving aside the problems of accurately measuring respiratory centre output, it is effectively impossible to determine the direction of causality, i.e. whether a low ventilatory response leads to hypercapnia or hypercapnia results in a low ventilatory response.

Ventilatory responses to hypoxia are also usually impaired in patients with chronic airflow obstruction.[137] Although interpretation is again compromised by adverse respiratory mechanics, the responses of both ventilation and mouth occlusion pressure to hypoxia are significantly less in chronically hypoxaemic patients than in better oxygenated patients with airway obstruction of similar severity, suggesting the possibility of adaptation to chronic hypoxia.[138]

9.10 RESPIRATORY FAILURE IN CHRONIC OBSTRUCTIVE PULMONARY DISEASE

9.10.1 Definitions and adaptations

In qualitative terms respiratory failure is an inability to maintain normal pulmonary gas exchange; an operational definition[139] sets arbitrary limits of a PaO_2 less than 60 mmHg with or without $PaCO_2$ greater than 49 mmHg at sea level and in the absence of a primary metabolic alkalosis. Hypoxaemia without hypercapnia is sometimes designated type 1 respiratory failure and hypercapnic respiratory failure, of which COPD is the commonest cause (also known as ventilatory failure), is designated as type 2.

Patients with severe airflow limitation when relatively 'well' may have levels of PaO_2 as low as 40–50 mmHg (5–6 kPa), but similar levels developing acutely in a normal subject (or in asthma) would rapidly impair the function of vital organs. In the chronic state, various compensatory mechanisms reduce the impact of the low PaO_2; these include changes in cardiac output, the oxygen dissociation curve, haemoglobin and tissue metabolism.

9.10.2 Acute exacerbations of chronic obstructive pulmonary disease

9.10.2.1 Pulmonary gas exchange

When, in a patient with COPD, an acute insult such as a bronchial infection occurs, the PaO_2 falls and $PaCO_2$ may rise. The worsening hypoxaemia is due primarily to deterioration in $\dot{V}_A/\dot{Q}$ matching, amplified by a decrease in mixed venous oxygen tension resulting from increased oxygen consumption.[140] At lower values of PaO_2, the steepness of the oxygen dissociation curve dictates that even a

small fall will considerably reduce the supply of oxygen to the tissues. For the same reasons a modest increment in the inspired oxygen concentration and in the PaO_2 can considerably increase the margin of safety and the amount of oxygen available to the tissues.[139] In general, the threat to life from *untreated* respiratory failure comes from hypoxaemia and not hypercapnia.[141] When breathing room air, the inverse relationship between alveolar PCO_2 and PO_2, together with the likely increased $AaPO_2$, dictate that the PaO_2 will fall to life-threatening levels before the $PaCO_2$ becomes narcotic. In the classic study by McNicol and Campbell of a large number of patients admitted to hospital with *untreated* respiratory failure due to an exacerbation of COPD, an initial $PaCO_2$ value greater than 80 mmHg (10.7 kPa) was found only once (Fig. 9.16).[141] The danger of uncontrolled oxygen is that it can provide the false security of a raised PaO_2 or SaO_2 at the same time, allowing the $PaCO_2$ to rise to dangerous levels (see below).

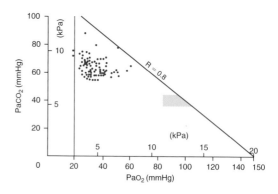

Figure 9.16 Arterial blood gases while breathing room air in patients presenting to hospital with respiratory failure due to acute exacerbations of chronic obstructive pulmonary disease (COPD) (data of McNicol and Campbell[141]). The values are plotted on a CO_2–O_2 diagram (cf. Fig. 2.9 in Chapter 2). The diagonal line represents possible alveolar gas tensions in a steady state with a respiratory exchange ratio (R) of 0.8; the horizontal distance between each point and the R-line then represents the calculated alveolar–arterial PO_2 difference ($AaPO_2$). The shaded area is the normal range and the vertical line at PaO_2 of 20 mmHg indicates the likely lowest PaO_2 compatible with survival. Note that most patients had $PaCO_2$ between 8 kPa and 10.7 kPa; higher values of $PaCO_2$ are virtually impossible, unless the patient has received oxygen to breathe.

9.10.2.2 Acid–base changes

In the study of McNicol and Campbell, 22 of 76 patients presenting with hypercapnic respiratory failure had initial values of arterial pH greater than 7.40 when, even with a chronic respiratory acidosis, a pH a little less than normal might be expected and an acute increase in $PaCO_2$ would reduce it further (see Chapter 4, Section 4.5.2).[141] More marked acidaemia is seen in more severe exacerbations, and eventually a metabolic acidosis is superimposed on respiratory acidosis. The level of acidaemia on admission is well recognized as a useful guide to prognosis in acute exacerbations of COPD, with values of $[H^+]$ exceeding 55 nM (pH <7.26) associated with an adverse outcome.[142] If pH is frankly alkaline, a coexisting primary metabolic alkalosis is likely. When this is seen in patients with respiratory failure and chronic airflow obstruction, the drug therapy should be carefully scrutinized, as such patients are particularly prone to develop a metabolic alkalosis when treated with drugs such as diuretics and corticosteroids, which promote renal excretion of hydrogen and chloride ions with retention of bicarbonate.[143] An additional alkalosis will tend to potentiate the disturbance of gas exchange by depressing ventilation and thus encouraging persistent hypercapnia.

An apparent metabolic alkalosis can be seen in patients with acute-on-chronic respiratory failure receiving ventilatory support. If, in a patient previously adapted to a high PCO_2, ventilation is increased to produce a more normal $PaCO_2$, the pH may rise alarmingly (Fig. 9.17). What then

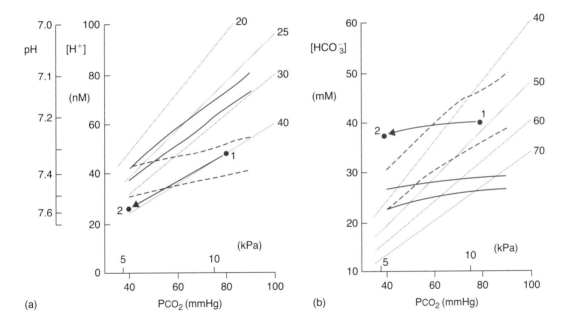

Figure 9.17 Effect of acutely lowering $PaCO_2$ by assisted ventilation in a subject with mainly chronic respiratory acidosis. The acid–base values are plotted on diagrams relating (a) $[H^+]$ to PCO_2 and (b) $[HCO_3^-]$ to PCO_2, and the graphs show 'confidence bands' for patients with acute (solid lines) and chronic (broken lines) respiratory acidosis, as in Fig. 4.11 in Chapter 4. Initially (1) the patient's values represent a chronic respiratory acidosis; when the $PaCO_2$ is lowered acutely to normal (2), the values follow a line parallel to the acute band. The actual values are:

	PCO_2 (mmHg)	$[H^+]$ (nM)	pH	$[HCO_3^-]$ (mM)
1	80	48	7.32	40
2	40	25.6	7.59	37.5

In isolation, the values at (2) suggest a primary metabolic alkalosis, but they actually represent an acute respiratory alkalosis superimposed on a chronic respiratory acidosis.

appears to be a metabolic alkalosis is actually a lag in excretion of bicarbonate ions (via the kidneys) behind elimination of CO_2 (via the lungs), i.e. an acute respiratory alkalosis superimposed on a chronic respiratory acidosis, masquerading as a primary metabolic alkalosis. The same pattern is sometimes seen even without mechanical ventilation in the early days of recovery from an episode of acute-on-chronic respiratory failure when delayed excretion of bicarbonate ions may be encouraged by use of diuretics or steroids. A logical approach to this situation is the cautious use of a carbonic anhydrase inhibitor, which produces a metabolic acidosis, thus removing some of the bicarbonate, encouraging a fall in $PaCO_2$ and a corresponding rise in PaO_2.

9.10.2.3 Respiratory mechanics and recovery from exacerbations

Most studies of the acute functional changes in exacerbations of COPD have compared measurements during hospital admission with convalescence and later. Unlike asthma, the fall in FEV_1 during an exacerbation of COPD is modest, with the abnormal gas exchange tending to dominate and to determine therapy. Increasing resistance of the small airways associated with inflammation, oedema and secretions exacerbates expiratory flow limitation, resulting in greater dynamic hyperinflation and higher operating tidal lung volumes.[51,144] Consequently FRC and RV increase, while VC and IC decrease; TLC shows no significant change.[144] Improvement in airway function can continue for as long as 6 weeks following an exacerbation,[51] and pulmonary gas exchange improves pari passu.[144] Improvement can also be monitored using forced oscillation, but FEV_1 has a superior signal-to-noise ratio.[145]

9.10.3 Effects of oxygen therapy

The potential adverse effects of uncontrolled oxygen therapy in acute exacerbations of COPD have been recognized since the 1950s, but, even in 2007, the risk is often ignored.[146] In a study of a large number of patients admitted to hospital with exacerbations, there was an inverse relationship between the initial arterial pH and PaO_2, i.e. patients

with relatively better oxygenation tended to have a more severe respiratory acidosis.[147] This apparently paradoxical finding results from prior treatment with uncontrolled oxygen in the emergency department or ambulance bringing the patient to hospital.[146]

The mechanism(s) of the acute respiratory acidosis induced by oxygen remain uncertain. Some evidence favours the 'classical' explanation of reduced ventilatory drive[148,149] and an overall reduction in ventilation while breathing oxygen, while other studies suggest that this traditional explanation is inadequate, as the fall in total ventilation when oxygen is administered is small, unsustained and related inconsistently to the rise in $PaCO_2$. The alternative hypothesis proposes an alteration in ventilation/perfusion matching due to increased inspired oxygen. Increasing the alveolar PO_2 releases compensatory vasoconstriction in poorly ventilated alveoli, thereby depriving some of the better ventilated alveoli of their perfusion and increasing the physiological dead space and V_D/V_T ratio.[150,151] In terms of the Riley–Cournand three-compartment model of gas exchange (see Chapter 2, Section 2.3.4), the increase in dead space ventilation occurs at the expense of ventilation of the (ideal) alveolar compartment, resulting in a higher $PaCO_2$, without necessarily any change in the total ventilation. Possibly, both mechanisms contribute to varying degrees in different individuals.

Whatever the mechanism of oxygen-induced hypercapnia, the practical message is that caution is required with uncontrolled oxygen, especially in patients with pre-existing hypercapnia, and especially in the unstable state in the first 48–72 hours of an exacerbation. The compromise in such situations is to aim for only modest enrichment of the inspired air. Some favour use of low-flow oxygen via nasal cannulae, but it is important to appreciate that, although the oxygen flow is thus controlled, the concentration inspired by the patient (F_IO_2) is not; it can vary considerably, both between and within individuals, depending on severe factors, including the rate of oxygen consumption and the pattern of breathing.[152] An accurate F_IO_2 can be delivered using a mask based on the Venturi principle, in which the concentration breathed by the patient is independent of oxygen flow rate (within fairly wide limits). In these devices the oxygen is driven through a nozzle, the size of which determines the concentration delivered to the patient: the higher the input flow of oxygen, the more air is entrained around the nozzle, maintaining a constant proportionality at the patient's mouth and nose. The concentrations of 24.5 per cent, 28 per cent and 35 per cent were originally chosen by Campbell to facilitate easy assessment of pulmonary gas exchange and calculation of the AaPO$_2$; under normal atmospheric conditions, these F$_I$O$_2$ values equate to inspired oxygen tensions (P$_I$O$_2$, BTPS) of 175 mmHg, 200 mmHg and 250 mmHg respectively, compared with the sea level atmospheric P$_I$O$_2$ (BTPS) of 150 mmHg. It should be noted that the 24.5 per cent O$_2$ delivered by the most commonly used mask represents an enrichment of the inspired air of only an additional 3.5 per cent.

9.10.4 Effects of non-invasive ventilation

The use of intubation and artificial ventilation in selected patients has been standard practice for severe exacerbations of COPD for many years, but this is needed much less frequently since the introduction of non-invasive ventilation (NIV) via a tight-fitting facemask or other interface. Non-invasive ventilation has been shown in several studies to improve outcome in comparison with 'standard care'.[153] It results in improved blood gases by increasing ventilation rather than by any effect on $\dot{V}_A/\dot{Q}$ relationships,[154] and it allows higher inspired oxygen concentrations to be given safely. Its use is associated with a reduction in the work of breathing, related partly to reducing the inspiratory threshold load associated with dynamic hyperinflation and PEEP$_i$.[155]

Longer-term domiciliary nocturnal NIV is less well established in COPD than in chronic ventilatory failure due to skeletal and neuromuscular conditions (see Chapter 16, Section 16.61 and Chapter 20, Section 20.4.3.1) but can result in improved daytime blood gases.[156–158] Its use is associated with less hyperinflation and reductions in FRC and RV.[157] There appears to be no detectable improvement in respiratory muscle function,[159] but the reduction in plasma bicarbonate resulting from increased CO$_2$ excretion overnight[160] may remove a factor depressing spontaneous breathing when this resumes during the day.

9.11 EXERCISE

9.11.1 Overview

The most important symptom limiting exercise in patients with COPD is breathlessness, at least in those with more severe airway obstruction, but leg fatigue is also a contributor, particularly in those with less severe disease and particularly in exercise tests that involve cycling rather than walking.[161–163] Impaired cardiac function and circulatory limitation are less common, although relative tachycardia is frequently found due to deconditioning secondary to reduced activity.

Breathlessness results largely from the combination of an increased load imposed by adverse respiratory mechanics and impaired capacity of the respiratory muscles. Both the load and the capacity are affected adversely by hyperinflation, which tends to increase on exercise due to the greater ventilatory demand and consequently increasing expiratory flow limitation. The resulting dynamic hyperinflation is a key factor determining the limits to exercise, the nature and severity of breathlessness, the deterioration of gas exchange and the effects of therapy.[50,163,164] Compensatory mechanisms, such as changes in shape of the chest wall and shortening of the diaphragmatic muscle fibres, may limit the consequences of hyperinflation if they develop gradually, but they break down and may be overwhelmed during exercise.

9.11.2 Respiratory mechanics during exercise

Dynamic hyperinflation (DH) is often present at rest in patients with COPD, and it is likely to increase further on exercise. In essence, DH represents a compensatory adaptation to expiratory flow limitation, as, in principle, higher expiratory tidal flows can be achieved at volumes closer to full inflation (see Fig. 9.3). Consequently EELV and end inspiratory lung volume (EILV) increase and the 'operating volumes' during breathing are closer to TLC than at rest (see Fig. 9.8). The tidal volume itself may increase little as its upper extreme is constrained by the point of full inflation. Despite the 'compensation' of DH, expiratory flow at the higher volumes may still be flow-limited over a larger proportion of the tidal volume than at rest.[165] Since TLC itself does not change significantly during exercise, measurement of inspiratory capacity (IC = TLC − EELV) gives a valid index of the extent of DH.[52] DH is inevitably accompanied by a reduction in dynamic compliance of the lungs, due to the shape of their pressure–volume relationship (see Chapter 1, Section 1.2.1). Any increase in tidal volume has a similar effect, and both factors (DH and increased tidal volume) increase the work of breathing.[166] At the same time, the pressure-generating capacity of the inspiratory muscles is less at the higher operating lung volumes and therefore greater diaphragmatic activation is needed to achieve a given output.[167]

The alternative way of increasing ventilation on exercise is by a more rapid breathing frequency. This again increases the load on the inspiratory muscles as they are required to contract more frequently. Additionally, because of the abnormally slow expiration through narrowed airways, the shorter expiratory time with higher breathing frequencies curtails expiration, which may exacerbate hyperinflation,[50] with further adverse effects on the load/capacity ratio of the inspiratory muscles (see Fig. 9.7).

In one study of a large number of patients with COPD of varying severity, the average increase in EELV (reduction in IC) on exercise was about 0.4 L,[50] but the extent is very variable, with a general inverse correlation between the exercise-induced reduction in IC and the resting value.[50] The severity of breathlessness has been shown to be proportional to the decrease in IC during both steady-state exercise[168] and a 6-min walk.[169] EILV rises close to TLC in some patients at peak exercise,[167] and the level of breathlessness increases disproportionately once an apparently minimal value of IRV of about 0.5 L is reached.[170]

Exercise capacity is related closely to the severity of resting hyperinflation: peak $\dot{V}O_2$ during progressive exercise is inversely proportional to the resting IC or IC/TLC.[171,172] An increase in EELV (or decrease in IC) on exercise is not universal in COPD and is less likely to occur in people with more expiratory 'flow reserve' at rest.[173] Some patients maintain a relatively unchanged EELV at lower work rates, increasing more markedly towards the end of progressive exercise, while in others DH increases progressively with workload.[174]

9.11.3 Circulatory effects of exercise

Patients with COPD also have abnormal circulatory responses to exercise; in particular, there is often an abnormal rise in pulmonary arterial pressure and a tendency for the stroke volume to be smaller and the heart rate to be greater than normal at a given workload.[175] At the end of a symptom-limited progressive exercise test, however, cardiac output and heart rate are usually well below the expected maxima. Although such patients tend to be unfit, they are often incapable of sufficient exercise to cause anaerobic metabolism, so that an 'anaerobic threshold' may not be detectable, peak blood concentrations of lactate are less than normal, and the disproportionate rise of ventilation normally seen at higher levels of exercise may not occur.

9.11.4 Pulmonary gas exchange and arterial blood gases on exercise

In COPD with mild airway obstruction, matching of ventilation and perfusion may improve on exercise, with an increase in the overall mean $\dot{V}_A/\dot{Q}$ ratio and more even distribution of ventilation.[176] In more severe airway obstruction, oxygen desaturation is more common, with or without worsening hypercapnia. Early studies suggested that a fall in PaO_2 was a more consistent feature of emphysema,[177] but subsequent experience has shown that it is not a reliable discriminator. Hypoxaemia on exercise does not necessarily imply deteriorating $\dot{V}_A/\dot{Q}$ relationships, as other contributory factors include inadequate overall ventilation and the effect of decreased mixed venous PO_2 due to greater extraction of oxygen from the blood by the exercising muscles. The latter amplifies the effect of lung units with low $\dot{V}_A/\dot{Q}$ ratios.[178]

Dynamic hyperinflation also plays a major role in determining arterial blood gases on exercise, with the consequent restriction of tidal volume together with the increased physiological dead space reducing effective alveolar ventilation. The extent of DH on exercise has been shown to correlate with both the reduction in PaO_2 and the increase in $PaCO_2$.[172,179] The increase in $PaCO_2$ during exercise also correlates with the tendency to hypercapnia while breathing uncontrolled oxygen at rest.[179]

There are differences in gas exchange and blood gases between different types of exercise, which may be of clinical importance, as the results of cycle ergometry may not give an accurate picture of respiratory function during normal everyday activities. Comparisons of walk tests, e.g. 6-min walk (6 MW), shuttle walk, or progressive exercise on a treadmill with the results of cycling show that walking is associated with a higher peak $\dot{V}O_2$ but lower peak blood lactate, the latter presumably reflecting the bulk of the muscles employed.[180,181] Of importance, walking has been shown consistently to result in lower PaO_2 or SaO_2,[180–182] and consequently cycling tests may underestimate the severity of desaturation, a finding that has obvious implications for evaluating patients for ambulatory oxygen treatment. The precise mechanism of the greater desaturation when walking is uncertain, but less efficient gas exchange is implied by the finding of a higher V_D/V_T ratio, and either postural differences and their effect on FRC or differences in pulmonary haemodynamics may be relevant.[181]

9.11.5 Effects of therapy on exercise performance

The main way in which effective treatment improves exercise capacity and performance in COPD is by reducing ventilation and consequently reducing expiratory flow limitation and dynamic hyperinflation, or at least allowing exercise to continue for longer before their effects become limiting. This effect has been well demonstrated, e.g. during constant load exercise with treatment with long-acting bronchodilators, both anticholinergic drugs and β-agonists.[183,184] These agents increase IC, both at rest and on exercise, with consequently a larger tidal volume and lower EELV after a given period of exercise ('isotime') (Fig. 9.18). The 'signal' resulting from bronchodilatation is relatively greater with such measurements on exercise than that given by FEV_1 (although, as discussed in Section 9.5.1, increases in other spirometric volumes, e.g. IC and VC at rest, also allow better recognition of bronchodilator effects in COPD than FEV_1).

A similar mechanism underlies the beneficial effect of breathing oxygen on exercise, even in individuals with only mild hypoxaemia.[185] In those with more severe hypoxaemia, oxygen during exercise delays the development of DH and reduces breathlessness in proportion to the reduction in ventilation, albeit at the cost of rising $PaCO_2$.[186] The effects of bronchodilators and oxygen on constant work rate exercise are additive.[187] Although oxygen given only during recovery from exercise hastens the resolution of DH,[188] this does not necessarily alleviate breathlessness more rapidly.[188,189]

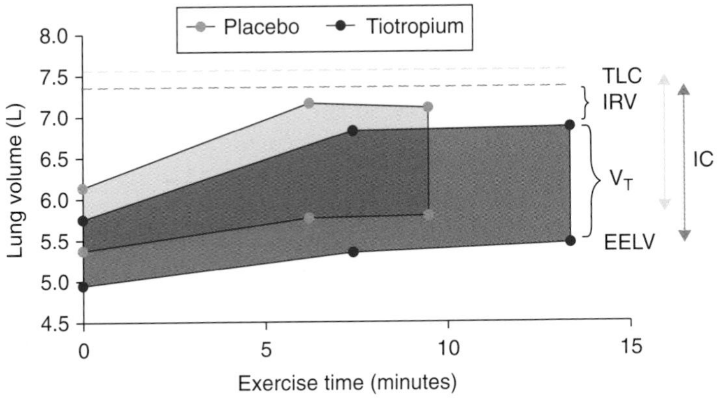

Figure 9.18 Effect of a bronchodilator (tiotropium, ●) compared with placebo (●) on 'operational lung volumes' in patients with chronic obstructive pulmonary disease (COPD) during constant workload exercise. A major effect of the bronchodilator is a reduction in dynamic hyperinflation and an increase in inspiratory capacity, which allows longer exercise duration. Redrawn from ref. 183 with permission from the American College of Chest Physicians.

EELV, end expiratory lung volume; IC, inspiratory capacity; IRV, inspiratory reserve volume; TLC, total lung capacity; V_T, tidal volume.

9.11.6　Effects of pulmonary rehabilitation and muscle training

The strength of both the respiratory and the peripheral muscles are important determinants of exercise capacity and symptoms in COPD.[161,190] Reductions in both the strength[191] and the endurance [192] of limb muscles have been shown and are probably related to the inactivity and deconditioning that develop as airway obstruction worsens. Exercise training has been shown to increase endurance, with a lower ventilation and consequently less dynamic hyperinflation for a given work rate.[193] The main mechanism by which training improves exercise performance is thus similar to that of other therapeutic interventions such as bronchodilators and oxygen. In addition to a reduction in ventilatory demand, however, there may also be a change in perception of the symptom.[194]

Pulmonary rehabilitation has been shown in many studies to improve exercise performance.[195] Although exercise training is probably the key factor, other components of a rehabilitation programme, which probably act synergistically, include improvements in nutrition, optimizing drug treatment, psychosocial support and patient education.

9.11.7　Relation of exercise performance to measurements at rest

In an individual with COPD, the prediction of exercise performance from resting lung function is not very accurate, but clear correlations are found across populations of patients with widely varying severity of disease. Thus, in progressive exercise testing, both maximum ventilation and maximum $\dot{V}o_2$ are related independently to the FEV_1[171,196] and to the severity of hyperinflation as expressed by the ratio IC/TLC.[171] Other factors that have been shown in different studies to relate independently to performance include D_Lco,[197] P_Imax[198] and bodyweight (as a percentage of ideal).[199] Similarly, the results of 6-min walk tests correlate with FEV_1, D_Lco, Kco,[200] P_Imax[201] and bodyweight.[202] Of potential clinical importance, even modest acute increases in weight impair performance.[203] Although changes in FEV_1 are sensitive to progression of mild to moderate COPD, the 6-min walk distance (6 MWD) becomes more sensitive in more advanced disease.[204] The

severity of arterial desaturation during walk tests is proportional to resting D_Lco[200,205] and resting Sao_2,[205] but it is not clearly related to either the distance walked or the severity of breathlessness.[200] Breathlessness during progressive exercise in patients with COPD is related closely to both ventilation and $\dot{V}o_2$.[206] As with measurements of ventilation, the severity of breathlessness correlates independently with mechanical function (FEV_1) and respiratory muscle function.[207]

9.12　EVOLUTION OF CHRONIC AIRFLOW OBSTRUCTION AND SENSITIVE TESTS

9.12.1　Rate of decline of FEV_1

Functional[10] and pathological[11] evidence shows that the major site of airway narrowing in patients with COPD is in the small conducting airways less than 2 mm in diameter. In health these contribute little to tests such as the FEV_1 or airway resistance, and extensive disease in this 'silent zone' can occur before it is recognizable by conventional tests. Even when the FEV_1 becomes detectably abnormal, many individuals remain untroubled by breathlessness; most patients presenting to hospital with symptoms due to chronic airway obstruction have an FEV_1 of 50 per cent or less of the predicted value. By the time this happens the disease may have been developing for 20 years.

Epidemiological studies show an average age-related decline of FEV_1 in healthy non-smoking individuals of about 30–40 mL per year; this is greater in smokers and correlates with the amount smoked.[208,209] A minority of smokers appear particularly susceptible to the effects of tobacco smoke and show an accelerated rate of decline leading to overt COPD (Fig. 9.19). The classic study of Fletcher and Peto suggested that this proportion was about 10–15 per cent of smokers,[208] but the more recent Copenhagen City Heart study suggests a higher figure of at least 25 per cent.[210] Although the Fletcher and Peto study showed no overall decline related to mucous hypersecretion, the Copenhagen data show an additional effect, at least when subjects with more advanced COPD were included.[211] Smokers who quit show a minimal improvement in FEV_1 (average 2%) but, more importantly, the

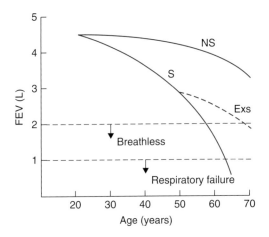

Figure 9.19 Schematic diagram of decline of forced expiratory volume in 1 s (FEV₁) with age in a healthy non-smoker (NS) and a susceptible smoker (S). Symptoms are usually not significant until FEV₁ has fallen to 50 per cent or so of its predicted value; respiratory failure becomes increasingly likely when FEV₁ falls to 1 L or less (cf. Fig. 9.14a). The rate of decline is slowed after cessation of smoking (Exs) and runs parallel to the non-smoker. Based on data of Fletcher and Peto.[208]

Table 9.3 Sensitive tests of 'small airway function' in chronic obstructive pulmonary disease (COPD)

Test	Reference
$\dot{V}_E$ max at low lung volumes	217
Moments analysis of forced spirogram	218
Density dependence of $\dot{V}_E$ max and/or resistance	219
Reduced VC and increased RV	220
Frequency dependence of dynamic compliance	221
Frequency dependence of resistance	222
Slope of phase III	223
Abnormal isotopic ventilation scans Widening of AaPo₂	224

AaPo₂, alveolar–arterial Po₂ difference; RV, residual volume; VC, vital capacity; $\dot{V}_E$ max, maximum expiratory flow.

subsequent rate of decline reverts to values comparable to those of non-smokers.[212]

Frequent physical activity by smokers appears to have a protective effect and is associated with a reduced rate of decline of FEV₁ in the population in general.[213] A consistent finding in several studies is that BHR to non-specific stimuli such as methacholine or histamine is associated with a more rapid rate of decline.[212,214,215] This observation is used in support of the so called 'Dutch hypothesis', which maintains that the airway obstruction associated with both asthma and COPD should be regarded similarly as expressions of a primary abnormality of the airways rather than as distinct conditions. This hypothesis remains controversial and on present knowledge it is not possible to distinguish cause and effect between the association of BHR and rapid decline of airway function: either BHR could predispose to deterioration, or early disease may be responsible for BHR.[216]

9.12.2 Sensitive tests of 'small airway function'

The relative insensitivity of the FEV₁ to early changes in COPD has stimulated the search for more sensitive tests that identify early disease in the small airways (Table 9.3). Although these tests are generally regarded as reflecting narrowing of the small airways, most are also affected by loss of lung recoil and should be regarded more correctly as tests of peripheral lung function.

9.12.2.1 Maximum expiratory flow at small lung volumes

In normal subjects, maximum flow at larger volumes is determined mainly by the diameter of the more central airways, but $\dot{V}_E$ max later in expiration more closely reflects damage in the more peripheral airways (see Chapter 1, Section 1.6.5.2). On an MEFV curve, low flows in the terminal portion producing a greater convexity towards the volume axis are therefore a characteristic early feature.[217] The FEF₂₅₋₇₅% VC (previously known as the maximum mid-expiratory flow, MMEF) is sometimes regarded as a specific test of 'small airway function', but, as discussed in Chapter 1, Section 1.6.5.9, this is not so and it is doubtful whether it conveys any more information than the conventional spirometric indices of FEV₁, (F) VC and their ratio.

9.12.2.2 Transit time analysis

The lung units with the lowest flow rates take the longest time to empty during forced expiration and, although their contribution to flow is small, their contribution to the mean transit time is disproportionately great; for this reason transit time analysis (see Chapter 1, Section 1.6.5.10) has been proposed for detecting early disease,[218] but its potential value has been little exploited.

9.12.2.3 Air and helium flow–volume curves

Comparison of MEFV curves breathing air and a helium/oxygen mixture to assess the density dependence of $\dot{V}_E$ max may be helpful for identifying narrowing of central airways but has not proved to be of value in predicting peripheral airway function in COPD.[219]

9.12.2.4 Reduced vital capacity

A spirometric variant that probably reflects disease of the small airways is a reduction in FEV_1 and VC, but with a normal FEV_1/VC ratio, together with an increased RV, increased RV/TLC but usually normal TLC.[220] This pattern has been described in sporadic reports but its frequency is uncertain.

9.12.2.5 Frequency dependence of compliance and resistance

Other tests reflect uneven distribution of ventilation resulting from the patchy nature of disease in the peripheral airways. In healthy subjects the compliance of the lungs during tidal breathing (dynamic compliance) is close to the static compliance (see Chapter 1, Section 1.2.5) but, even with mild airway disease, it becomes less than the static compliance and declines further as breathing frequency increases.[221] The assessment of the frequency dependence of dynamic compliance is, however, tedious, fraught with technical problems and impracticable on a large scale. Unevenness in the distribution of resistance of the small airways also predicates that resistance falls at higher breathing frequencies, because, with increasing frequency, ventilation is distributed preferentially via airways with lower resistance as frequency increases. The frequency dependence of airway resistance is more readily measurable than compliance, particularly using forced oscillation at various frequencies, a technique that offers one of the more practicable

methods for detecting early disease in the peripheral airways.[222]

9.12.2.6 Single-breath nitrogen test

Another useful technique in this context is the single-breath test for uneven ventilation (see Chapter 2, Section 2.1.9), which allows measurement of closing volume and the slope of phase III. In practice, the latter is the more useful index and is less subject to variation between observers.[223]

9.12.2.7 Isotope scans

Abnormal isotopic ventilation scans are seen in some smoking individuals with otherwise normal function, but normal regional distribution of ventilation can be seen in others even when FEV_1/VC or phase III are abnormal so that the significance of such findings is uncertain.[224]

9.12.2.8 Alveolar–arterial P_{O_2} difference

Widening of the AaP_{O_2} is non-specific but is seen with early airway disease. However, it requires blood sampling and cautious interpretation, as its relationship to the proportion of venous admixture is alinear and it increases if alveolar P_{O_2} rises, e.g. during transient hyperventilation (see Chapter 4, Section 4.4.2.4).

9.12.2.9 Value of 'small airway tests'

The main hope of these 'sensitive' tests was the early detection of changes in the small airways in COPD, with a view to reversing, or at least halting, the damage. In practice, however, their application has proved disappointing. Comparison with structure of the small airways in subsequently resected lungs has shown that changes in the respiratory and membranous bronchioles relate better to FEV_1 (even when relatively 'normal') than to flow volume or single-breath indices,[225] although the relationship is stronger when several different 'small airway' tests are abnormal.[226]

Long-term follow-up of smokers to detect those with accelerated decline of FEV_1 suggests that, if the initial FEV_1/VC ratio is normal, an abnormal single-breath nitrogen slope does not discriminate but it may improve the prediction of more rapid deterioration in subjects with an initially reduced FEV_1/VC.[227] On the other hand, initially low D_LCO and KCO do presage more rapid decline in FEV_1.[228]

9.12.3 Prediction of survival

In patients with established COPD across a broad range of severity, FEV_1 is generally the best single correlate of survival and mortality,[229,230] but, clearly, several other factors, related and unrelated to respiratory function, are also important. However, if patients within a narrow range of severity (usually defined by FEV_1, as % predicted) are studied it is not surprising that the predictive value of FEV_1 itself is weakened. Consequently, comparisons of the prognostic value of different indices and claims about which are 'the best' need to be tempered by the context of the particular population being studied. Thus, in patients with more advanced disease and respiratory failure, arterial Po_2 and Pco_2 are particularly important, as demonstrated by the classical trials of long-term oxygen treatment.[128,129] Other studies in patients with less severe disease have highlighted the prognostic value of the 6 MW distance[231] and the severity of breathlessness.[232] More accurate prognosis is possible by combining functional data including FEV_1 and exercise capacity with breathlessness and body mass index (BMI) to give a multidimensional index.[233,234] In patients with predominant and advanced emphysema the regional distribution of emphysema is a further important prognostic factor, with relatively more emphysema in the lower zones worsening the prognosis.[235]

9.13 CHRONIC OBSTRUCTIVE PULMONARY DISEASE PHENOTYPES

9.13.1 'Bronchial' and 'emphysematous' types of chronic obstructive pulmonary disease

It has been traditional to distinguish two main patterns of COPD with differing clinical, radiographic and functional features that correlate in general with pathological changes predominantly in the airways or the alveoli respectively.[5] Although typical examples of the two polar groups are seen, the majority of patients with COPD fall in between, with evidence

of both emphysema and bronchial/bronchiolar disease. Apart from the context of lung volume reduction surgery (LVRS; see Section 9.15), the distinction is usually of little relevance to the individual patient. Of greater clinical importance is to distinguish patients with largely 'fixed' airflow obstruction (many, but not all, of whom have emphysema) from those whose airway narrowing is more variable (i.e. patients likely to have asthma). The D_LCO and, more specifically, KCO are of value in this distinction but the two diagnoses are not mutually exclusive. Even in the presence of significant emphysema, asthma may coexist, as evidenced, for example, by marked variability of airway obstruction and a useful response to appropriate therapy such as corticosteroids.

Emphysema in the context used here implies the panacinar variety of at least moderate severity; the centrilobular or centriacinar form results from dilatation and destruction of respiratory bronchioles and is accompanied by more severe narrowing of the small airways.[11] Centrilobular emphysematous airspaces may themselves be an important cause of gas exchange abnormalities in COPD (see Section 9.6.3).[108]

The classical features of the emphysematous patient (type 'A' or 'pink puffer') include radiographic evidence of emphysema, greatly increased total lung capacity, and static compliance with markedly reduced lung recoil pressure; both the D_LCO and KCO are reduced, hypoxaemia at rest is only mild, and the arterial Pco_2 is less than average for the degree of airflow obstruction. The cardiac output is normal or low and the pulmonary vascular resistance is high, especially on exercise. At the other extreme, the patient with primary bronchial disease (type 'B' or 'blue bloater') is often obese, with a smaller increase in total lung capacity and less reduction in lung recoil pressure; the D_LCO is reduced but KCO is relatively preserved, the Pao_2 is severely reduced and often accompanied by polycythaemia, the $Paco_2$ is above average for the level of airflow limitation, and the cardiac output may be greater than normal.[5,106] Ventilatory responses to CO_2 are reduced in both groups, but more so in the bronchial type (who usually have resting hypercapnia). However, in patients with severe COPD, even with no CT evidence of emphysema, the D_LCO usually shows a reduction due to maldistribution of the inspired test gas, and an increased TLC with consequently reduced maximum lung recoil is seen.[236] A reduction in K_{CO} in COPD is more specific for emphysema, with a consistently good inverse relationship found with CT-derived measurements of the extent and severity of emphysema.[119,237] The relationship to CT-derived emphysema is strengthened further by combining indices of airway obstruction with K_{CO}.[238] The topographical distribution of emphysema also influences its effects on respiratory function. A stronger association is seen between reduced K_{CO} and upper rather than lower zone dominance, while the effects on airway function are relatively greater when emphysema preferentially affects the lower zones, presumably because the airway support by the surrounding alveoli is less in the basal regions in the upright position.[239]

9.13.2 α_1-Antitrypsin (AAT) phenotypes

The 'purest' examples of emphysema occur in patients with severe deficiency of AAT (usually Pi type ZZ) who can have radiographic and functional evidence of advanced disease at an early age. Since the effects of the deficiency are synergistic with those of cigarette smoking, which also causes bronchial disease, it is unusual even with AAT deficiency to find patients with no evidence of 'bronchitis'. This interaction with cigarette smoking also accounts for some of the wide range in severity of the functional abnormalities.[240] However, many non-smoking ZZ individuals,[241] and even some smokers,[240] have little or no functional abnormality.

Although severe AAT deficiency has proved very valuable as a model of the pathogenesis and functional consequences of emphysema, it accounts for only a very small proportion of patients with COPD. Intermediate levels of AAT, most often associated with the heterozygous Pi MZ, inevitably occur more frequently. The early suggestion that this much commoner partial deficiency might be responsible for emphysema in many patients with COPD has not been borne out. Epidemiological studies have shown that the MZ phenotype is associated with a slightly increased age-related decline of FEV_1.[242] Subtle changes in lung distensibility have been found in MZ individuals,[243] but their contribution to the overall COPD population is very small.[242]

9.14 EMPHYSEMATOUS BULLAE AND BULLECTOMY

Bullae can develop in otherwise healthy lungs, in which case they are usually of little functional consequence. The bigger dilemma is presented by bullae in patients with COPD, in whom prediction of the likely benefit of surgical treatment may be desirable. Removal of an area of dead space is rarely relevant, as bullae are usually not significantly ventilated or perfused (Fig. 9.20).[244] More commonly

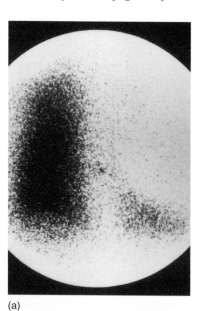

(a)

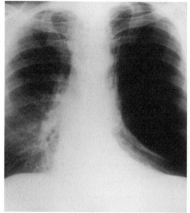

(b)

Figure 9.20 (a) Ventilation scan and (b) chest radiograph of a patient with a large emphysematous bulla, showing that the bulla is virtually unventilated.

the aim is to allow surrounding compressed healthy lung to regain useful function and to reduce the degree of hyperinflation. In general, the larger the bulla, the better the short- and long-term functional results.[245] Hypercapnia is not necessarily a contraindication to surgery,[244,246] but the outcome is poorer and the rate of subsequent postoperative decline in FEV_1 is much faster when severe generalized emphysema is present.[24] The best guides to the presence of generalized emphysema are the CO uptake (in particular the K_{CO}) and possibly the static pressure–volume curve. Since most bullae are unventilated, they merely occupy space within the lung, and these tests essentially assess the remainder of the lungs.[244,247] The pressure–volume curve is displaced upwards on the volume axis by the volume of the bulla, but its slope reflects the compliance of the rest of the lungs.

Bullectomy in appropriately selected patients usually improves some aspect of pulmonary function: most consistently there is a small rise in PaO_2, a fall in FRC and some increase in FEV_1, which may improve gradually over a year or more.[248] Unless the FEV_1 rises, useful symptomatic benefit is unlikely.[244] For the reasons discussed above, bullectomy results in no consistent changes in V_D/V_T ratio, CO diffusing capacity or static compliance.[244] The rise in PaO_2 is most easily explained by improved function of the surrounding 'squashed' lung that was previously contributing to the physiological shunt.

9.15 LUNG VOLUME REDUCTION SURGERY

9.15.1 Functional effects of lung volume reduction surgery (LVRS)

In the 1990s a resurgence of interest in LVRS for the treatment of COPD, and particularly emphysema, led to a number of case series reporting benefit. Consistent within these reports were increases in FEV_1, VC, PaO_2 and exercise performance, with reductions in TLC, RV, FRC and sometimes $PaCO_2$.[249–251] Improved oxygenation during sleep has also been reported.[252] These uncontrolled studies have subsequently been confirmed in large randomized controlled studies,[253,254] and improvements in exercise performance and breathlessness sustained in some individuals for up to 4 years have been

reported.[255] Improvements are seen in both progressive exercise and 6-min walk tests, and in a constant-load exercise test patients are able to continue longer or to maintain the same exercise with less breathlessness.[251]

9.15.2 Mechanisms of improvement post lung volume reduction surgery

Several studies have addressed the mechanism(s) of improvement in both static respiratory function and exercise performance. The best preoperative predictor of improvement in VC is the ratio RV/TLC, which reflects the mismatch in hyperinflated individuals between lung and chest wall size.[256–258] Much of the increase in FEV_1 follows the increase in VC pari passu, but in some patients the ratio FEV_1/VC also increases.[258] Improvements in the elastic recoil of the lungs have been reported, based mainly on the finding of a higher value of maximum lung recoil ($P_L$max) postoperatively. However, this is an inevitable consequence of a reduction in TLC, as the point of full inflation is set by a balance between the recoil of the lungs and chest wall and the force of inspiratory muscle contraction. When lung volume is reduced by surgical resection, this balance will occur at a lower volume at which the inspiratory muscles are able to exert greater force, distending the remaining lung to a greater extent than preoperatively and thus generating a higher $P_L$max (see Chapter 1, Section 1.2.1).

Following LVRS the inspiratory muscles would be expected to operate at a better mechanical advantage. Thus, the area of apposition of the diaphragm to the internal surface of the ribcage is greater at the reduced FRC, although there is little or no change in the curvature of the diaphragmatic dome.[259,260] Maximum inspiratory pressures are increased, whether recorded after voluntary or stimulated contraction,[261] and activation of the diaphragm and other inspiratory muscles during tidal breathing is reduced, which probably contributes to the reduced effort of breathing.[260] In addition, dynamic hyperinflation during exercise is less and the reduction correlates with lower symptom scores.[251,262] Thus, the overall mechanical effects of LVRS are both a reduction in the load to breathe (due to less DH) and an improvement in inspiratory muscle function, both direct consequences of the reduced operating lung volumes.

9.15.3 Selection criteria for lung volume reduction surgery

The functional benefits of LVRS vary considerably between individuals. Of the relevant prognostic criteria, the topographical distribution of emphysema is of particular importance, with generally better results reported when the distribution is heterogeneous and when it predominantly affects the upper rather than the lower lobes and the 'rind' rather than the 'core' of the lungs.[255,263,264] The distribution can be evaluated qualitatively or quantitatively by isotope perfusion[263] or CT scanning.[265] One important finding of the large American randomized controlled trial of LVRS was that patients with very severely impaired respiratory function had an unacceptably high early postoperative mortality, and the authors concluded that the procedure is generally contraindicated in patients with FEV_1 of 20 per cent predicted or less, together with either homogeneously distributed emphysema on CT scanning or D_LCO of 20 per cent predicted or less (implying very severe widespread emphysema).[265] Although an elevated resting arterial $PaCO_2$ (>45 mmHg) increases the risk,[266] this is not necessarily an absolute contraindication, as useful functional improvements may be seen.[267]

9.15.4 Bronchoscopic lung volume reduction

A recent refinement of surgical volume reduction is the use of bronchoscopic techniques in which one-way endobronchial valves are positioned with the aim of obstructing the segmental bronchi, leading to deflation of the lung subtended by that airway. In selected cases, similar results to LVRS have been described, with increases in spirometric volumes and exercise endurance associated with less dynamic hyperinflation,[268] but the effectiveness of valve insertion depends on the extent of collateral ventilation, which is more marked in emphysematous than healthy lungs.[103]

9.16   MACLEOD'S (SWYER JAMES) SYNDROME

The syndrome of unilateral hyperlucent lung is strictly a radiographic diagnosis and, not surprisingly, the functional features vary. Evidence of generalized airflow obstruction is often present. In one study of seven patients, all had reductions in the FEV_1/VC ratio with increases in RV and FRC; TLC measured plethysmographically was high or normal.[269] The resting PaO_2 was on average decreased and the $AaPO_2$ widened. The single-breath D_LCO and K_{CO} were normal or mildly reduced. Regional studies with radioactive xenon showed that the mean perfusion of the affected lung was 25 per cent of the total and ventilation during tidal breathing was approximately matched to perfusion. During exercise, excessive ventilation and heart rate were found; in a progressive test most patients stopped with values of ventilation well below the maximum predicted from the FEV_1 but with heart rates that were approaching predicted maxima. The authors therefore suggested that a low cardiac output, possibly due to impaired development of the pulmonary circulation, may impose a circulatory limit during exercise that is at least as important as the ventilatory impairment due to airflow obstruction.

9.17   OBLITERATIVE BRONCHIOLITIS

The terms 'obliterative bronchiolitis' (OB), 'constrictive bronchiolitis' and 'bronchiolitis obliterans' refer to a condition in which the walls of the membranous bronchioles are inflamed and fibrosed with resulting concentric narrowing and obliteration of their lumens. It occurs in a variety of settings,[270] including inhalation of fumes such as NO_2 and after ingestion of the Asian vegetable *Sauropus androgynus*,[271] and occasionally after severe viral respiratory infections. However, it is most commonly recognized after allogeneic bone marrow or haematopoietic stem cell transplantation (HSCT)[272,273] or lung transplantation.[274,275] In the condition known as panbronchiolitis, reported mainly from Japan, the pathological changes are predominantly in the respiratory bronchioles, but the functional picture of progressive airway obstruction is similar to that in OB.[276]

The functional recognition of OB is highly dependent on the context in which it develops. It is particularly common after lung transplantation, affecting 50–60 per cent of long-term survivors;[277] it appears to be rather less common, but develops earlier, after HSCT.[273] Frequent monitoring of respiratory function and the availability of sequential measurements aid recognition and early detection of the condition. These factors also account for the greater value of 'small airway' tests in this context compared with the overall population of patients with early or mild diffuse airway obstruction, in whom single cross-sectional measurements may be the only ones available.

The functional features of OB are largely non-specific, as predominant involvement of the peripheral airways is shared with the common chronic airway diseases (COPD, bronchiectasis, asthma). In established OB, reductions are seen in FEV_1, VC, FEV_1/VC and specific airway conductance. An increased TLC is, however, much less common than in patients with COPD or asthma; in some cases, especially after lung transplantation, any tendency for TLC to increase may be countered by coexistent restrictive conditions, including infection, lung injury or the effects of the operation itself (see Chapter 17, Section 17.2.1). The situation following single-lung transplantation (SLT) for COPD is, of course, likely to be different as the remaining hyperinflated lung will contribute to measurements of static lung volumes.

In transplant populations, the severity of the functional abnormality is used to grade OB or the bronchiolitis obliterans syndrome (BOS), with different criteria applied to the two main patient populations affected (Table 9.4). The grading is based largely on spirometric criteria, particularly FEV_1, with a lung function score (LFS) that combines FEV_1 and D_LCO also used in the haematological population.[273]

Many studies have investigated the value of different tests in early recognition of BOS. The varying signal-to-noise ratio of the commonly applied tests is very relevant. Of the commonly applied forced expiratory measurements, FEV_1, FEV_1/VC and measurements of mid expiratory flow (FEF_{50}, FEF_{25-75}) give similar information.[279] A reduction of 20 per cent in FEF_{25-75} may be detectable before a similar change in FEV_1, but the converse is also seen.[280] More sensitive for early detection is measurement of the distribution of ventilation using the single-breath nitrogen test (see Chapter 2, Section 2.1.9).[280,281] In established disease the slope of phase III correlates with spirometric abnormalities, including FEV_1 and FEV_1/VC.[282] However, in early disease it becomes demonstrably abnormal before the conventional spirometric volumes or

Table 9.4 Functional criteria for diagnosis of complications of transplantation

Grade	FEV_1 (% baseline)	
BOS post lung transplantation[278]		
0	>90	and FEF_{25-75} >75% baseline
0-p*	81–90	and/or FEF_{25-75} ≤75% baseline
1	66–80	
2	51–65	
3	≤50	
GVHD post-HSCT[273]		
0	>80 or LFS 2	
1	60–79 or LFS 3–5	
2	40–59 or LFS 6–9	
3	≤39 or LFS 10–12	

*0-p, 'potential BOS' stage.
BOS, bronchiolitis obliterans syndrome; FEF, forced expiratory flow; GVHD, graft versus host disease; HSCT, haematopoietic stem cell transplantation; LFS, 'lung function score', i.e. sum of forced expiratory volume in 1 s (FEV_1) (% predicted) and diffusing capacity (D_LCO) (% predicted), where >80% = 1; 70–79% = 2; 60–69% = 3; 50–59% = 4; 40–49% = 5; <40% = 6.

mid-expiratory flow,[280] and in heart–lung or bilateral lung recipients it may increase several months before the criteria for BOS 0-p are met.[280,282] Because of the contribution of the diseased native lung, the single-breath test is of little value after SLT; in this population, sequential measurement of FEV_1 is the most useful approach and is superior in both sensitivity and specificity to FEF_{25-75} for early detection of BOS.[283] The value of sequential measurements for early detection of disease depends importantly on their frequency and domiciliary spirometric measurements with transmission by telemetry may sometimes be valuable.[284] With the onset of BOS, the natural history in most patients is of progressive decline in FEV_1, with the steepest fall in the first few months.[284]

REFERENCES

1 Pride NB. The assessment of airflow obstruction. *Br J Dis Chest* 1971; **65**: 135–69.
2 Leaver DG, Tattersfield AE, Pride NB. Contributions of loss of lung recoil and of enhanced airways collapsibility to the airflow obstruction of chronic bronchitis and emphysema. *J Clin Invest* 1973; **52**: 2117–28.

3 Petty TL, Silvers GW, Stanford RE. Mild emphysema is associated with reduced elastic recoil and increased lung size but not with airflow limitation. *Am Rev Respir Dis* 1987; **136**: 867–71.

4 Hogg JC, Wright JL, Wiggs BR, *et al.* Lung structure and function in cigarette smokers. *Thorax* 1994; **49**: 473–8.

5 Burrows B, Fletcher CM, Heard BE, *et al.* The emphysematous and bronchial types of chronic airways obstruction. *Lancet* 1966; **1**: 830–35.

6 Hardie JA, Buist AS, Vollmer WM, *et al.* Risk of overdiagnosis of COPD in asymptomatic elderly never-smokers. *Eur Respir J* 2002; **20**: 1117–22.

7 Pauwels RA, Buist AS, Calverley PMA, Jenkins CR, Hurd SS. Global strategy for the diagnosis, management and prevention of chronic obstructive pulmonary disease. *Am J Respir Crit Care Med* 2001; **163**: 1256–76.

8 National Collaborating Centre for Chronic Conditions. Chronic obstructive pulmonary disease. *Thorax* 2004; **59** (suppl. 1).

9 Celli BR, MacNee W, Agusti A, *et al.* Standards for the diagnosis and treatment of patients with COPD: a summary of the ATS/ERS position paper. *Eur Respir J* 2004; **23**: 932–46.

10 Yanai M, Sekizawa K, Ohrui T, Sasaki H, Takishima T. Site of airway obstruction in pulmonary disease: direct measurement of intrabronchial pressure. *J Appl Physiol* 1992; **72**: 1016–23.

11 Hogg JC. Pathophysiology of airflow limitation in chronic obstructive pulmonary disease. *Lancet* 2004; **364**: 709–21.

12 Dayman H. Mechanics of airflow in health and in emphysema. *J Clin Invest* 1951; **30**: 1175–90.

13 Nakano Y, Muro S, Sakai H, *et al.* Computed tomographic measurements of airway dimensions and emphysema in smokers: correlation with lung function. *Am J Respir Crit Care Med* 2000; **162**: 1102–8.

14 Saetta M, Ghezzo H, Kim WD. Loss of alveolar attachments in smokers: a morphometric correlate of lung function impairment. *Am Rev Respir Dis* 1985; **132**: 894–900.

15 Kim WD, Eidelman DH, Izquierdo JL, *et al.* Centrilobular and panlobular emphysema in smokers: two distinct morphological and functional entities. *Am Rev Respir Dis* 1991; **144**: 1385–90.

16 Hogg JC, Chu F, Utokaparch S, *et al.* The nature of small airway obstruction in chronic obstructive pulmonary disease. *N Engl J Med* 2004; **350**: 2645–53.

17 Jordanoglou J, Pride NB. A comparison of maximum inspiratory and expiratory flow in health and lung disease. *Thorax* 1968; **23**: 38–45.

18 Mead J. The lung's 'quiet zone'. *N Engl J Med* 1970; **282**: 1318–19.

19 Hasegawa M, Nasuhara Y, Onodera Y, *et al.* Airflow limitation and airway dimensions in chronic obstructive pulmonary disease. *Am J Respir Crit Care Med* 2006; **173**: 1309–15.

20 Macklem PT, Fraser RG, Brown WG. Bronchial pressure measurements in emphysema and bronchitis. *J Clin Invest* 1965; **44**: 897–905.

21 Kelly CA, Gibson GJ. Relation between FEV_1 and peak expiratory flow in patients with chronic airflow obstruction. *Thorax* 1988; **43**: 335–6.

22 Aggarwal AN, Gupta D, Jindal SK. The relationship between FEV_1 and peak expiratory flow in patients with airway obstruction is poor. *Chest* 2006; **130**: 1454–61.

23 Burrows B, Strauss RH, Niden AH. Chronic obstructive lung disease: III. Interrelationships of pulmonary function data. *Am Rev Respir Dis* 1965; **91**: 861–8.

24 Krowka MJ, Enright PL, Rodarte JR, Hyatt RE. Effect of effort on measurement of forced expiratory volume in one second. *Am Rev Respir Dis* 1987; **136**: 829–33.

25 Jayamanne DS, Epstein H, Goldring RM. Flow–volume contour in COPD: correlation with pulmonary mechanics. *Chest* 1980; **77**: 749–57.

26 Morris MJ, Lane DJ. Tidal expiratory flow patterns in airflow obstruction. *Thorax* 1981; **36**: 135–42.

27 Hyatt RE. The interrelationship of pressure, flow and volume during various respiratory manoeuvres in normal and emphysematous patients. *Am Rev Respir Dis* 1961; **83**: 676–83.

28 D'Angelo E, Prandi E, Marrazzini L, Milic Emili J. Dependence of maximal flow volume curves on time course of proceeding inspiration in patients with chronic obstructive lung disease. *Am Rev Respir Dis* 1994; **150**: 1581–6.

29 Koulouris NG, Valta P, Lavoie A, *et al.* A simple method to detect expiratory flow limitation during spontaneous breathing. *Eur Respir J* 1995; **8**: 306–13.

30 Koulouris NG, Dimopoulou I, Valta P, *et al.* Detection of expiratory flow limitation during exercise in COPD patients. *J Appl Physiol* 1997; **82**: 723–31.

31 Eltayara L, Becklake MR, Velta CA, Milic Emili J. Relationship between chronic dyspnoea and expiratory flow limitation in patients with chronic obstructive pulmonary disease. *Am J Respir Crit Care Med* 1996; **154**: 1726–34.

32 Eltayara L, Ghezzo H, Milic Emili J. Orthopnoea and tidal expiratory flow limitation in patients with stable COPD. *Chest* 2001; **119**: 99–104.

33 Baydur A, Wilkinson L, Mehdian R, Bains B, Milic Emili J. Extrathoracic expiratory flow limitation in obesity and obstructive and restrictive disorders. *Chest* 2004; **125**: 98–105.

34 Dellaca RL, Duffy N, Pompilio PP, *et al.* Expiratory flow limitation detected by forced oscillation and negative expiratory pressure. *Eur Respir J* 2007; **29**: 363–74.

35 Van Noord JA, Clement J, van de Woestijne KP, Demedts M. Total respiratory resistance and reactance in patients with asthma, chronic bronchitis and emphysema. *Am Rev Respir Dis* 1991; **143**: 922–7.

36 Pelzer AM, Thompson ML. Body plethysmographic measurements of airway conductance in obstructive pulmonary disease. *Am Rev Respir Dis* 1969; **99**: 194–204.

37 Finucane KE, Colebatch HJH. Elastic behaviour of the lung in patients with airways obstruction. *J Appl Physiol* 1969; **26**: 330–38.

38 Gibson GJ, Pride NB, Davis J, Schroter RC. Exponential description of the static pressure–volume curve of normal and diseased lungs. *Am Rev Respir Dis* 1979; **120**: 799–811.

39 Colebatch HJH,Greaves IA, Ng CKY. Pulmonary mechanics in diagnosis, in *Mechanisms of Airways Obstruction in Human Respiratory Disease* (eds de Kock MA, Nadel JA and Lewis CM), Balkema, Cape Town, 1979, pp. 25–47.

40 Paré PD, Brooks LA, Bates J, *et al.* Exponential analysis of the lung pressure–volume curve as a predictor of pulmonary emphysema. *Am Rev Respir Dis* 1982; **126**: 54–61.

41 Gugger M, Gould G, Sudlow MF, Wraith PK, MacNee W. Extent of pulmonary emphysema in man and its relation to the loss of elastic recoil. *Clin Sci* 1991; **80**: 353–8.

42 Osborne S, Hogg JC, Wright JL, Coppin C, Paré PD. Exponential analysis of the pressure–volume curve: correlation with mean linear intercept and emphysema in human lungs. *Am Rev Respir Dis* 1988; **137**: 1083–8.

43 Silvers GW, Petty TL, Stanford RE. Elastic recoil changes in early emphysema. *Thorax* 1980; **35**: 490–95.

44 Dykstra BJ, Scanlon PD, Kester MM, Beck KC, Enright PL. Lung volumes in 4,774 patients with obstructive lung disease. *Chest* 1999; **115**: 68–74.

45 Paré PD, Wiggs BJR, Coppin CA. Errors in the measurement of total lung capacity in chronic obstructive lung disease. *Thorax* 1983; **38**: 468–71.

46 Hutchison DCS, Barter CE, Martelli NA. Errors in the measurement of vital capacity. *Thorax* 1973; **28**: 584–7.

47 Leith DE, Brown R. Human lung volumes and the mechanisms that set them. *Eur Respir J* 1999; **13**: 468–72.

48 Morris MJ, Madgwick RG, Lane DJ. Difference between functional residual capacity and elastic

equilibrium volume in patients with chronic obstructive pulmonary disease. *Thorax* 1996; **51**: 415–19.

49 Ferguson GT. Why does the lung hyperinflate? *Proc Am Thorac Soc* 2006; **3**: 176–9.

50 O'Donnell DE, Revill SM, Webb KA. Dynamic hyperinflation and exercise intolerance in chronic obstructive pulmonary disease. *Am J Respir Crit Care Med* 2001; **164**: 770–77.

51 Stevenson NJ, Walker PP, Costello RW, Calverley PMA. Lung mechanics and dyspnoea during exacerbations of chronic obstructive pulmonary disease. *Am J Respir Crit Care Med* 2005; **172**: 1510–16.

52 Yan S, Kaminski D, Sliwinski P. Reliability of inspiratory capacity for estimating end-expiratory lung volume changes during exercise in patients with chronic obstructive pulmonary disease. *Am J Respir Crit Care Med* 1997; **156**: 55–9.

53 Gibson GJ, Clark E, Pride NB. Static transdiaphragmatic pressures in normal subjects and in patients with chronic hyperinflation. *Am Rev Respir Dis* 1981; **124**: 685–9.

54 Byrd RB, Hyatt RE. Maximal respiratory pressures in chronic obstructive lung disease. *Am Rev Respir Dis* 1968; **98**: 848–56.

55 Decramer M, Demedts M, Rochette F, Billiet L. Maximal transrespiratory pressures in obstructive lung disease. *Clin Respir Physiol* 1980; **16**: 479–90.

56 Similowski R, Yan S, Gauthier A, Macklem PT, Bellemare F. Contractile properties of the human diaphragm during chronic hyperinflation. *N Engl J Med* 1991; **325**: 917–23.

57 Levine S, Kaiser L, Leferovich J, Tikunov B. Cellular adaptations in the diaphragm in chronic obstructive pulmonary disease. *N Engl J Med* 1997; **337**: 1799–806.

58 Levine S, Gregory C, Nguyen T, *et al.* Bioenergetic adaptation of individual human diaphragmatic myofibers to severe COPD. *J Appl Physiol* 2002; **92**: 1205–13.

59 Orozco-Levi M, Gea J, Lloreta JL, *et al.* Subcellular adaptation of the human diaphragm in chronic obstructive pulmonary disease. *Eur Respir J* 1999; **13**: 371–8.

60 Rochester DF, Braun NMT. Determinants of maximal inspiratory pressure in chronic obstructive pulmonary disease. *Am Rev Respir Dis* 1985; **132**: 42–7.

61 Man WD, Hopkinson NS, Harraf F, *et al.* Abdominal muscle and quadriceps strength in chronic obstructive pulmonary disease. *Thorax* 2005; **60**: 718–22.

62 Ferreira IM, Brooks D, Lacasse Y, Goldstein RS. Nutritional support for individuals with COPD: a meta-analysis. *Chest* 2000; **117**: 672–8.

63 Lotters F, van Tol B, Kwakkel G, Gosselink R. Effects of controlled inspiratory muscle training in patients

with COPD: a meta-analysis. *Eur Respir J* 2002; **20**: 570–76.

64 Hill K, Jenkins SC, Philippe D, *et al*. High-intensity inspiratory muscle training in COPD. *Eur Respir J* 2006; **27**: 1119–28.

65 Gilmartin JJ, Gibson GJ. Abnormalities of chest wall motion in patients with chronic airflow obstruction. *Thorax* 1984; **39**: 264–71.

66 Ninane V, Rypens F, Yernault J-C, De Troyer A. Abdominal muscle use during breathing in patients with chronic airflow obstruction. *Am Rev Respir Dis* 1992; **146**: 16–21.

67 Citterio G, Agostoni E, Del Santo A, Marazzini L. Decay of inspiratory muscle activity in chronic airway obstruction. *J Appl Physiol* 1981; **51**: 1388–97.

68 Aldrich TK, Hendler JM, Vizioli LD, *et al*. Intrinsic positive end-expiratory pressure in ambulatory patients with airways obstruction. *Am Rev Respir Dis* 1993; **147**: 845–9.

69 De Troyer A. Effect of hyperinflation on the diaphragm. *Eur Respir J* 1997; **10**: 708–13.

70 Singh B, Eastwood PR, Finucane KE. Volume displaced by diaphragm motion in emphysema. *J Appl Physiol* 2001; **91**: 1913–23.

71 Gorman RB, McKenzie DK, Pride NB, Tolman JF, Gandevia SC. Diaphragm length during tidal breathing in patients with chronic obstructive pulmonary disease. *Am J Respir Crit Care Med* 2002; **166**: 1461–9.

72 Bellemare F, Grassino A. Force reserve of the diaphragm in patients with chronic obstructive pulmonary disease. *J Appl Physiol* 1983; **55**: 8–13.

73 Pardy RL, Roussos C. Endurance of hyperventilation in chronic airflow limitation. *Chest* 1983; **83**: 744–50.

74 Kyroussis D, Johnson LC, Hamnegard C-H, Polkey MI, Moxham J. Inspiratory muscle maximum relaxation rate measured from submaximal sniff nasal pressure in patients with severe COPD. *Thorax* 2002; **57**: 254–7.

75 Mador MJ, Kufel TJ, Pineda LA, Sharma GK. Diaphragmatic fatigue and high-intensity exercise in patients with chronic obstructive pulmonary disease. *Am J Respir Crit Care Med* 2000; **161**: 118–23.

76 Kesten S, Rebuck AS. Is the short-term response to inhaled beta-adrenergic agonist sensitive or specific for distinguishing between asthma and COPD? *Chest* 1994; **105**: 1042–5.

77 Calverley PMA, Burge PS, Spencer S, *et al*. Bronchodilator reversibility testing in chronic obstructive pulmonary disease. *Thorax* 2003; **58**: 659–64.

78 American Thoracic Society. ATS standardization of spirometry: 1994 update. *Am J Respir Crit Care Med* 1995; **152**: 1107–36.

79 Corris PA, Neville E, Nariman S, Gibson GJ. Dose response study of inhaled salbutamol powder in chronic airflow obstruction. *Thorax* 1983; **38**: 292–6.

80 Belman MJ, Botnick WC, Shin JW. Inhaled bronchodilators reduce dynamic hyperinflation during exercise in patients with chronic obstructive pulmonary disease. *Am J Respir Crit Care Med* 1996; **153**: 967–75.

81 Newton MF, O'Donnell DE, Forkert L. Response of lung volumes to inhaled salbutamol in a large population of patients with severe hyperinflation. *Chest* 2002; **121**: 1042–50.

82 O'Donnell DE, Fluge T, Gerken F, *et al*. Effects of tiotropium on lung hyperinflation, dyspnoea and exercise tolerance in patients with COPD. *Eur Respir J* 2004; **23**: 832–40.

83 O'Donnell DE, Sciurba F, Celli B, *et al*. Effect of fluticasone propionate/salmeterol on lung hyperinflation and exercise endurance in COPD. *Chest* 2006; **130**: 647–56.

84 Pepin V, Brodeur J, Lacasse Y, *et al*. Six-minute walking versus shuttle walking: responsiveness to bronchodilation in chronic obstructive pulmonary disease. *Thorax* 2007; **62**: 291–8.

85 James AL, Finucane KE, Ryan G, Musk AW. Bronchial responsiveness, lung mechanics, gas transfer and corticosteroid response in patients with chronic airflow obstruction. *Thorax* 1988; **43**: 916–22.

86 Callahan CM, Dittus RS, Katz BP. Oral corticosteroid therapy for patients with stable chronic obstructive pulmonary disease. *Ann Intern Med* 1991; **114**: 216–23.

87 Pauwels RA, Lofdahl, C-G, Laitinen LA, *et al*. Long term treatment with inhaled budesonide in persons with mild chronic obstructive pulmonary disease who continue smoking. *N Engl J Med* 1999; **340**: 1948–53.

88 Burge PS, Calverley PM, Jones PW, *et al*. Randomized, double blind, placebo controlled study of fluticasone propionate in patients with moderate to severe chronic obstructive pulmonary disease: the ISOLDE trial. *Br Med J* 2000; **320**: 1297–303.

89 Postma DS, Boezen HM. Rationale for the Dutch hypothesis. *Chest* 2004; **126**: 96–104S.

90 Ramsdale EH, Morris MM, Roberts RS, Hargreave FE. Methacholine bronchial responsiveness in chronic bronchitis: relationship to airflow obstruction and cold air responsiveness. *Thorax* 1984; **39**: 912–18.

91 Riess A, Wiggs B, Verburgt L, *et al*. Morphologic determinants of airway responsiveness in chronic smokers. *Am J Respir Crit Care Med* 1996; **154**: 1444–9.

92 Van Schoor J, Joos GF, Panwels RA. Indirect bronchial hyperresponsiveness in asthma: mechanisms, pharmacology and implications for clinical research. *Eur Respir J* 2000; **16**: 514–33.

93 Sterk PJ, Bel EH. The shape of the dose–response curve to inhaled bronchoconstrictor agents in asthma and in chronic obstructive pulmonary disease. *Am Rev Respir Dis* 1991; **143**: 1433–7.

94 Cheung D, Schot R, Zwinderman AH, *et al.* Relationship between loss in parenchymal elastic recoil pressure and maximal airway narrowing in subjects with alpha1-antitrypsin deficiency. *Am J Respir Crit Care Med* 1997; **155**: 135–40.

95 Schichilone N, Marchese R, Catalano F, *et al.* Bronchodilatory effect of deep inspiration is absent in subjects with mild COPD. *Chest* 2004; **125**: 2029–35.

96 Tashkin DP, Altose MD, Connett JE, *et al.* Methacholine reactivity predicts changes in lung function over time in smokers with early chronic obstructive pulmonary disease. The Lung Health Study Research Group. *Am J Respir Crit Care Med* 1996; **153**: 1802–11.

97 Brutsche MH, Downs SH, Schindler C, *et al.* Bronchial hyperresponsiveness and the development of asthma and COPD in asymptomatic individuals: SAPALDIA cohort study. *Thorax* 2006; **61**: 671–7.

98 Ramsdale ED, Morris MM, Hargreave FE. Interpretation of the variability of peak flow rates in chronic bronchitis. *Thorax* 1986; **41**: 771–6.

99 Chester EH, Schwartz HJ, Fleming GM. Adverse effect of propranolol on airway function in non-asthmatic chronic obstructive lung disease. *Chest* 1981; **79**: 540–44.

100 Salpeter S, Ormiston T, Salpeter E. Cardioselective beta-blockers for chronic obstructive pulmonary disease. *Cochrane Database Syst Rev* 2005; (4): CD003566.

101 Van der Woude HJ, Zaagsma J, Postma DS, *et al.* Detrimental effects of beta-blockers in COPD: a concern for nonselective beta-blockers. *Chest* 2005; **127**: 818–24.

102 Fregonese L van Veen HPAA, Sterk PJ, Stolk J. Ventilation inhomogeneity in alpha1-antitrypsin-deficient emphysema. *Eur Respir J* 2006; **28**: 323–9.

103 Cetti EJ, Moore AJ, Geddes DM. Collateral ventilation. *Thorax* 2006; **61**: 371–3.

104 Terry PB, Traystman RJ, Newball HH, Batra G, Menkes HA. Collateral ventilation in man. *N Engl J Med* 1978; **298**: 10–15.

105 Higuchi T, Reed A, Oto T, *et al.* Relation of interlobar collaterals to radiological heterogeneity in severe emphysema. *Thorax* 2006; **61**: 409–13.

106 Burrows B, Kettel LJ, Niden AH, *et al.* Patterns of cardiovascular dysfunction in chronic obstructive lung disease. *N Engl J Med* 1972; **286**: 912–18.

107 West JB. Causes of carbon dioxide retention in lung disease. *N Engl J Med* 1971; **284**: 1232–6.

108 West JB. Gas exchange when one lung region inspires from another. *J Appl Physiol* 1971; **30**: 479–87.

109 Wagner PD, Dantzker DR, Dueck R, *et al.* Ventilation–perfusion inequality in chronic obstructive pulmonary disease. *J Clin Invest* 1977; **59**: 203–16.

110 Barbera JA, Ramirez J, Roca J, *et al.* Lung structure and gas exchange in mild chronic obstructive pulmonary disease. *Am Rev Respir Dis* 1990; **141**: 895–901.

111 Hunt JM, Copland J, McDonald CF, *et al.* Cardiopulmonary response to oxygen therapy in hypoxaemic chronic airflow limitation. *Thorax* 1989; **44**: 930–36.

112 Lane DJ, Howell JBL, Giblin B. Relation between airways obstruction and CO_2 tension in chronic obstructive airways disease. *Br Med J* 1968; **3**: 707–9.

113 Bégin P, Grassimo A. Inspiratory muscle dysfunction and chronic hypercapnia in chronic obstructive pulmonary disease. *Am Rev Respir Dis* 1991; **143**: 905–12.

114 Gorini M M, Misuri G, Corrado A, *et al.* Breathing pattern and carbon dioxide retention in severe chronic obstructive pulmonary disease. *Thorax* 1996; **51**: 677–83.

115 Chan CS, Bye PTP, Woolcock AJ, Sullivan CE. Eucapnia and hypercapnia in patients with chronic airflow limitation. *Am Rev Respir Dis* 1990; **141**: 861–5.

116 Calverley PMA, Leggett RJ, McElderry L, Flenley DC. Cigarette smoking and secondary polycythaemia in hypoxic cor pulmonale. *Am Rev Respir Dis* 1982; **125**: 507–10.

117 Chetty KG, Light RW, Stansbury DW, Milne N. Exercise performance of polycythaemia chronic obstructive pulmonary disease patients: effects of phlebotomy. *Chest* 1990; **98**: 1073–7.

118 Morrison NF, Abboud RT, Ramadan F, *et al.* Comparison of single breath carbon monoxide diffusing capacity and pressure–volume curves in detecting emphysema. *Am Rev Respir Dis* 1989; **139**: 1179–87.

119 Gould GA, Redpath AT, Ryan M, *et al.* Lung CT density correlates with measurements of airflow limitation and the diffusing capacity. *Eur Respir J* 1991; **4**: 141–6.

120 Morrison NJ, Abboud RT, Muller NL, *et al.* Pulmonary capillary blood volume in emphysema. *Am Rev Respir Dis* 1990; **141**: 53–61.

121 Douglas NJ, Calverley PMA, Leggett RJE, *et al.* Transient hypoxaemia during sleep in chronic bronchitis and emphysema. *Lancet* 1979; **1**: 1–4.

122 Douglas NJ, Flenley DC. Breathing during sleep in patients with obstructive lung diseases. *Am Rev Respir Dis* 1990; **141**: 1055–70.

123 O'Donoghue FJ, Catcheside PG, Ellis EE, *et al.* Sleep hypoventilation in hypercapnic chronic obstructive pulmonary disease: prevalence and associated factors. *Eur Respir J* 2003; **21**: 977–84.

124 Stradling JR, Lane DJ. Nocturnal hypoxaemia in chronic obstructive pulmonary disease. *Clin Sci* 1983; **64**: 213–22.

125 Little SA, Elkholy MM, Chalmers GW, *et al.* Predictors of nocturnal oxygen desaturation in patients with COPD. *Respir Med* 1999; **93**: 202–7.

126 Chaouat A, Weitzenblum E, Kessler R, *et al.* Outcome of COPD patients with mild daytime hypoxaemia with or without sleep-related oxygen desaturation. *Eur Respir J* 2001; **17**: 848–55.

127 Toraldo DM, Nicolardi G, De Nuccio F, Lorenzo R, Ambrosino N. Pattern of variables describing desaturator COPD patients, as revealed by cluster analysis. *Chest* 2005; **128**: 3828–37.

128 Nocturnal Oxygen Therapy Trial Group. Continuous or nocturnal oxygen therapy in hypoxaemic chronic obstructive lung disease: a clinical trial. *Ann Intern Med* 1980; **93**: 391–8.

129 Medical Research Council Working Party. Long term domiciliary oxygen therapy in chronic hypoxic cor pulmonale complicating chronic bronchitis and emphysema. *Lancet* 1981; **1**: 681–6.

130 Connaughton JJ, Catterall JR, Elton RA, Stradling JR, Douglas NJ. Do sleep studies contribute to the management of patients with severe chronic obstructive pulmonary disease? *Am Rev Respir Dis* 1988; **138**: 341–4.

131 Laurenco RV, Miranda JM. Drive and performance of the ventilatory apparatus in chronic obstructive lung disease. *N Engl J Med* 1968; **279**: 52–9.

132 Lane DJ, Howell JBL. The relationship between sensitivity to carbon dioxide and clinical features in patients with chronic airways obstruction. *Thorax* 1970; **25**: 150–58.

133 Altose MD, McCauley WC, Kelson SG, Cherniack NS. Effects of hypercapnia and flow resistive loading on respiratory activity in chronic airways obstruction. *J Clin Sci* 1977; **59**: 500–507.

134 Gribbin HR, Gardiner IT, Heinz GJ, *et al.* The role of impaired inspiratory muscle function in limiting the ventilatory response to CO_2 in chronic airflow obstruction. *Clin Sci* 1983; **64**: 487–95.

135 Murciano D, Aubier M, Bussi S, *et al.* Comparison of oesophageal, tracheal and mouth occlusion pressure in patients with chronic obstructive pulmonary disease during acute respiratory failure. *Am Rev Respir Dis* 1982; **126**: 837–41.

136 Montes de Oca M, Celli BR. Mouth occlusion pressure, CO_2 response and hypercapnia in severe chronic obstructive pulmonary disease. *Eur Respir J* 1998; **12**: 666–71.

137 Kepron W, Cherniack RM. The ventilatory response to hypercapnia and to hypoxaemia in chronic obstructive lung disease. *Am Res Respir Dis* 1973; **108**: 843–50.

138 Bradley CA, Fleetham JA, Anthonisen NR. Ventilatory control in patients with hypoxaemia due to obstructive lung disease. *Am Rev Respir Dis* 1979; **120**: 21–30.

139 Campbell EJM. The management of acute respiratory failure in chronic bronchitis and emphysema. *Am Rev Respir Dis* 1967; **96**: 626–39.

140 Barbera JA, Roca J, Ferrer A, *et al.* Mechanisms of worsening gas exchange during acute exacerbations of chronic obstructive pulmonary disease. *Eur Respir J* 1997; **10**: 1285–91.

141 McNicol MW, Campbell EJM. Severity of respiratory failure: arterial blood gases in untreated patients. *Lancet* 1965; **1**: 336–41.

142 Jeffrey AA, Warren PM, Flenley DC. Acute hypercapnic respiratory failure in patients with chronic obstructive lung disease: risk factors and use of guidelines for management. *Thorax* 1992; **47**: 34–40.

143 Robin ED. Abnormalities of acid–base regulation in chronic pulmonary disease with special reference to hypercapnia and extracellular alkalosis. *N Engl J Med* 1963; **268**: 917–22.

144 Parker CM, Voduc N, Aaron SD, Webb KA, O'Donnell DE. Physiological changes during symptom recovery from moderate exacerbations of COPD. *Eur Respir J* 2005; **26**: 420–28.

145 Johnson MK, Birch M, Carter R, Kinsella J, Stevenson RD. Measurement of physiological recovery from exacerbation of chronic obstructive pulmonary disease using within-breath forced oscillometry. *Thorax* 2007; **62**: 299–306.

146 Joosten SA, Koh MS, Bu X, Smallwood D, Irving LB. The effects of oxygen therapy in patients presenting to an emergency department with exacerbations of chronic obstructive pulmonary disease. *Med J Aust* 2007; **186**: 235–8.

147 Plant PK, Owen JL, Elliott MW. One year period prevalence study of respiratory acidosis in acute exacerbations of COPD: implications for the provision of non-invasive ventilation and oxygen administration. *Thorax* 2000; **55**: 550–54.

148 Dunn WF, Nelson SB, Hubmayr RD. Oxygen-induced hypercarbia in obstructive pulmonary disease. *Am Rev Respir Dis* 1991; **144**: 526–30.

149 Robinson TD, Freiberg DB, Regnis JA, Young IH. The role of hypoventilation and ventilation–perfusion redistribution in oxygen-induced hypercapnia during acute exacerbations of chronic obstructive pulmonary disease. *Am J Respir Crit Care Med* 2000; **161**: 1524–9.

150 Aubier M, Murciano D, Milic Emili J, *et al*. Effects of the administration of O_2 on ventilation and blood gases in patients with chronic obstructive pulmonary disease during acute respiratory failure. *Am Rev Respir Dis* 1980; **122**: 747–54.

151 Sassoon CSH, Hassell KT, Mahutte CK. Hyperoxic-induced hypercapnia in stable chronic obstructive pulmonary disease. *Am Rev Respir Dis* 1987; **135**: 907–11.

152 Bazuaye EA, Stone TN, Corris PA, Gibson GJ. Variability of inspired oxygen concentration with nasal cannulas. *Thorax* 1992; **47**: 609–11.

153 Lightowler JV, Wedzicha JA, Elliott MW, *et al*. Non-invasive positive pressure ventilation to treat respiratory failure resulting from exacerbations of chronic obstructive pulmonary disease. Cochrane systematic review and meta-analysis. *Br Med J* 2003; **326**: 185–7.

154 Diaz O, Iglesia R, Ferrer M, *et al*. Effects of non-invasive ventilation on pulmonary gas exchange and hemodynamics during acute hypercapnic exacerbations of chronic obstructive pulmonary disease. *Am J Crit Care Med* 1997; **156**: 1840–45.

155 Appendini L, Patessio A, Zanaboni S. Physiologic effects of positive end-expiratory pressure and mask pressure support during exacerbations of chronic obstructive pulmonary disease. *Am J Respir Crit Care Med* 1994; **149**: 1069–76.

156 Clini E, Sturani C, Rossi A, *et al*. The Italian multicentre study on non-invasive ventilation in chronic obstructive pulmonary disease patients. *Eur Respir J* 2002; **20**: 529–38.

157 Diaz O, Begin P, Torrealba B, Jover E, Lisboa C. Effects of non-invasive ventilation on lung hyperinflation in stable hypercapnic COPD. *Eur Respir J* 2002; **20**: 1490–98.

158 Windisch W, Kostic S, Dreher M, Virchow JC, Sorichter S. Outcome of patients with stable COPD receiving controlled non-invasive positive pressure ventilation aimed at a maximal reduction of $PaCO_2$. *Chest* 2005; **128**: 657–62.

159 Schonhofer B, Polkey MI, Suchi S, Kohler D. Effect of home mechanical ventilation on inspiratory muscle strength in COPD. *Chest* 2006; **130**: 1834–8.

160 Windisch W, Dreher M Storre JH, Sorichter S. Nocturnal non-invasive positive pressure ventilation: physiological effects on spontaneous breathing. *Respir Physiol Neurobiol* 2006; **150**: 251–60.

161 Hamilton AL, Killian KJ, Summers E, Jones NL. Muscle strength, symptom intensity, and exercise capacity in patients with cardiorespiratory disorders. *Am J Respir Crit Care Med* 1995; **152**: 2021–31.

162 Man WD, Soliman MG, Gearing J, *et al*. Symptoms and quadriceps fatigability after walking and cycling in chronic obstructive pulmonary disease. *Am J Respir Crit Care Med* 2003; **168**: 562–7.

163 Calverley PMA. Dynamic hyperinflation. *Proc Am Thorac Soc* 2006; **3**: 239–44.

164 O'Donnell DE. Hyperinflation, dyspnea, and exercise intolerance in chronic obstructive pulmonary disease. *Proc Am Thorac Soc* 2006; **3**: 180–84.

165 Babb TG, Viggiano R, Hurley B, Staats B, Rodarte JR. Effect of mild-to-moderate airflow limitation on exercise capacity. *J Appl Physiol* 1991; **70**: 223–30.

166 Sliwinski P, Kaminski D, Zielinski H, Yan S. Partitioning of the elastic work of inspiration in patients with COPD during exercise. *Eur Respir J* 1998; **11**: 416–21.

167 Sinderby C, Spahija J, Beck J, *et al*. Diaphragm activation during exercise in chronic obstructive pulmonary disease. *Am J Respir Crit Care Med* 2001; **163**: 1637–41.

168 Puente-Maestu L, Garcia de Pedro J, Martinez-Abad Y, *et al*. Dyspnea, ventilatory pattern, and changes in dynamic hyperinflation related to the intensity of constant work rate exercise in COPD. *Chest* 2005; **128**: 651–6.

169 Marin JM, Carrizo SJ, Gascon M, *et al*. Inspiratory capacity, dynamic hyperinflation, breathlessness, and exercise performance during the 6-minuted-walk test in chronic obstructive pulmonary disease. *Am J Respir Crit Care Med* 2001; **163**: 1395–9.

170 O'Donnell DE. Impacting patient-centered outcomes in COPD: breathlessness and exercise tolerance. *Eur Respir Rev* 2006; **15**: 37–41.

171 Albuquerque AL, Nery LE, Villaca DS, *et al*. Inspiratory fraction and exercise impairment in COPD patients GOLD stages II–III. *Eur Respir J* 2006; **28**: 939–44.

172 Diaz O, Villafranca C, Ghezzo H, *et al*. Breathing pattern and gas exchange at peak exercise in COPD patients with or without tidal flow limitation at rest. *Eur Respir J* 2001; **17**: 1120–27.

173 Alverti A, Stevenson N, Dellaca RL, *et al*. Regional chest wall volumes during exercise in chronic obstructive pulmonary disease. *Thorax* 2004; **59**: 210–16.

174 Vogiatzis I, Georgiadou O, Golemati S, *et al*. Patterns of dynamic hyperinflation during exercise and recovery in patients with severe chronic obstructive pulmonary disease. *Thorax* 2005; **60**: 723–9.

175 Light RW, Mintz HM, Linden GS, Brown SE. Hemodynamics of patients with severe chronic obstructive pulmonary disease during progressive upright exercise. *Am Rev Respir Dis* 1984; **130**: 391–5.

176 Barbera JA, Roca J, Ramirez J, *et al.* Gas exchange during exercise in mild chronic obstructive pulmonary disease: correlation with lung structure. *Am Rev Respir Dis* 1991; **144**: 520–25.

177 Jones NL. Pulmonary gas exchange during exercise in patients with chronic airway obstruction. *Clin Sci* 1966; **31**: 39–50.

178 Danztker DR, D'Alonzo GE. The effect of exercise on pulmonary gas exchange in patients with severe chronic obstructive pulmonary disease. *Am Rev Respir Dis* 1986; **134**: 1135–9.

179 O'Donnell DE, D'Arsigny C, Fitzpatrick M, Webb KA. Exercise hypercapnia in advanced chronic obstructive pulmonary disease: the role of lung hyperinflation. *Am J Respir Crit Care Med* 2002; **166**: 663–8.

180 Christensen CC, Ryg MS, Edvardsen A, Skjonsberg OH. Effect of exercise mode on oxygen uptake and blood gases in COPD patients. *Respir Med* 2004; **98**: 656–60.

181 Palange P, Forte S, Onorati P, *et al.* Ventilatory and metabolic adaptations to walking and cycling in patients with COPD. *J Appl Physiol* 2000; **88**: 1715–20.

182 Turner SE, Eastwood PR, Cecins NM, Hillman DR, Jenkins SC. Physiologic responses to incremental and self-paced exercise in COPD: a comparison of three tests. *Chest* 2004; **126**: 766–73.

183 Maltais F, Hamilton A, Marciniuk D, *et al.* Improvements in symptom-limited exercise performance over 8h with once daily tiotropium in patients with COPD. *Chest* 2005; **128**: 1168–78.

184 O'Donnell DE, Vodue N, Fitzpatrick M, Webb KA. Effect of salmeterol on the ventilatory response to exercise in chronic obstructive pulmonary disease. *Eur Respir J* 2004; **24**: 86–94.

185 Somfay A, Porszasz J, Lee SM, Casaburi R. Dose–response effect of oxygen on hyperinflation and exercise endurance in nonhypoxaemic COPD patients. *Eur Respir J* 2001; **18**: 77–84.

186 O'Donnell DE, D'Arsigny C, Webb KA. Effects of hyperoxia on ventilatory limitation during exercise in advanced chronic obstructive pulmonary disease. *Am J Respir Crit Care Med* 2001; **163**: 892–8.

187 Peters MM, Webb KA, O'Donnell DE. Combined physiological effects of bronchodilators and hyperoxia on exertional dyspnoea in normoxic COPD. *Thorax* 2006; **61**: 559–67.

188 Stevenson NJ, Calverley PMA. Effect of oxygen on recovery from maximal exercise in patients with chronic obstructive pulmonary disease. *Thorax* 2004; **59**: 668–72.

189 Nandi K, Smith AA, Crawford A, *et al.* Oxygen supplementation before or after submaximal exercise in patients with chronic obstructive pulmonary disease. *Thorax* 2003; **58**: 670–73.

190 Lotters F, Van Tol B, Kwakkel G, Gosselink R. Effects of controlled inspiratory muscle training in patients with COPD: a meta-analysis. *Eur Respir J* 2002; **20**: 570–76.

191 Bernard S, LeBlanc P, Whittom F, *et al.* Peripheral muscle weakness in patients with chronic obstructive pulmonary disease. *Am J Respir Crit Care Med* 1998; **158**: 629–34.

192 Couillard A, Maltais F, Saey D, *et al.* Exercise-induced quadriceps oxidative stress and peripheral muscle dysfunction in patients with chronic obstructive pulmonary disease. *Am J Respir Crit Care Med* 2003; **167**: 1664–9.

193 Porszasz J, Emtner M, Goto S, *et al.* Exercise training decreases ventilatory requirements and exercise-induced hyperinflation at submaximal intensities in patients with COPD. *Chest* 2005; 128: 2025–34.

194 O'Donnell DE, Bertley JC, Chau LK, Webb KA. Qualitative aspects of exertional breathlessness in chronic airflow limitation: pathophysiologic mechanisms. *Am J Respir Crit Care Med* 1997; **155**: 109–15.

195 Troosters T, Casaburi R, Gosselink R, Decramer M. Pulmonary rehabilitation in chronic obstructive pulmonary disease. *Am J Respir Crit Care Med* 2005; **172**: 19–38.

196 Carter R, Peavler M, Zinkgraf S, Williams J, Fields S. Predicting maximal exercise ventilation in patients with chronic obstructive pulmonary disease. *Chest* 1987; **92**: 253–9.

197 Dillard TA, Piantadosi S, Rajagopal KR. Determinants of maximum exercise capacity in patients with chronic airflow obstruction. *Chest* 1989; **96**: 267–71.

198 Loiseau A, Dubreuil C, Loiseau P, *et al.* Exercise tolerance in chronic obstructive pulmonary disease: importance of active and passive components of the ventilatory system. *Eur Respir J* 1989; **2**: 522–7.

199 Gray-Donald K, Gibbons L, Shapiro SH, Martin JG. Effect of nutritional status on exercise performance in patients with chronic obstructive pulmonary disease. *Am Rev Respir Dis* 1989; **140**: 1544–8.

200 Mak VHF, Bugler JR, Roberts CM, Spiro SG. Effects of arterial oxygen desaturation on six minute walk distance, perceived effort and perceived

breathlessness in patients with airflow limitation. *Thorax* 1993; **48**: 33–6.

201 Wijkstra PJ, TenVergert EM, van der Mark TW, *et al.* Relation of lung function, maximal inspiratory pressure, dyspnoea and quality of life with exercise capacity in patients with chronic obstructive pulmonary disease. *Thorax* 1994; **49**: 468–72.

202 Schols AMWJ, Mostert R, Soeters PB, Wouters EFM. Body composition and exercise performance in patients with chronic obstructive pulmonary disease. *Thorax* 1991; **46**: 695–9.

203 Swinburn CR, Cooper BG, Mould H, Corris PA, Gibson GJ. Adverse effect of additional weight on exercise against gravity in patients with chronic obstructive airways disease. *Thorax* 1989; **44**: 716–20.

204 Casanova C, Cote CG, Marin JM, *et al.* The 6-minute walking distance: long term follow up in patients with COPD. *Eur Respir J* 2007; **29**: 535–40.

205 D'Urzo AD, Mateika J, Bradley TD, *et al.* Correlates of arterial oxygenation during exercise in severe chronic obstructive pulmonary disease. *Chest* 1989; **95**: 13–17.

206 Silverman M, Barry J, Hellerstein H, Janos J, Kelsen S. Variability of the perceived sense of effort in breathing during exercise in patients with chronic obstructive pulmonary disease. *Am Rev Respir Dis* 1988; **137**: 206–9.

207 Mahler DA, Harver A. A factor analysis of dyspnoea ratings, respiratory muscle strength and lung function in patients with chronic obstructive pulmonary disease. *Am Rev Respir Dis* 1992; **145**: 467–70.

208 Fletcher CM, Peto R. The natural history of chronic airflow obstruction. *Br Med J* 1977; **1**: 1645–8.

209 Peat JK, Woolcock AJ, Cullen K. Decline of lung function and development of chronic airflow limitation: a longitudinal study of non-smokers and smokers in Busselton, Western Australia. *Thorax* 1990; **45**: 32–7.

210 Lokke A, Lange P, Scharling H, Fabricius P, Vestbo J. Developing COPD: a 25 year follow up study of the general population. *Thorax* 2006; **61**: 935–9.

211 Vestbo J, Prescott E, Lange P, *et al.* Association of chronic mucus hypersecretion with FEV_1 decline and COPD morbidity. *Am J Respir Crit Care Med* 1996; **153**: 1530–35.

212 Scanlon PD, Connett JE, Waller LA, *et al.* Smoking cessation and lung function in mild-to-moderate chronic obstructive pulmonary disease: the Lung Health Study. *Am J Respir Crit Care Med* 2000; **161**: 381–90.

213 Garcia-Aymerich J, Lange P, Benet M, Schnohr P, Anto JM. Regular physical activity modifies smoking-related lung function decline and reduces risk of chronic obstructive pulmonary disease: a population-based cohort study. *Am J Respir Crit Care Med* 2007; **175**: 458–63.

214 Rijcken B, Schouten JP, Xu X, *et al.* Airway hyper-responsiveness to histamine associated with accelerated decline in FEV_1. *Am J Respir Crit Care Med* 1995; **151**: 1377–82.

215 O'Connor GT, Sparrow D, Weiss ST. A prospective longitudinal study of methacholine airway responsiveness as a predictor of pulmonary function decline: the Normative Aging Study. *Am J Respir Crit Care Med* 1995; **152**: 87–92.

216 Vestbo J, Hogg JC. Convergence of the epidemiology and pathology of COPD. *Thorax* 2006; **61**: 86–8.

217 Knudson RJ, Burrows B, Lebowitz MD. The maximal expiratory flow volume curve: its use in the detection of ventilatory abnormalities in a population study. *Am Rev Respir Dis* 1976; **114**: 871–9

218 Pride NB. Analysis of forced expiration: a return to the recording spirometer? *Thorax* 1979; **34**: 144–9.

219 Paré PD, Brooks LA, Coppin CA, *et al.* Density dependence of maximal expiratory flow and its correlation with small airway disease in smokers. *Am Rev Respir Dis* 1985; **131**: 521–6.

220 Stanescu D. Small airways obstruction syndrome. *Chest* 1999; **116**: 231–3.

221 Woolcock AJ, Vincent NJ, Macklem PT. Frequency dependence of compliance as a test for obstruction in the small airways. *J Clin Invest* 1969; **48**: 1097–106.

222 Goldman MD, Saadeh C, Ross D. Clinical application of forced oscillation to assess peripheral airway function. *Respir Physiol Neurobiol* 2005; **148**: 179–94

223 Buist AS, Ross BB. Quantitative analysis of the alveolar plateau in the diagnosis of early airway obstruction. *Am Rev Respir Dis* 1973; **108**: 1078–87.

224 Barter SJ, Cunningham DA, Lavender JP, *et al.* Abnormal ventilation scans in middle aged smokers: comparison with tests of overall lung function. *Am Rev Respir Dis* 1985; **132**: 148–51.

225 Matsuba K, Shirakusa T, Kuwano, K, Hayashi S, Shigematsu N. Small airways disease in patients without chronic air-flow limitation. *Am Rev Respir Dis* 1987; **136**: 1106–11.

226 Wright JL, Lawson LM, Pare PD, *et al.* The detection of small airways disease. *Am Rev Respir Dis* 1984; **129**: 989–94.

227 Stanescu D, Sanna A, Veriter C, Robert A. Identification of smokers susceptible to development

of chronic airflow limitation: a 13-year follow-up. *Chest* 1998; **114**: 416–25.

228 Cauberghs M, Clement J, van de Woestijne KP. Functional alterations accompanying a rapid decline in ventilatory function. *Am Rev Respir Dis* 1993; **147**: 379–84.

229 Anthonisen NR, Wright EC, Hodgkin JE. Prognosis in chronic obstructive pulmonary disease. *Am Rev Respir Dis* 1986; **133**: 14–20.

230 Hansen EF, Phanareth K, Laursen LC, Kok-Jensen A, Dirksen A. Reversible and irreversible airflow obstruction as predictor of overall mortality in asthma and chronic obstructive pulmonary disease. *Am J Respir Crit Care Med* 1999; **159**: 1267–71.

231 Pinto-Plata VM, Cote C, Cabral H, Taylor J, Celli BR. The 6-min walk distance: change over time and value as a predictor of survival in severe COPD. *Eur Respir J* 2004; **23**: 28–33.

232 Nishimura K, Isumi T, Tsukino M, Oga T. Dyspnea is a better predictor of 5-year survival than airway obstruction in patients with COPD. *Chest* 2002; **121**: 1434–40.

233 Celli BR, Cote CG, Marin JM, *et al.* The body-mass index, airflow obstruction, dyspnea, and exercise capacity index in chronic obstructive pulmonary disease. *N Engl J Med* 2004; **350**: 1005–12.

234 Celli BR, Calverley PMA, Rennard SI, *et al.* Proposal for a multidimensional staging system for chronic obstructive pulmonary disease. *Respir Med* 2005; **99**: 1546–54.

235 Martinez FJ, Foster G, Curtis JL, *et al.* Predictors of mortality in patients with emphysema and severe airflow obstruction. *Am J Respir Crit Care Med* 2006; **173**: 1326–34.

236 Gelb AF, Zamel N, Hogg JC, Muller NL, Schein MJ. Pseudophysiologic emphysema resulting from severe small-airways disease. *Am J Respir Crit Care Med* 1998; **158**: 815–19.

237 Baldi S, Miniati M, Bellini CR, *et al.* Relationship between extent of pulmonary emphysema by high-resolution computed tomography and lung elastic recoil in patients with chronic obstructive pulmonary disease. *Am J Respir Crit Care Med* 2000; **164**: 585–9.

238 Cerveri I, Dore R, Corsico A, *et al.* Assessment of emphysema in COPD: a functional and radiologic study. *Chest* 2004; **125**: 1714–18.

239 Parr DG, Stoel, BC, Stolk J, Stockley RA. Pattern of emphysema distribution in alpha-1-antitrypsin deficiency influences lung function impairment. *Am J Respir Crit Care Med* 2004; **170**: 1172–8.

240 DeMeo DL, Sandhaus RA, Barker AF, *et al.* Determinants of airflow obstruction in severe alpha-1-antitrypsin deficiency. *Thorax* 2007; **62**: 806–13.

241 Seersholm N, Kok-Jensen A. Clinical features and prognosis of life time non-smokers with severe alpha-1-antitrypsin deficiency. *Thorax* 1998; **53**: 265–8.

242 Dahl M, Tybjaerg-Hansen A, Lange P, Vestbo J, Nordestgaard BG. Change in lung function and morbidity from chronic obstructive pulmonary disease in alpha-1-antitrypsin MZ heterozygotes: a longitudinal study of the general population. *Ann Intern Med* 2002; **136**: 270–79.

243 Tattersall SF, Pereira RP, Hunter D, *et al.* Lung distensibility and airway function in intermediate $alpha_1$ antitrypsin deficiency (PiMZ). *Thorax* 1979; **34**: 637–46.

244 Pride NB, Barter CE, Hugh Jones P. The ventilation of bullae and the effect of their removal on thoracic gas volumes and tests of overall pulmonary function. *Am Rev Respir Dis* 1973; **107**: 83–98.

245 Baldi S, Palla A, Mussi A, *et al.* Influence of bulla volume on postbullectomy outcome. *Can Respir J* 2001; **8**: 233–8.

246 Potgieter PD, Benatar SR, Hewitson RP, Ferguson AD. Surgical treatment of bullous lung disease. *Thorax* 1981; **36**: 885–90.

247 Gould GA, Redpath AT, Ryan M, *et al.* Parenchymal emphysema measured by CT lung density correlates with lung function in patients with bullous disease. *Eur Respir J* 1993; **6**: 698–704.

248 Palla A, Desideri M, Rossi G, *et al.* Elective surgery for giant bullous emphysema: a 5-year clinical and functional follow-up. *Chest* 2005; **128**: 2043–50.

249 Gelb AF, McKenna RJ, Brenner M, *et al.* Contribution of lung and chest wall mechanics following emphysema resection. *Chest* 1996; **110**: 11–17.

250 Sciurba FC, Rogers RM, Keenan RJ, *et al.* Improvement in pulmonary function and elastic recoil after lung-reduction surgery for diffuse emphysema. *N Engl J Med* 1996; **334**: 1095–9.

251 Martinez FJ, de Oca MM, Whyte RI, *et al.* Lung-volume reduction improves dyspnea, dynamic hyperinflation, and respiratory muscle function. *Am J Respir Crit Care Med* 1997; **155**: 1984–90.

252 Krachman SL, Chatila W, Martin UJ, *et al.* Effects of lung volume reduction surgery on sleep quality and nocturnal gas exchange in patients with severe emphysema. *Chest* 2005; **128**: 3221–8.

253 Fishman A, Martinez F, Naunheim K, *et al.* A randomized trial comparing lung-volume-reduction surgery with medical therapy for severe emphysema. *N Engl J Med* 2003; **348**: 2059–73.

254 Berger RL, Wood KA, Cabral HJ, *et al.* Lung volume reduction surgery: a meta-analysis of randomized clinical trials. *Treat Respir Med* 2005; **4**: 201–9.

255 Naunheim KS, Wood DE, Mohsenifar Z, *et al*. Long-term follow-up of patients receiving lung-volume-reduction surgery versus medical therapy for severe emphysema by the National Emphysema Treatment Trial Research Group. *Ann Thorac Surg* 2006; **82**: 431–43.

256 Fessler HE, Permutt S. Lung volume reduction surgery and airflow limitation. *Am J Respir Crit Care Med* 1998; **157**: 715–22.

257 Ingenito EP, Loring SH, Moy ML, *et al*. Physiological characterization of variability in response to lung volume reduction surgery. *J Appl Physiol* 2003; **94**: 20–30.

258 Fessler HE, Scharf SM, Permutt S. Improvement in spirometry following lung volume reduction surgery. *Am J Respir Crit Care Med* 2002; **165**: 34–40.

259 Cassart M, Hamacher J, Verbandt Y, *et al*. Effects of lung volume reduction surgery for emphysema on diaphragm dimensions and configuration. *Am J Respir Crit Care Med* 2001; **163**: 1171–5.

260 Gorman RB, McKenzie DK, Butler JE, Tolman JF, Gandevia SC. Diaphragm length and neural drive after lung volume reduction surgery. *Am J Crit Care Med* 2005. 172; 1259–66.

261 Laghi F, Jubran A, Topeli A, *et al*. Effect of lung volume reduction surgery on diaphragmatic neuromechanical coupling at 2 years. *Chest* 2004; **125**: 2188–95.

262 O'Donnell DE, Webb KA, Bertley JC, Chau LKL, Conlan AA. Mechanisms of relief of exertional breathlessness following unilateral bullectomy and lung volume reduction surgery in emphysema. *Chest* 1996 ; **110**: 18–27.

263 Wang SC, Fischer KC, Slone RM, *et al*. Perfusion scintigraphy in the evaluation for lung volume reduction surgery: correlation with clinical outcome. *Radiology* 1997; **205**: 243–8.

264 Nakano Y, Coxson HO, Bosan S, *et al*. Core to rind distribution of severe emphysema predicts outcome of lung volume reduction surgery. *Am J Respir Crit Care Med* 2001; **164**: 2195–9.

265 National Emphysema Treatment Trial Research Group. Patients at high risk of death after lung-volume-reduction surgery. *N Engl J Med* 2001; **345**: 1075–83.

266 Szekely LA, Oelberg DA, Wright C, *et al*. Preoperative predictors of operative morbidity and mortality in COPD patients undergoing bilateral lung volume reduction surgery. *Chest* 1997; **111**: 550–58.

267 O'Brien GM, Furukawa S, Kuzma AM, Cordova F, Criner GJ. Improvements in lung function, exercise, and quality of life in hypercapnic COPD patients after lung volume reduction surgery. *Chest* 1999; **115**: 75–84.

268 Hopkinson NS, Toma TP, Hansell DM, *et al*. Effect of bronchoscopic lung volume reduction on dynamic hyperinflation and exercise in emphysema. *Am J Respir Crit Care Med* 2005; **171**: 453–60.

269 Warrell DA, Hughes JMB, Rosenzweig DY. Cardiopulmonary performance at rest and during exercise in seven patients with increased transradiancy of one lung (Macleod's syndrome). *Thorax* 1970; **29**: 587–97.

270 Schlesinger C, Veeraraghavan S, Koss MN. Constructive (obliterative) bronchiolitis. *Curr Opin Pulm Med* 1998; **4**: 288–93.

271 Hsiue TR, Guo YL, Chen KW, *et al*. Dose–response relationship and irreversible obstructive ventilatory defect in patients with consumption of *Sauropus androgynus*. *Chest* 1998; **113**: 71–6.

272 Krowka MJ. Lung function and the complications of bone marrow transplantation. *Chest* 1992; **101**: 1186.

273 Soubani AO, Uberti JP. Bronchiolitis obliterans following haematopoietic stem cell transplantation. *Eur Respir J* 2007; **29**: 1007–19.

274 Burke CM, Theodore J, Dawkins KD, *et al*. Post transplant obliterative bronchiolitis and other late lung sequelae in human heart–lung transplantation. *Chest* 1984; **86**: 824–9.

275 Estenne M, Hertz MI. Bronchiolotis obliterans after human lung transplantation. *Am J Respir Crit Care Med* 2002; **166**: 440–44.

276 Homma S, Sakamoto S, Kawabata M, *et al*. Comparative clinicopathology of obliterative bronchiolitis and diffuse panbronchiolitis. *Respiration* 2006; **73**: 481–7.

277 Boehler A, Kesten S, Weder W, Speich R. Bronchiolitis obliterans after lung transplantation: a review. *Chest* 1998; **114**: 1411–26.

278 Estenne M, Maurer JR, Boehler A, *et al*. Bronchiolitis obliterans syndrome 2001: an update of the diagnostic criteria. *J Heart Lung Transplant* 2002; **21**: 297–310.

279 Chacon RA, Corris PA, Dark JH, Gibson GJ. Tests of airway function in detecting and monitoring treatment of obliterative bronchiolitis after lung transplantation. *J Heart Lung Transplant* 2000; **19**: 263–9.

280 Estenne M, Van Muylem A, Knoop C, Antoine M. Detection of obliterative bronchiolitis after lung transplantation by indexes of ventilation distribution. *Am J Respir Crit Care Med* 2000; **162**: 1047–51.

281 Arens R, McDonough JM, Zhao H, *et al*. Altered lung mechanics after double-lung transplantation. *Am J Respir Crit Care Med* 1998; **158**: 1403–9.

282 Reynaud-Gaubert M, Thomas P, Badier M, *et al.* Early detection of airway involvement in obliterative bronchiolitis after lung transplantation: functional and bronchoalveolar lavage cell findings. *Am J Respir Crit Care Med* 2000; **161**: 1924–9.

283 Lama VN, Murray S, Mumford JA, *et al.* Prognostic value of bronchiolitis obliterans syndrome stage O-p in single-lung transplant recipients. *Am J Respir Crit Care Med* 2005; **172**: 379–83.

284 Lama VN, Murray S, Lonigro RJ, *et al.* Course of FEV(1) after onset of bronchiolitis obliterans syndrome in lung transplant recipients. *Am J Respir Crit Care Med* 2007; **175**: 1192–8.

10

Bronchiectasis and Cystic Fibrosis

The main abnormality of mechanical respiratory function in both cystic fibrosis (CF) and generalized, non-CF bronchiectasis is diffuse airway obstruction, with many functional features shared with chronic obstructive pulmonary disease (COPD). At first glance it may appear strange that conditions characterized anatomically by bronchial dilatation are associated with functional evidence of airway narrowing. The explanation of the paradox lies in the different generations of airways affected, with the dilatation occurring in larger, more proximal airways (visible to the naked eye and on plain radiography or computer tomography (CT) scanning) while the functional abnormality is due to narrowing of the smaller airways.

10.1 BRONCHIECTASIS

10.1.1 Abnormalities of respiratory mechanics

Abnormal function is demonstrable in most patients with clinically significant bronchiectasis, although at presentation to hospital, spirometric measurements often show only mild abnormalities, even in patients with symptoms for many years.[1] In very mild disease, abnormalities may be subtle and not apparent on routine spirometry. However, tests for uneven ventilation will often show evidence of generalized disease of the smaller airways, even when imaging techniques suggest that bronchiectasis is localized.

The typical functional abnormalities are nonspecific, with reductions in maximum flows, FEV_1/VC and airway conductance and an increase

in residual volume.[2] Plethysmographic measurements usually show an increase in TLC in patients with more severe airway obstruction;[2] as in any condition associated with diffuse airway obstruction, volume measurements by gas dilution are likely to underestimate TLC and may give the erroneous impression of a combined obstructive and restrictive ventilatory defect. The mechanism(s) of airway obstruction are not fully established; as in COPD, abnormal collapsibility of the central airways may contribute.[3] CT studies have suggested that localized emphysema may be relevant in some individuals.[4,5] Scans show decreased lung attenuation, particularly in the areas affected most severely by bronchiectasis. However, the reduced attenuation does not correlate with overall carbon monoxide (CO) diffusing capacity (D_LCO),[5] and KCO is normal in most patients.[4] The amount of excessive airway secretions is not related to the severity of airway obstruction functionally.[5] The mechanical constraints imposed by more severe airway obstruction result in expiratory flow limitation (EFL), demonstrable by the negative expiratory pressure technique; as in COPD, this is an important determinant of breathlessness.[6]

10.1.2 Abnormalities of gas exchange

The distribution of ventilation, as assessed by either the single-breath or the multiple-breath nitrogen washout, is abnormal even in relatively mild disease.[7] Arterial hypoxaemia is frequent in patients with significant airflow obstruction; there may be an increase in the 'anatomical' shunt, which has been attributed to communications between the pulmonary and bronchial circulations.[8] With severe generalized airway obstruction, carbon dioxide (CO_2) retention and cor pulmonale are likely.

A study of the regional distribution of radio-active xenon[9] showed reduced ventilation of the bronchiectactic regions, usually accompanied by some reduction in perfusion, although the defects of perfusion were less well defined. Defects were also frequent in the non-ectatic regions, a finding compatible with generalized airway narrowing.

10.1.3 Effects of surgery for bronchiectasis

Functional changes in patients who have undergone surgery for bronchiectasis are usually related to the extent of any persisting disease rather than to the resection itself. In the absence of residual disease, the removal of one or two lobes in childhood produces no significant abnormality of lung volumes in adult life,[2] but in many such individuals childhood resection of bronchiectatic areas was incomplete and functional abnormalities persist or deteriorate in adult life.

10.1.4 Ciliary dysmotility and Young's syndrome

As severe respiratory infections in infancy have become less common in advanced countries, other causes of bronchiectasis have become more apparent. In addition to CF (see Section 10.2), these include congenital and acquired immune deficiency states and abnormalities of mucociliary clearance. The latter comprise disorders of ciliary function (primary ciliary dyskinesia) and of the mucus lining the airway (e.g. Young's syndrome).

Historically, the rate of mucociliary clearance was measured by external monitoring of the clearance of inhaled radiolabelled particles (e.g. an aerosol of technetium-labelled microspheres) over a measured distance of the trachea.[10] More simply, abnormalities of mucociliary clearance can be identified or excluded using the saccharin test,[11] in which a small particle of saccharin is placed on the inferior turbinate of one nostril and the time from placing the particle to the subject tasting the saccharin is recorded. Normally this is less than 30 min; if it exceeds 60 min, clearance is definitely abnormal. These tests do not distinguish abnormalities of ciliary function from those due to the composition of respiratory mucus. Ciliary function can be assessed directly by brushing nasal cilia and measuring ciliary beat frequency (CBF) using photometric[12] or other methods. The investigation is usually combined with a qualitative assessment of ciliary beating and with ultrastructural examination. The normal CBF is quoted as 12–14 Hz, but there is considerable variation even within individuals.[13] In primary ciliary abnormalities the frequency is greatly reduced and a large proportion of cilia are seen to have dyskinetic motion. It should, however, be noted that a secondary reduction in CBF may be seen in the presence of respiratory infection and bronchiectasis of other causes.[13]

The characteristic functional abnormalities of patients with ciliary dyskinesia,[14,15] or Young's syndrome,[16] are similar to those with other causes of bronchiectasis, i.e. an obstructive ventilatory defect with varying degrees of acute reversibility. Sequential measurements in patients with ciliary dyskinesia show that, unlike CF, airway obstruction is not rapidly progressive.[15]

10.2 CYSTIC FIBROSIS

Although CF was formerly a disease confined to childhood, the better prognosis in recent years means that increasing numbers of adults in their twenties or thirties with CF are now seen, but by that age many have severely abnormal respiratory function. The functional picture is of airflow obstruction, increasing as the disease progresses so that functional indices expressed as per cent predicted usually decline with age. In younger individuals without clinical pulmonary disease and with virtually normal spirometry, evidence of mild airway obstruction is demonstrable using tests such as V_{max} at small lung volumes or indices of gas exchange abnormality such as a widened alveolar–arterial P_{O_2} difference (AaP_{O_2}) or increased dead space/tidal volume ratio (V_D/V_T).[17] Forced oscillation appears to be less sensitive in CF than in asthma.[18]

10.2.1 Abnormalities of respiratory mechanics

One noteworthy difference from the usual functional pattern in patients with chronic airway obstruction, and common to several series of patients with CF, is that TLC, even when measured by plethysmography, is often normal or sometimes reduced.[19] The absence of an increase in TLC might be due to relative alveolar hypoplasia, for which there is some pathological evidence, and/or to areas of lung fibrosis consequent on repeated infections. The static pressure–volume (PV) curve of the lungs shows a shift to the left, with lower values of lung recoil pressure at a given per cent TLC, but the slope of the curve, representing lung compliance, remains normal;[20] this pattern is similar to that seen in asthma (see Chapter 11, Section 11.1.1). The chest wall appears to adapt differently to the pulmonary hyperinflation in the two sexes, with females showing relatively more expansion of the ribcage, while male patients accommodate the expansion more by shortening of the diaphragm.[21] Expiratory flow limitation (EFL) is often demonstrable at rest, particularly in older individuals with more markedly reduced FEV_1, leading to more severe hyperinflation and reduced inspiratory capacity. The presence of EFL correlates well with more severe breathlessness.[22]

10.2.2 Bronchodilator and bronchoconstrictor effects

Bronchodilators produce the expected modest increase in FEV_1,[23,24] but, at least, in one study, they had no apparent benefit for exercise capacity.[24] Many individuals with CF show bronchial hyperresponsiveness (BHR) to non-specific stimuli.[25] This is probably due mainly to the greatly thickened walls of the peripheral airways, which are much thicker than the walls of equivalent airways in COPD.[26] In general the BHR correlates with reduced FEV_1, but it can also be seen in some individuals without established airway obstruction.[23]

10.2.3 Respiratory muscle function

Malnutrition is common in CF and might be expected to lead to respiratory muscle weakness. Reductions in maximum respiratory processes have been reported in some[27] but not all studies and, in general, the function and bulk of the respiratory muscles are better preserved than non-respiratory muscles.[28,29] Interpretation of the maximum inspiratory pressure (P_Imax) may be complicated by

hyperinflation (elevated functional residual capacity, FRC). Improvements in P_Imax have been reported following parenteral nutrition[30] and respiratory muscle training,[31,32] but this is not necessarily accompanied by improved exercise performance.

10.2.4 Abnormalities of gas exchange

Maldistribution of ventilation and mismatching of ventilation to perfusion produce the expected consequences for gas exchange, with an increase in physiological dead space and physiological shunt. As with other causes of bronchiectasis, there is an apparent increase in some patients in the intrapulmonary 'anatomical' shunt. This is demonstrable by the failure of PaO_2 to increase to the normal value of 550 mmHg after a period of breathing pure oxygen[33] and by use of the multiple inert gas technique to study detailed distributions of ventilation and perfusion.[34] The mechanism is not clear, but possibilities include multiple areas of atelectasis consequent on retention of tenacious sputum or the presence of small 'true' right-to-left shunts.

As CF is not accompanied by widespread alveolar destruction, abnormalities of D_LCO are usually mild. In individuals with more severe airway obstruction, the single-breath D_LCO may be reduced due to maldistribution of the test gas, but Kco is usually normal.[4] Kco may, however, fail to show the normal rise when the subject changes from the sitting to supine posture,[35] possibly because of an elevated pulmonary arterial pressure resulting from hypoxic vasoconstriction.

Elevation of $PaCO_2$ occurs with advanced airway obstruction and in the pre-transplant era implied an ominous prognosis. Patients with end-stage CF and hypercapnia frequently develop a primary metabolic alkalosis, which complicates the chronic respiratory acidosis. For a given $PaCO_2$, patients with CF have a more alkaline pH than those with advanced COPD. This tendency to alkalosis is related to the combination of low body $[Cl^-]$ and $[Na^+]$, as well as to the hypoalbuminaemia commonly seen in advanced CF.[36] There is no evidence of defective respiratory control in CF. Although the ventilatory response to CO_2 may be impaired, this is a consequence of the mechanical abnormality and the mouth occlusion pressure response to CO_2 is normal.[37]

10.2.5 Breathing during sleep in cystic fibrosis

As with COPD, arterial desaturation is common during sleep, particularly rapid-eye-movement (REM) sleep.[38] In general, nocturnal SaO_2 is related to awake blood gases as well as to the severity of airway obstruction as assessed by FEV_1.[39,40] Consequently, some individuals with more severe airway obstruction may show marked nocturnal desaturation despite relatively mild blood gas abnormality awake.[39]

10.2.6 Exercise in cystic fibrosis

The limits to progressive exercise in CF may be either ventilatory or peripheral, the latter related to the sensation of effort by the exercising muscles.[41] In general, individuals with more severe airway narrowing are more likely to be limited by breathlessness, and those with milder disease are more likely to be limited by leg discomfort, as occurs in healthy subjects.[42] Over a range of severity, peak oxygen uptake correlates with FEV_1.[42,43]

Exercise ventilation is excessive for the workload because of the increased dead space and V_D/V_T.[44,45] The physiological shunt may decrease because of improved $\dot{V}_A/\dot{Q}$ matching on exercise. Thus, despite a fall in mixed venous oxygenation, arterial blood gases and SaO_2 may change little,[34,46] unless airway obstruction is severe, when a fall in oxygenation and a rise in $PaCO_2$ are likely.[47] Use of supplemental oxygen during exercise in individuals who show desaturation increases exercise duration[48] and oxygen post-exercise can accelerate the recovery of the high heart rate and ventilation.[49]

10.2.7 Prognostic value of respiratory function tests in cystic fibrosis

The FEV_1 has been shown to be the strongest independent predictor of mortality in patients with CF not undergoing lung transplantation.[50,51] Although maximum exercise capacity also correlates with survival, it offers no additional prognostic information.[50] In a large study of survival of adult patients, the cut-off value of FEV_1 giving optimal sensitivity and specificity was 55 per cent of predicted: 96 per cent of the population with greater values survived for 5 years, while 54 per cent of those with lower

Table 10.1 Factors associated with more rapid decline in forced expiratory volume in 1 s (FEV_1) in cystic fibrosis

Factor	Reference
Female sex	54
ΔF508 homozygosity	54
Malnutrition	53
Pancreatic insufficiency	54
Glucose intolerance/diabetes	55, 56
Colonization with *Pseudomonas* spp.	53
Colonization with *Burkholderia* spp.	57, 58
High sputum elastase concentration	59

values died.[50] The rate of decline of FEV_1 is a more powerful predictor of mortality than a single measurement.[52] The annual rate of decline of FEV_1 is also used widely as a guide to the optimal timing of lung transplantation.[53] Several factors have been shown to influence the average annual rate of decline of FEV_1 (Table 10.1). Over the past 30 years, as the prognosis of the condition and survival have increased steadily, the average rate of decline of FEV_1 in young adults has concomitantly decreased,[60] such that conclusions based on the literature of even 10 years ago may no longer be valid.

REFERENCES

1 King PT, Holdsworth SR, Freezer NJ, Villanueva E, Holmes PW. Characterisation of the onset and presenting clinical features of adult bronchiectasis. *Respir Med* 2006; **100**: 2183–9.

2 Landau LI, Phelan PD, Williams HE. Ventilatory mechanics in patients with bronchiectasis starting in childhood. *Thorax* 1974; **29**: 304–12.

3 Fraser RG, Macklem PT, Brown WG. Airway dynamics in bronchiectasis. *Am J Roentgenol* 1965; **93**: 821–35.

4 Loubeyre P, Paret M, Revel D, Wiesendanger T, Brune J. Thin-section CT detection of emphysema associated with bronchiectasis and correlation with pulmonary function tests. *Chest* 1996; **109**: 360–65.

5 Roberts HR, Wells AU, Milne DG, *et al.* Airflow obstruction in bronchiectasis: correlation between computed tomography features and pulmonary function tests. *Thorax* 2000; **55**: 198–204.

6 Koulouris NG, Retsou S, Kosmas E, *et al.* Tidal expiratory flow limitation, dyspnoea and exercise capacity in patients with bilateral bronchiectasis. *Eur Respir J* 2003; **21**: 743–8.

7 Cherniack NS, Carton RW. Factors associated with respiratory insufficiency in bronchiectasis. *Am J Med* 1966; **41**: 562–71.

8 Pande JN, Jain BP, Gupta RG, Guleria JA. Pulmonary ventilation and gas exchange in bronchiectasis. *Thorax* 1971; **26**: 727–33.

9 Bass H, Henderson JA.M, Heckscher T, *et al.* Regional structure and function in bronchiectasis. *Am Rev Respir Dis* 1968; **97**: 598–609.

10 Yeates DB, Aspin N, Levison H, *et al.* Mucociliary tracheal transport rates in man. *J Appl Physiol* 1975; **39**: 487–95.

11 Stanley P, MacWilliam L, Greenstone M, Mackey IS, Cole PJ. Efficacy of a saccharin test for screening to detect abnormal mucociliary clearance. *Br J Dis Chest* 1984; **78**: 62–5.

12 Rutland J, Cole PJ. Non-invasive sampling of nasal cilia for measurement of beat frequency and study of ultrastructure. *Lancet* 1980; **ii**: 564–5.

13 Veale D, Rodgers AD, Griffiths CJ, Ashcroft T, Gibson GJ. Variability in ciliary beat frequency in normal subjects and in patients with bronchiectasis. *Thorax* 1993; **48**: 1018–20.

14 Mossberg B, Afzelius BA, Eliasson R, Camner P. On the pathogenesis of obstructive lung disease: a study on the immotile-cilia syndrome. *Scand J Respir Dis* 1978; **59**: 55–65.

15 Hellinckx J, Demedts M, De Boeck K. Primary ciliary dyskinesia: evolution of pulmonary function. *Eur J Pediatr* 1998; **157**: 422–6.

16 De Iongh R, Ing A, Rutland J. Mucociliary function, ciliary ultrastructure and ciliary orientation in Young's syndrome. *Thorax* 1992; **47**: 184–7.

17 Lamarre A, Reilly BJ, Bryan AC, Levison H. Early detection of pulmonary function abnormalities in cystic fibrosis. *Paediatrics* 1972; **50**: 291–8.

18 Lebecque P, Stanescu D. Respiratory resistance by the forced oscillation technique in asthmatic children and cystic fibrosis patients. *Eur Respir J* 1997; **10**: 891–5.

19 Ries AL, Sosa G, Prewitt L, Friedman PJ, Harwood IR. Restricted pulmonary function in cystic fibrosis. *Chest* 1988; **94**: 575–9.

20 Zapletal A, Desmond KJ, Demizio D, Coates AL. Lung recoil and the determination of airflow limitation in cystic fibrosis and asthma. *Pediatr Pulmonol* 1993; **15**: 13–18.

21 Bellemare F, Jeanneret A. Sex differences in thoracic adaptation to pulmonary hyperinflation in cystic fibrosis. *Eur Respir J* 2007; **29**: 98–107.

22 Holland AE, Denehy L, Wilson JW. Does expiratory flow limitation predict chronic dyspnoea in adults with cystic fibrosis? *Eur Respir J* 2006; **28**: 96–101.

23 Van Haren EHJ, Lammers J-WJ, Festen J, van Herwaarden CLA. Bronchial vagal tone and responsiveness to histamine, exercise and bronchodilators in adult patients with cystic fibrosis. *Eur Respir J* 1992; **5**: 1083–8.

24 Dodd JD, Barry SC, Daly LE, Gallagher CG. Inhaled beta-agonists improve lung function but not maximal exercise capacity in cystic fibrosis. *J Cystic Fibrosis* 2005; **4**: 101–5.

25 Eggleston PA, Rosenstein BJ, Stackhouse CM, Alexander MF. Airway hyperreactivity in cystic fibrosis: clinical correlates and possible effects on the course of the disease. *Chest* 1988; **94**: 360–65.

26 Tiddens HA, Koopman LP, Lambert RK, *et al.* Cartilaginous airway wall dimensions and airway resistance in cystic fibrosis lungs. *Eur Respir J* 2000; **15**: 735–42.

27 Mier A, Rodington A, Brophy C, Hudson M, Green M. Respiratory muscle function in cystic fibrosis. *Thorax* 1990; **45**: 750–52.

28 Marks J, Pasterkamp H, Tal A, Leahy F. Relationships between respiratory muscle strength, nutritional status and lung volume in cystic fibrosis and asthma. *Am Rev Respir Dis* 1986; **133**: 414–17.

29 Pinet C, Cassart M, Scillia P, *et al.* Function and bulk of respiratory and limb muscles in patients with cystic fibrosis. *Am J Respir Crit Care Med* 2003; **168**: 989–94.

30 Mansell AL, Andersen JE, Muttart CR, *et al.* Short-term pulmonary effects of total parenteral nutrition in children with cystic fibrosis. *J Pediatr* 1984; **104**: 700–705.

31 Asher MI, Pardy RL, Coates AL, Thomas E, Macklem PT. The effects of inspiratory muscle training in patients with cystic fibrosis. *Am Rev Respir Dis* 1982; **126**: 855–9.

32 Enright S, Chatham K, Ionescu AA, Unnithan VB, Shale DJ. Inspiratory muscle training improves lung function and exercise capacity in adults with cystic fibrosis. *Chest* 2004; **126**: 405–11.

33 Moss AJ, Desilets CT, Higashino SM, *et al.* Intrapulmonary shunts in cystic fibrosis. *Pediatrics* 1968; **41**: 438–45.

34 Dantzker DR, Patten GA, Bower JA. Gas exchange at rest and during exercise in adults with cystic fibrosis. *Am Rev Respir Dis* 1982; **125**: 400–405.

35 O'Brodovich HM, Mellins RB, Mansell AL. Effects of growth on the diffusion constant for carbon monoxide. *Am Rev Respir Dis* 1982; **125**: 670–73.

36 Holland AE, Wilson JW, Kotsimbos TC, Naughton MT. Metabolic alkalosis contributes to acute hypercapnic respiratory failure in adult cystic fibrosis. *Chest* 2003; **124**: 490–93.

37 Bureau MA, Lupien L, Begin R. Neural drive and ventilatory strategy of breathing in normal children and in patients with cystic fibrosis and asthma. *Pediatrics* 1981; **68**: 187–94.

38 Spier S, Rivlin J, Hughes D, Levison H. The effect of oxygen on sleep, blood gases and ventilation in cystic fibrosis. *Am Rev Respir Dis* 1984; **129**: 712–18.

39 Frangolias DD, Wilcox PG. Predictability of oxygen saturation during sleep in patients with cystic fibrosis: clinical, spirometric, and exercise parameters. *Chest* 2001; **119**: 434–41.

40 Milross MA, Piper AJ, Norman M, *et al.* Predicting sleep-disordered breathing in patients with cystic fibrosis. *Chest* 2001; **120**: 1239–45.

41 Lands LC, Heigenhauser GJF, Jones NL. Analysis of factors limiting maximal exercise performance in cystic fibrosis. *Clin Sci* 1992; **83**: 391–7.

42 Moorcroft AJ, Dodd ME, Morris J, Webb AK. Symptoms, lactate and exercise limitation at peak cycle ergometry in adults with cystic fibrosis. *Eur Respir J* 2005; **25**: 1050–56.

43 Hebestreit H, Kieser S, Rudiger S, *et al.* Physical activity is independently related to aerobic capacity in cystic fibrosis. *Eur Respir J* 2006; **28**: 734–9.

44 Cerney FJ, Pullano TP, Cropp GJA. Cardiorespiratory adaptations to exercise in cystic fibrosis. *Am Rev Respir Dis* 1982; **126**: 217–20.

45 Thin AG, Dodd JD, Gallagher CG, Fitzgerald MX, Mcloughlin P. Effect of respiratory rate on airway deadspace ventilation during exercise in cystic fibrosis. *Respir Med* 2004; **98**: 1063–70.

46 Henke KG, Orenstein DM. Oxygen saturation during exercise in cystic fibrosis. *Am Rev Respir Dis* 1984; **129**: 708–11.

47 Coates AL, Canny G, Zinman R, *et al.* The effects of chronic airflow limitation, increased dead space and the pattern of ventilation on gas exchange during maximal exercise in advanced cystic fibrosis. *Am Rev Respir Dis* 1988; **138**: 1524–31.

48 McKone EF, Barry SC, FitzGerald MX, Gallagher CG. The role of supplemental oxygen during submaximal exercise in patients with cystic fibrosis. *Eur Respir J* 2002; **20**: 134–42.

49 Shah AR, Keens TG, Gozal D. Effect of supplemental oxygen on supramaximal exercise performance and recovery in cystic fibrosis. *J Appl Physiol* 1997; **83**: 1641–7.

50 Moorcroft AJ, Dodd ME, Webb AK. Exercise testing and prognosis in adult cystic fibrosis. *Thorax* 1997; **52**: 291–3.

51 Belkin RA, Henig NR, Singer LG, *et al.* Risk factors for death of patients with cystic fibrosis awaiting lung transplantation. *Am J Respir Crit Care Med* 2006; **173**: 659–66.

52 Milla CE, Warwick WJ. Risk of death in cystic fibrosis patients with severely compromised lung function. *Chest* 1998; **113**: 1230–34.

53 Rosenbluth DB, Wilson K, Ferkol T, Schuster DP. Lung function decline in cystic fibrosis patients and timing for lung transplantation referral. *Chest* 2004; **126**: 412–19.

54 Corey M, Edwards L, Levison H, Knowles M. Longitudinal analysis of pulmonary function decline in patients with cystic fibrosis. *J Pediatr* 1997; 131, 809–14.

55 Milla CE, Warwick WJ, Moran A. Trends in pulmonary function in patients with cystic fibrosis correlate with the degree of glucose intolerance at baseline. *Am J Respir Crit Care Med* 2000; **162**: 891–5.

56 Rosenecker J, Hofler R, Steinkamp G, *et al.* Diabetes mellitus in patients with cystic fibrosis: the impact of diabetes mellitus on pulmonary function and clinical outcome. *Eur J Med Res* 2001; **6**: 345–50.

57 Courtney JM, Dunbar KEA, McDowell A, *et al.* Clinical outcome of Burkholderia cepacia complex infection in cystic fibrosis adults. *J Cystic Fibrosis* 2004; **3**: 93–8.

58 Kalish LA, Waltz DA, Dovey M, *et al.* Impact of *Burkholderia dolosa* on lung function and survival in cystic fibrosis. *Am J Respir Crit Care Med* 2006; **173**: 421–5.

59 Mayer-Hamblett N, Aitken ML, Accurso FJ, *et al.* Association between pulmonary function and sputum biomarkers in cystic fibrosis. *Am J Respir Crit Care Med* 2007; **175**: 822–8.

60 Que C, Cullinan P, Geddes D. Improving rate of decline of FEV_1 in young adults with cystic fibrosis. *Thorax* 2006; **61**: 155–7.

Asthma

The defining criteria for asthma include variability of airway narrowing and a heightened bronchial response to various inhaled agents, the phenomenon known as 'bronchial hyperresponsiveness' (BHR). Asthma is sometimes regarded as 'reversible' airway obstruction, but reliance on this term is potentially misleading, as reversibility is often incomplete and, even when in apparent remission, many patients with asthma show a degree of persistent airway narrowing, however subtle. As asthma is defined essentially in functional terms, it is one of the rare situations in which tests of respiratory function may be diagnostic in addition to playing their more usual role of assessing and quantifying abnormalities of function.

11.1 STATICS

11.1.1 Elastic properties of the lungs

The static pressure–volume (PV) curve in asthma characteristically shows a displacement to the left (Fig. 11.1), such that at any absolute or relative lung volume, recoil pressure is reduced compared with normal.[1,2] Unlike the pattern seen in emphysema, however, the static compliance over the tidal breathing range is usually normal and the general shape of the curve is preserved, with the exponent K of a monoexponential function fitted to the curve normal or only slightly increased.[1] The precise cause of

the changes in the PV curve remains elusive. In general, patients with more persistent airflow obstruction show more marked loss of recoil.[2] Although in theory this might reflect emphysema, the degree of abnormality is not related to either carbon monoxide (CO) uptake or computer tomography (CT) evidence of emphysema.[2] A more likely explanation for the reduction in lung recoil in asthma is the phenomenon of stress relaxation of the lungs,[3] together, possibly, with an increased ability of the inspiratory muscles to expand the thorax due to the greater neural drive to the muscles.[4]

11.1.2 Abnormalities of lung volumes

As with other diffuse airway diseases, both RV and functional residual capacity (FRC) increase in the face of airway narrowing. The 'operating lung volumes' over the tidal breathing range are consequently higher than normal. An increase in TLC is a consistent finding in asthmatic subjects with chronic airway obstruction in the stable state. It is also seen in many asymptomatic adult patients with a history of childhood asthma, even with little or no airway obstruction on spirometric criteria.[5] In some earlier studies, part of the reported increase in TLC may have been artefactual related to errors in plethysmography (see Chapter 1, Section 1.3.3), but more recent studies using slower panting frequencies confirm a true increase. An increased TLC is also demonstrable by radiographic measurements during

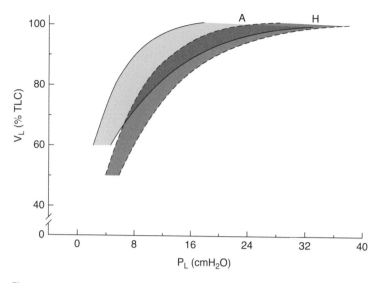

Figure 11.1 Ranges of static pressure–volume curves in groups of asthmatic (A) and healthy (H) subjects with volume plotted as per cent actual total lung capacity (TLC). In relation to the relative lung volume there is a reduction in lung recoil pressure in the patients but little or no change in slope of the curve over the tidal range (static compliance). Redrawn with permission from ref. 1.

P_L, lung recoil pressure; V_L, lung volume.

acute spontaneous asthma.[6] On the other hand, most measurements performed during short-term challenge studies, e.g. with methacholine, show no significant change in TLC,[7] although increases have been reported occasionally with other forms of bronchial challenge.[8] The difference between the acute challenge situation and the spontaneous exacerbation may relate to the timescale over which an increase in TLC is likely to develop.

11.1.3 Respiratory muscle function

Although the increased airway resistance of asthma is greater on expiration than inspiration, it is the inspiratory muscles that bear the main load. In addition, because of the lung hyperinflation, they are required to work with an impaired mechanical advantage. Nevertheless, respiratory muscle function in asthma is generally well preserved, although in some individuals it may be impaired due to chronic steroid treatment.[9,10] Minor reductions in maximum inspiratory pressure ($P_I$max) measured at FRC are seen in association with the hyperinflation, and improvement after bronchodilator with an accompanying reduction in FRC has been described.[11] Even in acute attacks, however, $P_I$max is well preserved in most patients.[12] Doubtless, respiratory

muscle fatigue occurs in life-threatening asthma, but no confirmatory measurements are available.

11.2 AIRWAY STRUCTURE AND FUNCTION

11.2.1 Airway structure

Asthma is characterized structurally by increased thickness of the airway walls. This has been described in patients dying from asthma and in asthmatic subjects dying from other causes, as well as in patients with a history of asthma undergoing lung resection for other reasons, e.g. bronchial carcinoma. Increased bronchial wall thickness is found throughout the bronchial tree and, in general, is more marked in fatal asthma. Thickening of the wall affects large and small airways, including membranous bronchioles.[13,14] Importantly, however, the diameter of the airway lumen is generally preserved despite thickening of the wall, at least in milder disease.[15] Airway 'remodelling' in asthma, defined as changes in the compositional content and organization of the cellular and molecular constituents of the airway wall,[16] is not a recent discovery as most of the structural changes have been recognized for

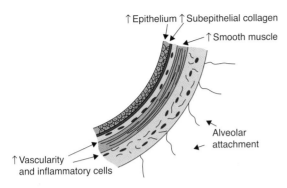
↑Epithelium ↑Subepithelial collagen
↑Smooth muscle
Alveolar attachment
↑Vascularity and inflammatory cells

Figure 11.2 Diagrammatic representation of factors contributing to increased airway wall thickness in asthma.

nearly a century. The remodelling affects all the constituent layers of the airway wall (Fig. 11.2):[16] the epithelium is increased in volume by more goblet cells and greater vascularity; the subepithelial collagen layer (lamina reticularis) is characteristically thickened; the smooth muscle mass is increased by a combination of greater size (hypertrophy) and number (hyperplasia) of smooth muscle cells, with in addition an increase in the extracellular matrix between the muscle cells;[17] and, finally, the adventitia that makes up the largest proportion of the airway wall, comprising connective tissue, lymphatics and small vessels, is also thickened.

It is generally assumed that the greater airway wall thickness has an adverse affect on respiratory function, particularly by enhancing the effect of a stimulus to bronchoconstriction (see below) and also by reducing the distensibility of the airway, as can be demonstrated by measurements of airway conductance in relation to lung elastic recoil.[17] There are, however, also some theoretical advantages, related in particular to the greater stiffness of the airway wall, which is likely to make it less compressible during forceful expiration; this may be particularly relevant at the 'choke point' during forced expiration (see Chapter 1, Section 1.6.5.4), thereby helping to maintain maximum expiratory flow.[16]

11.2.2 Airway function

Many individuals with mild asthma have normal spirometric volumes during remission but, as with early chronic obstructive pulmonary disease

(COPD), abnormal function of the peripheral airways may be detectable using more sensitive techniques. Thus, direct measurements of peripheral airway resistance during fibre-optic bronchoscopy have shown marked increases in patients with mild asymptomatic asthma despite normal FEV_1 and specific airway conductance.[18] In patients with symptomatic airway obstruction, routine tests of airway function show the anticipated features of reduced FEV_1, FEV_1/VC, maximum expiratory flows at all volumes, and increased RV and airway resistance. None of these is specific for asthma.

Various studies have attempted to identify patterns of abnormality of airway function that distinguish asthma from COPD, in particular from emphysema. Because emphysema is associated with more marked reduction in elastic recoil, a disproportionate effect on maximum expiratory flow might be expected. As a group, the ratio of maximum expiratory flow at 50 per cent VC to airway conductance is lower in emphysema than in asthma, but there is too much overlap between groups to make this a useful discriminator[19] and in practice single indices of maximum flow or airway resistance fail to differentiate the two conditions.

Unless a large acute improvement is found after bronchodilator, routine tests performed on a single occasion are not usually diagnostic in asthma. Much more revealing than a large battery of tests are repeated simple measurements: e.g. a patient whose FEV_1/VC is 1.5/2.5 at one clinic visit and who, a week later, with or without a change in treatment, has values of 2.5/4.0 is clearly asthmatic. Frequent monitoring of airway function is easily obtainable by having patients make their own measurements of peak expiratory flow (PEF) at home two or four times a day (Fig. 11.3). Clearly this has the advantage of allowing measurements when symptoms are at their worst, such as in the middle of the night or on rising in the morning. It is not unusual for a patient with very labile asthma to have relatively normal spirometry in an outpatient clinic in the afternoon and yet to have been waking at 4.00 a.m. each day with orthopnoea and severe distress due to asthma. The patient's symptoms can easily be dismissed or even attributed to episodes of left ventricular failure unless objective evidence is obtained.

Marked diurnal variation of airway function is characteristic of asthma. Although the mechanism is not clear, this variation is essentially an exaggeration of that found in healthy subjects. In general, the fall in PEF at night or in the early morning is related to the severity of impairment of daytime function and also to the degree of daytime bronchial hyper-responsiveness to methacholine.[20] In shift workers who sleep by day, the pattern reverses, with the

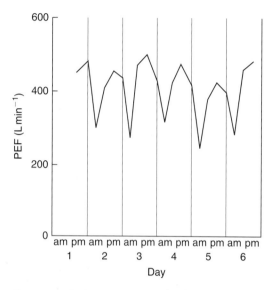

Figure 11.3 Peak expiratory flow (PEF) recorded four times daily in an asthmatic patient, showing the characteristic variability and morning dip.

lowest values of airway function in the evening. The characteristic 'morning dip' of airway function occurs to varying degrees in most asthmatic subjects; its symptomatic consequences become evident in those with the largest variation in function. Unusually large variation of PEF has also been shown to relate to the absence of a maximum (plateau) response to bronchial challenge,[21] which itself may imply an increased likelihood of life-threatening attacks (see Chapter 1, Section 1.6.8.2).

As with other causes of diffuse airway obstruction, patients with significant airway obstruction develop dynamic, in addition to static, hyperinflation and this increases further on exercise (see Chapter 9, Section 9.11.2).[22] Dynamic hyperinflation also occurs during methacholine-induced bronchoconstriction, even without expiratory flow limitation (EFL), suggesting that EFL per se is not necessarily the trigger to its development.[23]

The relation between airway function and symptoms in asthma is only approximate (Fig. 11.4). Mildly abnormal spirometry is often demonstrable during clinical remission and, similarly, a high frequency of spirometric abnormalities[24] and/or bronchial hyperresponsiveness[25] or increased diurnal variation of PEF[26] can be found in completely asymptomatic adults who have a history of asthma in childhood. Furthermore, many people with asthma are remarkably well adjusted to quite severe

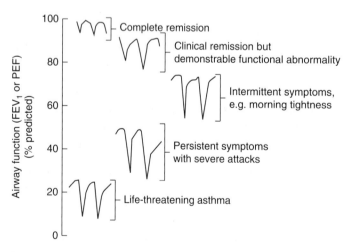

Figure 11.4 Schematic relations between airway function and symptoms in asthma with forced expiratory volume in 1 s (FEV$_1$) and peak expiratory flow (PEF) recorded four times a day over 48 h. Many asymptomatic asthmatic patients (clinical remission) have demonstrably abnormal function. When symptoms are intermittent, the severity may be seriously underestimated unless measurements are made at the time of symptoms, usually in the early morning. Severe life-threatening attacks usually develop against a background of instability and poor control.

degrees of persistent airflow obstruction when this shows little variation. An important factor determining both the symptoms and the severity of gas exchange disturbance in asthma is the rate at which the airway narrowing has developed; e.g. a patient whose FEV_1 falls from a normal value of 4 L to 1.5 L over a couple of days is likely to be seriously ill, whereas another who has adapted physiologically and psychologically to an optimal FEV_1 of 1.5 L may be leading a normal life. By the time a patient requires hospital admission with acute severe asthma, the level of airway function is likely to be grossly reduced, with FEV_1 that may be only 10 per cent or so of the normal value.

11.2.3 Effects of bronchodilators

One standard definition of asthma specifies airway narrowing that varies over short periods of time, either spontaneously or as the result of treatment. But this begs the questions by how much, and over how short a period? There are no arbitrary levels applicable in all cases to allow ready answers to these questions. As a group, people with asthma show larger acute increases in spirometric volumes after bronchodilator than either normal subjects or those with chronic airway disease of other aetiology. A relatively large acute bronchodilator response is seen even when pre-bronchodilator function is relatively normal,[27] but there is a 'ceiling' effect, in that if airway function is almost normal, there is little further room for improvement. By contrast, bronchodilators may also have little effect when asthma is very severe; the largest improvements are seen between these extremes (Fig. 11.5). Although arbitrary percentage or absolute increases in FEV_1 after bronchodilator (e.g. 15% ± 200 mL) are sometimes used as criteria to diagnose or exclude asthma, they can mislead and should not be applied rigidly. Occasionally, a large increase (e.g. 0.5 L or more) is diagnostic; more commonly, a smaller increase is suggestive and a repeat on a second occasion may be supportive. Very little increase may be seen in severe asthma – but equally a 20 per cent increase when the FEV_1 is only 0.5 L is often found in non-asthmatic chronic airflow obstruction.

Airway resistance or conductance and measurements during forced expiration usually move in the same direction with deterioration or improvement

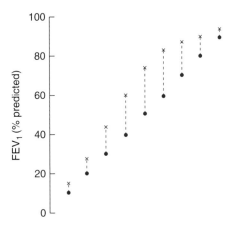

Figure 11.5 Schematic diagram of acute effects of an inhaled bronchodilator in a patient with varying severity of asthma. The improvement in forced expiratory volume in 1 s (FEV_1; broken line) is likely to be greatest when the pre-bronchodilator value is moderately reduced. When it is close to normal there is less scope for improvement, and in severe asthma the effect is also reduced.

of asthma, but they are not necessarily closely related. Sometimes, e.g. in bronchodilator drug studies, play is made of the different 'sensitivity' of various tests, but in practice the signal-to-noise ratio and innate variability of each measurement both within and between subjects favour the FEV_1 and vital capacity. Large proportional changes in maximum expiratory flows at low lung volumes after bronchodilator are particularly problematic as their interpretation is complicated by any change in VC. It is not unusual in patients with more severe airway obstruction to see a larger increase in VC than in FEV_1 after bronchodilator. On the basis of these measurements, patients are sometimes classified as either 'flow responders' or 'volume responders', the evidence suggesting that volume responses in particular reflect dilatation of smaller airways.[28] Studies using CT scanning have shown that an increase in diameter of medium-sized airways is related more closely to volume recruitment, i.e. an increase in VC, than to an increase in FEV_1.[4] The differential effects of bronchodilators on FEV_1 and VC are analogous to post-bronchoconstrictor measurements when the reduction in VC may be independent of the reduction in FEV_1, particularly in individuals with more severe asthma.[29] An important effect of volume recruitment by dilatation of smaller airways is a reduction in dynamic hyperinflation, which is demonstrable by plethysmography.[30] Clearly, however, this method of evaluating bronchodilator responses is impracticable for use in large numbers of subjects.

The predominant sites of action of different types of bronchodilator drugs may differ, although conclusions based on comparing the results of different tests of airway function require caution. It is reasonable to attribute large changes in airway conductance with little change in 'small airway' tests (such as $\dot{V}_E$max at small lung volumes) to predominant constriction or dilatation of the more central airways. However, in clinically significant diffuse airway obstruction, large changes in calibre of the smaller airways are also reflected by changes in airway resistance. In normal subjects, studies of the sites of action of bronchodilator drugs suggest that anticholinergic agents have their main effects in the more proximal airways (which would correspond to the known distribution of parasympathetic innervation), while sympathomimetic agents probably act more generally.[31] In asthmatic airways, however, the respective sites of action are less distinct and anticholinergic agents may act more generally in the bronchial tree.[32] The route of administration may also be relevant as some evidence suggests that systemically administered drugs have a relatively greater effect on tests of 'small airway' function in asthma than when the drug is given by inhalation.[33]

In some patients with moderate or severe chronic and apparently largely irreversible airway obstruction, the characteristic variability of asthma comes to light only after a course of oral corticosteroids. In such patients regular measurements of FEV_1 and/or PEF are essential in order to identify a true improvement in airway function.

11.3 BRONCHIAL HYPERRESPONSIVENESS

11.3.1 Nature of bronchial responsiveness in asthma

The phenomenon of BHR in asthma has been recognized for 60 years, but the precise mechanism(s) responsible remain uncertain. In individuals with asthma, BHR can be demonstrated using many different types of stimulus. These include chemical agents that mimic the effects of the parasympathetic nervous system (methacholine), substances that are released naturally from mast cells (histamine), exogenous irritants (sulphur dioxide, citric acid), breathing cold dry air, and exercise (see Section 11.9.2). Often the clinical correlates of BHR are recognized by the patient (e.g. when developing wheezing and chest tightness in response to a frosty morning or a smoky atmosphere, to inhaled drugs, or after coughing, yawning or laughing). The same phenomenon may be evident to the experienced clinical physiologist, who recognizes that repeat measurements of FEV_1 result in progressively deteriorating performance, frequently accompanied by bouts of coughing.

Bronchial responsiveness is related closely to, but not necessarily identical with, a clinical diagnosis of asthma.[34] Increased bronchial responses to nonspecific stimuli are seen in other situations, e.g. after viral upper respiratory tract infections (see Chapter 13, Section 13.1), while occasional patients with asthma according to all other criteria fail to show BHR. In general, however, the relationship is close. On average, the degree of BHR is greater than in COPD, although there is appreciable overlap.[35] Unlike the situation in COPD, there is no clear relation of BHR in asthma to baseline airway calibre,[36] but the relation to spontaneous variation of airway function is clearer in asthma than in COPD.[35] The other major difference between the responses in the two conditions is the range of potential stimuli, which is much greater in patients with asthma than in COPD, who are generally less responsive to challenges that cause release of mediators as opposed to direct smooth muscle agonists.[37]

11.3.2 Pattern of bronchial responsiveness

The most commonly used agent for bronchial challenge is methacholine, with the response usually measured by simple indices such as the concentration provoking a 20 per cent reduction in FEV_1 (PC_{20}; see Chapter 1, Section 1.6.8.2). Alternatively, dose–response curves to the inhaled stimulus can be analysed in a manner akin to dose–response relationships in vitro, i.e. in terms of a threshold response (sensitivity) and the slope of the response (reactivity).[38] An important feature

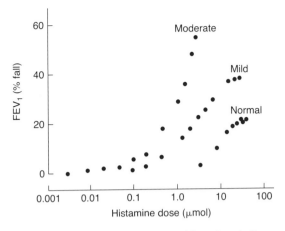

Figure 11.6 Dose–response curves to histamine challenge in three individuals, two with asthma and one normal. Both of the asthmatic people show hyperresponsiveness in comparison with the normal subject. The patient with mild asthma and the normal subject show a plateau response, whereas the patient with moderate asthma shows no plateau despite a fall in forced expiratory volume in 1 s (FEV$_1$) greater than 50 per cent. Redrawn from ref. 39, with permission from the American Thoracic Society.

of the dose–response relationship in normal subjects is the development of a plateau FEV$_1$ as the dose of stimulus is increased (Fig. 11.6).[39,40] Some patients with asthma fail to show such a plateau as the dose is increased, suggesting that they lack a mechanism present in healthy subjects that limits airway narrowing. Clinically, this may have important implications if progressive airway narrowing were to continue unchecked. It has, for example, been shown that the absence of a plateau response in some asthmatic individuals is associated with greater spontaneous diurnal variation of airway function.[21] It is possible that each of the three features of the dose–response curve – i.e. threshold (left shift), reactivity (slope) and maximal response – are determined by separate mechanisms.[16] Exaggerated narrowing (i.e. absence of a plateau) could reflect either progressive bronchoconstriction of all airways or closure of some (or both mechanisms). Most healthy subjects develop a plateau after only modest airway narrowing.[40] It has been suggested that asthmatic subjects who show a disproportionate reduction in VC on challenge may be those who develop more marked airway closure and have the propensity to uncontrolled airway narrowing during challenge.[29]

11.3.3 Effects of deep inspiration on airway function

A further striking functional abnormality of asthma related to bronchial hyperresponsiveness is the effect of a deep inspiration (DI). In healthy subjects, DI has a bronchodilating effect,[41] and it also counters methacholine-induced bronchoconstriction.[42] Since these effects are greatly attenuated in asthma, it has been proposed that an important cause of BHR relates to the impaired ability of DI to stretch the smooth muscle of asthmatic airways.[42] Furthermore, DI not only fails to relieve bronchoconstriction in patients with asthma but also sometimes has the paradoxical effect of provoking greater bronchoconstriction. The potential mechanisms of these intriguing responses and their relation to BHR have been the subject of many studies over the past 20 years.

The effect of DI can be assessed using either tests of forced expiration or airway resistance/conductance. With forced expiratory tests, expiratory flow is compared at iso-lung volume following full and incomplete ('partial') inspirations to obtain a maximum/partial (M/P) flow ratio. A value of M/P greater than 1 implies bronchodilatation post-DI and a value less than 1 implies bronchoconstriction. In patients with stable asthma, Lim et al. showed that M/P was related inversely to the severity of airway obstruction (i.e. patients with more severe airway obstruction showed a reduction in maximum expiratory flow after DI); on the other hand, with asthma induced by histamine to provoke equally severe airway obstruction, M/P was greater than 1, i.e. DI resulted in bronchodilatation.[43] The same authors also showed that the time course of recovery from the effects of DI is longer for the bronchoconstriction seen in spontaneous asthma than for the bronchodilatation occurring after induced asthma. The authors suggested that the mechanisms and sites of each process were likely to vary in the two different situations. In a subsequent study, the same group, studying patients during and after a spontaneous exacerbation of asthma, again showed a greater constrictor effect of DI (M/P <1) in patients with more severe airway obstruction, but within an individual, as the function improved, the bronchoconstrictor effect diminished, suggesting that the improvement was related to resolution of airway inflammation following treatment of the acute attack (Fig. 11.7).[44]

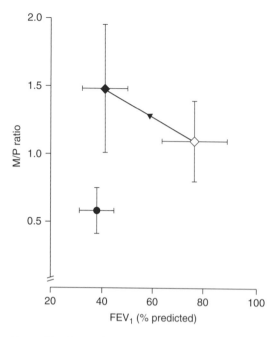

Figure 11.7 Comparison of maximum/partial (M/P) ratios (mean ± standard deviation, SD) in subjects with severe spontaneous asthma (●) and before (◇) and after (◆) histamine-induced bronchoconstriction. Note that M > P with induced asthma but M < P in spontaneous asthma. Redrawn from ref. 43, with permission from the American Thoracic Society.

FEV_1, forced expiratory volume in 1 s.

Subsequent work on the effects of DI after bronchial challenge in healthy subjects has highlighted not only the bronchodilator effect (DI reversing induced bronchoconstriction) but also a 'bronchoprotective' effect,[45] with preceding DI protecting against the effects of challenge. The latter may be the more important effect[46] and is reduced or absent even in mild asthma. If either healthy individuals[47] or asthmatic subjects[48] avoid DI before bronchial challenge testing, their responsiveness is appreciably increased. Nevertheless, normal subjects who avoid DI pre-challenge are still less responsive than patients with asthma.[49,50]

The amount of bronchodilatation after DI following methacholine-induced bronchoconstriction predicts the level of maximum bronchoconstriction, emphasizing the potential link between DI and what is probably the most important aspect of BHR: those individuals with the greatest reduction in FEV_1 after challenge show a smaller bronchodilator effect of DI.[51] Treatment with inhaled steroids

changes the position of the methacholine dose–response curve, shifting it to the right (lower sensitivity), and also improves the bronchodilator effect of DI in mild asthma. Some evidence also suggests that inhaled steroid treatment can re-establish a maximum plateau response to challenge, thus potentially protecting against unlimited airway narrowing.[52]

11.3.4 Potential mechanisms of bronchial hyperresponsiveness in asthma

Several hypotheses have been proposed to explain both the non-specific BHR and the abnormal responses to DI shown by patients with asthma. Any combination of the following may be relevant.

11.3.4.1 Airway and parenchymal hysteresis

Froeb and Mead proposed that the effects of the preceding volume history (e.g. taking deep inspirations) on airway calibre may differ substantially, depending on the relative magnitudes of airway and parenchymal hysteresis (Fig. 11.8).[53] Hysteresis is a phenomenon displayed by all elastic structures and is related to the energy losses that occur when tissues are stretched, such that the elastic properties displayed during stretching differ from those during subsequent relaxation; in other words, the pressure–volume relationship differs during inspiration and expiration. This applies to both the alveoli (parenchyma) and the airways, with the hysteresis of each potentially varying independently. During DI both the airway smooth muscle and the lung parenchyma are stretched. As both structures show hysteresis, when the stress of the DI is removed with a return to resting lung volume, the tension in both the lung parenchyma and the airways is reduced to less than it was pre-stretch. If hysteresis of the lung parenchyma is considerable, elastic recoil is greatly reduced on expiration following DI, thus allowing the airway smooth muscle to shorten and narrow the airway. On the other hand, if DI disproportionately decreases the tension in the airway muscle itself, the airway would dilate, despite a small decrease in lung recoil. The net effect on the airway thus depends on the balance between the relative hysteresis of the parenchyma and the airways.[54]

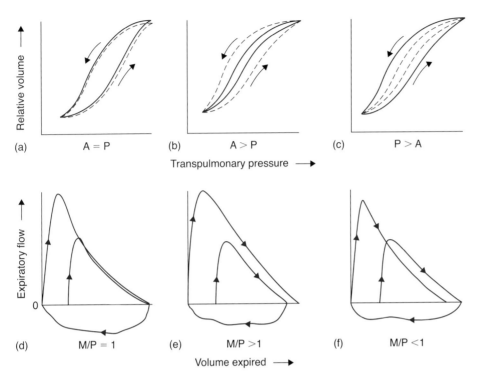

Figure 11.8 Effects of hysteresis of airways (A) and lung parenchyma (P) on maximum/partial (M/P) ratio. (a–c) Schematic pressure–volume curves of airways (broken lines) and parenchyma (solid lines), with volume of each plotted on a relative scale. (d–f) Resulting maximum and partial expiratory flow–volume curves. If airway hysteresis exceeds parenchymal as in (b), airway size during expiration following full inspiration is relatively greater for a given transpulmonary pressure and consequently, as in (e), maximum expiratory flow is greater than after incomplete inspiration (i.e. M/P >1). Conversely, if parenchymal hysteresis exceeds airway (c), airway size is relatively smaller after full inspiration and M/P <1 (f). If hysteresis of airways and parenchyma is similar (a), deep inspiration has no effect on expiratory flow (d).

Hysteretic behaviour is shown by a single alveolus, but in the intact lung the situation is more complex, as a major factor is the number of alveoli contributing to volume change; at the same overall lung volume this is likely to differ on inspiration and expiration. Since airway calibre depends on both the intrinsic properties of the airway and elastic support by the surrounding alveoli, the net effect on airway function will depend on the relative magnitudes of airway and parenchymal hysteresis. Hysteresis increases during bronchoconstriction as the tone of the contractile elements of the airways and parenchyma increases. If airway hysteresis is greater than parenchymal hysteresis, airway volume will be greater during expiration than inspiration and therefore maximum expiratory flow will be greater after DI than before, i.e. M/P >1. If, on the other hand, parenchymal hysteresis exceeds airway hysteresis,

airway calibre at a given lung volume will be less after than before DI, i.e. M/P <1. This hypothesis has proved very helpful in understanding many of the results in the literature, such as those of Lim and colleagues.[43,44] In acute spontaneous asthma and in stable patients with more severe airway obstruction in whom DI induces bronchoconstriction (M/P <1), parenchymal hysteresis is presumably greater than airway hysteresis. On the other hand, with methacholine-induced bronchoconstriction, when DI generally induces bronchodilatation, airway hysteresis exceeds parenchymal, i.e. M/P >1. Lim and colleagues argued that in spontaneous asthma more peripheral airways are likely to be involved and their effect is encompassed within 'parenchymal hysteresis'. However, the precise structural elements involved are not clear. The relative hysteresis hypothesis is clearly only a partial explanation for BHR and the effects of DI and it does not allow detailed exploration of the underlying cellular mechanisms.

11.3.4.2 Abnormalities of smooth muscle structure and function

At first sight, the increased mass of bronchial smooth muscle in asthma would be expected to increase the force of muscle contraction, but this is not necessarily the case, as proliferation of the muscle might actually impair its contractility.[55] The velocity of muscle shortening might also increase,[16] an effect potentially amplified by decreased tethering (support) by the surrounding alveoli (see below). Studies in vitro, however, do not suggest a greater ability of asthmatic airways to develop force.[16]

The contractility of airway smooth muscle depends on cyclical changes in its length. In the airway this is accomplished by normal tidal breathing together with occasional deep inspiration. An impaired ability of deep inspiration to stretch airway smooth muscle might reside in the muscle itself or might result from inability to transmit and apply the requisite force to the muscle. It has been suggested that the airway muscle itself may be stiffened by the deposition of connective tissue in the various layers of the airway, including between the muscle cells themselves, thereby attenuating the ability of tidal breathing and deep inspiration to stretch the muscle. This would lead to a failure to break the 'cross bridges' between actin and myosin filaments of the muscle, thus stiffening the airway and encouraging a 'frozen' state.[16,56] Collagenous thickening of the basement membrane is a well-recognized feature of the asthmatic airway; this might in theory reduce the effectiveness of muscle shortening and could therefore be protective of airway calibre. Recent data on the effects of bronchial thermoplasty, in which smooth muscle disruption is deliberately induced, support an important role for abnormal smooth muscle behaviour in determining BHR.[57]

11.3.4.3 Overall geometry of the airway

The considerable thickening of the airway wall seen in asthma does not necessarily encroach on the lumen in the resting state,[15,55] but, in theory, it would greatly amplify the effect of a bronchoconstrictor. Airway wall thickening is also likely to increase the heterogeneity of airway narrowing and consequently the propensity to closure. However, in patients with no significant pre-challenge airway obstruction, there are no consistent relationships between BHR and airway geometry, and in particular no clear relation to airway thickness as assessed by CT,[58] although such a relationship has been shown in patients with spirometric evidence of pre-challenge airway narrowing.[59]

11.3.4.4 Altered airway/parenchymal relationship

The restraining effect of the surrounding alveoli may be responsible for the plateau airway response seen in healthy subjects challenged by methacholine. In asthma, inflammatory changes in the adventitia surrounding the airway could greatly impair this restraining effect on airway narrowing (see Fig. 11.2), such that no plateau effect on bronchoconstriction is seen when asthmatic patients undergo bronchial challenge.[60] This would greatly increase the likelihood of airway closure and might be relevant to those asthmatic individuals who show a disproportionate reduction in VC during challenge testing.[29] The loss of such a 'geometric buffer' would be particularly apparent at lower lung volumes where the pressure distending the airways is less; it is therefore relevant that the degree of airway narrowing in response to a bronchoconstrictor is markedly increased at such lung volumes.[16] On the other hand, dynamic hyperinflation would offer partial protection against this effect of peribronchial inflammation, which effectively uncouples the airways from the surrounding lung parenchyma.

11.3.5 Clinical use of bronchial challenge tests

11.3.5.1 Non-specific inhalational challenges

It is unusual for a non-smoking healthy subject to have a PC_{20} of less than 8 mg methacholine per millilitre; most asthmatic subjects in remission have values between 1 mg ml^{-1} and 8 mg ml^{-1}, while troublesome asthma is often associated with values below 1 mg ml^{-1}. The level of BHR in an individual tends to increase during periods when asthma is more troublesome, even if there is little change in the level of airway function at the time of challenge. Consequently, in individuals who are sensitive to seasonal allergens it may vary with the season. The decline in BHR following an episode of acute severe asthma is delayed well after improvement of the FEV$_1$ and continues for a period once FEV$_1$ has reached a stable value.[61] The severity of BHR may be relevant to the cause and outcome of acute severe asthma. For example, it has been shown that patients requiring ventilatory support during an acute attack have greater BHR in remission than those not requiring assisted ventilation.[62]

In practice, the clinical situation in which tests of BHR are most useful is in patients with suspected asthma with atypical symptoms, e.g. so-called 'cough variant asthma' with relatively normal lung function. Demonstration of abnormal responsiveness to methacholine is useful in this context, although confirmation of the diagnosis also requires a therapeutic response.[63] In general, compared with patients with typical asthma, those with cough variant asthma are more likely to have a demonstrable maximum response plateau on challenge.[21]

For assessing the response to challenge, airway function can be measured by spirometric measurements or by airway resistance, the latter measured either plethysmographically or by forced oscillation; the results correlate reasonably well.[64] Despite the effect of DI transiently attenuating methacholine-induced bronchoconstriction, most clinical testing utilizes FEV$_1$ for simplicity and consistency of performance. Measurements of expiratory flow at particular lung volumes are no more sensitive than FEV$_1$, at least in recognition of exercise-induced asthma (EIA).[65]

11.3.5.2 Specific inhalational challenges

Bronchial challenge testing using specific agents to which the individual may have been sensitized has been employed widely in experimental studies although, apart from the specific area of occupational asthma, it is little used in clinical practice. When testing for specific sensitivity, the FEV$_1$ is usually followed for several hours to detect any late response in addition to the immediate response. The results should be compared with those in an identical procedure using only the carrier in which the putative allergen is administered. Such tests are rarely performed using the common allergens that provoke responses in atopic subjects.

A wide variety of chemicals have been shown to be potential bronchoconstrictors in various occupations. When investigating for suspected occupational asthma, the initial investigation usually involves having the patient make frequent recordings of PEF throughout the working day, while exposed to the potential agent, and continuing the measurements at home in the evening as reactions are often late rather than immediate.[66] Having in this way confirmed a problem, it may then be necessary to identify the specific chemical responsible by exposing the subject in a controlled fashion. However, it can be difficult to judge the appropriate dose and, rather than give a potentially large dose by direct inhalation from a nebulizer or insufflator, an alternative is to mimic the working situation by the subject painting, soldering, spraying or shaking the suspect substance.[67] The actual measurement made is rarely critical, as fairly gross changes are being sought and FEV$_1$ or PEF usually suffices. If possible, a control test using an inert substance should also be performed.

11.3.5.3 Oral challenge tests

Oral challenge tests are undertaken less frequently than inhalational tests, but they have an important role in a few patients, particularly in relation to possible adverse effects of drugs in asthma. As with inhalation challenge, the agents may be either specific (drugs that produce idiosyncratic reactions in only a few patients) or non-specific (drugs that in sufficient dose produce adverse reactions in all asthmatic subjects). Of the former, the analgesic and anti-inflammatory drugs are the most important. Patients with analgesic-induced asthma are almost always sensitive to aspirin, but the pattern of response to other drugs varies between individuals. It may be important for a patient's management to establish which analgesics can safely be taken, and this is best done under controlled conditions with close supervision. It is usually unnecessary (and may be unwise) to use aspirin itself if the history is clear, but challenges with other analgesics (preferably with a placebo control) may be appropriate. The FEV$_1$ should be followed for at least 2 h as the effects may sometimes be delayed.[68]

Of the non-idiosyncratic reactions, the adverse effects of β-sympathetic antagonists are the most important. Their effect is dose-related and can be minimized by using a cardioselective agent, although the wisest counsel is to avoid β-blockers if possible in any patient with a convincing recent or remote history of asthma. Occasionally there are compelling reasons for their use, or the history of asthma is less than definite, and then the effects of a test dose of a cardioselective β-blocker can be observed by following FEV_1 for 4 h after a single dose. The effect of a β-blocker in an individual is, however, not constant and, as with inhalation challenge, it is likely to become more evident if control of the asthma deteriorates: even if an insignificant response to a single test dose is found, it is advisable to continue regular monitoring of PEF by the patient at home for a few weeks if regular treatment is commenced.

As a precaution, a $β_2$-agonist should be immediately available for nebulization at the time of any challenge tests.

11.4 DECLINE OF FEV_1 AND PERSISTENT AIRWAY OBSTRUCTION IN ASTHMA

A degree of persistent airway obstruction is common in asthma and usually is readily apparent using simple spirometric measurements of FEV_1 and vital capacity.[69] When mild, the patient may be asymptomatic between exacerbations, but more severe persistent airway narrowing is accompanied by chronic shortness of breath. In young or middle-aged adults evidence of airway obstruction is more likely in those who had more severe asthma in childhood.[70,71]

Persistent airway narrowing and the use of the term 'COPD' in this context is often a semantic matter. In general in asthma, the more carefully one assesses respiratory function, the more frequently some evidence of persistent airway narrowing is found. It is more appropriate to designate this in purely functional terms as 'chronic airway (airflow) obstruction' rather than as 'COPD', as the latter term may be taken to imply a second diagnosis. Of course, since both asthma and COPD are common conditions, the combination is found not infrequently, particularly in smokers. It may

then be impossible to apportion the contributions to persistent airway obstruction of the two conditions. Studies comparing populations diagnosed with either asthma or COPD have shown that, for a similar level of airway obstruction (i.e. equivalent FEV_1), those with asthma tend to have relatively less hyperinflation with lower RV and FRC and consistently better preserved carbon monoxide diffusing capacity (D_LCO) and K_CO;[71,72] the arterial PO_2 also tends to be a little higher on average in subjects with asthma.[72] As a group, patients with asthma have a larger acute bronchodilator response in terms of increase in FEV_1 than those with COPD, but, as discussed above, the considerable overlap makes this an unhelpful diagnostic criterion unless the increase in FEV_1 is large.

Population studies have shown that the rate of decline of FEV_1 of adult individuals with asthma is on average greater than in non-asthmatic subjects.[73,74] Risk factors for more rapid decline in patients with asthma include smoking, atopy and greater BHR.[75] Persistent exposure to occupational agents[76] and genetic predisposition[77] may also contribute in some individuals. Recent studies have shown that long-term treatment with inhaled steroids can reduce the rate of decline of FEV_1 of patients with asthma.[78,79]

11.5 TESTS OF GAS EXCHANGE

11.5.1 Chronic stable asthma

Conventional tests for inequalities of ventilation in asthma show no distinguishing features when compared with other types of airway obstruction. In mild or moderate stable asthma the PaO_2 is usually close to normal and on average higher than in patients with COPD with an equivalent severity of airway obstruction.[72] Since, however, hypocapnia is common in patients with mild[78,80] or even no[81] airway obstruction, an increase in the $AaPO_2$ is common.

Studies of gas exchange in stable asthma using the multiple inert gas elimination technique (MIGET) show evidence of $\dot{V}/\dot{Q}$ mismatching even in mild asthma.[82] The abnormalities are apparent mainly in relation to the distribution of perfusion; an increased dispersion of $\dot{V}_A/\dot{Q}$ ratios in relation to perfusion is due mainly to low $\dot{V}_A/\dot{Q}$ areas reflecting parts of the lung that are perfused but poorly ventilated.[83] In some individuals, the distribution of $\dot{V}_A/\dot{Q}$ ratios is bimodal, with a more distinct population of lung units with very low $\dot{V}_A/\dot{Q}$ ratios, which may represent alveoli distal to obstructed small airways, which retain slow ventilation via collateral channels.[84]

Local adjustment of perfusion to ventilation occurs, which minimizes the effects on blood gases of bronchoconstriction.[85] Consequently, defects of ventilation on lung scanning are usually matched by defects of lung perfusion.[86] Occasionally, the defects of perfusion scanning alone may be sufficiently well-defined to cause diagnostic confusion with pulmonary embolism.

11.5.2 Acute severe asthma

By the time an asthmatic patient is admitted to hospital with acute severe asthma, airway narrowing is usually very severe. Since most patients with acute severe asthma were previously relatively well, and because there is often little time for adjustments to the severe physiological insult, abnormal blood gases have much more serious implications than in the typical patient with respiratory failure due to an exacerbation of COPD. The abnormalities of distribution of ventilation and perfusion in acute severe asthma are essentially an exaggeration of those seen in milder chronic asthma,[87] with distribution of

perfusion typically bimodal and an appreciable proportion supplying lung units with low $\dot{V}_A/\dot{Q}$ ratios, but little or no 'anatomical' shunt.[88]

During recovery, improvement in $\dot{V}_A/\dot{Q}$ matching tends to lag behind improvement in mechanical function and continues after FEV_1 has returned to normal values,[89] a feature that is recognizable in clinical practice by delayed correction of PaO_2 and $AaPO_2$.

There are general relationships between the severity of asthma (as assessed by FEV_1) and abnormality of blood gases (Figs 11.9 and 11.10). The classic study of McFadden and Lyons,[80] together with general experience, suggests that PaO_2 less than 60 mmHg (8 kpa) and/or any rise in $PaCO_2$ are ominous signs in acute asthma. Since $PaCO_2$ is usually less than normal in this situation, even a normal value may be serious, as it can herald rapid deterioration. In one large series of severe acute asthma,[90] a raised $PaCO_2$ was present initially in as many as 61 of 229 episodes. In the majority, hypercapnia responded rapidly to emergency treatment so that assisted ventilation was required in only five of the episodes.

The most common acid–base disturbance is respiratory alkalosis, but this is superseded by respiratory acidosis if $PaCO_2$ rises. A complicating metabolic acidosis is quite common in more severe asthma. A combined metabolic and respiratory acidosis was seen in half the hypercapnic patients in the

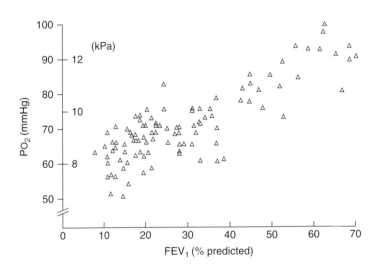

Figure 11.9 Relationship of PaO_2 (breathing air) to forced expiratory volume in 1 s (FEV_1) in patients with asthma of varying severity. Hypoxaemia is relatively mild unless asthma is severe; a PaO_2 of 60 mmHg or less indicates a very severe attack. Redrawn with permission from: McFadden ER, Lyons HA. Arterial blood gas tension in asthma. *N Engl J Med* 1968; **278**: 1027–32. Copyright © 1968 Massachusetts Medical Society. All rights reserved.

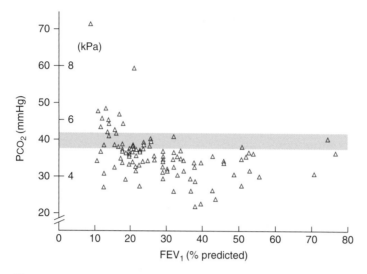

Figure 11.10 Relationship of P_{aCO_2} to forced expiratory volume in 1 s (FEV_1) in patients with asthma of varying severity. In mild or moderate asthma the P_{aCO_2} is usually low. A high (and often also a normal) value indicates a very severe attack. The shaded area shows the normal range. Redrawn with permission from: McFadden ER, Lyons HA. Arterial blood gas tension in asthma. *N Engl J Med* 1968; **278**: 1027–32. Copyright © 1968 Massachusetts Medical Society. All rights reserved.

previously mentioned series of 229 episodes.[91] This picture was associated with particularly severe hypoxaemia and an increased anion gap (presumably due to accumulation of lactate resulting from anaerobic metabolism).

11.6 CARBON MONOXIDE DIFFUSING CAPACITY

The older literature using steady-state methods of measuring D_LCO often reported low values in asthma, with improvement as airway obstruction resolved. These findings are explicable in terms of improving $\dot{V}_A/\dot{Q}$ matching with treatment. These techniques are, however, now virtually obsolete and the standard single-breath method for measurement of D_LCO and KCO more consistently shows normal or increased values in asthma.[92,93] Indeed, in clinical practice, patients with asthma represent one of the two most common groups with supranormal values (the other being obesity).[94] In part, the raised KCO reflects uptake of CO in the better-ventilated alveoli, which tend also to be the better perfused because of locoregional compensatory mechanisms. This does not, however, explain an increase in total D_LCO, which is probably due mainly to relatively better

perfusion of the upper zones of the lungs in asthma compared with normal subjects. This in turn may result from either a mild increase in pulmonary arterial pressure or a more negative pleural pressure generated during inspiration as a consequence of the airway narrowing (or both).[92] The former hypothesis is supported by the finding that D_LCO in normal subjects increases at altitude, presumably due to the increase in pulmonary arterial pressure; the latter hypothesis is supported by the demonstration of increases in D_LCO in healthy subjects breathing via an artificial resistance.[95]

Whatever the mechanism, the normality or supranormality of D_LCO and KCO offers a very useful distinguishing feature in patients with chronic airway obstruction due to asthma from the pattern in COPD and emphysema, where both values are usually markedly reduced. Conversely, if a patient with 'COPD' is found to have normal values, the possibility of asthma should be seriously considered.

11.7 VENTILATORY CONTROL

The ventilatory response to carbon dioxide (CO_2) is usually impaired in patients with moderate or severe airway obstruction and increases as asthma improves.[96] Mouth occlusion pressure responses, however, are more often normal or, when airway narrowing is marked, increased.[97] In a classic study, Rebuck and Read showed that patients who developed hypercapnia during an acute attack failed to show the anticipated increase in ventilatory response to CO_2 in remission.[96] Similar findings have been reported with both the ventilatory and the airway occlusion pressure responses to hypoxia in patients with near-fatal asthma.[98] It is also noteworthy that patients who develop hypercapnia during a severe attack are likely to develop it again in a subsequent episode.[90] It therefore appears that constitutional sensitivity to CO_2 and/or hypoxia may be important factors in the development of life-threatening asthma, and innate sensitivity to CO_2 may influence whether or not hypercapnia is likely in an acute attack.

Since in most patients with asthma ventilatory control is normal, it is often assumed that uncontrolled oxygen therapy in an acute attack is safe. In very severe asthma, however, hypercapnia may develop or worsen with uncontrolled oxygen.[99] Consequently, in any situation where CO_2 retention is established or incipient, caution with the administration of oxygen is advisable. In general, 35 per cent oxygen via a Venturi mask represents a reasonable compromise in acute asthma, as it is both safe and adequate.[100]

11.8 RESPIRATORY FUNCTION DURING SLEEP

Patients with asthma characteristically show exaggerated circadian variation in lung function with nadir values in the early morning. In many this is associated with nocturnal or early morning symptoms, and nocturnal asthma is sometimes defined by a large decrease in FEV_1 or peak flow, e.g. more than 15 per cent between bedtime and awakening. This pattern is an exaggeration of the normal diurnal variation in airway function, with sleep itself also playing a role. Airway resistance tends to be higher in stages 3 and 4 of non-REM sleep (slow-wave sleep).[101] Patients with nocturnal asthma also show greater bronchial hyperresponsiveness at 4.00 a.m. than when awake.[102] In healthy subjects, FRC decreases in sleep compared with wakefulness and, despite having hyperinflation when awake, patients with asthma tend to show a greater reduction in FRC, such that its value during sleep is similar to normal.[103]

Hyperinflation in awake patients is regarded as an adaptive mechanism that assists in maintaining airway patency, and the apparent absence of this mechanism during sleep suggests that the mechanical interaction between the airways and lung parenchyma is altered in sleep. Irvin et al. have shown how this potentially important change in the interaction of airways and parenchyma during sleep may result from inflammatory changes in the small airways.[104] They studied patients with nocturnal asthma by plethysmography while asleep and awake. When the patients were awake, increasing lung volume by applying negative pressure around the chest had the expected effect of reducing resistance, but restoring FRC during sleep to pre-sleep values had no such effect. Detailed bronchoscopic and biopsy studies have shown a parallel increase in inflammatory activity in the early hours of the morning.[105] This may account for the findings by 'uncoupling' the lung parenchymal support to the small airways.

11.9 RESPIRATORY FUNCTION DURING EXERCISE

11.9.1 Changes during exercise

Most interest in exercise function in patients with asthma has focused on exercise-induced asthma (EIA), a phenomenon that usually develops a few minutes after a short burst of exercise. Performance during a progressive exercise study, at least in patients with little or no airway obstruction, is usually relatively normal, with $\dot{V}O_2$max related more closely to the level of habitual activity than to either the FEV_1 or bronchial responsiveness.[106] In patients with more marked airway obstruction, similar mechanical constraints on exercise performance operate as in COPD. Depending on the severity of the airway narrowing and the intensity of the exercise, varying degrees of expiratory flow limitation and consequent dynamic hyperinflation (see Chapter 9, Section 9.11.2) may occur,[107] although this tends to be more labile in asthma than COPD, due to variation in bronchial motor tone.[108] Bronchodilatation during exercise is a characteristic feature of many patients with asthma that may protect against excessive flow limitation.[109] Bronchodilatation is seen, for example, even in patients with a spontaneous exacerbation or with bronchoconstriction following allergen challenge[109]

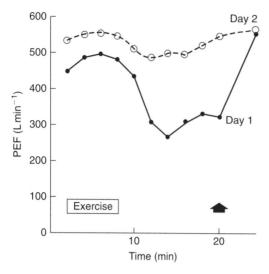

Figure 11.11 Characteristic pattern of exercise-induced asthma. Peak expiratory flow (PEF) is plotted against time during and after 6 min running on a treadmill. On day 1, no premedication has been given; PEF shows a slight increase during exercise, followed by a marked fall within 5 min of the end of exercise. At 20 min a bronchodilator aerosol has been administered. On day 2, the bronchodilator has been given before exercise and this virtually abolishes the exercise-induced fall in PEF.

or following the bronchoconstriction associated with a previous bout of exercise.[110]

During moderate intensity exercise, PaO_2 is usually well maintained or may increase.[111] However, during high-intensity exhausting exercise, a reduction in oxygenation may be seen; this is more evident in terms of decrease in SaO_2 than PaO_2, although some subjects also show a reduction in the latter.[107]. Where a reduction in PaO_2 occurs, this is associated with an increased $AaPO_2$. The reduction in SaO_2 is due additionally to a pH-related shift of the oxygen dissociation curve that accompanies the metabolic acidosis of heavy exercise and results in a lower SaO_2 for a given PaO_2.[107]

11.9.2 Exercise-induced asthma

Exercise-induced asthma typically develops gradually after about 10 min of fairly strenuous exercise and is best demonstrated by discontinuing exercise after 6–8 min and following PEF or FEV_1 (Fig. 11.11). The severity of airway obstruction usually reaches a maximum 15–20 min after the start of exercise and then recovers gradually. Exercise-induced

asthma is most easily demonstrated in younger subjects, probably mainly because of their greater fitness and capacity to exercise, since a $\dot{V}O_2$ of about 75 per cent of the normal maximum sustained for a few minutes is necessary. It is well recognized that certain types of exercise, such as running outdoors, are particularly likely to provoke asthma, whereas swimming is rarely a problem.[112]

The mechanism of EIA has been the subject of many studies, with emphasis in recent years on cooling and drying of the airway mucosa as the inspired air is warmed and humidified.[113] There is still debate over whether changes in temperature or hydration of the airway are more important.[114] The thermal hypothesis of EIA relates not only to cooling of the airway but also to the rapid rewarming after exercise associated with reactive hyperaemia of the bronchial microvasculature and oedema of the airway wall. The osmotic hypothesis proposes that evaporation of water during exercise from the airway initiates events leading to contraction of bronchial smooth muscle via release of mediators from various airway cells; the effect of smooth muscle contraction may be amplified by airway oedema.[114] The finding that inspiring hot dry air can result in severe EIA favours the osmotic rather than thermal mechanism.[115] This hypothesis also fits with the clinical observation that exercise in a humid atmosphere such as a swimming pool is less likely to provoke asthma than when dry air is breathed. A mechanism involving release of bronchoconstrictor mediators is favoured by the inhibitory effects of mediator antagonists as well as bronchodilators; the inhibitory effects of vasodilators such as nitrates and calcium channel antagonists may also be explained on the basis of improved water delivery to the airway mucosa.[114]

Following development of, and recovery from, EIA, a 'refractory period' is seen in many subjects for about 2 h; during this time the bronchoconstrictor response to a further exercise test is attenuated or abolished. EIA can develop during prolonged exercise,[116] but with subsequent recovery so that many asthmatic subjects recognize their ability to 'run through' attacks in this way. Alternatively, they can avoid EIA by a warm-up period of exercise, which can reduce refractoriness without causing serious bronchoconstriction.[117] Refractoriness appears not to be dependent on the smooth muscle itself, as subjects remain responsive to histamine while refractory to exercise. Cross-refractoriness between exercise and osmotic or hyperventilation-induced asthma suggests that mediator-related mechanisms may be common to all three types of stimuli.[118]

The development of EIA is accompanied by the expected deterioration of pulmonary gas exchange with increased $\dot{V}_A/\dot{Q}$ mismatching, resulting in a widened $AaPO_2$ and arterial hypoxaemia,[119] findings similar to those after challenge with methacholine or allergen. A surprising finding in a detailed study of EIA following high-intensity exercise, was that gas exchange was impaired post-exercise, not only in those subjects who showed frank bronchoconstriction (i.e. reduction in FEV_1), but also in those who did not. In the latter group, however, the gas exchange disturbance took longer to develop. The authors postulated that it resulted from smooth muscle contraction and inflammatory narrowing of the peripheral airways; although the effects were not detected using FEV_1, there was a sustained reduction in the vital capacity consistent with closure of small airways.[120]

In the laboratory, EIA is conveniently demonstrated using either a cycle ergometer or a treadmill; a rapid incremental work rate protocol or high-intensity constant work rate are equally useful.[121] An important practical issue related to EIA relates to professional athletes: regulations such as those of the International Olympic Committee approve the use of inhaled β-agonists only in individuals with objective evidence of asthma or 'exercise-induced bronchoconstriction'. In this population, the relation between suggestive symptoms and a positive exercise challenge is relatively weak, and exercise protocols may not be sufficiently sensitive to identify abnormalities in all affected athletes. Use of eucapnic voluntary hyperventilation is recommended as an alternative challenge method. This involves hyperventilating dry air containing 5 per cent CO_2 at room temperature for 6 min at a target ventilation of 30 times the subject's FEV_1. A reduction in FEV_1 of 10 per cent or more of the pre-test value is considered positive.[122] This appears to be more sensitive for detecting BHR in athletes than exercise protocols and is easier to standardize.[123] It has been suggested that BHR occurring in some elite athletes may reflect not asthma but, rather, injury to the airways as a consequence of the very high ventilation achieved during exercise.[124]

11.10 ALLERGIC BRONCHOPULMONARY ASPERGILLOSIS

Allergic bronchopulmonary aspergillosis is virtually confined to asthmatic individuals, and the functional pattern is essentially that of asthma, although with generally less reversible airway obstruction than is seen in uncomplicated asthma. Features associated with the condition include episodes of pulmonary collapse with consolidation leading to permanent scarring and bronchiectasis. Not surprisingly, therefore, patients with aspergillosis compared with other asthmatic individuals tend to show less acute reversibility to bronchodilator and a slightly lower D_LCO.[125]

11.11 BYSSINOSIS

Byssinosis is considered here since in its acute form it resembles occupational asthma. The characteristic symptom is chest tightness, which is accompanied by measurable falls in FEV_1 over the working day, typically maximal on the first day of the week. Most affected individuals show BHR to non-specific challenge, e.g. with histamine.[126] Long-term effects are related to smoking as well as to cotton dust,[127,128] but those patients showing larger across-shift changes in FEV_1 also show a more rapid annual decline.[129] The D_LCO and KCO are usually well preserved at least in non-smokers, implying that significant emphysema is not a feature.[130]

REFERENCES

1 Colebatch HJH, Greaves IA, Ng CKY. Pulmonary mechanics in diagnosis, in *Mechanisms of Airways Obstruction in Human Respiratory Diseases* (eds deKock MA, Nadel JA and Lewis CM), Balkena, Cape Town, 1979, pp. 25–47.
2 Gelb AF, Licuanan J, Shinar CM, Zamel N. Unsuspected loss of lung elastic recoil in chronic persistent asthma. *Chest* 2002; **121**: 715–21.
3 Rodarte JR, Noredin G, Miller C, Brusasco V, Pellegrino R. Lung elastic recoil during breathing at increased lung volume. *J Appl Physiol* 1999; **87**: 1491–5.

4 Brown RH, Pearse DB, Pyrgos G, *et al*. The structural basis of airways hyperresponsiveness in asthma. *J Appl Physiol* 2006; **101**: 30–39.

5 Merkus PJFM, van Essen-Zandvliet EEM, Kouwenberg KM, *et al*. Large lungs after childhood asthma. *Am Rev Respir Dis* 1993; **148**: 1484–9.

6 Blackie SP, Al-Majed S, Staples CA, Hilliam C, Paré PD. Changes in total lung capacity during acute spontaneous asthma. *Am Rev Respir Dis* 1990; **142**: 79–83.

7 Lougheed MD, Lam M, Forkert L, Webb KA, O'Donnell DE. Breathlessness during acute bronchoconstriction in asthma: pathophysiologic mechanisms. *Am Rev Respir Dis* 1993; **148**: 1452–9.

8 Pellegrino R, Brusasco V. On the causes of lung hyperinflation during bronchoconstriction. *Eur Respir J* 1997; **10**: 468–75.

9 Decramer M, Lacquet LM, Fagard R, Rogiers P. Corticosteroids contribute to muscle weakness in chronic airflow obstruction. *Am J Respir Crit Care Med* 1994; **150**: 11–16.

10 Gallagher CG. Respiratory steroid myopathy. *Am J Respir Crit Care Med* 1994; **150**: 4–6.

11 Weiner P, Suo J, Fernandez E, Cherniack RM. The effect of hyperinflation on respiratory muscle strength and efficacy in healthy subjects and patients with asthma. *Am Rev Respir Dis* 1990; **141**: 1501–5.

12 Lavietes MH, Grocela JA, Maniatis P, *et al*. Inspiratory muscle strength in asthma. *Chest* 1988; **93**: 1043–8.

13 Carroll N, Elliot J, Morton A, James A. The structure of large and small airways in nonfatal and fatal asthma. *Am Rev Respir Dis* 1993; **147**: 405–10.

14 Kuwano K, Bosken CH, Pare PD, *et al*. Small airways dimensions in asthma and in chronic obstructive pulmonary disease. *Am Rev Respir Dis* 1993; **148**: 1220–25.

15 Sciurba FC. Physiologic similarities and differences between COPD and asthma. *Chest* 2004; **126**: 117–24S.

16 McParland BE, Macklem PT, Paré PD. Airway wall remodelling: friend or foe? *J Appl Physiol* 2003; **95**: 426–34.

17 Brown NJ, Salome CM, Berend N, Thorpe CW, King GG. Airway distensibility in adults with asthma and healthy adults, measured by forced oscillation technique. *Am J Respir Crit Care Med* 2007; **176**: 129–37.

18 Wagner EM, Liu MC, Weinmann GG, Pernutt S, Bleecker ER. Peripheral lung resistance in normal and asthmatic subjects. *Am Rev Respir Dis* 1990; **141**: 584–8.

19 Mellisant CF, Van Noord JA, van de Woestijne KP, Demedts M. Comparison of dynamic lung function indices during forced and quiet breathing in upper airway obstruction, asthma and emphysema. *Chest* 1990; **98**: 77–83.

20 Martin RJ, Cicutto LC, Ballard RD. Factors related to the nocturnal worsening of asthma. *Am Rev Respir Dis* 1990; **141**: 33–8.

21 Kang H, Koh YY, Yoo Y, *et al*. Maximal airway response to methacholine in cough-variant asthma: comparison with classic asthma and its relationship to peak expiratory flow variability. *Chest* 2005; **128**: 3881–7.

22 Kosmas EN, Milic-Emili J, Polychronaki A, *et al*. Exercise-induced flow limitation, dynamic hyperinflation and exercise capacity in patients with bronchial asthma. *Eur Respir J* 2004; **24**: 378–84.

23 Tantucci E, Ellafi M, Duguet A, *et al*. Dynamic hyperinflation and flow limitation during methacholine-induced bronchoconstriction in asthma. *Eur Respir J* 1999; **14**: 295–301.

24 Martin AJ, Landau LI, Phelan PD. Lung function in young adults who had asthma in childhood. *Am Rev Respir Dis* 1980; **122**: 609–16.

25 Godden DJ, Ross S, Abdalla M, *et al*. Outcome of wheeze in childhood. *Am J Respir Crit Care Med* 1994; **149**: 106–12.

26 Boulet LP, Turcotte H, Brochu A. Persistence of airway obstruction and hyperresponsiveness in subjects with asthma remission. *Chest* 1994; **105**: 1024–31.

27 Lorber DB, Kaltenborn W, Burrows B. Responses to isoproterenol in a general population sample. *Am Rev Respir Dis* 1978; **118**: 855–61.

28 Pare PD, Lawson LM, Brooks LA. Patterns of response to inhaled bronchodilators in asthmatics. *Am Rev Respir Dis* 1983; **127**: 680–85.

29 Gibbons WJ, Sharma A, Lougheed D, Macklem PT. Detection of excessive bronchoconstriction in asthma. *Am J Respir Crit Care Med* 1996; **153**: 582–9.

30 Smith HR, Irvin CG, Cherniack RM. The utility of spirometry in the diagnosis of reversible airways obstruction. *Chest* 1992; **101**: 1577–81.

31 Ingram RH, Wellman JJ, McFadden ER, *et al*. Relative contributions of large and small airways to flow limitation in normal subjects before and after atropine and isoproterenol. *J Clin Invest* 1977; **59**: 696–703.

32 Partridge MR, Saunders KB. Site of action of ipratropium bromide and clinical and physiological determinants of response in patients with asthma. *Thorax* 1981; **36**: 530–33.

33 Tashkin DP, Trevor E, Chopra SK, Taplin GV. Sites of airway dilatation in asthma following inhaled versus subcutaneous terbutaline. *Chest* 1980; **68**: 14–26.

34 Pattermore PK, Asher MI, Harrison AC, *et al*. The interrelationship among bronchial hyperresponsiveness, the diagnosis of asthma and asthma symptoms. *Am Rev Respir Dis* 1990; **142**: 549–54.

35 Brand PLP, Postma DS, Kerstjens HAM, et al. Relation of airway hyperresponsiveness to respiratory symptoms and diurnal peak flow variation in patients with obstructive lung disease. Am Rev Respir Dis 1991; 143: 916–21.

36 Yan K, Salome CM, Woolcock AJ. Prevalence and nature of bronchial hyperresponsiveness in subjects with chronic obstructive pulmonary disease. Am Rev Respir Dis 1985; 132: 25–9.

37 Van Schoor J, Pauwels R, Joos G. Indirect bronchial hyperresponsiveness: the coming of age of a specific group of bronchial challenges. Clin Exp Allergy 2005; 35: 250–61.

38 Orehek J, Gayrard P. Les tests de provocation bronchique non-specifiques dans l'asthme. Bull Eur Physiopathol Respir 1976; 12: 565–98.

39 Woolcock AJ, Salome CM, Yan K. The shape of the dose–response curve to histamine in asthmatics and normal subjects. Am Rev Respir Dis 1984; 130: 71–5.

40 Moore BJ, Hilliam CC, Verburgt LM, et al. Shape and position of the complete dose–response curve for inhaled methacholine in normal subjects. Am J Respir Crit Care Med 1996; 154: 642–8.

41 Nadel JA, Tierney DF. Effect of a previous deep inspiration on airway resistance in man. J Appl Physiol 1961; 16: 717–19.

42 Fish JE, Ankin MG, Kelly JF, Peterman VI. Regulation of bronchomotor tone by lung inflation in asthmatic and non-asthmatic subjects. J Appl Physiol 1981; 50: 1079–86.

43 Lim TK, Pride NB, Ingram RH Jr. Effects of volume history during spontaneous and acutely induced airflow obstruction in asthma. Am Rev Respir Dis 1987; 135: 591–6.

44 Lim TK, Ang SM, Rossing TH, Ingenito EP, Ingram RH Jr. The effects of deep inhalation on maximal expiratory flow during intensive treatment of spontaneous asthmatic episodes. Am Rev Respir Dis 1989; 140: 340–43.

45 Malmberg P, Larsson K, Sundblad BM, Zhiping W. Importance of the time interval between FEV_1 measurements in a methacholine provocation test. Eur Respir J 1993; 6: 680–86.

46 Scichilone N, Permutt S, Togias A. The lack of the bronchoprotective and not the bronchodilatory ability of deep inspiration is associated with airway hyperresponsiveness. Am J Respir Crit Care Med 2001; 163: 413–19.

47 Skloot G, Permutt S, Togias A. Airway hyperresponsiveness in asthma: a problem of limited smooth muscle relaxation with inspiration. J Clin Invest 1995; 96: 2393–403.

48 King GG, Moore BJ, Seow CY, Pare PD. Airway narrowing associated with inhibition of deep inspiration during methacholine inhalation in asthmatics. Am J Respir Crit Care Med 2001; 164: 216–18.

49 Burns GP, Gibson GJ. Airway hyperresponsiveness in asthma. Am J Respir Crit Care Med 1998; 158: 203–6.

50 Brusasco V, Pellegrino R. Complexity of factors modulating airway narrowing in vivo: relevance to assessment of airway hyperresponsiveness. J Appl Physiol 2003; 95: 1305–13.

51 Pellegrino R, Violante B, Brusasco V. Maximal bronchoconstriction in humans: relationship to deep inhalation and airway sensitivity. Am J Respir Crit Care Med 1996; 153: 115–21.

52 Cockcroft DW. Deep inhalation bronchodilation and oral corticosteroids in asthma. Chest 2006; 130: 7–8.

53 Froeb HF, Mead J. Relative hysteresis of the dead space and lung in vivo. J Appl Physiol 1968; 25: 244–8.

54 Wang L, Paré PD. Deep inspiration and airway smooth muscle adaptation to length change. Respir Physiol Neurobiol 2003; 137: 169–78.

55 James AL, Wenzel S. Clinical relevance of airway remodelling in airway diseases. Eur Respir J 2007; 30: 134–55.

56 Fredberg JJ. Frozen objects, small airways, big breaths and asthma. J Allergy Clin Immunol 2000; 106: 615–24.

57 Cox G, Miller JD, McWilliams A, Fitzgerald JM, Lam S. Bronchial thermoplasty for asthma. Am J Respir Crit Care Med 2006; 173: 965–9.

58 Little SA, Sproule MW, Cowan MD, et al. High resolution computed tomographic assessment of airway wall thickness in chronic asthma: reproducibility and relationship with lung function and severity. Thorax 2002; 57: 247–53.

59 Boulet LP, Laviolette M, Turcotte H, et al. Bronchial subepithelial fibrosis correlates with airway responsiveness to methacholine. Chest 1997; 112: 45–52.

60 Macklem PT. A theoretical analysis of the effect of airway smooth muscle load on airway narrowing. Am J Respir Crit Care Med 1996; 153: 83–9.

61 Whyte MKB, Choudry NB, Ind PW. Bronchial hyperresponsiveness in patients recovering from acute severe asthma. Respir Med 1993; 87: 29–35.

62 Pouw EM, Koeter GH, de Monchy JGR, Homan AJ, Sluiter HJ. Clinical assessment after a life-threatening attack of asthma; the role of bronchial hyperreactivity. Eur Respir J 1990; 3: 861–6.

63 Irwin RS, French CT, Smyrnios NA, Curley FJ. Interpretation of positive results of a methacholine inhalation challenge and 1 week of inhaled bronchodilator use in diagnosis and treating cough-variant asthma. Arch Intern Med 1997; 157: 1981–7.

64 Evans TM, Rundell KW, Beck KC, Levine AM, Baumann JM. Airway narrowing measured by spirometry and impulse oscillometry following

room temperature and cold temperature exercise. *Chest* 2005; **128**: 2412–19.

65 Dickinson JW, Whyte GP, McConnell AK, Nevill AM, Harries MG. Mid-expiratory flow versus FEV$_1$ measurements in the diagnosis of exercise induced asthma in elite athletes. *Thorax* 2006; **61**: 111–14.

66 Burge PS. Single and serial measurements of lung function in the diagnosis of occupational asthma. *Eur J Respir Dis* 1982; **63** (suppl. 123): 47.

67 Pepys J, Hutchcroft BJ. Bronchial provocation tests. *Am Rev Respir Dis* 1975; **112**: 829–59.

68 Smith AP. Response of aspirin-allergic patients to challenge by some analgesics in common use. *Br Med J* 1971; **2**: 494–6.

69 Brown PJE, Greville HW, Finucane KE. Asthma and irreversible airflow obstruction. *Thorax* 1984; **39**, 131–6.

70 Rasmussen F, Taylor DR, Flannery EM, *et al.* Risk factors for airway remodelling in asthma manifested by a low postbronchodilator FEV$_1$/vital capacity ratio: a longitudinal population study from childhood to adulthood. *Am J Respir Crit Care Med* 2002; **165**: 1480–88.

71 Boulet LP, Turcotte H, Hudon C, Carrier G, Maltais F. Clinical, physiological and radiological features of asthma with incomplete reversibility of airflow obstruction compared with those of COPD. *Can Respir J* 1998; **5**: 270–77.

72 Fabbri LM, Romagnoli M, Corbetta L, *et al.* Differences in airway inflammation in patients with fixed airflow obstruction due to asthma or chronic obstructive pulmonary disease. *Am J Respir Crit Care Med* 2003; **167**: 418–24.

73 Lange P, Parner J, Vestbo J, Schnohr P, Jensen G. A 15-year follow-up study of ventilatory function in adults with asthma. *N Engl J Med* 1998; **339**: 1194–200.

74 James AL, Palmer LJ, Kicic E, *et al.* Decline in lung function in the Busselton Health Study: the effects of asthma and cigarette smoking. *Am J Respir Crit Care Med* 2005; **171**: 109–14.

75 Ulrik CS. Outcome of asthma: longitudinal changes in lung function. *Eur Respir J* 1999; **13**: 904–18.

76 Anees W, Moore VC, Burge PS. FEV$_1$ decline in occupational asthma. *Thorax* 2006; **61**: 751–5.

77 Jongepier H, Boezen HM, Dijkstra A, *et al.* Polymorphisms of the ADAM33 gene are associated with accelerated lung function decline in asthma. *Clin Exp Allergy* 2004; **34**: 757–60.

78 Lange P, Scharling H, Ulrik CS, Vestbo J. Inhaled corticosteroids and decline of lung function in community residents with asthma. *Thorax* 2006; **61**: 100–104.

79 O'Byrne PM, Pedersen S, Busse WW, *et al.* Effects of early intervention with inhaled budesonide on lung function in newly diagnosed asthma. *Chest* 2006; **129**: 1478–85.

80 McFadden ER, Lyons HA. Arterial blood gas tension in asthma. *N Engl J Med* 1968; **278**: 1027–32.

81 Osborne CA, O'Connor BJ, Lewis A, *et al.* Hyperventilation and asymptomatic chronic asthma. *Thorax* 2000; **55**: 1016–22.

82 Echazarreta AL, Gomez FP, Ribas J, *et al.* Pulmonary gas exchange responses to histamine and methacholine challenges in mild asthma. *Eur Respir J* 2001; **17**: 609–14.

83 Wagner PD, Hedenstierna G, Bylin G. Ventilation–perfusion irregularity in asymptomatic asthma. *Am Rev Respir Dis* 1987; **118**: 511–24.

84 Wagner PD, Dantzker DR, Lacovoni VE, *et al.* Ventilation–perfusion irregularity in asymptomatic asthma. *Am Rev Respir Dis* 1978; **118**: 511–24.

85 Harris RS, Winkler T, Tgavalekos N, *et al.* Regional pulmonary perfusion, inflation, and ventilation defects in bronchoconstricted patients with asthma. *Am J Respir Crit Care Med* 2006; **174**: 245–53.

86 Woolcock AJ, McRae J, Morris JC, Read J. Abnormal pulmonary blood flow distribution in bronchial asthma. *Aust Ann Med* 1966; **15**: 196–203.

87 Rodriguez-Roisin R, Ballester E, Roca J, Torres A, Wagner PD. Mechanisms of hypoxaemia in patients with status asthmaticus requiring mechanical ventilation. *Am Rev Respir Dis* 1989; **139**: 732–9.

88 Roca J, Ramis L, Rodriguez-Roisin R, *et al.* Serial relationships between ventilation–perfusion inequality and spirometry in acute severe asthma requiring hospitalization. *Am Rev Respir Dis* 1988; **137**: 1055–61.

89 Ferrer A, Roca J, Wagner PD, Lopez FA, Rodriguez-Roisin R. Airway obstruction and ventilation–perfusion relationships in acute severe asthma. *Am Rev Respir Dis* 1993; **147**: 579–80.

90 Mountain RD, Sahn SA. Clinical features and outcome in patients with acute asthma presenting with hypercapnia. *Am Rev Respir Dis* 1988; **138**: 535–9.

91 Mountain RD, Heffner JE, Brackett NC, Sahn SA. Acid–base disturbances in acute asthma. *Chest* 1990; **98**: 651–5.

92 Collard P, Njinou B, Nejadnik B, Keyeux A, Frans A. Single breath diffusing capacity for carbon monoxide in stable asthma. *Chest* 1994; **105**: 1426–9.

93 Akesson U, Dahlstrom JA, Wollmer P. Changes in transfer factor of the lung in response to bronchodilatation. *Clin Physiol* 2000; **20**: 14–18.

94 Saydain G, Beck KC, Decker PA, Cowl CT, Scanlon PD. Clinical significance of elevated diffusing capacity. *Chest* 2004; **125**: 446–52.

95 Keens TG, Mansell A, Krastins IRB, *et al.* Evaluation of the single breath diffusion capacity in asthma and cystic fibrosis. *Chest* 1979; **76**: 41–4.

96 Rebuck AS, Read J. Patterns of ventilatory response to carbon dioxide during recovery from severe asthma. *Clin Sci* 1971; **41**: 13–21.

97 Zachon H, Despas PJ, Anthonisen N. Occlusion pressure responses in asthma and chronic obstructive pulmonary disease. *Am Rev Respir Dis* 1976; **114**: 917–27.

98 Kikuchi Y, Okabe S, Tamura G, *et al.* Chemosensitivity and perception of dyspnea in patients with a history of near-fatal asthma. *N Engl J Med* 1994; **330**: 1329–34.

99 Chien JW, Ciufo R, Novak R, *et al.* Uncontrolled oxygen administration and respiratory failure in acute asthma. *Chest* 2000; **117**: 728–33.

100 Ford DJ, Rothwell RPG. 'Safe oxygen' in acute asthma: prospective trial using 35% Ventimask prior to admission. *Respir Med* 1989; **83**: 189–94.

101 Bellia V, Cuttitta G, Insalaco G, Visconti A, Bonsignore G. Relationship of nocturnal bronchoconstriction to sleep stages. *Am Rev Respir Dis* 1989; **140**: 363–7.

102 Martin RJ, Cicutto LC, Ballard RD. Factors related to the nocturnal worsening of asthma. *Am Rev Respir Dis* 1990; **141**: 33–8.

103 Ballard RD, Irvin CG, Martin RJ, *et al.* Influence of sleep on lung volume in asthmatic patients and normal subjects. *J Appl Physiol* 1990; **68**: 2034–41.

104 Irvin CG, Pak J, Martin RJ. Airway–parenchyma uncoupling in nocturnal asthma. *Am J Respir Crit Care Med* 2000; **161**: 50–56.

105 Kraft M, Djukanovic R, Wilson S, Holgate ST, Martin RJ. Alveolar tissue inflammation in asthma. *Am J Respir Crit Care Med* 1996; **154**: 1505–10.

106 Garfinkel SK, Kesten S, Chapman KR, Rebuck AS. Physiologic and nonphysiologic determinants of aerobic fitness in mild to moderate asthma. *Am Rev Respir Dis* 1992; **145**: 741–5.

107 Haverkamp HC, Dempsey JA, Miller JD, *et al.* Gas exchange during exercise in habitually active asthmatic subjects. *J Appl Physiol* 2005; **99**: 1938–50.

108 Johnson BD, Scanlon PD, Beck KC. Regulation of ventilatory capacity during exercise in asthmatics. *J Appl Physiol* 1995; **79**: 892–901.

109 Crimi E, Pellegrino R, Smeraldi A, Brusasco V. Exercise-induced bronchodilation in natural and induced asthma: effects on ventilatory response and performance. *J Appl Physiol* 2002; **92**: 2353–60.

110 Haverkamp HC, Dempsey JA, Miller JD, *et al.* Repeat exercise normalizes the gas-exchange impairment induced by a previous exercise bout in asthmatic subjects. *J Appl Physiol* 2005; **99**: 1843–52.

111 Feisal KA, Fuleihan FJ. Pulmonary gas exchange during exercise in young asthmatic patients. *Thorax* 1979; **34**: 393–6.

112 Anderson SD, Silverman M, König P, Godfrey S. Exercise induced asthma. *Br J Dis Chest* 1975; **69**: 1–39.

113 Strauss RH, McFadden ER, Ingram RH, Deal EC, Jaeger JJ. Influence of heat and humidity on the airway obstruction induced by exercise in asthma. *J Clin Invest* 1978; **61**: 433–40.

114 Anderson SD, Daviskas E. The mechanism of exercise-induced asthma is ... *J Allergy Clin Immunol* 2000; **106**: 453–9.

115 Argyros GJ, Phillips YY, Rayburn DB, Rosenthal RR, Jaeger JJ. Water loss without heat flux in exercise-induced bronchospam. *Am Rev Respir Dis* 1993; **147**: 1419–24.

116 Suman OE, Babcock MA, Pegelow DF, Jarjour NN, Reddan WG. Airway obstruction during exercise in asthma. *Am J Respir Crit Care Med* 1995; **152**: 24–31.

117 Reiff DB, Choudry NB, Pride NB, Ind PW. The effect of prolonged submaximal warm-up exercise on exercise-induced asthma. *Am Rev Respir Dis* 1989; **139**: 479–84.

118 Godfrey S, Bar-Yishay E. Exercise-induced asthma revisited. *Respir Med* 1993; **87**: 331–44.

119 Young IH, Corte P, Schoeffel RE. Pattern and time course of ventilation–perfusion inequality in exercise-induced asthma. *Am Rev Respir Dis* 1982; **125**: 304–11.

120 Haverkamp HC, Dempsey JA, Miller JD, *et al.* Repeat exercise normalizes the gas-exchange impairment induced by a previous exercise bout in asthmatic subjects. *J Appl Physiol* 2005; **99**: 1843–52.

121 De Fuccio MB, Nery LE, Malagui C, *et al.* Clinical role of rapid-incremental tests in the evaluation of exercise-induced bronchoconstriction. *Chest* 2005; **128**: 2435–42.

122 Anderson SD, Argyros GJ, Magnussen H, Holzer K. Provocation by eucapnic voluntary hyperpnoea to identify exercise induced bronchoconstriction. *Br J Sports Med* 2001; **35**: 344–7.

123 Rundell KW, Anderson SD, Spiering BA, Judelson DA. Field exercise vs. laboratory eucapnic voluntary hyperventilation to identify airway hyperresponsiveness in elite cold weather athletes. *Chest* 2004; **125**: 909–15.

124 Holzer K, Douglass JA. Exercise induced bronchoconstriction in elite athletes: measuring the fall. *Thorax* 2006; **61**: 94–6.

125 Malo JL, Inouye T, Hawkins R, *et al.* Studies in chronic allergic bronchopulmonary aspergillosis. *Thorax* 1977; **32**: 275–80.

126 Fishwick D, Fletcher AC, Pickering CAC, Niven RM, Faragher EB. Lung function, bronchial reactivity,

atopic status and dust exposure in Lancashire cotton mill operatives. *Am Rev Respir Dis* 1992; **145**: 1103–8.

127 Fishwick D, Fletcher AM, Pickering CA, Niven RM, Faragher EB. Lung function in Lancashire cotton and man made fibre spinning mill operatives. *Occup Environ Med* 1996; **53**: 46–50.

128 Su YM, Su JR, Sheu JY, Loh CH, Liou SH. Additive effect of smoking and cotton dust exposure on respiratory symptoms and pulmonary function of cotton textile workers. *Ind Health* 2003; **41**: 109–15.

129 Glindmeyer HW, Lefante JL, Jones RN, Rando RJ, Weill H. Cotton dust and across-shift change in FEV_1 as predictors of annual change in FEV_1. *Am J Respir Crit Care Med* 1994; **149**: 584–90.

130 Honeybourne D, Pickering CAC. Physiological evidence that emphysema is not a feature of byssinosis. *Thorax* 1986; **41**: 6–11.

Central Airway Obstruction and Bronchial Carcinoma

12.1 UPPER AIRWAY OBSTRUCTION

12.1.1 Mechanisms of narrowing of the central airway

Localized narrowing of the central airway is much less common than the various forms of diffuse airway obstruction discussed in Chapters 9–11. The distinction on clinical features alone is not always easy but it has obvious therapeutic implications. This section describes the consequences of narrowing at the level of the pharynx, larynx, extra- and intrathoracic trachea, and right and left main bronchi. The site of the abnormality affects the functional pattern. In particular, whether the obstruction is within or without the thorax determines whether the main effects are on expiratory or inspiratory flow. The pressure surrounding the intrathoracic airway is pleural pressure, whereas around the extrathoracic airway the pressure is close to atmospheric. The precise anatomical site of the demarcation between the two is not clear, and the mobility of the trachea in the longitudinal direction implies a grey area in the region of the thoracic inlet where a varying pattern may be seen.

Narrowing of the airway can be both structural and functional. One example of functional narrowing is the reduced pharyngeal calibre resulting from ineffective action of the pharyngeal dilator muscles during sleep in individuals with obstructive sleep apnoea (see Chapter 16, Section 16.2). Less obvious dynamic effects may also occur either within, or 'downstream' of, a structural narrowing, which will exaggerate the differences between inspiratory and expiratory flows (see below and Fig. 12.1).

12.1.2 Effects of upper airway obstruction on mechanical function

12.1.2.1 Airway resistance

The resistance of the airway (R_{AW}) is dominated by the calibre of the narrowest part of the bronchial tree, which, in normal subjects during quiet breathing, is the central airway. Consequently, measurements of R_{AW} and conductance are particularly sensitive to narrowing of the trachea or larynx. In most patients with tracheal narrowing, airway or total pulmonary resistance is markedly increased.[1–3] Since, however, resistance is measured at low flows, any dynamic effects may be considerably underestimated. If the measurement is made at higher flows, a disproportionate rise may be seen.[1] Consequently, measurement of R_{AW} at rest can underestimate the load imposed with the increased flows on exercise,[4] corresponding to the well-recognized tendency for stridor to become more obvious on exercise or during hyperventilation at rest.

12.1.2.2 Maximum flow–volume curves with extrathoracic airway narrowing

The most characteristic features of 'upper' airway obstruction are seen with narrowing of the

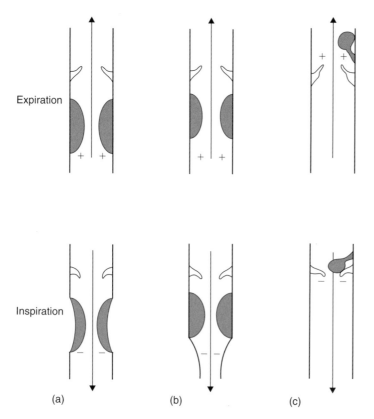

Figure 12.1 Possible mechanisms of inspiratory dynamic narrowing in patients with extrathoracic airway obstruction. Upper diagrams represent forced expiration and lower diagrams forced inspiration (airflow indicated by arrows). In (a) and (b) there is a subglottic stenosis; during expiration the tracheal pressure is above atmospheric (+), but the unusually negative pressure necessary during forceful inspiration may produce additional dynamic narrowing either within the lesion itself (a) or on its downstream (alveolar) side (b). Rarely a supraglottic pedunculated tumour (c) may be sucked into the airstream during inspiration.

extrathoracic airway. These can be closely mimicked in normal subjects by imposing a resistance at the mouth. The resulting pressure, volume and flow relationships are discussed in detail in Chapter 1, Section 1.6.5.6, and the maximum flow–volume curve in the model situation (see Fig. 1.35 in Chapter 1) should be compared with the examples from patients in Figs 12.2 and 12.3. In simple terms, increased resistance of the extrathoracic airway reduces those maximum flows that are most dependent on effort; these are maximum inspiratory flow throughout the VC and maximum expiratory flow ($\dot{V}_E$max) at higher lung volumes. During forceful expiration the additional resistance that needs to be overcome means that less pressure than normal is dissipated in dynamic

compression of the intrathoracic airways. Because of the shape of the isovolume pressure–flow curves at different lung volumes (see Fig. 1.35 in Chapter 1), this results in reduced $\dot{V}_E$max only at higher lung volumes, with the later part of the maximum expiratory flow–volume (MEFV) curve retaining a normal contour. The characteristic appearance of maximum flow–volume curves with extrathoracic airway obstruction thus, in effect, resembles that produced by an overall reduction in the driving pressure. The appearances may therefore be similar to those seen with respiratory muscle weakness (see Chapter 20, Section 20.2.1.3), but the distinction is usually clear in the clinical context, or it can be made by checking maximum static respiratory pressures or R_{AW}.

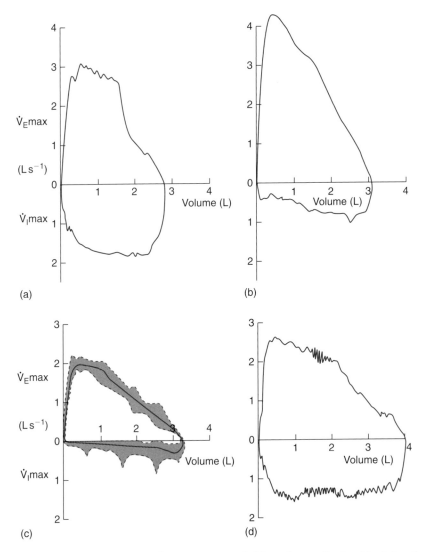

Figure 12.2 Maximum flow–volume curves recorded from three patients with obstruction of the extrathoracic airway. (a) External compression of the trachea by a large neurofibroma; the peak on the expiratory curve is blunted and maximum inspiratory flows are reduced throughout the vital capacity. Forced expiratory volume in 1s (FEV_1) = 2.4 L, forced inspiratory volume in 1s (FIV_1) = 1.2 L, $\dot{V}_E max_{50}/\dot{V}_I max_{50}$ = 1.8. (b) A patient with bilateral vocal cord paralysis associated with Shy–Drager syndrome; the expiratory curve is normal but there is a gross reduction of maximum inspiratory flow indicating a predominantly dynamic effect, probably within the hypotonic larynx. $\dot{V}_E max_{50}/\dot{V}_I max_{50}$ = 4.5. (c) Reductions in both expiratory and inspiratory flows with very marked oscillations (amplitude indicated by broken lines); the oscillations and discrepancy between expiration and inspiration again suggest a marked dynamic effect. This patient had a large carcinoma of the epiglottis which presumably had a ball-valve-like effect during inspiration (cf. Fig. 12.1c). FEV_1 = 2.5 L, FIV_1 = 0.45 L, $\dot{V}_E max_{50}/\dot{V}_I max_{50}$ = 10. (d) The same patient as in (c) after a course of radiotherapy. Flows are generally improved and the mid-vital capacity (VC) ratio is more normal, but increased oscillations and the typical pattern of extrathoracic airway obstruction remain. FEV_1 = 2.5 L, FIV_1 = 1.75 L, $\dot{V}_E max_{50}/\dot{V}_I max_{50}$ = 1.3.

$\dot{V}_E max_{50}$, maximum expiratory flow at 50 per cent vital capacity; $\dot{V}_I max_{50}$, maximum inspiratory flow at 50 per cent vital capacity.

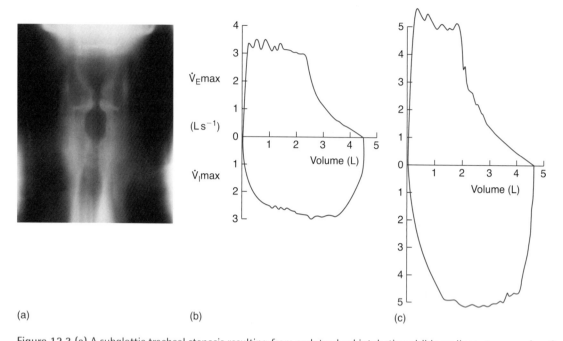

(a)   (b)   (c)

Figure 12.3 (a) A subglottic tracheal stenosis resulting from endotracheal intubation visible on linear tomography of the trachea. (b,c) The patient's maximum flow–volume curves before and after dilatation. The peak expiratory flow (PEF) remains blunted after dilatation, indicating that some narrowing remains; the curvature of the maximum expiratory flow–volume (MEFV) curve at lower volumes also suggests mild diffuse intrathoracic airway narrowing (the patient had been a smoker). Corresponding changes in spirometry and mid-vital capacity (VC) flow ratio were $FEV_1 = 2.75 \rightarrow 4.21$, $\dot{V}_E max_{50}/\dot{V}_I max_{50} 1.07 \rightarrow 0.54$. (Note the relative insensitivity of FEV_1 in this situation.)

FEV_1, forced expiratory volume in 1s; $\dot{V}_E max_{50}$, maximum expiratory flow at 50 per cent vital capacity; $\dot{V}_I max_{50}$, maximum inspiratory flow at 50 per cent vital capacity.

Similar flow–volume curves could in theory result simply from inadequate effort due to poor cooperation, but here the hallmark is lack of consistency on repeat measurements.

In some cases there is an unusually large discrepancy between the effects on maximum expiratory and inspiratory flow–volume curves, with a dramatic reduction of $\dot{V}_I max$, even sometimes with completely normal $\dot{V}_E max$ at all lung volumes (e.g. Fig. 12.2b). Such a pattern implies a pronounced dynamic effect with additional narrowing during forced inspiration. This can occasionally be seen with a pedunculated tumour in the larynx acting like a 'ball valve' and being sucked into the airstream on inspiration (Figs 12.1c and 12.2c). More commonly, dynamic changes occur within the structurally narrowed area itself,[5] if this is not completely rigid (Fig. 12.1a). When gas molecules pass from a wider to a narrower tube, their linear velocity has to be increased and the accelerating force is accompanied by a fall in pressure along the walls of the narrowed segment, encouraging further dynamic narrowing (a phenomenon known as the Bernouilli effect). A third possible dynamic mechanism of narrowing relates to the airway 'downstream' from the obstruction, i.e. on the alveolar side of the narrowed airway during inspiration (Fig. 12.1b), where additional narrowing might occur due to the unusually negative intraluminal pressures necessary to overcome the structural narrowing upstream. The normal adult trachea, however, is sufficiently well stabilized for this not to be a major factor, but it is more likely if there is any tracheal damage,[6] e.g. tracheomalacia. It also occurs more commonly in the more compliant (less rigid) trachea of infants, in whom the clinical counterpart is croup, a common manifestation of upper airway obstruction in young children.

General inspection of the contour of the flow–volume curves is often the best guide to the presence of obstruction of the extrathoracic airway. Marked oscillations of flow are sometimes evident if large dynamic effects occur. As a quantitative index, the mid-VC flow ratio ($\dot{V}_E max_{50}/\dot{V}_I max_{50}$) is more precise. This is close to unity in normal subjects and is considerably reduced with diffuse intrathoracic airflow obstruction. With extrathoracic lesions the ratio may be similar to normal if the narrowing is very severe and 'fixed', i.e. if dynamic factors are not important; more typically it exceeds 1 because of disproportionate reduction of inspiratory flow.[5]

12.1.2.3 Effects of breathing helium–oxygen mixture

Comparison of flow–volume curves breathing air and a helium–oxygen mixture (heliox) is sometimes helpful in the recognition of upper airway obstruction. The low-density heliox normally reduces resistance and increases flow in the central airways, where it is turbulent and therefore more dependent on gas density. An unusually large effect of helium might therefore be expected in patients with central airway narrowing, but, in practice, proportional increases in $\dot{V}_E max$ with helium are similar to normal. Occasionally, when obstruction is very severe, the increase in $\dot{V}_E max$ may actually be less than normal.[7] This paradoxical finding may simply reflect less turbulence of flow when it is severely limited.

12.1.2.4 Detection of upper airway narrowing in patients with coexisting chronic obstructive pulmonary disease

A particular problem arises with the recognition of additional upper airway obstruction in patients with diffuse intrathoracic airflow obstruction such as chronic obstructive pulmonary disease (COPD). In this situation greater dynamic compression inside the chest makes $\dot{V}_E max$ less dependent on effort than normal. Consequently, upper airway obstruction is less easy to recognize on flow–volume curves.[8] In effect, narrowing of the extrathoracic airway is often self-imposed by patients with COPD by breathing through pursed lips.

12.1.2.5 Central intrathoracic airway narrowing

With narrowing of the lower, intrathoracic trachea, the characteristic flow–volume curves are rather different (Figs 12.4 and 12.5). The appearances resemble those of extrathoracic narrowing to the extent that expiratory flows at high lung volumes are markedly reduced, but they share with the more common causes of intrathoracic obstruction (e.g. COPD, asthma) a proportionally greater reduction in expiratory than inspiratory flow such that the mid-VC ratio ($\dot{V}_E max_{50}/\dot{V}_I max_{50}$) is low. The MEFV curve may show a small early peak, due to emptying of the upper airway proximal to the narrowing, followed characteristically by a plateau or near-plateau of flow over a large part of the VC.

12.1.2.6 Effects of central airway narrowing on other tests of respiratory mechanics

The foregoing analysis of the mechanisms involved should help understanding of the abnormalities of simple tests in subjects with upper airway obstruction. Any of the following clues should alert the observer to the possibility of obstruction of the central airway:

• Disproportionate impairment of forced inspiratory measurements: the forced inspiratory volume in 1s (FIV_1) can be measured easily with a spirometer and is characteristically less than the forced expiratory volume in 1s (FEV_1) with extrathoracic obstruction;[10] in healthy subjects or the 'usual' types of airflow obstruction, FIV_1 exceeds FEV_1.
• An unexpectedly high R_{AW} (especially with a relatively normal FEV_1).
• An unusually low peak expiratory flow (PEF) in comparison with the FEV_1.[11] Since the FEV_1 effectively integrates maximum expiratory flows over both effort-dependent and effort-'independent' portions of the MEFV curve, it is relatively insensitive to narrowing of the central airway. Peak expiratory flow, which is completely effort-dependent, is reduced to a much greater extent.

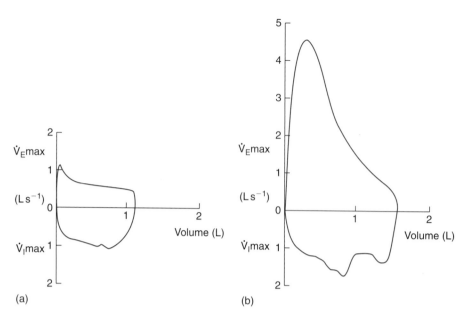

Figure 12.4 Maximum flow–volume curves of a patient with a carcinoma of the lower trachea before (a) and after (b) radiotherapy. The initial flow–volume curve (a) suggests narrowing of the intrathoracic trachea: $FEV_1 = 0.751$, $FIV_1 = 1.11$, $\dot{V}_Emax_{50}/\dot{V}_Imax_{50} = 0.56$. The improvement after treatment (b) is evident; the relatively poor inspiratory flows were unexplained.

FEV_1, forced expiratory volume in 1s; FIV_1, forced inspiratory volume in 1s; $\dot{V}_Emax_{50}$, maximum expiratory flow at 50 per cent vital capacity; V_Imax_{50}, maximum inspiratory flow at 50 per cent vital capacity.

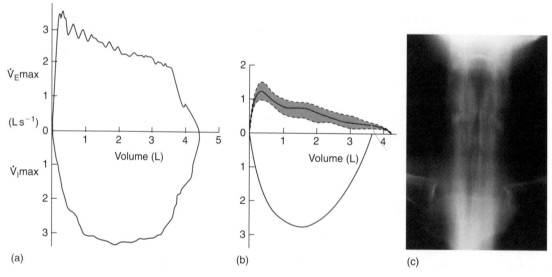

Figure 12.5 Two unusual causes of central intrathoracic airway obstruction. (a) Flow–volume curves of a patient with tracheal compression from maga-oesophagus. $\dot{V}_Emax_{50}/\dot{V}_Imax_{50} = 0.69$. (b) Curves of a patient with relapsing polychondritis affecting the major airways. $FEV_1 = 0.8$ L, $FIV_1 = 1.5$ L, $\dot{V}_Emax_{50}/\dot{V}_Imax_{50} = 0.21$. Marked oscillations of expiratory flow were evident, indicating a pronounced dynamic effect. Tomography of the trachea (c) showed extensive narrowing of both the extrathoracic airway (including the larynx) and intrathoracic trachea, but the flow–volume curves indicated that central intrathoracic airway narrowing was the dominant functional abnormality. (b) and (c) reproduced from: Gibson GJ, Davis P. Respiratory complications of relapsing polychondritis. *Thorax* 1974; **29**: 726–31, with permission from the BMJ Publishing Group.

FEV_1, forced expiratory volume in 1s; FIV_1, forced inspiratory volume in 1s; $\dot{V}_Emax_{50}$, maximum expiratory flow at 50 per cent vital capacity; V_Imax_{50}, maximum inspiratory flow at 50 per cent vital capacity.

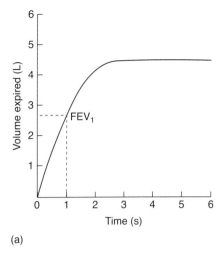
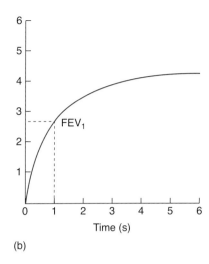

(a)   (b)

Figure 12.6 (a) The 'straight' spirogram of central airway obstruction recorded from the patient whose flow–volume curve is illustrated in Fig. 12.5a. Note that lung emptying is complete in 3 s (normal). (b) Spirogram of a patient with a similar forced expiratory volume in 1 s (FEV$_1$) to (a), but with the curvature seen with the 'usual' airflow obstruction associated with asthma or chronic obstructive pulmonary disease (COPD). Note that lung emptying is still continuing at 6 s.

• The 'straight' forced expiratory spirogram (Fig. 12.6):[1] since with upper airway narrowing the MEFV curve typically shows a near-plateau of $\dot{V}_E$max in the early part of expiration (Figs 12.2–12.5), the ratio of expired volume to time (i.e. flow) is virtually constant over this period so that the spirogram (volume versus time) shows a straight line, in contrast to the usual curvature. This appearance of the spirogram is, however, closely mimicked in some patients with severe chronic diffuse airflow obstruction, where it corresponds to a flow–volume curve with an initial sharp peak (which contributes little to expired volume), followed by a very slow expiration with low and only very slowly diminishing flow rates.

Note that the latter three points above do not necessarily aid the distinction between extrathoracic and intrathoracic location of the offending lesion – for this, comparison of expiratory and inspiratory measurements is more relevant. Of simple tests, PEF is the most sensitive to central airway narrowing, but until the airway diameter is reduced to less than 10 mm, any abnormality is difficult to detect. With further narrowing, the relation between diameter and flow is very steep,[2,12] so that only minor decreases in airway calibre can produce rapid functional and clinical deterioration.

The VC of patients with central airway narrowing is usually well preserved until the obstruction becomes so severe that the patient can no longer sustain the effort necessary to complete a full expiration. The TLC is also usually normal, but a large difference between helium dilution and plethysmographic estimates may be seen, particularly when upper airway resistance is markedly increased. A discrepancy between the two estimates of TLC can result from artefactual overestimation of plethysmographic volumes in the presence of a markedly increased R$_{AW}$ (see Chapter 1, Section 1.3.3).[13]

12.1.3 Effects on gas exchange and exercise

Maldistribution of ventilation has been reported in some patients but is most likely related to coexistent generalized airway disease,[5] as occasional patients are seen with severe and extensive central airway narrowing and normal results of tests of 'small airway' function, such as the slope of phase III of the single-breath nitrogen test.[9,14]

Severe obstruction of the upper airway is an important, if infrequent, cause of hypercapnia, which can develop insidiously and may be unrecognized clinically. Unlike patients with typical chronic airflow obstruction, elevation of the Pa$_{CO_2}$, when it occurs, is usually the result of 'pure' hypoventilation, i.e. there is no significant ventilation/perfusion mismatching or widening of the $AaPO_2$ gradient. The usual risks associated with hypercapnia apply, however, and checking the $PaCO_2$ is a wise precaution in any patient with severe obstruction of the upper airway, especially if surgical treatment is contemplated.

Exercise capacity is likely to be limited in the presence of significant obstruction of the upper airway, but few studies have been reported. There is no evidence of deteriorating pulmonary gas exchange,[4] but if hypercapnia is present at rest, it is likely to worsen on exercise due to progressive hypoventilation.[9] Again, the functional consequences can be mimicked by normal subjects breathing through a narrow orifice at the mouth: such studies on exercise show underventilation with a rising $PaCO_2$ and falling PaO_2 but no widening of $AaPO_2$.[4]

12.1.4 Causes of tracheal and laryngeal narrowing

The commoner pathological abnormalities that produce the functional pattern of central airway obstruction include tracheal stenosis and tumours, large goitres and bilateral vocal cord palsy. The evidence on unilateral cord palsy is less certain, but a mild reduction of $\dot{V}_I$max with an increase in the mid-VC ratio has been reported in some patients.[15]

12.2 BRONCHIAL CARCINOMA

12.2.1 Generalized and localized airway obstruction

In most cases conventional lung function tests in patients with bronchial carcinoma reflect the level of general airway function rather than specific effects of the tumour. Since both bronchial carcinoma and COPD are due mainly to cigarette smoking, diffuse airway obstruction is extremely common in patients with lung cancer. For reasons that are unclear, the risk of developing bronchial carcinoma increases with increasing severity in COPD, even after adjusting for age and smoking history.[16]

Occasionally, if the tumour occupies a strategic position, its direct effects may dominate the functional picture. For example, involvement of the

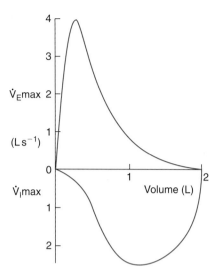

Figure 12.7 Maximum flow–volume curves from a patient with narrowing of the right main bronchus caused by a carcinoma. Delayed emptying and filling of the right lung during forced expiratory and inspiratory manoeuvres lead to disproportionately low flows at end expiration and end inspiration. The appearance on expiration is indistinguishable from the more 'usual' generalized intrathoracic airflow obstruction, but the inspiratory abnormality is more specific and is a useful diagnostic pointer if the appearance is consistent on repeated measurements.

main carina produces the pattern of central intrathoracic airway narrowing, while complete occlusion of a main bronchus can produce severe volume restriction due to collapse of a whole lung. Severe narrowing of the right or left main bronchus can be difficult to detect with routine tests of lung mechanics, because the flow signal at the mouth is 'swamped' by air expired from the unaffected side. It may, however, be detectable on a flow–volume curve as marked slowing at the end of forced inspiration and expiration (Fig. 12.7). This appearance is more readily identifiable at the end of forceful inspiration as the expiratory appearance is not dissimilar to that seen with the diffuse airway obstruction of COPD or asthma. The inspiratory pattern needs to be distinguished, however, from simple inability to maintain maximum effort throughout inspiration. The effect on the forced expiratory spirogram is to produce a rather subtle biphasic appearance due to markedly asynchronous emptying of the two lungs.[17] Once a main

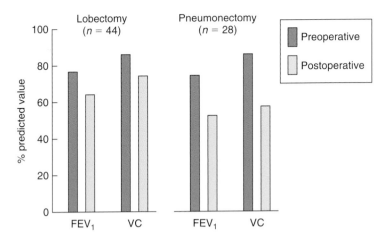

Figure 12.8 Average values of forced expiratory volume in 1s (FEV$_1$) and vital capacity (VC) (each expressed as per cent of predicted value) measured preoperatively and 4 months postoperatively in 44 patients who underwent lobectomy and in 28 patients who underwent pneumonectomy.

bronchus is occluded or virtually occluded, there may simply be an apparent loss of volume with a 'parallel shift' of the MEFV curve.[18]

12.2.2 Effects of lung resection

Thoracotomy alone inevitably produces a temporary reduction in lung volume, even without lung resection. This effect gradually resolves over 2–3 months, and between 3 months and 1 year there is little further change.[19] Average values of FEV$_1$ and VC from a series of patients before and 4 months after either lobectomy or pneumonectomy are shown in Fig. 12.8. As would be anticipated, changes after pneumonectomy are appreciably greater than those after lobectomy. This and other series show mean proportional reductions of VC of approximately 15 per cent and 35 per cent after lobectomy and pneumonectomy respectively. Changes in other static lung volumes (RV, TLC) are proportionately less than those in VC.

The effect of lung resection on carbon monoxide diffusing capacity (D$_L$CO) is more complex, as its value is dependent not only on the volume of gas-containing lung present but also on the volume of blood in the pulmonary capillaries, which in turn is dependent on pulmonary blood flow. After removal of a lung, the vessels of the remaining lung have to accommodate all the cardiac output, which at rest changes little. The rate of CO uptake per unit volume of functioning lung

(i.e. KCO) therefore increases and as a result the overall D$_L$CO changes relatively less than does gaseous lung volume.[20,21] Even after lobectomy this effect is apparent as a small average rise in KCO. Maximum exercise performance, as assessed by symptom-limited V̇O$_2$max also tends to be relatively better preserved than lung volume.[21,22]

12.2.3 Prediction of postoperative respiratory function

An important factor in any decision about surgery for bronchial carcinoma relates to the likely functional outcome – are the patient's reserves of lung function sufficient not only for survival but for a tolerable existence after removal of a lobe or lung? The average values for pre- and postoperative FEV$_1$ and VC illustrated in Fig. 12.8 conceal considerable variation between individuals (Fig. 12.9), mirroring variation in the contribution to preoperative function of the lobe or lung resected. Clearly, the removal of a lung that is completely collapsed due to a tumour obstructing a main bronchus would not be expected to produce much change in respiratory function postoperatively. On the other hand, resection of a lobe or lung containing a small peripheral tumour would probably be associated with considerable loss of function. It is well recognized that the presence of a lung cancer may have more profound effects on the function of the affected lung than might be anticipated

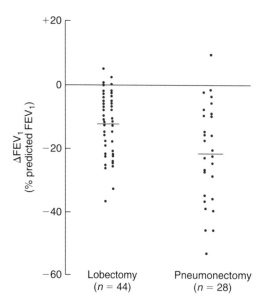

Figure 12.9 Individual values of change in forced expiratory volume in 1s (FEV$_1$) (ΔFEV$_1$, expressed as a percentage of predicted FEV$_1$) in the patients whose group mean values are shown in Fig. 12.8, emphasizing the considerable variation between individuals. Note that with pneumonectomy the values of ΔFEV$_1$ range from virtually zero to more than 50 per cent predicted FEV$_1$.

from the chest radiograph and, ideally, account needs to be taken of this when estimating the likely postoperative function. The variable function of the lobe or lung to be removed implies that estimation of postoperative function requires a method of quantifying its preoperative contribution. Historically, various methods have been used for this purpose, including bronchospirometry and balloon occlusion of the pulmonary artery, but these have been superseded by radioisotopic and other imaging techniques.

Isotope scanning in patients with lung cancer was used initially as a guide to the likely resectability of a bronchial tumour, but its use for this indication has now been abandoned in favour of computed tomography (CT) and related techniques. Lung scans are, however, still useful as quantitative guides to unilateral lung function, particularly in candidates for possible pneumonectomy. In combination with preoperative functional measurements such as FEV$_1$, a scan can, with reasonable accuracy, be used to estimate the likely postoperative values. This approach has

been used in several studies over the past 30 years.[21] The principle is illustrated in Fig. 12.10. Lung cancers can produce surprisingly large defects of both perfusion and ventilation (Fig. 12.11) and in most cases the defects appear well matched. The mechanisms may vary and include not only obvious candidates, such as obstruction of an airway or pulmonary vessel, but also reflex effects. In combination with preoperative measurements of respiratory function, a ventilation or perfusion lung scan predicts post-pneumonectomy FEV$_1$ and VC (Fig. 12.12) and V̇o$_2$max on exercise with reasonable accuracy.[20,23,24] Although it has also been used to estimate postoperative D$_L$CO,[19] for the reasons outlined above the prediction of D$_L$CO using the simple equation illustrated in Fig. 12.10 would be expected to be less accurate than for lung volumes and this is borne out in practice.[20]

Estimation of post-lobectomy function using lung scans has also been attempted;[19,25] oblique images of ventilation and/or perfusion help in delineating specific lobes, but prediction is likely to be less accurate than for pneumonectomy. Since, however, on average the effects of lobectomy are appreciably less than those of pneumonectomy, precise estimation of the consequences is less important unless preoperative respiratory function is severely compromised. An alternative method that has been proposed for estimating post-lobectomy function is simply to take account of the number of lung segments that are likely to require removal and to multiply the preoperative functional index by the proportion of segments remaining.[26] This allows a maximum likely effect of lobectomy to be estimated but takes no account of the contribution to function of the segments removed.

12.2.4 Prediction of postoperative morbidity and mortality

There has been considerable interest in using either preoperative function or estimated postoperative function to identify patients with a high risk of postoperative morbidity or mortality. Many studies have evaluated the predictive value of different tests, including spirometry,[27,28] D$_L$CO[29] and exercise testing.[28,30] Latterly, considerable emphasis has been placed on the potential value of exercise testing, which has the clear advantage of evaluating both cardiac and pulmonary reserve.[31]

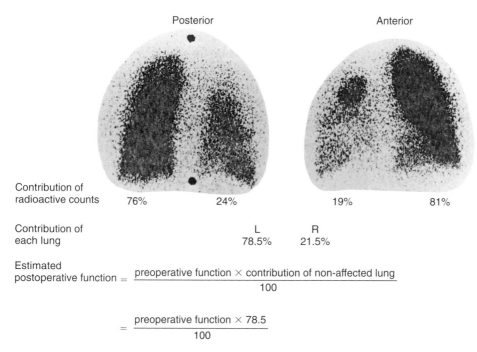

Posterior   Anterior

Contribution of
radioactive counts   76%   24%   19%   81%

Contribution of   L   R
each lung   78.5% 21.5%

Estimated
postoperative function $= \dfrac{\text{preoperative function} \times \text{contribution of non-affected lung}}{100}$

$$= \dfrac{\text{preoperative function} \times 78.5}{100}$$

Figure 12.10 Principle of estimation of post-pneumonectomy function using preoperative lung scan: it is assumed that the contribution of the lung to be resected to the index being calculated (e.g. forced expiratory volume in 1s, FEV_1) is related to the proportional perfusion or ventilation. Average values for proportional function are taken from posterior and anterior scintigrams.

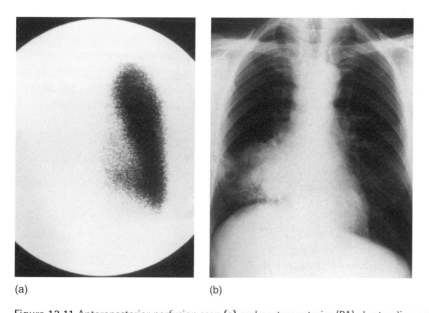

(a)   (b)

Figure 12.11 Anteroposterior perfusion scan **(a)** and posteroanterior (PA) chest radiograph **(b)** with a bronchial carcinoma affecting the right intermediate bronchus. The scan shows effectively complete absence of perfusion of the right lung. A ventilation scan showed a similar absence of function.

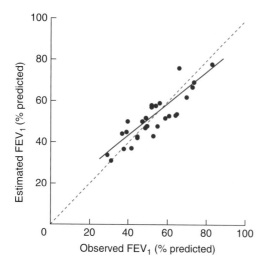

Figure 12.12 Comparison of forced expiratory volume in 1s, (FEV$_1$) estimated from preoperative value and perfusion lung scan and FEV$_1$ measured 4 months after pneumonectomy in 28 patients. Solid line represents regression and broken line identity. Redrawn from: Corris PA *et al.* Use of radionuclide scanning in the preoperative estimation of pulmonary function after pneumonectomy. *Thorax* 1987; **42**: 285–91, with permission from the BMJ Publishing Group.

In practice, however, it is probably necessary only in borderline cases as simple measurements suffice in the majority.[32] With spirometry, estimated postoperative values are generally better predictors than unqualified preoperative values. One widely used criterion is that pneumonectomy is contraindicated if the estimated postoperative FEV$_1$ is less than 0.8 L. This has been tested prospectively with some success.[33] Such a value is likely to imply very severe generalized airway obstruction, but it is more appropriate to express the estimate of postoperative function in relation to that predicted for the individual. A more recently proposed estimated postoperative FEV$_1$ above which pneumonectomy can be performed with low morbidity is 40 per cent of the predicted value. On the other hand, if the estimated value is less than 30 per cent of predicted, the risks of mortality or severe persisting morbidity are sufficiently high to be prohibitive in most patients. There are, however, a number of patients in the 'grey area' with estimated postoperative FEV$_1$ approximately 30–40 per cent of predicted, where the decision will

always be difficult; here, other factors such as age, motivation and comorbidity need to be taken carefully into account. In such patients additional measurements, including D$_L$CO and exercise testing are likely to be helpful. The guidelines published by the British Thoracic Society suggest that no further tests are required for lobectomy if the preoperative FEV$_1$ (post-bronchodilator) is more than 1.5 L and for pneumonectomy if preoperative FEV$_1$ is more than 2 L, provided that there is no coexistent interstitial lung disease or unexpected disability due to breathlessness.[32] People with lower values should in addition have D$_L$CO and SaO$_2$ measured, plus a quantitative isotope perfusion scan to estimate postoperative FEV$_1$ if pneumonectomy is being considered. If the decision remains unclear, an exercise test is advised, either formal progressive cardiopulmonary exercise testing or a shuttle walk test.[34] Desaturation during exercise of more than 4 per cent predicts an increased risk of postoperative complications,[35] as does a $\dot{V}O_2$max of less than 50 per cent predicted.[36]

Respiratory function may improve after other types of treatment of bronchial carcinoma, particularly when the tumour is occluding or almost occluding one or other main bronchus. Improvements in FEV$_1$, VC and Vmax have been reported in such situations using various forms of local treatment, including phototherapy,[37] endobronchial radiotherapy[38] and the insertion of tracheobronchial stents.[39] The improvements are accompanied by better ventilation and perfusion of the affected lung, with radioisotopic $\dot{V}$ and $\dot{Q}$ scans usually showing increases of similar magnitude.

REFERENCES

1   Shim C, Corro P, Park CC, Williams MH. Pulmonary function studies in patients with upper airway obstruction. *Am Rev Respir Dis* 1972; **106**: 233–8.

2   Van Noord JA, Wellens W, Clarysse I, *et al.* Total respiratory resistance and reactance in patients with upper airway obstruction. *Chest* 1987; **92**: 475–80.

3   Horan T, Mateus S, Beraldo P, *et al.* Forced oscillation technique to evaluate tracheostenosis in patients with neurologic injury. *Chest* 2001; **120**: 69–73.

4   Al-Bazzaz F, Grillo H, Kazemi H. Response to exercise in upper airway obstruction. *Am Rev Respir Dis* 1975; **111**: 631–40.

5 Miller RD, Hyatt RE. Evaluation of obstructing lesions of the trachea and larynx by flow–volume curves. *Am J Respir Dis* 1973; **108**: 476–81.

6 Gibson GJ, Pride NB, Empey DW. The role of inspiratory dynamic compression in upper airway obstruction. *Am Rev Respir Dis* 1973; **108**: 1352–60.

7 Lavelle TE, Rotman HH, Weg JG. Isoflow–volume curves in the diagnosis of upper airway obstruction. *Am Rev Respir Dis* 1978; **117**: 845–52.

8 Robertson DR, Swinburn CR, Stone TN, Gibson GJ. Effects of an external resistance on maximum flow in chronic obstructive lung disease: implications for recognition of coincident upper airway obstruction. *Thorax* 1989; **44**: 461–8.

9 Gibson GJ, Davis P. Respiratory complications of relapsing polychondritis. *Thorax* 1974; **29**: 726–31.

10 Bonnet Y, Lissac J, Pocidalo JJ. L'exploration fonctionelle pulmonaire des stenoses laryngo-tracheales secondaires a la tracheotomie. *Poumon Coeur* 1962; **18**: 59–72.

11 Empey DW. Assessment of upper airways obstruction. *Br Med J* 1972; **3**: 503–5.

12 Miller RD, Hyatt RE. Obstructing lesions of the larynx and trachea. *Mayo Clin Proc* 1969; **44**: 145–61.

13 Yernault J-C, Englert M, Sergysels R, DeCoster A. Upper airway stenosis: a physiologic study. *Am Rev Respir Dis* 1973 ; **108**: 996–1000.

14 Simonsson B, Maimberg R. Differentiation between localized and generalized airway obstruction. *Thorax* 1964; **19**: 416–19.

15 Cormier Y, Kashima H, Summer W, Menkes H. Airflow in unilateral vocal cord paralysis before and after Teflon injection. *Thorax* 1978; **33**: 57–61.

16 Purdue MP, Gold L, Jarvholm B, *et al.* Impaired lung function and lung cancer incidence in a cohort of Swedish construction workers. *Thorax* 2007; **62**: 51–6.

17 Gascoigne AD, Corris PA, Dark JH, Gibson GJ. The biphasic spirogram: a clue to unilateral narrowing of a mainstem bronchus. *Thorax* 1990; **45**: 637–8.

18 Gelb AF, Tashkin DP, Epstein JD, Szeftel A, Fairshter R. Physiologic characteristics of malignant unilateral mainstem bronchial obstruction: diagnosis and Nd–YAG laser treatment. *Am Rev Respir Dis* 1988; **138**: 1382–5.

19 Markos J, Mullan BP, Hillman DR, *et al.* Preoperative assessment as a predictor of mortality and morbidity after lung resection. *Am Rev Respir Dis* 1989; **139**: 902–10.

20 Corris PA, Ellis DA, Hawkins T, Gibson GJ. Use of radionuclide scanning in the preoperative estimation of pulmonary function after pneumonectomy. *Thorax* 1987; **42**: 285–91.

21 Brunelli A, Xiume F, Refai M, *et al.* Evaluation of expiratory volume, diffusion capacity, and exercise tolerance following major lung resection. *Chest* 2007; **131**: 141–7.

22 Nugent AM, Steele IC, Carragher AM, *et al.* Effect of thoracotomy and lung resection on exercise capacity in patients with lung cancer. *Thorax* 1999; **54**: 334–8.

23 Olsen GN, Block AJ, Tobias JA. Prediction of post-pneumonectomy pulmonary function using quantitative macroaggregate lung scanning. *Chest* 1974; **66**: 13–16.

24 Win T, Tasker AD, Groves AM, *et al.* Ventilation–perfusion scintigraphy to predict postoperative pulmonary function in lung cancer patients undergoing pneumonectomy. *Am J Roentgenol* 2006; **187**: 1260–65.

25 Tisi GM. Preoperative evaluation of pulmonary function. *Am Rev Respir Dis* 1979; **119**: 293–310.

26 Zieher BG, Gross TJ, Kern JA, *et al.* Predicting postoperative pulmonary function in patients undergoing lung resection. *Chest* 1995; **108**: 68–72.

27 Kearney DJ, Lee TH, Reilly JJ, DeCamp MM, Sugarbaker DJ. Assessment of operative risk in patients undergoing lung resection: importance of predicted pulmonary function. *Chest* 1994; **105**: 753–9.

28 Richter Larsen K, Svendsen UG, Milman N, Brenoe J, Petersen BN. Exercise testing in the preoperative evaluation of patients with bronchogenic carcinoma. *Eur Respir J* 1997; **10**: 1559–65.

29 Ferguson MK, Little L, Rizzo L, *et al.* Diffusing capacity predicts morbidity and mortality after pulmonary resection. *J Thorac Cardiovasc Surg* 1988; **96**: 894–900.

30 Brutsche MH, Spiliopoulos A, Bolliger CT, *et al.* Exercise capacity and extent of resection as predictors of surgical risk in lung cancer. *Eur Respir J* 2000; **15**: 828–32.

31 Weisman IM. Cardiopulmonary exercise testing in the preoperative assessment for lung resection surgery. *Semin Thorac Cardiovasc Surg* 2001; **13**: 116–25.

32 British Thoracic Society, Society of Cardiothoracic Surgeons of Great Britain, Ireland Working Party. BTS guidelines: guidelines on the selection of patients with lung cancer for surgery. *Thorax* 2001; **56**: 89–108.

33 Boysen PG, Harris JO, Block AJ, Olsen GN. Preoperative evaluation for pneumonectomy using perfusion scanning. *Chest* 1981; **80**: 163–6.

34 Win T, Jackson A, Groves AM, *et al.* Comparison of shuttle walk with measured peak oxygen consumption in patients with operable lung cancer. *Thorax* 2006; **61**: 57–60.

35 Ninan M, Sommers KE, Landreneau RG, *et al.* Standardised exercise oximetry predicts postpneumonectomy outcome. *Ann Thorax Surg* 1997; **64**: 328–33.

36 Win T, Jackson A, Sharples L, *et al.* Cardiopulmonary exercise tests and lung cancer surgical outcome. *Chest* 2005; **127**: 1159–65.

37 Gilmartin JJ, Veale D, Cooper BG, *et al.* Effects of laser treatment on respiratory function in malignant narrowing of the central airway. *Thorax* 1987; **42**: 578–82.

38 Goldman JM, Bulman AS, Rathmell AJ, *et al.* Physiological effect of endobronchial radiotherapy in patients with major airway occlusion by carcinoma. *Thorax* 1993; **48**: 110–14.

39 Wilson GE, Walshaw MJ, Hind CR. Treatment of large airway obstruction in lung cancer using expandable metal stents inserted under direct vision via the fibreoptic bronchoscope. *Thorax* 1996; **51**: 248–52.

13

Respiratory Infections and Acute Respiratory Distress Syndrome

13.1 UPPER RESPIRATORY TRACT INFECTIONS

The symptoms of viral upper respiratory tract infections in otherwise healthy individuals may conceal more generalized involvement of the peripheral airways. Although simple spirometric volumes are often unaffected,[1] abnormal peripheral airway function may be detectable during a flu-like illness or even during simple colds caused by rhino- or other viruses. The abnormalities are subtle: frequency dependence of compliance may be demonstrable[2] and, especially in smokers, comparison of flow–volume curves breathing air and low-density helium may show abnormal function.[3]

With influenza, mild reduction of lung volumes and, more consistently, reduced PaO_2, with widening of alveolar–arterial PO_2 difference ($AaPO_2$), have been reported.[4] Total airway resistance remains within the normal range,[5,6] but a small increase may become evident retrospectively on repeat testing.[6] A detectable reduction in FEV_1/VC is unusual,[4] but there is a more consistent reduction in maximum expiratory flow ($\dot{V}_E max$) at low lung volumes.[6] Even if baseline airway function is normal during a viral infection, an increase in non-specific bronchial responsiveness may be demonstrable on challenge.[5,6] Healthy subjects may develop more severe maximum airway narrowing on challenge with methacholine without necessarily any change in PC_{20} (see Chapter 1, Section 1.6.8.2).[7] These results

have obvious implications for studies of bronchial responsiveness, where account needs to be taken of the effects of any recent viral infection. As might be expected, the effects of viral infection are more marked in subjects with even mild asthma, in whom a decrease in baseline FEV_1 as well as an increase in bronchial responsiveness is demonstrable.[8]

Sequential measurement of maximum respiratory pressures shows evidence of transient mild respiratory muscle weakness,[9] usually asymptomatic in previously healthy subjects but potentially more important in those with pre-existing respiratory muscle weakness.[10]

The demonstration of abnormal function during naturally acquired viral respiratory infections has led to studies of the effects of influenza immunization. Use of live attenuated influenza vaccine in healthy subjects may reduce maximum expiratory flows at low lung volumes[11] and increase bronchial responsiveness, although the increase is less than occurs with spontaneous symptomatic infections.[12] A small reduction in FEV_1 has been reported in patients with established airflow obstruction,[11] but this is not a universal finding.[13]

13.2 PNEUMONIA

In acute pneumonia a mild reduction of lung volumes is common in previously healthy individuals.[14] A variable degree of hypoxaemia is present, its severity depending on the extent of the consolidation[15] and the presence of pre-existing disease, in particular airflow obstruction. Radioisotope scans usually show a greater reduction of ventilation than perfusion of the affected lung.[16] The reduced perfusion presumably results from vasoconstriction due to regional hypoxia. Such local adjustment helps to minimize the gas exchange disturbance, but residual mismatching of ventilation ($\dot{V}_A$) and perfusion ($\dot{Q}$) is still sufficient to lower the PaO_2. Detailed study of the distribution of ventilation and perfusion using the multiple inert gas elimination technique (MIGET) shows a combination of intrapulmonary shunt and $\dot{V}_A/\dot{Q}$ mismatching; both are more severe in patients with more extensive pneumonia who require ventilatory support.[17] Breathing 100 per cent oxygen produces no change in the shunt but a wider dispersion of $\dot{V}_A/\dot{Q}$ ratios consistent with release of hypoxic pulmonary vasoconstriction.[17]

Carbon monoxide diffusing capacity (D_LCO) has been measured infrequently in acute pneumonia, but a reduction persisting for several weeks has been reported following lobar pneumonia[18] and legionnaires' disease.[19]

In 'atypical' pneumonia caused by viruses or mycoplasma there may be both loss of volume and airway narrowing, with a mild reduction of the FEV_1/VC ratio and maldistribution of ventilation with an increased slope of phase III and a widened $AaPO_2$.[20] Recovery of spirometric volumes is notably slower after mycoplasma than pneumococcal pneumonia.[14]

In severe fulminating pneumonia, maintenance of adequate oxygenation is often difficult, even with high inspired oxygen concentrations, and the functional abnormalities are then similar to those found in other causes of the acute respiratory distress syndrome (see Section 13.5).

Follow-up studies of patients after the severe acute respiratory syndrome (SARS) have shown that most survivors have regained normal lung volumes 6 months later, although D_LCO remained low in a minority. The most frequent abnormalities were related to exercise capacity, which was often still impaired at 6 months, in terms of both a reduced 6-min walk distance and maximal performance in progressive exercise testing.[21,22] The exercise intolerance was disproportionate to any abnormalities of static respiratory function. Possible contributory factors include deconditioning and steroid treatment.

13.3 TUBERCULOSIS

One study in miliary tuberculosis showed a mild restrictive ventilatory defect, with, usually, a normal FEV_1/VC ratio; reduction in the steady-state D_LCO was proportional to the reduction in VC.[23] Long-term functional effects of tuberculosis have been recognized for many years and a high prevalence of chronic airway obstruction is particularly common, even after successful treatment.[24] The reduction in FEV_1 is usually proportionally greater than the reduction in VC, with a low FEV_1/VC ratio. The subsequent decline in spirometric volumes is likely to be greater than normal and any further episode of active disease further exacerbates the decline.[25]

13.4 HUMAN IMMUNODEFICIENCY VIRUS INFECTION

Several studies have examined the clinical and prognostic value of respiratory function in patients infected by the human immunodeficiency virus (HIV). With widespread pneumonia, as occurs commonly with opportunistic infections, particularly *Pneumocystis carinii*, there is a restrictive ventilatory defect with reductions in single-breath D_LCO and KCO.[26,27] The severity of hypoxaemia is variable, depending on the extent of the pneumonia; characteristically it worsens with widening of the $AaPO_2$ on exercise.[28] Both the resting D_LCO[26] and desaturation on exercise[29] are sufficiently sensitive to make *Pneumocystis* pneumonia very unlikely if the values are normal. However, these features are, of course, non-specific and are also seen with bacterial pneumonia and tuberculosis.[30,31] Recovery of D_LCO following *Pneumocystis* infection is only gradual and may continue for 3 months or more.[27]

Serial measurements of D_LCO for early identification of complications of HIV infection are of limited value, but, on average, lower values are predictive of subsequent opportunist infection and more rapid progression to full-blown acquired immunodeficiency syndrome (AIDS).[32,33] The mechanism(s) of the reduced D_LCO seen in some patients with HIV infection even in the absence of overt infection are unclear. In some patients the abnormality may be due to subclinical infection and in others to non-infective alveolitis. It does not appear to be attributable directly to pulmonary HIV infection, as patients in whom the virus can be identified in cells obtained by bronchoalveolar lavage have similar values to those with HIV-negative lavaged cells.[34] Separation of D_LCO into its membrane and capillary blood volume (V_c) components suggests that reduction of the latter is the prominent abnormality,[33] possibly reflecting early emphysema. Generalized airway obstruction develops in many patients with established AIDS and smoking may act synergistically in its development.[34] Patients may show increased bronchial responsiveness, demonstrable by large responses to bronchoconstrictors or bronchodilators.[35] As with many chronic illnesses, a large proportion of people with HIV develop respiratory muscle weakness; this correlates well with breathlessness in this population.[36] Correspondingly, the maximum workload achieved in progressive exercise by otherwise disease-free individuals with HIV infection is often impaired. This is accompanied by an abnormally steep response of heart rate in relation to $\dot{V}O_2$, suggesting circulatory limitation due to either occult cardiac disease[37] or deconditioning.[38]

13.5 ACUTE RESPIRATORY DISTRESS SYNDROME

Acute respiratory distress syndrome (ARDS) represents the more severe end of the spectrum of acute lung injury (ALI). Both can result from a number of diverse conditions, which include the effects of trauma, infection in the lung or sepsis elsewhere, fat embolism, aspiration, oxygen toxicity and drug overdose, all of which share similar radiographic and functional features. The main functional characteristic is extreme difficulty in maintaining adequate arterial oxygenation. The severity of the gas exchange disturbance is readily assessed in terms of the ratio of PaO_2 to the fractional concentration of oxygen in the inspired air (PaO_2/F_IO_2). This index has the advantage of being relatively independent of the F_IO_2 (see Chapter 4, Section 4.4.2.5). A value of 200 (PaO_2 in mmHg) or less is regarded as one of the criteria for the diagnosis of ARDS, while a value of 300 or less is consistent with ALI.[39]

The pathological features include a combination of interstitial and alveolar oedema, microatelectasis, vascular congestion and haemorrhage,

microthrombi and formation of hyaline membranes; a variable degree of pulmonary fibrosis develops if the patient survives. In the earliest stages, hypoxaemia and hypocapnia may be demonstrable before any radiographic change is seen. As the radiograph becomes abnormal, the hypoxaemia and respiratory alkalosis worsen and the effect of enriching the inspired air with oxygen has progressively less effect. The physiological shunt is greatly increased and the failure to correct the PaO_2 on high oxygen concentrations is indicative of an abnormal 'anatomical' shunt, demonstrable by the multiple inert gas technique.[40,41] In this situation the shunt is due to the large number of alveoli that are perfused but completely unventilated because of alveolar filling. Anatomical shunts of 30 per cent or more of the cardiac output are often seen and, in addition, there is increased blood flow to a population of alveoli with very low $\dot{V}_A/\dot{Q}$ ratios. Administration of 100 per cent oxygen increases the anatomical shunt due to absorption atelectasis.[41] Measurements in the prone position compared with supine show improvements in the PaO_2/F_IO_2, at least in the early stages of the condition.[42–44] Adoption of the prone position is accompanied by increases in functional residual capacity (FRC) and lung compliance[45] and is a recommended therapeutic manoeuvre in patients in whom adequate oxygenation cannot be sustained by other means.[46]

Respiratory mechanics in patients with ARDS have been studied intensively. Functional residual capacity and TLC determined by inert gas dilution typically show gross reductions,[47] and pulmonary compliance is correspondingly reduced.[48] The latter is regarded as the mechanical hallmark of the condition and largely reflects loss of alveoli due to fluid filling. Decreases of FRC of 50 per cent or more are found. At first sight it seems surprising that the chest wall 'allows' FRC to fall so markedly to values that are in effect less than the normal residual volume. The likely explanation relates to the concomitant large increase in intrapulmonary fluid volume, which implies an unusually large discrepancy between total thoracic volume and lung gas volume (Fig. 13.1). If account is taken of replacement of thoracic gas by fluid, it is likely that lung recoil at FRC is less than normal and hence that lung tissue gives less than normal support to the intrapulmonary airways. This may also be relevant to the

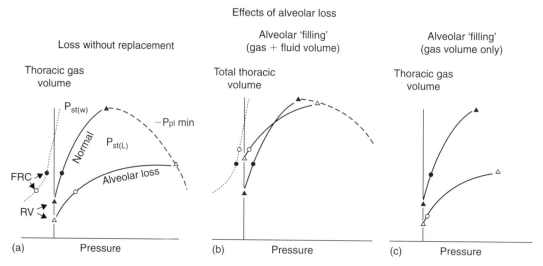

Figure 13.1 Schematic static lung pressure–volume (PV) curves (solid lines) for a normal complement of alveoli (solid symbols) and for a reduction in number of functioning units by 50 per cent (open symbols). If there is no replacement of the lost alveoli **(a)**, the curve shows a contraction by 50 per cent on the volume axis. The functioning lung units are more distended than normal close to the new total lung capacity (TLC) because of the improved mechanical advantage of the inspiratory muscles (whose maximum activity is represented here by the broken line, which is the mirror image of the minimum pleural surface pressure (P_{pl}) that the inspiratory muscles can generate during maximum static efforts at various lung volumes). If no change in the PV curve of the chest wall is assumed (static recoil pressure of chest wall, $P_{st(w)}$, dotted line), lung recoil pressure ($P_{st(L)}$) at functional residual capacity (FRC) (○) would be greater than normal. More correctly, the PV relationship of the chest wall should be plotted in relation to the volume of the *total* thoracic contents; usually the error in relating pressure *to thoracic gas volume alone* matters little, but if the lost alveoli are replaced by indistensible fluid or tissue, the error is significantly greater. **(b)** It is assumed that the volume (at TLC) of the lost alveoli has been so replaced and this is included in the total thoracic volume plotted (also included is a small contribution from the 'normal' lung tissue volume). The new FRC (total volume, ○) is now greater than normal (●) and the recoil pressure of the remaining functioning alveoli is less than normal. If this 'real' situation is assessed in the conventional way by plotting only *gas* volume **(c)**, the FRC appears to be disproportionately reduced; the low lung recoil pressure at FRC has serious implications for airway closure and alveolar collapse. (This model analysis ignores the lower inflection on the PV curve due to derecruitment/recruitment of alveoli.)

RV, residual volume.

finding that airway resistance is increased in patients with ARDS.[49]

A characteristic feature of the pressure–volume (PV) curve of the lungs in ARDS, particularly on inspiration, is a marked inflection at low lung volumes, due to progressive recruitment of alveoli that had collapsed during the preceding deflation (Fig. 13.2). The curve therefore has a more sigmoid shape than normal; this is evident particularly on the inspiratory (inflation) curve but may also be apparent on the expiratory (deflation) curve,[50] leading to greater hysteresis between the two curves due to the cyclical opening and closing of alveoli. This sequence appears to be particularly

damaging to the lungs, as also is overdistension of the reduced number of alveoli contributing to the volume change.[46] These considerations have led to a strategy of assisted ventilation, in which the lung PV curve is used as a guide to the volume range over which the patient breathes. In principle, alveolar recruitment should be optimized and the lungs protected from ventilator-induced lung injury by maintaining inflation between the lower and upper inflection points on the PV curve,[51] a strategy that can be applied automatically by modern ventilators. As a consequence, the tidal volume is curtailed and, in a landmark study,[52] a strategy of low tidal volume ventilation (6 mL per kg bodyweight) was shown to

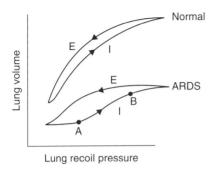

Figure 13.2 Schematic inspiratory (I) and expiratory (E) pressure–volume curves of lungs in a normal subject and a patient with acute respiratory distress syndrome (ARDS) (thoracic gas volume only). Hysteresis is much greater in ARDS, and the curve has a sigmoid shape over the tidal breathing range due to collapse and inspiratory reopening of airways and alveoli. Lung injury is minimized by ventilation over the range between the inflection points A and B.

confer better survival rates than a 'standard' approach in which a conventional tidal volume (12 mL/kg) was used. There is, however, a physiological cost to this strategy, as maintaining ventilation with a very small tidal volume and rapid frequency has adverse effects on the elimination of carbon dioxide (CO_2), due to the irreducible dead space and therefore higher dead space/tidal volume (V_D/V_T) ratio. The consequence is 'permissive hypercapnia', accompanied by respiratory acidosis, a moderate degree of which is usually accepted. A 'safe' level of acidosis has not been defined but the usual aim is to maintain arterial pH above 7.20.[46]

Once the alveoli have collapsed during deflation, very high pressures are required to reopen them and it is less damaging to forestall the collapse at the end of expiration if possible. Alveolar collapse is discouraged by maintaining a positive intrathoracic pressure so that the airway pressure never falls to atmospheric. This is achieved during artificial ventilation by the ventilator maintaining a positive end expiratory pressure (PEEP); in non-ventilated patients the same principle is applied by supplying continuous positive airway pressure (CPAP) via a tight-fitting facemask. The effect of positive airway pressure is to move the functioning alveoli higher up their individual PV curves, discouraging the tendency to collapse towards the end of expiration. Functional residual capacity (gas volume) consequently increases, leading to

better oxygenation by reducing intrapulmonary shunting and improving $\dot{V}_A/\dot{Q}$ matching.[39] Positive end expiratory pressure might, however, be deleterious if it reduced cardiac output due to the positive intrathoracic pressure impeding venous return. In practice decreases in cardiac output are usually small and outweighed by the improved oxygenation so that overall delivery of oxygen to the tissues increases.[40] Some patients with ARDS spontaneously develop 'intrinsic PEEP' (as is also seen in patients with severe chronic obstructive pulmonary disease, COPD). This may help to improve PaO_2, although it appears to be less effective than externally applied PEEP, perhaps because the latter is distributed more evenly throughout the lungs.[53]

Clinical and radiographic recovery from ARDS is not necessarily accompanied by the attainment of normal respiratory function.[54] Both restrictive and obstructive ventilatory defects have been described on long-term follow-up; reductions in D_LCO and KCO[54,55] and impaired gas exchange on exercise[56] are more frequent and may be permanent. More marked persistent reductions are seen in people who had more severe and prolonged acute disease, as indicated by wider $AaPO_2$, higher pulmonary artery pressure, longer duration of treatment with high inspired oxygen concentrations, and use of systemic corticosteroids during the acute illness.[54,57]

REFERENCES

1 Puhakka T, Lavonius M, Varpula M, *et al.* Pulmonary imaging and function in the common cold. *Scand J Infect Dis* 2001; **33**: 211–14.
2 Blair HT, Greenberg SB, Stevens PM, *et al.* Effects of rhinovirus infection on pulmonary function of healthy human volunteers. *Am Rev Respir Dis* 1976; **114**: 95–102.
3 Fridy WW, Ingram RH, Hierholzer JC, Colman MT. Airways function during mild viral respiratory illnesses. *Ann Intern Med* 1974; **80**: 150–55.
4 Johanson WG, Pierce AK, Sanford JP. Pulmonary function in uncomplicated influenza. *Am Rev Respir Dis* 1969; **100**: 141–6.
5 Empey DW, Laitinen LA, Jacobs, L, *et al.* Mechanisms of bronchial hyperreactivity in normal subjects after upper respiratory tract infection. *Am Rev Respir Dis* 1976; **113**: 131–9.

6 Little JW, Hall WJ, Douglas RG, *et al.* Airway hyper-reactivity and peripheral airway dysfunction in influenza A infection. *Am Rev Respir Dis* 1978; **118**: 295–303.

7 de Kluijver J, Grunberg K, Sont JK, *et al.* Rhinovirus infection in nonasthmatic subjects: effects on intrapulmonary airways. *Eur Respir J* 2002; **20**: 274–9.

8 Grunberg K, Timmers MC, de Klerk EP, Dick EC, Sterk PJ. Experimental rhinovirus 16 infection causes variable airway obstruction in subjects with atopic asthma. *Am J Respir Crit Care Med* 1999; **160**: 1375–80.

9 Mier-Jedrzejowicz A, Brophy C, Green M. Respiratory muscle weakness during upper respiratory tract infections. *Am Rev Respir Dis* 1988; **138**: 5–7.

10 Poponick JM, Jacobs I, Supinski G, DiMarco AF. Effect of upper respiratory tract infection in patients with neuromuscular disease. *Am J Respir Crit Care Med* 1997; **156**: 659–64.

11 Zeck R, Solliday N, Kehoe T, Berlin B. Respiratory effects of live influenza virus vaccine. *Am Rev Respir Dis* 1976; **114**: 1061–7.

12 Laitinen LA, Elkin RB, Empey DW, *et al.* Bronchial hyperresponsiveness in normal subjects during attenuated influenza viral infection. *Am Rev Respir Dis* 1991; **143**: 358–61.

13 Wongsurakiat P, Maranetra KN, Gulprasutdilog P, *et al.* Adverse effects associated with influenza vaccination in patients with COPD: a randomized controlled study. *Respirology* 2004; **9**: 550–56.

14 Laitinen LA, Miettinen AK, Kuosma E, Huhtala L, Lehtomaki K. Lung function impairment following mycoplasmal and other acute pneumonias. *Eur Respir J* 1992; **5**: 670–74.

15 Levin KP, Hanusa BH, Rotondi A, *et al.* Arterial blood gas and pulse oximetry in initial management of patients with community-acquired pneumonia. *J Gen Intern Med* 2001; **16**: 590–98.

16 Kjellman B. Regional lung function studied with Xe^{133} in children with pneumonia. *Acta Paediatr Scand* 1967; **56**: 467–76.

17 Gea J, Roca J, Torres A, *et al.* Mechanisms of abnormal gas exchange in patients with pneumonia. *Anesthesiology* 1991; **75**: 782–9.

18 Colp CR, Park SS, Williams MH. Pulmonary function studies in pneumonia. *Am Rev Respir Dis* 1962; **85**: 808–15.

19 Jonkers RE, Lettinga KD, Peis Rijcken TH, *et al.* Abnormal radiological findings and a decreased carbon monoxide transfer factor can persist long after the acute phase of *Legionella pneumophila* pneumonia. *Clin Infect Dis* 2004; **38**: 605–11.

20 Benusiglio LN, Stalder H, Junod AF. Time course of lung function changes in atypical pneumonia. *Thorax* 1980; **35**: 586–92.

21 Hui DS, Joynt GM, Wong KT, *et al.* Impact of severe acute respiratory syndrome (SARS) on pulmonary function, functional capacity and quality of life in a cohort of survivors. *Thorax* 2004; **60**: 401–9.

22 Yu CCW, Li AM, So RCH, *et al.* Longer term follow up of aerobic capacity in children affected by severe acute respiratory syndrome (SARS). *Thorax* 2006; **61**: 240–46.

23 Sharma SK, Pande JN, Singh YN, *et al.* Pulmonary function and immunologic abnormalities in miliary tuberculosis. *Am Rev Respir Dis* 1992; **145**: 1167–71.

24 Menezes AMB, Hallal PC, Perez-Padilla R, *et al.* Tuberculosis and airflow obstruction: evidence from the PLATINO study in Latin America. *Eur Respir J* 2007; **30**: 1180–85.

25 Hnizdo E, Singh T, Churchyard G. Chronic pulmonary function impairment caused by initial and recurrent pulmonary tuberculosis following treatment. *Thorax* 2000; **55**: 32–8.

26 Shaw RJ, Roussak C, Forster SM, *et al.* Lung function abnormalities in patients infected with human immunodeficiency virus with and without overt pneumonitis. *Thorax* 1988; **43**: 436–40.

27 Mitchell DM, Fleming J, Pinching AJ, *et al.* Pulmonary function in human immunodeficiency virus infection: a prospective 18 month study of serial lung function in 474 patients. *Am Rev Respir Dis* 1992; **146**: 745–51.

28 Chouaid C, Maillard D, Housset, B, *et al.* Cost effectiveness of non-invasive oxygen saturation measurement during exercise for the diagnosis of *Pneumocystis carinii* pneumonia. *Am Rev Respir Dis* 1993; **147**: 1360–63.

29 Sauleda J, Gea J, Aran X, *et al.* Simplified exercise test for the initial differential diagnosis of *Pneumocystis carinii* pneumonia in HIV antibody positive patients. *Thorax* 1994; **49**: 112–14.

30 Mitchell DM, Fleming J, Harris JRW, Shaw RJ. Serial pulmonary function tests in the diagnosis of *P. carinii* pneumonia. *Eur Respir J* 1993; **6**: 823–7.

31 Kvale PA, Rosen MJ, Hopewell PC, *et al.* A decline in the pulmonary diffusing capacity does not indicate opportunistic lung disease in asymptomatic persons infected with the human immunodeficiency virus. *Am Rev Respir Dis* 1993; **148**: 390–95.

32 Nieman RB, Fleming J, Coke RJ, Harris JRW, Mitchell DM. Reduced carbon monoxide transfer factor in human immunodeficiency virus type I infection as a predictor for faster progression to AIDS. *Thorax* 1993; **48**: 481–5.

33 Diaz PT, King MA, Pacht ER, *et al.* The pathophysiology of pulmonary diffusion impairment in human immunodeficiency virus infection. *Am J Respir Crit Care Med* 1999; **160**: 272–7.

34 Norris KA, Morris S, Patil S, Fernandes E. Pneumocystis colonization, airway inflammation, and pulmonary function decline in acquired immunodeficiency syndrome. *Immunol Res* 2006; **36**: 175–87.

35 O'Donnell CR, Bader MB, Zibrak JD, Jensen WA, Rose RM. Abnormal airway function in individuals with the acquired immunodeficiency syndrome. *Chest* 1988; **94**: 945–8.

36 Schulz L, Nagaraja HN, Rague N, Drake J, Diaz PT. Respiratory muscle dysfunction associated with human immunodeficiency virus infection. *Am J Respir Crit Care Med* 1997; **155**: 1080–84.

37 Johnson JE, Anders GT, Blanton HM, *et al.* Exercise dysfunction in patients seropositive for the human immunodeficiency virus. *Am Rev Respir Dis* 1990; **141**: 618–22.

38 Stringer WW. Mechanisms of exercise limitation in HIV+ individuals. *Med Sci Sports Exerc* 2000; **32**: S412–21.

39 Bernard GR, Artigas A, Brigham KL, *et al.* The American–European consensus conference on ARDS. *Am J Respir Crit Care Med* 1994; **149**: 818–24.

40 Ralph DD, Robertson HT, Weaver LJ, *et al.* Distribution of ventilation and perfusion during positive end-expiratory pressure in the adult respiratory distress syndrome. *Am Rev Respir Dis* 1985; **131**: 54–60.

41 Rodriguez-Roisin R, Roca J. Update '96 on pulmonary gas exchange pathophysiology in pneumonia. *Semin Respir Infect* 1996; **11**: 3–12.

42 Pelosi P, Brazzi L, Gattinoni L. Prone position in acute respiratory distress syndrome. *Eur Respir J* 2002; **20**: 1017–28.

43 Voggenreiter G, Aufmkolk M, Stiletto RJ, *et al.* Prone positioning improves oxygenation in post-traumatic lung injury: a prospective randomized trial. *J Trauma* 2005; **59**: 333–41.

44 Lee DL, Chiang HT, Lin SL, *et al.* Prone-position ventilation induces sustained improvement in oxygenation in patients with acute respiratory distress syndrome who have a large shunt. *Crit Care Med* 2002; **30**: 1446–52.

45 Pelosi P, Croci M, Calappi E, *et al.* Prone positioning improves pulmonary function in obese patients during general anesthesia. *Anesth Analg* 1996; **83**: 578–83.

46 Leaver SK, Evans TW. Acute respiratory distress syndrome. *Br Med J* 2007; **335**: 389–94.

47 Pontoppidan H, Geffin B, Lowenstein E. *Acute Respiratory Failure in the Adult*, Little, Brown, Boston, MA, 1973.

48 Katz JA, Zinn SE, Ozanne GM, Fairley HB. Pulmonary, chest wall and lung–thorax elastances in acute respiratory failure. *Chest* 1981; **81**: 304–11.

49 Tantucci C, Corbeil C, Chasse M, *et al.* Flow and volume dependence of respiratory system flow resistance in patients with adult respiratory distress syndrome. *Am Rev Respir Dis* 1992; **145**: 355–60.

50 Matamis D, Lemaire F, Harf A, *et al.* Total respiratory pressure–volume curves in the adult respiratory distress syndrome. *Chest* 1984; **86**: 58–66.

51 Terragni PP, Rosboch GL, Lisi A, Viale AG, Ranieri VM. How respiratory system mechanics may help in minimising ventilator-induced lung injury in ARDS patients. *Eur Respir J* 2003; **42** (suppl.): 15–21s.

52 Acute Respiratory Distress Syndrome Network. Ventilation with lower tidal volumes as compared with traditional tidal volumes for acute lung injury and the acute respiratory distress syndrome. *N Engl J Med* 2000; **342**: 1301–8.

53 Brandolese R, Broseghini C, Polese G, *et al.* Effects of intrinsic PEEP in pulmonary gas exchange in mechanically ventilated patients. *Eur Respir J* 1993; **6**: 358–63.

54 Hert R, Albert RK. Sequelae of the adult respiratory distress syndrome. *Thorax* 1994; **49**: 8–13.

55 Orme J Jr, Romney JS, Hopkins RO, *et al.* Pulmonary function and health-related quality of life in survivors of acute respiratory distress syndrome. *Am J Respir Crit Care Med* 2003; **167**: 690–94.

56 Neff TA, Stocker R, Frey HR, Stein S, Russi EW. Long-term assessment of lung function in survivors of severe ARDS. *Chest* 2003; **123**: 845–53.

57 Herridge MS, Cheung AM, Tansey CM, *et al.* One year outcomes in survivors of the acute respiratory distress syndrome. *N Engl J Med* 2003; **348**: 683–93.

14

Diffuse Parenchymal Lung Disease

14.1 GENERAL PATTERN OF FUNCTIONAL ABNORMALITY

In a classic description of the patterns of functional abnormality in lung disease, Baldwin et al. in 1949 described a group of patients with 'pulmonary insufficiency' characterized by small lung volumes and no evidence of airflow obstruction.[1] The more severely affected patients also had arterial hypoxaemia that typically worsened on exercise. Chest radiography showed evidence of pulmonary fibrosis, and the pattern was recognized as characteristic of diffuse alveolar disease. It seemed likely that the basic defect of gas exchange was impaired diffusion and this, together with the alveolar wall thickening demonstrable, histologically led Austrian et al. to coin the term 'alveolar–capillary block syndrome',[2] encouraging the image of a physical barrier between air and blood impeding uptake of oxygen. However, subsequently, Finley et al. calculated that very considerable thickening of the alveolar–capillary membrane would be necessary in order for a significant gradient of P_{O_2} to develop between the alveoli and the distal end of the pulmonary capillaries, i.e. for oxygen uptake to be limited by diffusion.[3] They argued that hypoxaemia in the 'alveolar–capillary block syndrome' was due instead to mismatching of ventilation $(\dot{V}_A)$ and perfusion $(\dot{Q})$.

A large number of conditions are grouped under the heading of this chapter, mostly characterized by varying combinations of diffuse fibrosis and inflammatory changes in the alveolar walls. The typical restrictive ventilatory defect that accompanies most of them comprises reductions in VC and TLC; the RV is usually normal or only slightly reduced, with the result that TLC (% predicted) is relatively greater than VC (% predicted) and the RV/TLC ratio tends to be high. Typically, the FEV_1 is reduced in proportion to, or slightly less than, the VC so that the FEV_1/VC ratio is normal or high; airway resistance or conductance is normal in absolute terms but, since the volume at which it is measured is reduced, specific airway conductance (SG_{AW}) may be greater than normal. In analysing the mechanisms of the volume changes it is important to remember the role of the chest wall and that in many conditions the volume of lung tissue is increased; both of these factors may influence the measured gaseous volumes.

A 'restrictive' ventilatory defect is seen also after surgical removal of lung tissue and, since the effects of diffuse alveolar disease show some similarities to loss of functioning alveoli, the consequences of pneumonectomy and lobectomy are first reviewed briefly. The typical functional consequences of diffuse alveolar disease are most clearly developed in patients with idiopathic pulmonary fibrosis (IPF; also known as cryptogenic fibrosing alveolitis) and, as the archetypal example, this is discussed in some detail, with subsequent descriptions emphasizing ways in which other conditions differ. There is sometimes a tendency to assume that a restrictive ventilatory defect with a low carbon monoxide diffusing capacity (D_LCO) implies a diagnosis of IPF, but it should be emphasized that the functional pattern is in no way specific.

14.2 SURGICAL REMOVAL OF LUNG TISSUE

Interpretation of the effects of pneumonectomy or lobectomy may be complicated by the lung removed (and sometimes that remaining) being abnormal. Early studies were of the removal of lungs largely destroyed by tuberculosis.[4,5] A clearer picture might be expected if pulmonary function is compared before and after surgery for bronchial carcinoma, but the effects of the tumour on respiratory function (see Chapter 12, Section 12.2.1) may complicate comparison.

In general, lung volumes after pneumonectomy tend to be larger than would be expected for a single lung. This applies to VC (see Fig. 12.8 in Chapter 12),[4–6] but more so to TLC, as the residual volume remains close to the value expected for two lungs,[5,6] presumably because of the influence of the chest wall. The relative overdistension of the surviving lung ('compensatory emphysema') can also be appreciated radiographically as mediastinal displacement or herniation across the midline. There is no evidence that pneumonectomy causes true destructive emphysema. If inspiratory muscle forces can be transmitted normally to the surviving lung, some degree of overdistension would be expected because at full inflation the muscles would be acting at a better mechanical advantage than normal (see Fig. 1.7d in Chapter 1). The maximum lung recoil pressure (P_Lmax) at the reduced TLC would then be greater than normal. Although the asymmetry of the situation makes prediction uncertain, there is some evidence from both pneumonectomy[4] and lobectomy[7] that P_Lmax is indeed increased after lung resection. Normally, however, healthy lungs are almost fully distended at TLC (i.e. the lung pressure–volume (PV) relationship is very shallow) and, therefore, little increase in volume would be expected as a result of a greater distending force. The extent of increase in TLC of the remaining lung after pneumonectomy suggests an additional long-term alteration in its distensibility ('stress relaxation').

The single-breath D_LCO after lung resection is reduced relatively less than lung volume, with a consequent increase in KCO, because the remaining lung has a large capillary blood volume relative to its gas volume.[8] A corollary of this effect is that, with a disease in which the number of gas-containing lung units is effectively reduced, an apparently 'normal' KCO may conceal some impairment of the function of the remaining ventilated alveoli.

Following pneumonectomy, both ventilation and perfusion are approximately twice the values expected for one lung, but there is little effect on the distribution of ventilation in the surviving lung.[9] As would be predicted from vascular pressure–flow relations in normal human lungs, doubling the blood flow through the surviving pulmonary vascular bed produces little change in pressure at rest.[10] The rise of pulmonary arterial pressure on exercise is, however, abnormally large; the pulmonary blood flow (i.e. cardiac output) is generally normal for the workload, provided that the remaining lung is healthy.[10] The ventilation for a given workload on exercise may be excessive but returns towards normal with time.[6]

The effects of lobectomy are generally minor with only small reductions in lung volumes (see Fig. 12.8 in Chapter 12) and no significant changes in indices of gas exchange.[8]

14.3 IDIOPATHIC PULMONARY FIBROSIS AND RELATED CONDITIONS

Diffuse pulmonary alveolitis or fibrosis of unknown aetiology has gone under various names, including Hamman–Rich syndrome, fibrosing alveolitis and usual interstitial pneumonia (UIP). Reclassification defined the 'idiopathic interstitial pneumonias' in terms mainly of the dominant histopathological appearances.[11] Idiopathic pulmonary fibrosis, associated with the pathological appearance recognized as UIP, is distinguished on histological criteria from other patterns including desquamative interstitial pneumonia (DIP), respiratory bronchiolitis interstitial lung disease (RBILD), lymphocytic interstitial pneumonia and the new category 'non-specific interstitial pneumonia' (NSIP). The NSIP pattern, which generally carries a more favourable prognosis, is seen particularly in association with certain collagen-vascular diseases (see Chapter 25), but it also occurs alone. The older and broader term 'cryptogenic fibrosing alveolitis' (CFA), used especially in the UK literature, encompasses patients with UIP and NSIP. The functional features of the two conditions are usually indistinguishable.

14.3.1 Static mechanical function

The major mechanical abnormality in IPF is a reduction in pulmonary compliance with an increase in recoil pressures (Fig. 14.1). The reduced

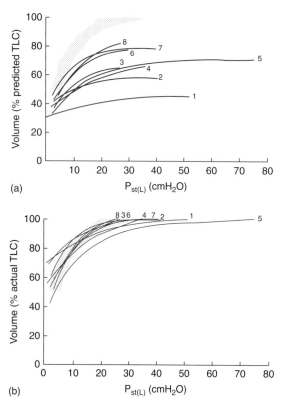

(a)

(b)

Figure 14.1 Static expiratory pressure–volume curves in eight patients with idiopathic pulmonary fibrosis (IPF), showing lung recoil pressure ($P_{st(L)}$) plotted against (a) absolute lung volume (% predicted total lung capacity (TLC), which takes account of variations in body size but not lung size) and (b) relative lung volume (% measured TLC). The stippled area represents the normal range. (a) Recoil pressures are increased at all volumes and maximum lung recoil pressure ($P_L$max) is greater than normal. (b) Recoil pressures remain higher than normal at volumes close to TLC due to the inappropriately large distending forces that the inspiratory muscles can apply to shrunken lungs. Reproduced from ref. 12 with permission from the American Thoracic Society.

lung distensibility constrains the tidal volume so that the characteristically increased ventilation is achieved by an unusually rapid frequency of breathing. In general, the smaller the VC, the smaller the tidal volume and the more rapid the breathing frequency.[13]

In theory the reduced compliance might result from either uniform stiffening of all the alveoli or a reduction in the number of functioning alveoli due to filling by inflammatory cells or replacement with indistensible fibrous tissue.[12,14] The structural appearances of the lungs support the latter mechanism, as the disease is characteristically patchy, with areas of relative normality interspersed with grossly abnormal areas. In such a situation the remaining functioning alveoli might be assessed more appropriately by replotting the PV relationship with lung volume related not to the predicted TLC (which corrects only for differences in body size) but to the actual TLC (which attempts to correct for differences in lung size – Fig. 14.1b). When plotted in this way, the curves appear more normal, but this is inevitable as they are 'forced' through 100 per cent on the volume scale. They remain more clearly abnormal at volumes close to TLC, where lung recoil pressure is disproportionately high. As explained above (see Section 14.2), an increased recoil pressure at full inflation does not imply a specific mechanism of lung shrinkage. The only way such a high recoil pressure can be generated is with an inappropriately strong effort by the inspiratory muscles, which are acting at an unusually good mechanical advantage at the restricted TLC (see Fig. 1.7d in Chapter 1). The values of $P_L$max found in pulmonary fibrosis are compatible with normal inspiratory muscle function at that thoracic volume.[15] The compliance in pulmonary fibrosis is often reduced disproportionately to the lung volume, i.e. specific compliance (C_L/FRC) is low. This does not necessarily imply a reduction in alveolar distensibility since other factors influence the measurement when the lungs have 'shrunk': first, because of the influence of the chest wall, the FRC is not reduced by the same proportion as other lung volumes and the surviving alveoli will therefore be operating on a less compliant part of their individual PV curves; second, it is conventional to measure compliance over a standard volume range (e.g. 0.5 L) or over the tidal breath, and if the number of functioning alveoli is reduced the measurement will extend up to a much less compliant volume range (Fig. 14.2).

An alternative approach to analysis of the PV curve is by fitting a monoexponential function and deriving the shape factor K. This reflects the elastic behaviour of the functioning alveoli and, in principle, is independent of lung volume (see Chapter 1, Section 1.2.2). Values of K in fibrosing alveolitis are usually normal or only mildly reduced,[14,16,17] implying that decreased distensibility of the ventilated alveoli plays a minor role in the restriction of lung volumes seen in this condition. For practical purposes, lung distensibility can be inferred, and progress followed, using lung volume measurements – ideally TLC, but in the absence of airway disease VC suffices. Formal measurement of the PV curve gives additional useful information only occasionally. If the cause of volume restriction is unclear and if extrapulmonary factors such as muscle weakness may be involved, measurement of $P_L$max may help to determine the predominant mechanism. A reduced lung compliance is not specific for intrapulmonary disease, as it is also seen with weakness and other extrapulmonary causes of volume restriction. The PV curve may also be useful in the patient with a borderline restrictive defect, where the demonstration of a clearly increased $P_L$max may help to distinguish a mild but real acquired reduction of volume due to pulmonary disease from lungs that are normal but constitutionally smaller than the average predicted volume. In some patients maximum respiratory pressures are mildly impaired compared with normal,[18] but the inspiratory muscles are usually still able to generate an abnormally negative pressure at full inflation, resulting in a high $P_L$max.

Many patients with IPF are chronic smokers, and coexistent emphysema is not uncommon. In some individuals the tendency to hyperinflation associated with emphysema counters the restricting tendency of pulmonary fibrosis, resulting in values of TLC and VC that remain normal despite severe disease.[19,20]

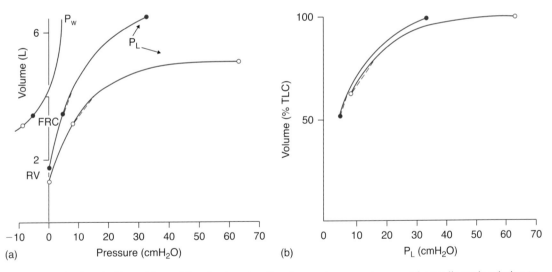

Figure 14.2 Predicted effect of loss of functioning alveoli on lung volumes and measured compliance in relation to (a) absolute volume and (b) relative lung volume (% total lung capacity, TLC). Closed circles represent premorbid situation and open circles the effect of reduction of alveoli by 25 per cent, assuming the pressure–volume (PV) curve of the chest wall (P_L) is unaffected. Functional residual capacity (FRC) is determined by the balance of passive recoil of lungs and chest wall and therefore falls relatively less than other volumes (a). The tidal breathing range is therefore over a less distensible part of the PV curve of the remaining alveoli, and pulmonary compliance (the slope of the broken line) measured over a similar absolute volume range (a) is low even if volume is expressed as per cent of actual TLC (b).

P_L, lung recoil pressure; P_W, chest wall recoil pressure.

14.3.2 Airway function

Early descriptions of function in pulmonary fibrosis concentrated on static measurements and assumed that the airways were normal. Some later studies appeared to show functional evidence of narrowing of the small airways. Histological examination often shows inflammatory changes in and around small airways and, indeed, it would be surprising if the most peripheral bronchioles were not involved in an extensive local inflammatory or fibrotic process. However, histology does not provide evidence on whether the narrowed airways subtend functioning alveoli. Conversely, even structurally normal airways may be functionless if the alveoli they serve no longer contribute to ventilation. The more appropriate question to ask, therefore, is whether there is narrowing of airways to ventilated alveoli.

It is well recognized that specific airway conductance and the FEV$_1$/VC ratio in pulmonary fibrosis are often greater than normal, implying that airway calibre is increased in relation to lung volume. This is clear, for example, from the maximum expiratory flow–volume (MEFV) curve, which often shows a well-preserved peak flow and maximum flows that are greater than normal for the absolute lung volume. If, however, maximum expiratory flow ($\dot{V}_E$ max) is related to the relative lung volume (i.e. as % VC), then values are often close to normal. One important determinant of airway calibre is lung recoil, which supplies the force distending the intrathoracic airways. Airway conductance (G_{AW}) and $\dot{V}_E$ max are high in fibrosis because recoil pressure is increased in relation to absolute lung volume (Fig. 14.1a). A similar relationship between $\dot{V}_E$ max and lung recoil pressure might therefore be expected in pulmonary fibrosis and normal subjects. Some studies have, however, shown that $\dot{V}_E$ max is reduced in relation to recoil pressure (despite being high in relation to lung volume), suggesting that the small airways are narrowed,[21,22] but further consideration shows that this conclusion is not necessarily valid. The effects of lung shrinkage on airway function depend importantly on the distribution of the non-functioning alveoli (Fig. 14.3). If, for example, a whole lobe were effectively destroyed, the airway supplying that lobe would be functionless and $\dot{V}_E$ max would be reduced in direct proportion to lung volume. But if the same number of 'lost' alveoli were scattered randomly throughout the lungs, individual airways would subtend both normal and functionless alveoli. Airway function would then appear supernormal in relation to the absolute lung volume. The real situation is probably somewhere between these extremes of (i) completely normal airway function (compatible with random loss of alveoli) and (ii) reduced function in proportion to the reduced volume, i.e. similar to lobectomy (Fig. 14.4). Only if $\dot{V}_E$ max is less than predicted by (ii), i.e. reduced relatively more than lung volume, can narrowing of *functioning* airways be inferred confidently. In most patients,

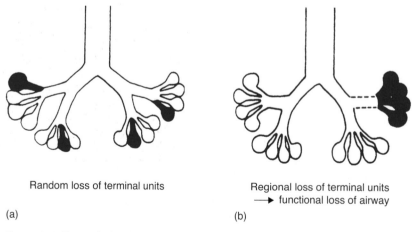

Random loss of terminal units

Regional loss of terminal units
⟶ functional loss of airway

(a) (b)

Figure 14.3 Theoretical effects of loss of peripheral lung units on airway function. Random loss of units (a) will have less effect on flow (or conductance) than loss of an equivalent number of units from a single region (b). In the latter case, airway function may be lost without airway disease (broken line).

$\dot{V}_E$max is normal or high in relation to the relative lung volume (i.e. % actual VC), implying well-preserved airway function.[12,23,24] In simpler terms this brings us back to the FEV_1/VC ratio: if this is reduced, narrowing of functioning airways is undoubtedly present; but if it is normal, no such inference can be made.

In summary, therefore, the mechanical function of the lungs in pulmonary fibrosis can largely be explained by the interactions between, on the one hand, shrunken lungs with a reduced complement of alveoli and, on the other hand, a chest wall,

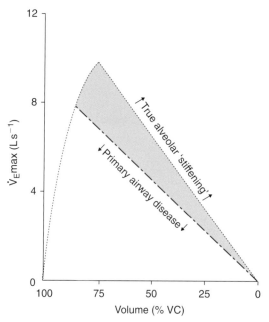

Figure 14.4 Schematic maximum expiratory flow–volume (MEFV) curves, illustrating the consequences of loss of 25 per cent of lung units, as might occur in idiopathic pulmonary fibrosis (IPF) if maximum expiratory flow ($\dot{V}_E$max) (Ls^{-1}) is related to the relative lung volume (% actual vital capacity, VC). Random loss of alveoli (as in Fig. 14.3a) should have virtually no effect and the curve will be indistinguishable from normal (dotted line). If airway function is lost in proportion to alveolar function (as in Fig. 14.3b), $\dot{V}_E$max at any per cent VC will be 25 per cent less than normal (dotted and dashed line). Values of $\dot{V}_E$max between these limits (shaded area) result from varying combinations of loss of alveolar and airway function. If $\dot{V}_E$max is reduced by more than 25 per cent, the functioning airways must be narrowed (and FEV_1/VC will be reduced).

FEV_1, forced expiratory volume in 1 s.

respiratory muscles and airways that remain appropriate for lungs of a more normal size.

14.3.3 Gas exchange function

The mechanisms of abnormal gas exchange in pulmonary fibrosis have been a matter of debate for 60 years. The 'alveolar–capillary block' concept[2] conjures up an image of a barrier to diffusion of gases, but impaired diffusion of oxygen probably plays only a limited role in the generation of hypoxaemia, at least under resting conditions, and mismatching of ventilation and perfusion are quantitatively more important. Maldistribution of ventilation and perfusion are demonstrable by an increased slope of phase III of the single-breath test and reduced efficiency of the washout of an intravenously infused gas.[25] As might be expected from the patchy nature of the disease, $\dot{V}_A/\dot{Q}$ mismatching occurs mainly at a local level within a lung region and would not necessarily be seen by comparison between regions.

The arterial blood gases typically show hypoxaemia with a widened alveolar–arterial PO_2 difference (AaPO_2) and increased venous admixture. The multiple inert gas elimination technique (MIGET) (see Chapter 2, Section 2.3.6) suggests that only a small proportion of the AaPO_2 at rest is due to diffusion impairment, but this increases on exercise.[26] Computation of the PaO_2 predicted from the distribution of $\dot{V}_A/\dot{Q}$ gives values at rest that slightly exceed those measured but this discrepancy, which reflects the additional effect of impaired oxygen diffusion, increases on exercise (Fig. 14.5). Limitation of oxygen diffusion will occur most readily in areas of lung with the lowest PO_2 gradient available to drive oxygen from alveoli into blood, i.e. in these lung units with lower than average $\dot{V}_A/\dot{Q}$ ratios. Thus, the two mechanisms of $\dot{V}_A/\dot{Q}$ mismatching and diffusion limitation effectively merge into one. Probably more important for diffusion of oxygen than the length of the diffusion pathway is the time available for equilibration of local alveolar and pulmonary capillary PO_2. Inevitably, this time is considerably reduced during exercise due to more rapid blood flow, particularly when (as in IPF) the capacity of the pulmonary capillary bed itself is diminished as a consequence of the disease.

Comparison of expired and arterial PCO_2 shows that the dead space/tidal volume (V_D/V_T) ratio is increased, often to a very considerable degree, because not only is the physiological dead space high but also V_T is constrained by mechanical factors. The $PaCO_2$ is usually less than normal in mild to moderate disease but can increase above normal in some patients with advanced disease.[27] There is no evidence of impaired sensitivity of the respiratory centres, and respiratory drive is usually greater than normal in proportion to the severity of the mechanical defect.[28]

Oxygen desaturation during sleep has often been reported in IPF; in general it is relatively mild and, as with patients with chronic obstructive pulmonary disease (COPD), the fall in oxygen saturation (SaO_2) is greater in those with lower awake values.[29,30]

14.3.4 Co-diffusing capacity

The D_LCO is virtually always reduced in IPF – indeed it is difficult to sustain the diagnosis if it is normal. The uptake of CO is reduced for a combination of reasons, including the smaller lung volume, maldistribution of inspired gas and pulmonary capillary damage. Overall, there is an

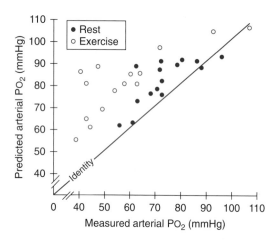

Figure 14.5 Arterial oxygen tension (PaO_2) predicted from ventilation/perfusion ($\dot{V}_A/\dot{Q}$) distributions measured by the multiple inert gas elimination technique (MIGET) plotted against measured PaO_2 in 15 patients with idiopathic pulmonary fibrosis (IPF) studied at rest (●) and on exercise (○). The predicted PaO_2 generally overestimates the measured value. The difference between them increases at lower PaO_2 and represents the additional reduction in PaO_2 due to limitation of oxygen diffusion. Redrawn from ref. 26 with permission from the American Thoracic Society.

inverse correlation between the D_LCO and pulmonary arterial pressure.[31] The KCO is also less than normal in most patients with established disease,[32] but in a few it remains normal.[33] It should, however, be remembered that in the context of fewer functioning alveoli a supernormal value might be expected, as is seen after lung resection (see Chapter 12, Section 12.2.2). The reductions in D_LCO and KCO correlate with the increase in $AaPO_2$ at rest and with the increase in pulmonary vascular resistance on exercise,[26] and CO uptake is therefore a good guide to the overall severity of gas exchange disturbance in IPF.

14.3.5 Exercise performance

The abnormalities of respiratory function during exercise in patients with IPF are essentially an exaggeration of those present at rest. Of different studies evaluating the limiting factor(s) to maximum exercise, some have concluded that mechanical factors, such as the size of the VC[34] and the maximum ventilation achievable, set the limit,[35] while others have found that impaired pulmonary gas exchange and/or circulatory dysfunction related to pulmonary vascular disease are more important.[36,37] Deconditioning and weakness of peripheral muscles may also be relevant in some individuals.[34]

The increased exercise ventilation results mainly from $\dot{V}_A/\dot{Q}$ mismatching and the consequent large physiological dead space. Ventilation is also inevitably increased by the pattern of rapid shallow breathing,[38] which causes the increased dead space to be ventilated more often than normal. The heart rate response to exercise is characteristically excessive and, although stroke volume is low, cardiac output is usually normal.[39] The small stroke volume is probably related to the reduced pulmonary vascular bed and pulmonary hypertension. The characteristic fall of PaO_2 on exercise is due in part to deteriorating $\dot{V}_A/\dot{Q}$ relationships; in addition, as discussed above, there is an increasing contribution from impaired diffusion of oxygen (Fig. 14.5).[26]

The 6-min walk distance (6 MWD) is sufficiently reproducible in patients with IPF for clinical use. It correlates well with measurements of $\dot{V}O_2 max$[40] and is used widely in monitoring progression of the disease as well as in assessing the value of ambulatory oxygen.

14.3.6 Relation of function to pathological, radiographic and clinical features

Despite uncertainty about the representativeness of lung biopsy specimens, several studies have reported correlations between the severity of alveolar wall fibrosis or cellularity/inflammation and tests of lung mechanics or gas exchange at rest and on exercise (Table 14.1). Although one study claimed that lung function tests can help to discriminate between predominant fibrosis or inflammation,[42] this was not borne out subsequently.[43–45] These functional–pathological correlations were all performed before the reclassification of IPF and its variants.[11] More recent comparisons of patients with UIP and NSIP histological patterns have, however, shown no clear functional distinctions between them.[46,47] In one large retrospective study of patients subsequently classified as having UIP or NSIP, the average TLC at presentation was slightly lower in the former group, but other lung volumes, $D_L CO$ and indices of gas exchange at rest and on exercise were similar.[46]

The pathological appearances that define RBILD and DIP are both associated strongly with smoking. In the absence of coexisting emphysema, however, the predominant functional pattern is restrictive rather than obstructive, despite the bronchiolocentric nature of the pathological changes in RBILD.[48,49] A reduction in $D_L CO$ is characteristic and improvement after smoking cessation has been reported in RBILD.[50] Striking hypoxaemia is sometimes seen in DIP.

In general, functional tests are more sensitive in IPF than the plain chest radiograph. A significant minority of patients with biopsy-proven disease have clear radiographs, but most of these have abnormal VC and/or $D_L CO$.[51] High-resolution computed tomography (HRCT) scanning is much more sensitive than plain radiography and relates better to functional abnormalities (Table 14.2). As with histological appearances, however, the severity or pattern of abnormal function does not distinguish between patients whose HRCT scans show dominance of one or other type of abnormality.[52–54] In individuals without coexistent emphysema the best functional correlate with CT severity in IPF is $D_L CO$ (Fig. 14.6). Despite the superiority of HRCT scanning over plain radiography, significant disease demonstrable by biopsy can occur in patients with suggestive functional abnormalities but a normal scan.[55]

In relation to clinical features, the severity of breathlessness during everyday activities is related inversely to both VC and $D_L CO$ and to the severity of desaturation on exercise.[56] Although oxygen

Table 14.1 Correlation coefficients of respiratory function with pathological severity of idiopathic pulmonary fibrosis (IPF)

Reference	n	Function	Desquamation	Cellularity	Fibrosis
42	23	VC		NS	-0.42^{*}
		$D_L CO$		NS	NS
		$\Delta AaPO_2$		0.56^{**}	0.85^{***}
43	26	VC		NS	-0.48^{*}
		Kco		NS	-0.58^{*}
		ΔSaO_2		NS	0.57^{*}
44	14	VC		NS	-0.60^{*}
		$D_L CO$		-0.62^{**}	-0.81^{***}
		Kco		NS	NS
		Exercise $AaPO_2$		NS	0.53^{*}
45	96 (27[†])	VC	$-0.55^{**\dagger}$	$-0.66^{**\dagger}$	NS
		$D_L CO$	-0.36^{**}	NS	NS
		Exercise $AaPO_2$	NS	NS	$0.59^{**\dagger}$

$^{*}P \leqslant 0.05$; $^{**}P < 0.01$; $^{***}P < 0.001$; [†]never smokers only.

$D_L CO$, carbon monoxide diffusing capacity; $\Delta AaPO_2$, change in alveolar–arterial PO_2 difference ($AaPO_2$) between rest and exercise; ΔSaO_2, change in oxygen saturation (SaO_2) between rest and exercise; Kco, Krogh factor; NS, non-significant; VC, vital capacity.

Modified with permission from ref. 41.

Table 14.2 Correlation coefficients of respiratory function with high-resolution computed tomography (HRCT) extent and pattern of idiopathic pulmonary fibrosis (IPF)

Reference	n	Function	Overall	Ground glass	Reticular
52, 53	54	VC	-0.37^{**}	-0.68^{*} ($n = 12$)	-0.76^{***}
		D_LCO	-0.68^{***}		
		KCO	-0.41^{**}		
		Exercise AaPo$_2$	0.45^{**} ($n = 33$)	0.73^{*} ($n = 11$)	0.55^{***} ($n = 37$)
54	39	VC	-0.46^{**}	-0.58^{***}	
		D_LCO	-0.40^{*}	NS	
		Exercise Pao$_2$	-0.6^{*} ($n = 13$)	-0.64^{**} ($n = 13$)	

$^{*}P < 0.05$; $^{**}P < 0.01$; $^{***}P < 0.001$.

AaPo$_2$, alveolar–arterial Po$_2$ difference; D_LCO, carbon monoxide diffusing capacity; KCO, Krogh factor; NS, non-significant; Pao$_2$, arterial oxygen tension; VC, vital capacity.
Modified from ref. 41.

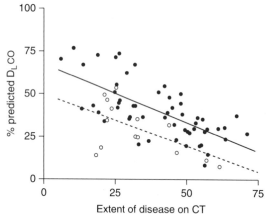

Figure 14.6 Inverse relation of carbon monoxide diffusing capacity (D_LCO) to extent of idiopathic pulmonary fibrosis (IPF) on high-resolution computed tomography (HRCT). Solid circles and regression line represent individuals without coexistent emphysema; open circles and broken line represent individuals with coexistent emphysema. Redrawn from ref. 52 with permission from the American Thoracic Society.

Table 14.3 Optimal functional predictors of survival in idiopathic pulmonary fibrosis (IPF)

	References
Single measurements	
(F)VC and/or TLC	59, 60
D_LCO	61, 62
Pao$_2$ at rest	63
Exercise capacity (6 MWD)	64, 65
ΔSao$_2$ on exercise	64, 66, 67
Change over 6–12 months	
Δ(F)VC	47, 62, 68, 69–71
ΔD_LCO	68, 71, 72
ΔAaPo$_2$ at rest	69

AaPo$_2$, alveolar–arterial Po$_2$ difference; D_LCO, carbon monoxide diffusing capacity; (F)VC, (forced) vital capacity; 6 MWD, 6-min walk distance; Pao$_2$, arterial oxygen tension; Sao$_2$, oxygen saturation; TLC, total lung capacity.

desaturation on exercise is one of the more sensitive functional tests, its reproducibility is rather poor[40] and in practice VC and D_LCO are the most appropriate measurements for evaluating the effects of treatment.

14.3.7 Functional predictors of prognosis

Despite treatment, most patients show declining function when this is studied over a 3-year period, with decreases in lung volumes and D_LCO more sensitive than resting gas exchange.[57] An improvement in VC or D_LCO after 3 months of treatment predicts a better long-term response.[58]

Tests of respiratory function are powerful predictors of long-term prognosis and survival in patients with IPF (Table 14.3). Lung volumes, D_LCO, measurements of gas exchange and exercise performance are broadly correlated in large populations of patients. When multivariate analyses are performed to identify which indices are independently associated with survival, sometimes one and sometimes another turns out as the most powerful. Also, the relative value of individual tests is likely to vary with the selection criteria used to identify the population and consequent variations in pathology and stage of disease. In general, change over a period of 6–12 months is more strongly predictive than a single measurement. The pathological appearances of NSIP have been shown in several studies to carry an appreciably better prognosis than those of UIP, but in multivariate analyses that include both histology and function the latter is more powerful and, once accounted for, the histological classification becomes insignificant.[72] Smoking contributes to the rate of decline, particularly of D_LCO,[73] and, presumably because of the effects of smoking, the FEV_1/VC ratio had independent predictive value in one study.[63]

Prediction of progress is of particular importance in relation to the optimal timing of lung transplantation. This has led to several studies, mainly retrospective, that have analysed the relative value of individual tests, measured on a single occasion or followed over a period. On the basis of these various studies Egan *et al.* proposed categorizing patients with 'limited' or 'advanced' disease depending on whether D_LCO was greater or less than 40 per cent of predicted and suggested that those in the latter category warranted consideration for transplantation.[74] They further proposed that 'limited' disease should be regarded as progressive if VC fell by more than 10 per cent over 6 months.

14.4 EXTRINSIC ALLERGIC ALVEOLITIS (HYPERSENSITIVITY PNEUMONITIS)

The abnormalities of respiratory mechanics in 'chronic' extrinsic alveolitis are generally similar to those of IPF, i.e. a typical restrictive ventilatory defect with reduced pulmonary compliance and increased lung recoil pressure.[75] As in IPF, the abnormalities of the PV curve are largely attributable to a reduction in the number of functioning alveoli.[76] A reduced value of the exponential parameter K has been reported in some individuals, and lower values are associated with a less good prognosis for improvement.[75] The D_LCO and K_{CO} are typically reduced, and D_LCO is generally more sensitive than lung volumes, at least in farmer's lung, in which it is related inversely to the radiographic abnormality.[77]

Even many years after acute episodes, D_LCO remains lower than in unaffected farmers.[78]

The frequency of an obstructive ventilatory defect is a matter of some dispute; in most patients with established fibrosis, indices of small airway function such as the closing volume and upstream conductance are within normal limits or are proportional to the reduction in volume.[76,79] Although small airway disease is demonstrable histologically, the abnormalities are typically seen in areas adjacent to diseased parenchyma, so that they make no contribution to the overall restrictive spirometric pattern.[80] Evidence of reduced attenuation on CT scans may be a more sensitive index of small airway dysfunction in this context and has been shown to correlate with the severity of 'air trapping' as indicated by an increased RV.[81] Frank emphysema is reported to occur more commonly in farmer's lung than in control farmers and may contribute to the reduced D_LCO in this condition[82] and also in chronic bird fancier's lung.[83]

Unequivocal functional evidence of airway narrowing (i.e. reduced FEV_1/VC) is more likely in the acute stages of the disease[79,84] or following inhalational challenge testing in a sensitized individual,[85] but a proportional reduction of FEV_1 and VC is the more usual pattern of response.[86,87] Following acute challenge, there is a deterioration in pulmonary gas exchange with reductions in PaO_2 and D_LCO and an increase in $AaPO_2$ at rest and on exercise.[87,88] Abnormal gas exchange on exercise post-challenge is more sensitive than at rest and may even identify responses in some otherwise asymptomatic farmers who may have subclinical disease.[87]

Cessation of exposure is associated with recovery of function in most individuals, although some abnormalities frequently persist, particularly in those with more chronic symptoms.[89] The rate of recovery of different tests varies, with PaO_2 increasing more rapidly than VC, and D_LCO increasing slowest of all, in some individuals continuing to improve for up to 2 years.[90]

14.5 SARCOIDOSIS

14.5.1 General functional pattern

The abnormalities of pulmonary function in patients with pulmonary sarcoidosis are generally less severe than in IPF, even in the face of marked

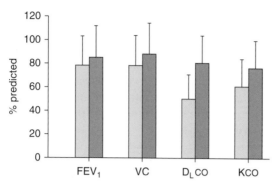

Figure 14.7 Mean ($\pm$ standard deviation, SD) values (% predicted) of spirometric volumes and carbon monoxide uptake at presentation from British Thoracic Society studies of 566 patients with cryptogenic fibrosing alveolitis (idiopathic pulmonary fibrosis, IPF) (light bars) and 149 patients with sarcoidosis and radiographic pulmonary shadowing (dark bars). Reproduced with permission from ref. 41.

radiographic shadowing (Fig. 14.7). In individuals with bilateral hilar lymphadenopathy (BHL) alone, lung function at rest is usually normal, with only a minority showing reductions in VC and D_LCO.[91] In patients presenting with diffuse pulmonary shadowing, the frequency of functional abnormality is greater and a mild restrictive ventilatory defect is common.[92]

14.5.2 Airway function

The frequency of airway obstruction varies in different series. One study suggested that this was the most frequent functional abnormality even at presentation,[93] but this was not confirmed in a large British Thoracic Society (BTS) multicentre study, where the definition of airway obstruction was based on a reduced FEV_1/VC ratio.[9] In this study only a small minority of non-smoking subjects had functional evidence of airway narrowing at presentation, but the frequency increased as the disease progressed. In a large Japanese study, evidence of airway narrowing was found in 8.8 per cent of subjects overall, particularly in males, smokers and subjects with more extensive radiographic disease.[94] In advanced fibrotic sarcoidosis, distortion of airways and the formation of bullae are common and airway obstruction may be severe.[95] A further contributor to airway obstruction in some individuals is localized stenosis of a proximal airway; such lesions

can be multiple[96] and occasionally produce the flow–volume pattern of central intrathoracic airway narrowing.[97] Airway obstruction is notably more common in black people,[98] in whom sarcoidosis overall tends to run a less benign course.

14.5.3 Respiratory muscle function

Granulomatous inflammation of skeletal muscle is well described in sarcoidosis and may underlie the reported reductions in respiratory muscle strength[99,100] and endurance.[101] Impaired inspiratory muscle function may contribute to the restrictive ventilatory defect and/or reduced exercise performance and breathlessness of some patients.[99,100]

14.5.4 Gas exchange function

Typically, the D_LCO is reduced a little more than VC, with KCO in the low normal range (Fig. 14.7).[92] The reduction in D_LCO is due to the membrane component (Dm) rather than the capillary blood volume (V_c).[102] The dominant cause of abnormal gas exchange is $\dot{V}_A/\dot{Q}$ mismatching, which results in hypoxaemia in more advanced cases. The development of pulmonary arterial hypertension is associated with severe hypoxaemia and a marked restrictive ventilatory defect in advanced disease.[103,104]

Abnormalities of gas exchange are exaggerated during exercise. Some reduction in maximum capacity, an abnormally high ventilatory response during submaximal exercise and an increased V_D/V_T ratio may be demonstrable, even in subjects with normal spirometry and clear chest radiograph.[105,106] However, abnormal gas exchange on exercise correlates well with impaired resting D_LCO, and widening of the $AaPO_2$ gradient is unlikely unless D_LCO is reduced.[105,107]

14.5.5 Functional, histological and radiographic correlations

Comparison of histological features and pulmonary function shows general relations between, on the one hand, the severity and extent of inflammatory changes in alveolar walls, thickening of the alveolar–capillary membrane and obliteration of alveolar architecture and, on the other hand, simple measurements such as VC, D_LCO and AaPO$_2$ on exercise.[108,109] Functional abnormalities relate less well to the density of pulmonary granulomas,[109] which presumably interfere less with pulmonary function.

Although the correlations between function and pathology are weak, they are better than those between function and chest radiography.[109] Not uncommonly, function is within normal limits in the face of florid radiographic abnormality, although in most instances radiographic improvement is associated with a measurable increase in VC.[92] High-resolution CT scanning, particularly on expiration, may show decreased attenuation that correlates with a raised residual volume, suggesting narrowing of the small airways.[110,111]

The relation between function and symptoms is closer than that between function and radiograph, and breathlessness is usually accompanied by measurably abnormal function.

14.5.6 Assessing progress and treatment

The VC and D_LCO are the usual measurements used for assessing the response to treatment with corticosteroids and following progress and there is no evidence that other indices are superior. Improvements in VC are not infrequently seen in the face of an unchanging chest radiograph. Simple functional tests have been criticized for a lack of sensitivity in sarcoidosis, but it is likely that they reflect the more significant pathological changes, whereas the radiographic picture may be dominated by less important abnormalities. The VC has been shown to be the most powerful functional predictor of long-term outcome in sarcoidosis.[112]

14.6 PNEUMOCONIOSES

The abnormalities of lung function in subjects exposed to fibrogenic dusts are among the most difficult to interpret. A major problem is that most affected individuals are middle-aged or elderly and inevitably a large proportion have been heavy smokers. Smoking alone may therefore be responsible for some of the changes found, or it may interact with the effects of dust in either additive or synergistic fashion. Some dusts produce not only alveolar fibrosis with effects visible radiographically

but also 'bronchitis', which may contribute to the functional abnormalities and be unrelated to radiographic shadowing. Also, in surveys of the functional effects of industrial dusts, the working population may not give a complete or representative picture of the effects of the dust, as more severely affected individuals may have retired or changed employment.

Of the commoner conditions, coal worker's pneumoconiosis (CWP) and silicosis are more often associated with overt evidence of airway obstruction than is asbestosis,[113] while with the latter, coexistent pleural disease (see Chapter 16, Section 16.4.2) may contribute to the functional abnormalities.

14.6.1 Asbestosis

In uncomplicated asbestosis the typical restrictive ventilatory defect and abnormalities of gas exchange are qualitatively similar to those of IPF. However, in relation to the severity of the radiographic abnormality[114] or the degree of volume restriction,[115] the D_LCO and pulmonary gas exchange tend to be better preserved in asbestosis than in IPF. Reductions in VC, TLC and D_LCO and desaturation on exercise all correlate with the profusion and extent of small irregular radiographic opacities.[116] Even in individuals with a clear plain chest radiograph, the extent of parenchymal fibrosis on HRCT scanning correlates with reduction in VC.[117,118] The presence of pleural disease adds to the restrictive defect,[118] but the combined effect of parenchymal and pleural disease on D_LCO and Kco is variable, as potentially counteracting influences apply, with pleural thickening tending to produce an increase in Kco.[119] In recent years evidence has accumulated of an additional effect of asbestos exposure on airway function, even in non-smokers. The prevalence of airway narrowing is greater in asbestos-exposed workers who have pleural plaques or pleural thickening than in those with a normal chest radiograph,[120] presumably because this reflects greater exposure. In those with radiographic evidence of asbestosis, the FEV$_1$/VC ratio is related to the profusion of opacities in a complex manner: there is a reduction with increasing profusion of mild to moderate severity but then an increase in the ratio with more severe asbestosis.[114] These findings have been attributed to increasing airway disease with greater exposure, but with the effect on airway function partially countered by greater elastic recoil associated with increasing alveolar fibrosis as asbestosis becomes more severe.[121] The additional effect of smoking is shown by a lower FEV_1/VC than in non-smokers with each radiographic score, and CT-demonstrable emphysema contributes to the reduced D_LCO in some smokers.[122]

14.6.2 Coal worker's pneumoconiosis

The effects of CWP depend on the radiographic category: abnormal function is the rule with the more extensive changes of complicated pneumoconiosis (progressive massive fibrosis, PMF), but in simple pneumoconiosis functional defects are much less frequent and less severe.

The most common ventilatory defect in coal miners is obstructive rather than restrictive.[123–125] Miners as a group have a slightly lower mean FEV_1 than comparable control groups, a finding that is most evident in subjects who have worked underground for long periods. It may be relevant that acute exposure during a normal working shift produces measurable decreases in FEV_1, VC and $\dot{V}_E$ max, especially in smokers.[126] In a large population, cumulative dust exposure has been shown to correlate negatively with FEV_1, VC and FEV_1/VC ratio, even in the absence of radiographically detectable pneumoconiosis.[127]

In simple CWP there is no clear relation between reduction of FEV_1 and increasing profusion of rounded radiographic opacities. The FEV_1 is usually more reduced in subjects with irregular opacities, a pattern that relates closely to smoking. In miners with simple CWP, the contribution of smoking to spirometric abnormalities greatly outweighs that of coal dust. In one survey of more than 8000 miners with simple CWP, an FEV_1/VC more than 2 standard deviations (SD) below predicted was found in only 6 per cent of non-smokers.[128] The authors calculated that the effect of smoking was on average five times greater than that of coal dust. Minor increases in residual volume have been demonstrated in non-smoking patients with simple CWP without spirometric abnormalities. Greater increases in RV and TLC are found when the FEV_1/VC ratio is low.[129] Small airway disease might be due either to intrinsic narrowing and distortion

resulting from deposition of coal dust, or to loss of airway support due to the characteristic 'focal' emphysema that accompanies the coal 'macule'. Relating $\dot{V}_E$ max to lung recoil pressure[130] suggests that both mechanisms may be relevant in different individuals. Subtle reductions in lung recoil pressure have been found even in subjects with category 1 changes.[131]

In subjects with significant airway obstruction, the expected mismatching of ventilation and perfusion occurs, widening $AaPO_2$ and lowering PaO_2. The D_LCO is usually within the normal range in simple CWP, although the mean values for groups of miners decline slightly but progressively from category 0 to 3.[132] There are also subtle differences between subjects with different types of opacity – in particular, lower mean values of D_LCO and KCO are found in miners whose radiographs show the pinhead (p) type of rounded opacity in comparison with the large q type,[133] but, nevertheless, most individual results are within normal limits. Lower values are seen in subjects with irregular opacities,[133] which are associated at autopsy with emphysema.

In complicated CWP the functional abnormalities are much more marked and there is a clearer relation between spirometric values and radiographic changes. Although airflow obstruction is generally more severe than in simple CWP, the TLC is usually 'inappropriately' normal, suggesting a combined obstructive and restrictive defect. Disturbances of gas exchange are also more consistently present and perfusion scans show obvious defects corresponding to radiographically visible large opacities or associated bullae.[134]

14.6.3 Silicosis

The functional effects of silica dust are generally intermediate between those of asbestos and coal dust: in particular, silica is more fibrogenic than coal dust, and this is reflected in a greater tendency to shrinkage of lung volumes, so that a restrictive ventilatory defect may be found, even in simple pneumoconiosis of more advanced stages.[135] Abnormalities of gas exchange, with increased dead space, arterial desaturation on exercise and impaired exercise tolerance, have also been shown in simple silicosis of category 2 or greater.[136]

In population studies of exposed workers, the reduction of spirometric volumes or $D_L CO$ is related to the profusion of radiographic and CT opacities.[137,138] The reductions in FEV_1 and FVC and their rate of decline correlate with the intensity of exposure.[139]

In complicated silicosis, the functional abnormalities become much more severe, with lung shrinkage, airflow limitation and markedly abnormal gas exchange.[135,140] A combined obstructive and restrictive ventilatory defect is characteristic,[137] and CT scanning suggests that much of the abnormality is attributable to the development of emphysema;[140–142] in non-smokers this is unlikely to be present without PMF.[140]

14.7 MISCELLANEOUS CONDITIONS

14.7.1 Langerhans' cell granulomatosis

In the early stages of Langerhans' cell granulomatosis (pulmonary histiocytosis X, eosinophil granuloma) the functional pattern usually shows a restrictive ventilatory defect with reduction in $D_L CO$.[143] Pulmonary hypertension is commoner than in other chronic lung diseases and apparently unrelated to the functional abnormality.[144] Exercise limitation is accompanied by an increased V_D/V_T and a pattern suggesting pulmonary vascular disease.[143] The natural history of the condition is usually progression to extensive 'honeycombing' with the formation of multiple cysts, frequently complicated by pneumothorax. In advanced cases with gross cystic change, spirometric evidence of airway narrowing is characteristic, together with a very low $D_L CO$, and the functional picture then resembles emphysema. Occasionally airway obstruction is the dominant functional feature at presentation.[145] The severity of airway obstruction and reduction in $D_L CO$ are the most significant functional determinants of survival.[146,147]

14.7.2 Pulmonary lymphangioleiomyomatosis

Lymphangioleiomyomatosis (LAM) is another condition in which diffuse nodular radiographic shadowing is accompanied by functional evidence of airway obstruction, which is present in about two-thirds of patients at diagnosis.[148] $D_L CO$ and $K CO$ are often markedly reduced and the functional pattern suggests emphysema, although TLC may remain within normal limits.[149] Measurements of the PV curve of the lungs show reduced lung recoil and an increase in pulmonary compliance, but relating maximum expiratory flow to lung recoil pressure suggests that 'intrinsic' airway narrowing also contributes to the reduced expiratory flow.[150] Exercise capacity is often greatly impaired[149,151] and is limited mainly by ventilatory factors due to the association of reduced capacity resulting from airway obstruction and greater ventilatory demand due to increased dead space ventilation.[149]

The rate of decline of FEV_1 is much more rapid than normal,[152,153] especially in those with lower $D_L CO$ and $K CO$,[153] and has been used as the index of outcome in studies of treatment.[152]

14.7.3 Cryptogenic organizing pneumonia

Cryptogenic organizing pneumonia (COP) is characterized radiographically by patchy shadows, which may be migratory, and histologically by intra-alveolar organizing pneumonia. The frequently associated obliteration of bronchioles gave rise to the alternative name of 'bronchiolitis obliterans organizing pneumonia' (BOOP), but COP is now the preferred term. Despite bronchiolar involvement, airway obstruction is not usually a functional feature; the pattern is essentially restrictive, with reduced FEV_1, VC and $D_L CO$, but the last is generally better preserved than in IPF.[154]

14.7.4 Alveolar proteinosis

In alveolar proteinosis many alveoli are partly or completely filled with proteinaceous material, which reduces the gas volumes of the lungs. The mechanical abnormality is a typical restrictive ventilatory defect with no evidence of airflow obstruction.[155,156] $D_L CO$ is reduced disproportionately to lung volume. A variable degree of arterial hypoxaemia is seen when breathing air and its severity is uninfluenced by posture.[157] Failure to correct the hypoxaemia by breathing 100 per cent oxygen is characteristic. The anatomical shunt presumably reflects continuing perfusion of fluid-filled alveoli, but $\dot{V}_A/\dot{Q}$ mismatching in alveoli that are partially filled may also contribute to the hypoxaemia when breathing room air. In one series an average 'anatomical' shunt of 20 per cent of the cardiac output was reported, and this accounted for most of the arterial hypoxaemia when breathing air.[155]

The most effective treatment of alveolar proteinosis is alveolar lavage, which results in increased lung volumes and D_LCO and reduces the shunt fraction, but even with apparent radiographic resolution function usually remains abnormal.[155] This probably reflects incomplete clearing of the alveolar material, but in some cases evolution to diffuse fibrosis has been observed.

14.7.5 Iatrogenic alveolitis and fibrosis

A large number of therapeutic drugs can injure the lungs, resulting in various clinicopathological patterns, with differing combinations of diffuse alveolar inflammation and fibrosis. The roles of respiratory function tests in this context are mainly in assessing the severity of functional impairment and in monitoring the development and progress of adverse effects.

With drugs that are used widely and that have a well-recognized propensity to injure the lung, pre-treatment measurement of spirometry, lung volumes and D_LCO is valuable as a baseline against which to compare later measurements in order to aid differential diagnosis and to detect adverse effects at an early stage. The value of periodic measurements (e.g. 6-monthly) for surveillance in asymptomatic individuals, however, is doubtful,[158,159] as reactions are likely to develop between measurements unless these are impracticably frequent.

Abnormal function before treatment is common in certain clinical scenarios and with certain drugs, e.g. amiodarone used for cardiac disease and methotrexate for rheumatoid disease. Some studies have suggested that abnormal pretreatment function is associated with a greater likelihood of an adverse effect, but this has not always been confirmed in larger studies,[160] and such an association may simply reflect earlier clinical recognition in individuals with initially compromised function.

For the recognition of alveolar reactions, a decline in D_LCO is usually the most sensitive

index, but inevitably this is relatively non-specific. Correction for haemoglobin may be particularly important in some conditions and with some drugs. One study of a large number of patients receiving low-dose long-term methotrexate for rheumatoid arthritis reported small (2–5%) but statistically significant reductions over 2 years in spirometric volumes and K_{CO} in otherwise asymptomatic individuals.[158] In the specific case of amiodarone, a significant minority of otherwise unaffected individuals show a reduction in D_LCO by as much as 20–30 per cent over the first few weeks of treatment, which stabilizes and is non-progressive.[161,162]

With radiation-induced pneumonitis and/or fibrosis the damage is maximal within the field irradiated, but it may sometimes extend further and result in more significant functional deficits. Again a restrictive ventilatory defect and disproportionate reduction in D_LCO may be seen, with the latter due in part to radiation-induced damage to the pulmonary capillaries.[163]

REFERENCES

1 Baldwin E de F, Cournand W, Richards DW. Pulmonary insufficiency: II. A study of thirty-nine cases of pulmonary fibrosis. *Medicine (Baltimore)* 1949; **28**: 1–25.
2 Austrian R, McClement JH, Renzetti AD, *et al.* Clinical and physiological features of some types of pulmonary diseases with impairment of alveolar capillary diffusion: a syndrome of alveolar capillary block. *Am J Med* 1951; **11**: 667–85.
3 Finley TN, Swenson EQ, Comroe JH. The cause of arterial hypoxaemia at rest in patients with 'alveolar-capillary block syndrome'. *J Clin Invest* 1962; **41**: 618–22.
4 McIlroy MB, Bates DV. Respiratory function after pneumonectomy. *Thorax* 1956; **11**: 303–11.
5 Gimeno F, Kraan JK, Orie NGM, Peset R. Pulmonary gas transfer 20 years after penumonectomy for pulmonary tuberculosis. *Thorax* 1977; **32**: 80–83.
6 Ogilvie C, Harris LH, Meecham J, Ryder G. Ten years after pneumonectomy for carcinoma. *Br Med J* 1963; **1**: 1111–15.
7 Berend N, Woolcock AJ, Martin GE. Effects of lobectomy on lung function. *Thorax* 1980; **35**: 145–50.
8 Corris PA, Ellis DA, Hawkins T, Gibson GJ. Use of radionuclide scanning in the preoperative estimation of pulmonary function after pneumonectomy. *Thorax* 1987; **42**: 285–91.

9   Anthonisen NR, Bass H, Heckscher T. [131]Xe studies of patients after pneumonectomy. *Scand J Respir Dis* 1968; **49**: 81–91.

10 Stanek V, Widimsky J, Hurych J, Petrickova J. Pressure, flow and volume changes during exercise within the pulmonary vascular bed in patients after pneumonectomy. *Clin Sci* 1969; **37**: 11–22.

11 American Thoracic Society, European Respiratory Society. ATS/ERS international multidisciplinary consensus classification of the idiopathic interstitial pneumonias. *Am J Respir Crit Care Med* 2002 **165**: 277–304.

12 Gibson GJ, Pride NB. Pulmonary mechanics in fibrosing alveolitis: the effects of lung shrinkage. *Am Rev Respir Dis* 1977; **116**: 637–47.

13 Javaheri S, Sicilian L. Lung function, breathing pattern and gas exchange in interstitial lung disease. *Thorax* 1992; **47**: 93–7.

14 Thompson MJ, Colebatch HJH. Decreased pulmonary distensibility in fibrosing alveolitis and its relation to decreased lung volume. *Thorax* 1989; **44**: 725–31.

15 De Troyer A, Yernault JC. Inspiratory muscle force in normal subjects and patients with interstitial lung disease. *Thorax* 1980; **35**: 92–100.

16 Gibson GJ, Pride NB, Davis J, Schroter RC. Exponential description of the static pressure–volume curve of normal and diseased lungs. *Am Rev Respir Dis* 1979; **120**: 799–811.

17 Hanley ME, King TE, Schwarz, M, *et al*. The impact of smoking on mechanical properties of the lungs in idiopathic pulmonary fibrosis and sarcoidosis. *Am Rev Respir Dis* 1991; **144**: 1102–6.

18 Gorini M, Spinelli A, Gianni R, *et al*. Neural respiratory drive and neuromuscular coupling during CO_2 rebreathing in patients with chronic interstitial lung disease. *Chest* 1989; **96**: 824–30.

19 Doherty MJ, Pearson MG, O'Grady EA, Pellegrini V, Calverley PM. Cryptogenic fibrosing alveolitis with preserved lung volumes. *Thorax* 1997; **52**: 998–1002.

20 Cottin V, Nunes H, Brillet PY, *et al*. Combined pulmonary fibrosis and emphysema: a distinct underrecognised entity. *Eur Respir J* 2005; **26**: 586–93.

21 Fulmer JD, Roberts WC, von Gal ER, Crystal RG. Small airways in idiopathic pulmonary fibrosis. *J Clin Invest* 1971; **60**: 595–610.

22 Ostrow D, Cherniack RM. Resistance to airflow in patients with diffuse interstitial lung disease. *Am Rev Respir Dis* 1973; **108**: 205–10.

23 Jayamanne DS, Epstein H, Goldring RM. The influence of lung volume on expiratory flow rates in diffuse interstitial lung disease. *Am J Med Sci* 1978; **275**: 329–36.

24 Pande JN. Interrelationships between lung volume, expiratory flow and lung transfer factor in fibrosing alveolitis. *Thorax* 1981; **36**: 858–62.

25 Ewan PW, Ronchetti R, Hughes JMB. Regional ventilation and ventilation–perfusion ratios in pulmonary fibrosis. *Prog Resp Res* 1975; **8**: 161–5.

26 Agusti AGN, Roca J, Gea J, *et al*. Mechanisms of gas-exchange impairment in idiopathic pulmonary fibrosis. *Am Rev Respir Dis* 1991; **143**: 219–25.

27 Nava S, Rubini F. Lung and chest wall mechanics in ventilated patients with end stage idiopathic pulmonary fibrosis. *Thorax* 1999; **54**: 390–95.

28 Renzi G, Milic Emili J, Grassino AE. The pattern of breathing in diffuse lung fibrosis. *Bull Eur Physiopathol Respir* 1982 **18**: 461–72.

29 Midgren B, Hansson L, Eriksson L, Airikkala P, Elmqvist D. Oxygen desaturation during sleep and exercise in patients with interstitial lung disease. *Thorax* 1987; **42**: 353–6.

30 Tatsumi K, Kumra H, Kunitomo F, Kuriyama T, Honda Y. Arterial oxygen desaturation during sleep in interstitial pulmonary disease. *Chest* 1989; **95**: 962–7.

31 Nadrous HF, Pellikka PA, Krowka MJ, *et al*. Pulmonary hypertension in patients with idiopathic pulmonary fibrosis. *Chest* 2005; **128**: 2393–9.

32 Rudd RM, Haslam PL, Turner-Warwick M. Cryptogenic fibrosing alveolitis. *Am Rev Respir Dis* 1981; **124**: 1–8.

33 Agusti C, Xaubet A, Roca J, Agusti AGN, Rodriguez-Roisin R. Interstitial pulmonary fibrosis with and without associated collagen vascular disease: results of a two year follow up. *Thorax* 1992; **47**: 1035–40.

34 Nishiyama O, Taniguchi H, Kondoh Y, *et al*. Quadriceps weakness is related to exercise capacity in idiopathic pulmonary fibrosis. *Chest* 2005; **127**: 2028–33.

35 Spiro SG, Dowdeswell IRG, Clark TJH. An analysis of submaximal exercise responses in patients with sarcoidosis and fibrosing alveolitis. *Br J Dis Chest* 1981; **75**: 169–80.

36 Harris-Eze AO, Sridhar G, Clemens RE, *et al*. Role of hypoxaemia and pulmonary mechanics in exercise limitation in interstitial lung disease. *Am J Respir Crit Care Med* 1996; **154**: 994–1001.

37 Hansen JE, Wasserman K. Pathophysiology of activity limitation in patients with interstitial lung disease. *Chest* 1996; **109**: 1566–76.

38 Jones NL, Rebuck AS. Tidal volume during exercise in patients with diffuse fibrosing alveolitis. *Bull Eur Physiopathol Respir* 1979; **15**: 321–7.

39 Bush A, Busst CM. Cardiovascular function at rest and on exercise in patients with cryptogenic fibrosing alveolitis. *Thorax* 1988; **43**: 276–83.

40 Eaton T, Young P, Milne D, Wells AU. Six-minute walk, maximal exercise tests: reproducibility in fibrotic interstitial pneumonia. *Am J Respir Crit Care Med* 2005; **171**: 1150–57.

41 Gibson GJ. Interstitial lung disease: pathophysiology and respiratory function. *Eur Respir Mon* 2000; **14**: 15–28.

42 Fulmer JD, Roberts WC, von Gal ER, Crystal RG. Morphologic–physiologic correlates of the severity of fibrosis and degree of cellularity in idiopathic pulmonary fibrosis. *J Clin Invest* 1979; **63**: 665–76.

43 Watters LC, King TE, Schwarz MI, *et al.* A clinical, radiographic and physiologic scoring system for the longitudinal assessment of patients with idiopathic pulmonary fibrosis. *Am Rev Respir Dis* 1986; **133**: 97–103.

44 Chinet T, Jaubert F, Dusser D, *et al.* Effects of inflammation and fibrosis on pulmonary function in diffuse lung fibrosis. *Thorax* 1990; **45**: 675–8.

45 Cherniack RM, Colby TV, Flint A, *et al.* Correlation of structure and function in idiopathic pulmonary fibrosis. *Am J Respir Crit Care Med* 1995; **151**: 1180–88.

46 Bjoraker JA, Ryu JH, Edwin MK, *et al.* Prognostic significance of histopathologic subsets in idiopathic pulmonary fibrosis. *Am J Respir Crit Care Med* 1998; **157**: 199–203.

47 Flaherty KR, Mumford JA, Murray S, *et al.* Prognostic implications of physiologic and radiographic changes in idiopathic interstitial pneumonia. *Am J Respir Crit Care Med* 2003; **168**: 543–8.

48 Moon J, du Bois RM, Colby TV, Hansell DM, Nicholson AG. Clinical significance of respiratory bronchiolitis on open lung biopsy and its relationship to smoking related interstitial lung disease. *Thorax* 1999; **54**: 1009–14.

49 Davies G, Wells AU, du Bois RM. Respiratory bronchiolitis associated with interstitial lung disease and desquamative interstitial pneumonia. *Clin Chest Med* 2004; **25**: 717–26.

50 Nakanishi M, Demura Y, Mizuno S, *et al.* Changes in HRCT findings in patients with respiratory bronchiolitis-associated interstitial lung disease after smoking cessation. *Eur Respir J* 2007; **29**: 453–461.

51 Epler GR, McLoud TC, Gaensler EA, *et al.* Normal chest roentgenograms in chronic diffuse infiltrative lung disease. *N Engl J Med* 1978 **298**: 934–9.

52 Wells AU, King AD, Rubens MB, *et al.* Lone cryptogenic fibrosing alveolitis: a functional–morphologic correlation based on extent of disease on thin-section computed tomography. *Am J Respir Crit Care Med* 1997; **155**: 1367–75.

53 Wells AU, Rubens MB, Du Bois RM, Hansell DM. Functional impairment in fibrosing alveolitis: relationship to reversible disease on thin section computed tomography. *Eur Respir J* 1997; **10**: 280–85.

54 Xaubet A, Agusti C, Luburich P, *et al.* Pulmonary function tests and CT scan in the management of idiopathic pulmonary fibrosis. *Am J Respir Crit Care Med* 1998; **158**: 431–6.

55 Orens JB, Kazerooni EA, Martinez FJ, *et al.* The sensitivity of high-resolution CT in detecting idiopathic pulmonary fibrosis proved by open lung biopsy: a prospective study. *Chest* 1995; **108**: 109–15.

56 Mahler DA, Harver S, Rosiello R, Daubenspeck JA. Measurement of respiratory sensation in interstitial lung disease: evaluation of clinical dyspnoea ratings and magnitude scaling. *Chest* 1989; **96**: 767–71.

57 Agusti C, Xaubet A, Agusti AGN, *et al.* Clinical and functional assessment of patients with idiopathic pulmonary fibrosis: results of a 3-year follow up. *Eur Respir J* 1994; **7**: 643–50.

58 Van Oortegem K, Wallaert B, Marquette CH, *et al.* Determinants of response to immunosuppressive therapy in idiopathic pulmonary fibrosis. *Eur Respir J* 1994; **7**: 1950–57.

59 Erbes R, Schaberg T, Loddenkemper R. Lung function tests in patients with idiopathic pulmonary fibrosis: are they helpful for predicting outcome? *Chest* 1997; **111**: 51–7.

60 Hubbard R, Johnston I, Britton J. Survival in patients with cryptogenic fibrosing alveolitis: a population-based cohort study. *Chest* 1998; **113**: 396–400.

61 Mogulkoc N, Brutsche MH, Bishop PW, *et al.* Pulmonary function in idiopathic pulmonary fibrosis and referral for lung transplantation. *Am J Respir Crit Care Med* 2001; **164**: 103–8.

62 Jegal Y, Kim DS, Shim TS, *et al.* Physiology is a stronger predictor of survival than pathology in fibrotic interstitial pneumonia. *Am J Respir Crit Care Med* 2005; **171**: 639–44.

63 Timmer SJ, Karamzaden AM, Yung GL, *et al.* 2002 Predicting survival of lung transplantation candidates with idiopathic interstitial pneumonia: does PaO$_2$ predict survival? *Chest* **122**: 779–84.

64 Hallstrand TS, Boitano LJ, Johnson WC, *et al.* The timed walk test as a measure of severity and survival in idiopathic pulmonary fibrosis. *Eur Respir J* 2005; **25**: 96–103.

65 Lederer DJ, Arcasoy SM, Wilt JS, *et al.* 2006 Six-minute-walk distance predicts waiting list survival in idiopathic pulmonary fibrosis. *Am J Respir Crit Care Med* **174**: 659–64.

66 Miki K, Maekura R, Hiraga T, *et al.* Impairments and prognostic factors for survival in patients with idiopathic pulmonary fibrosis. *Respir Med* 2003; **97**: 482–90.

67 Lama VN, Flaherty KR, Toews GB, *et al.* Prognostic value of desaturation during a 60 minute walk test in idiopathic interstitial pneumonia. *Am J Respir Crit Care Med* 2003; **168**: 1084–90.

68 Hanson D, Winterbauer RH, Kirtland SH, Wu R. Changes in pulmonary function test results after 1 year of therapy as predictors of survival in patients with idiopathic pulmonary fibrosis. *Chest* 1995; **108**: 305–10.

69 Collard HR, King TE Jr, Bartelson BB, *et al.* Changes in clinical and physiologic variables predict survival in idiopathic pulmonary fibrosis. *Am J Respir Crit Care Med* 2003; **168**: 538–42.

70 King TE Jr, Safrin S, Starko KM, *et al.* Analyses of efficacy end points in a controlled trial of interferon-gamma 1b for idiopathic pulmonary fibrosis. *Chest* 2005; **127**: 171–7.

71 Flaherty KR, Andrei AC, Murray S, *et al.* Idiopathic pulmonary fibrosis: prognostic value of changes in physiology and six-minute-walk test. *Am J Respir Crit Care Med* 2006; **174**: 803–9.

72 Latsi PI, du Bois RM, Nicholson AG, *et al.* Fibrotic idiopathic interstitial pneumonia: the prognostic value of longitudinal functional trends. *Am J Respir Crit Care Med* 2003; **168**: 531–7.

73 Schwartz DA, Helmers RA, Galvin JR, *et al.* Determinants of survival in idiopathic pulmonary fibrosis. *Am J Respir Crit Care Med* 1994; **149**: 450–54.

74 Egan JJ, Martinez FJ, Wells AU, Williams T. Lung function estimates in idiopathic pulmonary fibrosis: the potential for a simple classification. *Thorax* 2005; **60**: 270–73.

75 Sansores R, Perezpadilla R, Pare PD, Selma M. Exponential analysis of lung pressure–volume curve in patients with chronic pigeon breeders' lung. *Chest* 1992; **101**: 1352–6.

76 Schofield NM, Davies RJ, Cameron IR, Green M. Small airways in fibrosing alveolitis. *Am Rev Respir Dis* 1976; **113**: 729–35.

77 Cormier Y, Beanger J, Tardif A, Leblanc P, Laviolette M. Relationships between radiographic change, pulmonary function and bronchoalveolar lavage fluid lymphocytes in farmer's lung disease. *Thorax* 1986; **41**: 28–31.

78 Erkinjuntti-Pekkanen R, Kokkarinen JI, Tukiainen HO, *et al.* Long term outcome of pulmonary function in farmer's lung: a 14 year follow-up with matched controls. *Eur Respir J* 1997; **10**: 2046–50.

79 Warren CPW, Tse KS, Cherniack RM. Mechanical properties of the lung in extrinsic allergic alveolitis. *Thorax* 1978; **331**: 315–21.

80 Perez-Padilla R, Gaxiola M, Salas J, *et al.* Bronchiolitis in chronic pigeon breeder's disease. *Chest* 1996; **110**: 371–7.

81 Hansell DM, Wells AU, Padley SP, Muller NL. Hypersensitivity pneumonitis: correlation of individual CT patterns with functional abnormalities. *Radiology* 1996; **199**: 123–8.

82 Erkinjuntti-Pekkanen R, Rytkonen H, Kokkarinen JI, *et al.* 1998 Long-term risk of emphysema in patients with farmer's lung and matched control farmers. *Am J Respir Crit Care Med* **158**: 662–5.

83 Remy-Jardin M, Remy J, Wallaert B, Muller NL. Subacute and chronic bird breeder hypersensitivity pneumonitis: sequential evaluation with CT and correlation with lung function tests and bronchoalveolar lavage. *Radiology* 1993; **189**: 111–18.

84 Bourke SJ, Carter R, Anderson K, *et al.* Obstructive airways disease in non-smoking patients with pigeon fancier's lung. *Clin Exp Allergy* 1989; **19**: 629–32.

85 Hargreave FE, Pepys J. Allergic respiratory reactions in birdfanciers provoked by allergen inhalation provocation tests. *J Allergy Clin Immunol* 1972; **50**: 157–73.

86 Hendrick DJ, Marshall R, Faux JA, Krall J. Positive 'alveolar' responses to antigen inhalation provocation test: their validity and recognition. *Thorax* 1980; **35**: 415–27.

87 Schwaiblmair M, Beinert T, Vogelmeier C, Fruhmann G. Cardiopulmonary exercise testing following hay exposure challenge in farmer's lung. *Eur Respir J* 1997; **10**: 2360–65.

88 Ohtani Y, Kojima K, Sumi Y, *et al.* Inhalation provocation tests in chronic bird fancier's lung. *Chest* 2000; **118**: 1382–9.

89 Boyd G. Pulmonary function changes in pigeon fancier's lung. *Respir Med* 1990; **84**: 5–8.

90 Kokkarinen JI, Tukiainen HO, Terho EO. Recovery of pulmonary function in farmer's lung: a five year follow up study. *Am Rev Respir Dis* 1993; **147**: 793–6.

91 Winterbauer RH, Hutchinson JF. Use of pulmonary function tests in the management of sarcoidosis. *Chest* 1980; **78**: 640–47.

92 Gibson GJ, Prescott RJ, Muers MF, *et al.* British Thoracic Society sarcoidosis study: effects of long term corticosteroid treatment. *Thorax* 1996; **51**: 238–47.

93 Harrison BDW, Shaylor JM, Stokes TC, Wilkes AR. Airflow limitation in sarcoidosis – a study of pulmonary function in 107 patients with newly diagnosed disease. *Respir Med* 1991; **85**: 59–64.

94 Handa T, Nagai S, Fushimi Y, *et al.* Clinical and radiographic indices associated with airflow limitation in patients with sarcoidosis. *Chest* 2006; **130**: 1851–6.

95 Miller A, Teirstein AS, Jackler I, *et al.* Airway function in chronic pulmonary sarcoidosis with fibrosis. *Am Rev Respir Dis* 1974; **109**: 179–89.

96 Chambellan A, Turbie P, Nunes H, *et al.* Endoluminal stenosis of proximal bronchi in sarcoidosis: bronchoscopy, function, and evolution. *Chest* 2005; **127**: 472–81.

97 Hadfield JW, Page RL, Flower CDR, Stark JE. Localised airway narrowing in sarcoidosis. *Thorax* 1982; **37**: 443–7.

98 Sharma OP, Johnson R. Airway obstruction in sarcoidosis: a study of 123 nonsmoking black American patients with sarcoidosis. *Chest* 1988; **94**: 343–6.

99 Baydur A, Alsalek M, Louie SG, Sharma OP. Respiratory muscle strength, lung function, and dyspnea in patients with sarcoidosis. *Chest* 2001; **120**: 102–8.

100 Kabits H-J, Lang F, Walterspacher S, et al. Impact of impaired inspiratory muscle strength on dyspnea and walking capacity in sarcoidosis. *Chest* 2006; **130**: 1496–502.

101 Brancaleone P, Perez T, Robin S, Neviere R, Wallaert B. Clinical impact of inspiratory muscle impairment in sarcoidosis. *Sarcoidosis Vasc Diffuse Lung Dis* 2004; **21**: 219–27.

102 Lamberto C, Nunes H, Le Toumelin P, et al. Membrane and capillary blood components of diffusion capacity of the lung for carbon monoxide in pulmonary sarcoidosis. *Chest* 2004; **125**: 2061–8.

103 Sulica R, Teirstein AS, Kakaria S, et al. Distinctive clinical, radiographic, and functional characteristics of patients with sarcoidosis-related pulmonary hypertension. *Chest* 2005; **128**: 1483–9.

104 Handa T, Nagai S, Miki S, et al. Incidence of pulmonary hypertension and its clinical relevance in patients with sarcoidosis. *Chest* 2006; **129**: 1246–52.

105 Miller A, Brown LK, Sloane MF, Bhuptani A, Teirstein AS. Cardiorespiratory responses to incremental exercise in sarcoidosis patients with normal spirometry. *Chest* 1995; **107**: 323–9.

106 Delobbe A, Perrault H, Maitre J, et al. Impaired exercise response in sarcoid patients with normal pulmonary function. *Sarcoidosis Vasc Diffuse Lung Dis* 2002; **19**: 148–53.

107 Barros WG, Neder JA, Pereira CA, Nery LE. Clinical, radiographic and functional predictors of pulmonary gas exchange impairment at moderate exercise in patients with sarcoidosis. *Respiration* 2004; **71**: 367–73.

108 Huang CT, Heurich AE, Rosen Y, et al. Pulmonary sarcoidosis: roentgenographic, functional and pathologic correlations. *Respiration* 1979; **37**: 337–45.

109 Carrington CB, Gaensler EA, Mikos JP, et al. Structure and function in sarcoidosis. *Ann N Y Acad Sci* 1976; **278**: 265–82.

110 Davies CW, Tasker AD, Padley SP, Davies RJ, Gleeson FV. Air trapping in sarcoidosis on computed tomography: correlation with lung function. *Clin Radiol* 2000; **55**: 217–21.

111 Magkanas E, Voloudaki A, Bouros D, et al. Pulmonary sarcoidosis: correlation of expiratory high-resolution CT findings with inspiratory patterns and pulmonary function tests. *Acta Radiol* 2001; **42**: 494–501.

112 Mana J, Salazar A, Pujol R, Manresa F. Are the pulmonary function tests and the markers of activity helpful to establish the prognosis of sarcoidosis? *Respiration* 1996; **63**: 298–303.

113 Wang X, Yano E, Nonaka K, Wang M, Wang Z. Respiratory impairments due to dust exposure: a comparative study among workers exposed to silica, asbestos, and coalmine dust. *Am J Industr Med* 1997; **31**: 495–502.

114 Markos J, Musk AW, Finucane KE. Functional similarities of asbestosis and cryptogenic fibrosing alveolitis. *Thorax* 1988; **43**: 708–14.

115 Agusti AG, Roca J, Rodriguez-Roisin R, Xaubet A, Agusti-Vidal A. Different patterns of gas exchange response to exercise in asbestosis and idiopathic pulmonary fibrosis. *Eur Respir J* 1988; **1**: 510–16.

116 Lee YC, Singh B, Pang SC, et al. Radiographic (ILO) readings predict arterial oxygen desaturation during exercise in subjects with asbestosis. *Occup Environ Med* 2003; **60**: 201–6.

117 Neri S, Boraschi P, Antonelli A, Falaschi F, Baschieri L. Pulmonary function, smoking habits, and high resolution computed tomography (HRCT) early abnormalities of lung and pleural fibrosis in shipyard workers exposed to asbestos. *Am J Industr Med* 1996; **30**: 588–95.

118 Lebedova J, Diouha B, Rychia L, et al. Lung function impairment in relation to asbestos-induced pleural lesions with reference to the extent of the lesions and the initial parenchymal fibrosis. *Scand J Work Environment Health* 2003; **29**: 388–95.

119 Al Jarad N, Poulakis N, Peason MC, Rubens MB, Rudd RM. Assessment of asbestos-induced pleural disease by computed tomography: correlation with chest radiograph and lung function. *Respir Med* 1991; **85**: 203–8.

120 Kilburn KH, Warsaw RH. Abnormal lung function associated with asbestos disease of the pleura, the lung and both: a comparative analysis. *Thorax* 1991; **46**: 33–8.

121 Miller A, Lilis R, Godbald J, Chan E, Selikoff IJ. Relationship of pulmonary function to radiographic interstitial fibrosis in 2611 long-term asbestos insulators: an assessment of the International Labour Office profusion score. *Am Rev Respir Dis* 1992; **145**: 263–70.

122 Copley SJ, Lee YC, Hansell DM, et al. Asbestos-induced and smoking-related disease: apportioning pulmonary function deficit by using thin-section CT. *Radiology* 2007; **242**: 258–66.

123 Gevenois PA, Sergent G, De Maertelaer V, et al. Micronodules and emphysema in coal mine dust or

silica exposure: relation with lung function. *Eur Respir J* 1998; **12**: 1020–24.

124 Soutar CA, Hurley JF, Miller BG, Cowie HA, Buchanan D. Dust concentrations and respiratory risks in coalminers: key risk estimates from the British Pneumoconiosis Field Research. *Occup Environ Med* 2004; **61**: 477–81.

125 Akkoca YO, Eris Gulbay B, Saryal S, Karabiyikoglu G. Evaluation of the relationship between radiological abnormalities and both pulmonary function and pulmonary hypertension in coal workers' pneumoconiosis. *Respirology* 2007; **12**: 420–26.

126 Lapp NL, Hankinson JL, Burgess DB, O'Brien R. Changes in ventilatory function in coal miners after a work shift. *Arch Environ Health* 1972; **24**: 204–8.

127 Attfield MD, Hodous TK. Pulmonary function of US coal miners related to dust exposure estimates. *Am Rev Respir Dis* 1992; **145**: 605–9.

128 Kibelstis JA, Morgan EJ, Reger RB, *et al.* Prevalence of bronchitis and airway obstruction in American bituminous coal miners. *Am Rev Respir Dis* 1973; **108**: 886–93.

129 Morgan WKC, Burgess DB, Lapp NL, *et al.* Hyperinflation of the lungs in coal miners. *Thorax* 1971; **26**: 585–90.

130 Lapp NL, Seaton A. Lung mechanics in coal workers' pneumoconiosis. *Ann NY Acad Sci* 1972; **200**: 433–54.

131 Murphy DMF, Hall DR, Petersen MR, Lapp NL. The effects of coal workers' pneumoconiosis on lung mechanics. *Bull Eur Physiopathol Respir* 1978; **14**: 61–74.

132 Billiet L, van der Woestijne KP, Prignot J, Gyselin A. La capacityé; de diffusion pulmonaire chez le silicotique. *Acta Tuberc Belg* 1964; **55**: 255–8.

133 Cockcroft A, Berry G, Cotes JE, Lyons JP. Shape of small opacities and lung function in coal workers. *Thorax* 1982; **37**: 765–9.

134 Seaton A, Lapp NL, Chang CHJ. Lung perfusion scanning in coal workers' pneumoconiosis. *Am Rev Respir Dis* 1971; **103**: 338–49.

135 Ng T-P, Chan S-L. Lung function in relation to silicosis and silica exposure in granite workers. *Eur Respir J* 1992; **5**: 986–91.

136 Marek K, Kujawska A. L'influence des lesions pneumoconiotiques précoces sur la fonction respiratoire. *4th International Pneumoconiosis Conference*, Bucharest, 1971, p. 375.

137 Bégin R, Ostiguy G, Cantin A, Bergeron D. Lung function in silica-exposed workers: a relationship to disease severity assessed by CT scan. *Chest* 1988; **94**: 539–45.

138 Cowie RL, Mabena SK. Silicosis, chronic airflow limitation and chronic bronchitis in South African gold miners. *Am Rev Respir Dis* 1991; **143**: 80–84.

139 Hertzberg VS, Rosenman KD, Reilly MJ, Rice CH. Effect of occupational silica exposure on pulmonary function. *Chest* 2002; **122**: 721–8.

140 Kinsella M, Muller N, Vedal S, *et al.* Emphysema in silicosis: a comparison of smokers with non-smokers using pulmonary function testing and computed tomography. *Am Rev Respir Dis* 1990; **141**: 1497–500.

141 Cowie RL, Hay M, Thomas RG. Association of silicosis, lung dysfunction and emphysema in gold miners. *Thorax* 1993; **48**: 746–9.

142 Arakawa M, Gevenois PA, Saito Y, *et al.* Silicosis: expiratory thin-section CT assessment of airway obstruction. *Radiology* 2005; **236**: 1059–66.

143 Crausman RS, Jennings CA, Tuder RM, *et al.* Pulmonary histiocytosis X: pulmonary function and exercise pathophysiology. *Am J Respir Crit Care Med* 1996; **153**: 426–35.

144 Fartoukh M, Humbert M, Capron F, *et al.* Severe pulmonary hypertension in histiocytosis X. *Am J Respir Crit Care Med* 2000; **161**: 216–23.

145 Elliott JA. Severe airways obstruction as a presenting feature of pulmonary histiocytosis-X: a case report. *Br J Dis Chest* 1983; **77**: 299–302.

146 Delobbe A, Durieu J, Duhamel A, Wallaert B. Determinants of survival in pulmonary Langerhans' cell granulomatosis (histiocytosis X). Groupe d'Etude en Pathologie Interstitielle de la Societe de Pathologie Thoracique du Nord. *Eur Respir J* 1996; **9**: 2002–6.

147 Vassallo R, Ryu J, Schroeder D, Decker P, Limper A. Clinical outcomes of pulmonary Langerhans' cell histiocytosis in adults. *N Engl J Med* 2002; **346**: 484–90.

148 Ryu JH, Moss J, Beck GJ, *et al.* The NHLBI lymphangioleiomyomatosis registry: characteristics of 230 patients at enrollment. *Am J Respir Crit Care Med* 2006; **173**: 105–11.

149 Crausman RS, Jennings CA, Mortenson RL, *et al.* Lymphangioleiomyomatosis: the pathophysiology of diminished exercise capacity. *Am J Respir Crit Care Med* 1996; **153**: 1368–76.

150 Burger CD, Hyatt RE, Staats BA. Pulmonary mechanics in lymphangioleiomyomatosis. *Am Rev Respir Dis* 1991; **143**: 1030–33.

151 Taveira-DaSilva AM, Stylianou MP, Hedin CJ, *et al.* Maximal oxygen uptake and severity of disease in lymphangioleiomyomatosis. *Am J Respir Crit Care Med* 2003; **168**: 1427–31.

152 Taveira-DaSilva AM, Stylianou MP, Hedin CJ, Hathaway O, Moss J. Decline in lung function in patients with lymphangioleiomyomatosis treated with or without progesterone. *Chest* 2004; **126**: 1867–74.

153 Lazor R, Valeyre D, Lacronique H, *et al.* The Groupe d'Etudes et de Recherche sur les Maladies

'Orphelines' Pulmonaires. Low initial KCO pre-dicts rapid FEV1 decline in pulmonary lymphangi-oleiomyomatosis. *Respir Med* 2004; **98**: 536–41.

154 Guerry-Force ML, Muller NL, Wright JL, *et al.* A comparison of bronchiolitis obliterans with organizing pneumonia, usual interstitial pneumonia and small airways disease. *Am Rev Respir Dis* 1987; **135**: 705–12.

155 Rogers RM, Levin DC, Gray BA, Moseley LW. Physiologic effects of bronchopulmonary lavage in alveolar proteinosis. *Am Rev Respir Dis* 1978; **118**: 255–64.

156 Goldstein LS, Kavuru MS, Curtis-McCarthy P, *et al.* Pulmonary alveolar proteinosis: clinical fea-tures and outcomes. *Chest* 1998; **114**: 1357–62.

157 Lin F-C, Chen Y-C, Chang H-I, Chang S-C. Effect of body position on gas exchange in patients with idiopathic pulmonary alveolar proteinosis: no bene-fit of prone positioning. *Chest* 2005; **127**: 1058–64.

158 Cottin V, Tebib J, Massonnet B, Souquet PJ, Bernard JP. Pulmonary function in patients receiving long-term low-dose methotrexate. *Chest* 1996; **109**: 933–8.

159 Sunderji R, Kanji Z, Gin K. Pulmonary effects of low dose amiodarone: a review of the risks and rec-ommendations for surveillance. *Can J Cardiol* 2000; **16**: 1435–40.

160 Ohar JA, Jackson F Jr, Redd RM, Evans GR, Bedrossian CW. Usefulness of serial pulmonary function testing as an indicator of amiodarone toxicity. *Am J Cardiol* 1989; **64**: 1322–6.

161 Gleadhill IC, Wise RA, Schonfeld SA, *et al.* Serial lung function testing in patients treated with amio-darone: a prospective study. *Am J Med* 1989; **86**: 4–10.

162 Adams PC, Gibson GJ, Morley AR, *et al.* Amiodarone pulmonary toxicity: clinical and subclinical features. *Q J Med* 1986; **59**: 449–71.

163 Abratt RP, Morgan GW. Lung toxicity following chest irradiation in patients with lung cancer. *Lung Cancer* 2002; **35**: 103–9.

15

Pulmonary Vascular Disease

15.1 PULMONARY THROMBOEMBOLISM

The most specific functional information in patients with suspected pulmonary embolism (PE) is obtained from isotope scans. With the wide availability of spiral computed tomography (CT) scanning, isotope scans are used less often than hitherto, but they still have a role in clinical investigation (see below). Simple spirometric volumes (FEV_1, VC) are usually normal in uncomplicated pulmonary embolism, but they may be reduced if full inspiration is impeded by chest pain. Their main role is in differential diagnosis of acute breathlessness and in recognizing patients with coexisting airway obstruction (chronic obstructive pulmonary disease (COPD) or asthma). The characteristic pattern of arterial blood gases in acute pulmonary embolism is a reduction in both PaO_2 and $PaCO_2$ together with a respiratory alkalosis.

15.1.1 Gas exchange in acute pulmonary embolism

Detailed investigation of the distribution of ventilation and perfusion using the multiple inert gas elimination technique (MIGET)[1] and single photon emission computed tomography (SPECT)[2] in patients with acute PE shows uneven distribution of both alveolar ventilation ($\dot{V}_A$) and perfusion ($\dot{Q}$) with an abnormally wide dispersion of $\dot{V}_A/\dot{Q}$ ratios and an overall shift to a higher average $\dot{V}_A/\dot{Q}$

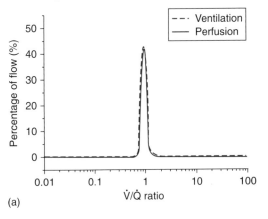

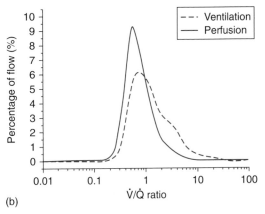

Figure 15.1 Distributions of ventilation and perfusion derived from single photon emission computed tomography (SPECT) scanning in a subject with pulmonary embolism (b) compared with normal (a). Note the broader distributions of both ventilation ($\dot{V}$) and perfusion ($\dot{Q}$) and the overall higher $\dot{V}/\dot{Q}$ ratio in the individual with pulmonary embolism. Redrawn from ref. 2 with permission from the American Thoracic Society.

(Fig. 15.1). The increase in overall $\dot{V}_A/\dot{Q}$ ratio corresponds to an increased physiological dead space, while the low $\dot{V}_A/\dot{Q}$ units contribute to arterial hypoxaemia. An additional factor, which acts synergistically with $\dot{V}_A/\dot{Q}$ inequality to reduce PaO_2, is a reduction in mixed venous PO_2 consequent on a reduced cardiac output.[1,3] There is no evidence of significant limitation to diffusion of oxygen, and increases in anatomical shunt are usually insignificant. The hypocapnia reflects an increase in alveolar and overall ventilation.

Arterial blood gas measurements have only a limited role in the diagnosis of PE: although a reduced PaO_2 is relatively sensitive, it is of course very non-specific. Because the reduced PaO_2 is associated with hypocapnia, the alveolar–arterial PO_2 difference ($AaPO_2$) may be markedly increased and is more sensitive than the PaO_2 alone.[4] However, even a normal $AaPO_2$ does not exclude acute PE,[5] and in practice no blood gas abnormalities are sufficiently specific to influence the diagnosis.[6,7] It has, however, been shown that a reduced initial oxygen saturation (SaO_2) below 95 per cent has predictive value in relation to the likelihood of subsequent complications (including mortality), whereas SaO_2 of 95 per cent or higher on room air at diagnosis is associated with a low probability of complications.[8]

Measurement of the physiological dead space has been suggested as a useful clinical test for detecting likely PE. The dead space/tidal volume (V_D/V_T) ratio is calculated using the Bohr equation (see Chapter 2, Section 2.1.2), with accurate measurement of tidal volume and mixed expired PCO_2 required in addition to the arterial value. Although the size of the dead space correlates with the size of perfusion defects demonstrable by scintigraphy,[9] in practice it is disappointing as a diagnostic test.[10]

Another test recommended in the older literature but no longer used is measurement of the so-called arterial–alveolar PCO_2 gradient ($aAPCO_2$). This is more appropriately described as the arterial to end tidal PCO_2 ($P_{et}CO_2$) gradient. Its theoretical justification is based on the fact that, in pulmonary vascular obstruction, the unperfused alveoli contribute no CO_2 to the mixed alveolar gas and therefore a gradient develops between the mean alveolar PCO_2 and the arterial PCO_2. In terms of the Riley–Cournand three-compartment model of gas exchange (see Chapter 2, Section 2.3.4), this is analogous to the increased physiological dead space. Although it is occasionally advocated as a useful clinical test for pulmonary embolism, in practice an abnormal value is non-specific as it is increased in chronic airway disease and other conditions in which maldistribution of ventilation makes the $P_{et}CO_2$ unrepresentative of the mean alveolar value.

Measuring the single-breath carbon monoxide diffusing capacity (D_LCO) may be impracticable in the acute stage of major pulmonary embolism but it can be obtained in less ill patients and shows a moderate reduction.[11,12]

15.1.2 Lung scintigraphy

For many years the mainstay of investigation of patients with suspected PE was ventilation and perfusion scanning using radioisotopes, and scintigraphy still has a role in excluding the diagnosis. In principle, the most specific diagnostic finding is typical wedge-shaped defects of perfusion with a normal distribution of ventilation (Fig. 15.2). Compensatory changes in the distribution of ventilation may, however, occur,[1] and subsequent pulmonary infarction can result in 'matched' defects that are much less specific diagnostically. Frequently, the picture is also clouded by coexisting chronic airway disease, which itself produces patchy distribution of ventilation and perfusion, although usually with less clearly defined defects and apparent matching on a macroscopic scale (see Fig. 9.13 in Chapter 9). In general, a completely normal perfusion scan is good evidence against significant PE,[13,14] although rare cases have been reported of extensive embolism in the face of an apparently normal scan.[15] Diagnostic accuracy is greatest when the $\dot{V}/\dot{Q}$ scan is evaluated alongside the pre-test clinical probability of PE, with both the clinical features and the scan appearances graded simply in terms of high, intermediate and low probability. Using this approach, and with pulmonary angiography as the final criterion, the authors of the Prospective Investigation of Pulmonary Embolism Diagnosis (PIOPED) study found that the combination of high clinical probability and a high probability scan was associated with a 95 per cent likelihood of PE, whereas with low clinical and scan probability the likelihood was only 4 per cent.[14]

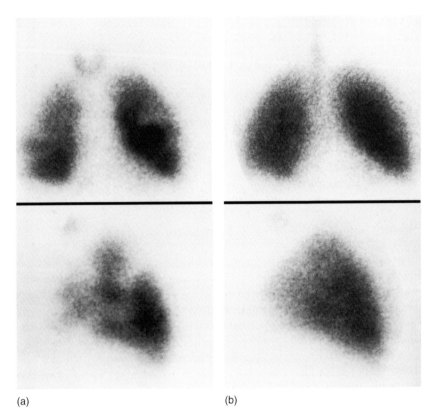

(a)   (b)

Figure 15.2 Anteroposterior (upper) and lateral (lower) (a) [99mTc] perfusion and (b) [81mKr] ventilation scans in a patient with pulmonary emboli. At least three clearly demarcated, wedge-shaped segmental defects of perfusion can be seen, but the distribution of ventilation is normal.

However, confident diagnosis is not possible in a large number of individuals with intermediate probability scans.

Several attempts have been made to automate quantitative measurements from lung scans, but to date none has been widely applied.[16,17] One of the difficulties with conventional isotope scans is their two-dimensional nature: studies with SPECT imaging (which provides three-dimensional scans) have suggested that this may be more sensitive and specific for diagnosing PE, and with a much lower radiation dose than spiral CT scanning.[18] This technique gives overall information on the distribution of ventilation and perfusion as well as three-dimensional regional information. In a recent SPECT study, the overall increase in the weighted median $\dot{V}/\dot{Q}$ value was found to be the most accurate diagnostic index of PE[2] (Fig. 15.1). Application

of SPECT technology seems likely to lead to a resurgence of interest in scintigraphic methods.

15.1.3 Chronic pulmonary thromboembolism

Patients with chronic pulmonary thromboembolism show similar functional features to those with acute embolism (i.e. hypoxaemia, hypocapnia, increased physiological dead space and reduced $D_L CO$). The mechanism of hypoxaemia is again increased dispersion of $\dot{V}_A/\dot{Q}$ ratios, amplified by a reduction in mixed venous oxygen tension.[19,20] Usually the $D_L CO$ and $K CO$ are impaired only modestly, possibly due to uptake of CO by the bronchial circulation, which develops anastomoses with the pulmonary circulation in embolized areas. A more markedly reduced $D_L CO$ (e.g. less than 50% predicted) in a patient with pulmonary hypertension should prompt a search for another cause such as pulmonary fibrosis.[21]

15.2 CHRONIC (PRIMARY) PULMONARY HYPERTENSION

Apart from differences in the scan appearances, the functional abnormalities in patients with pulmonary hypertension due to chronic thromboembolic disease and primary pulmonary hypertension are broadly similar.

15.2.1 Respiratory mechanics

Mechanical function of the lungs and thorax is usually within normal limits, although subtle abnormalities have been demonstrated in comparison with matched groups of healthy subjects. A small average reduction of VC has been reported in patients with primary pulmonary hypertension, but values are usually around 85–90 per cent predicted and within the normal reference range.[22,23] A modest reduction in maximum respiratory pressures was reported in one study;[24] the cause is not known, but this might contribute to the minor reduction of VC. However, TLC appears to be unaffected, while, on average, RV is slightly increased.[23] Evidence of mild airway obstruction was reported in one study of patients with more severe pulmonary hypertension, with a reduction in maximum expiratory flow particularly at low lung volumes, but without an increase in overall airway resistance, suggesting narrowing of the smaller airways.[23]

15.2.2 Co-diffusing capacity

Some reduction in the $D_L CO$ is almost universal in patients with clinically significant pulmonary hypertension.[22,25] The decrease in $D_L CO$ correlates with decreases in maximum oxygen uptake on exercise.[26] The transfer coefficient (KCO) is also characteristically reduced, as are both the membrane diffusing capacity (D_m) and the capillary blood volume (V_c) components of $D_L CO$.[27]

15.2.3 Pulmonary gas exchange

The characteristic abnormalities of pulmonary gas exchange in patients with pulmonary hypertension are hypoxaemia and hypocapnia. The latter reflects the increased ventilatory drive and persistent hyperventilation seen in these patients. Indeed, the severity of hypocapnia has been shown to relate independently to mortality from the condition.[28] Detailed studies of gas exchange have shown that hypoxaemia results from the combination of ventilation/perfusion mismatching and small intrapulmonary shunts, amplified by the low mixed venous oxygenation due to a low cardiac output.[29] On scintigraphic perfusion scanning, clear-cut defects are less obvious than with thromboembolic disease. Although minor irregularities are often seen (Fig. 15.3), the scan appearances may be helpful in distinguishing the two conditions.[30]

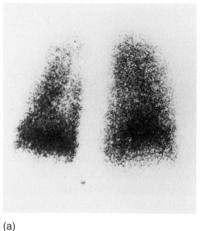 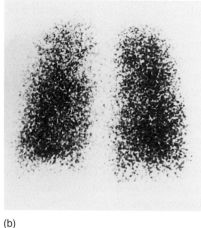

(a)   (b)

Figure 15.3 Posteroanterior ^{99m}Tc perfusion (a) and ^{133}Xe inhalation (b) scans in a patient with primary pulmonary hypertension. The inhalation scan is normal, but some unevenness of perfusion is visible. The perfusion defects are less clearly defined than in pulmonary emboli (cf. Fig. 15.2).

15.2.4 Exercise

During progressive exercise testing, patients with pulmonary hypertension characteristically show a marked reduction in maximum (peak) oxygen consumption ($\dot{V}O_2$max). At the break point of exercise, minute ventilation is close to that seen in healthy subjects due to the considerable hyperventilation, while at submaximal workloads ventilation is consistently excessive for the metabolic load (oxygen consumption or CO_2 output). Exercise is limited essentially by the cardiovascular system and, in particular, by the reduced stroke volume associated with increased pulmonary vascular resistance.[31,32] The rate of change of $\dot{V}O_2$ with increase in work rate is reduced in pulmonary hypertension compared with normal, due to the impaired circulatory response to exercise.[32] Hypocapnia and hypoxaemia persist during exercise and a further fall in oxygen saturation is commonly seen.[32]

The 6-min walk distance (6MWD) is used widely in assessing patients with pulmonary hypertension[33,34] and evaluating the effects of drug treatment.[35,36] As with progressive cardiopulmonary exercise testing, performance is limited by the restricted stroke volume,[34] and the MWD and $\dot{V}O_2$max correlate well.[33] The 6MWD and severity of hypocapnia have been shown to be the most important functional correlates of mortality in patients with pulmonary hypertension.[28,33]

15.2.5 Respiratory function during sleep

Oxygen desaturation during sleep is common in patients with pulmonary hypertension.[37,38] It may occur even among subjects who do not desaturate on exercise, but, inevitably, it is more common and more severe in those with arterial hypoxaemia when awake. In some individuals, particularly those with advanced disease, intermittent hypoxaemia during sleep is associated with periodic breathing of typical Cheyne–Stokes type.[39] The background conditions of low cardiac output, slowed circulation time and hyperventilation are the optimal setting in which Cheyne–Stokes respiration is likely to develop (see Chapter 6, Section 6.2.1). It can be corrected by increasing the inspired oxygen concentration,[39] or, more permanently, by successful lung transplantation.[40] Whether the presence of Cheyne–Stokes respiration has an adverse effect on the prognosis of pulmonary hypertension over and above that implied by the severity of the underlying condition is not known.

15.3 NON-THROMBOTIC PULMONARY EMBOLISM

Extensive fat embolism can result in the acute respiratory distress syndrome (ARDS), with poorly compliant lungs and extreme difficulty in maintaining oxygenation (see Chapter 13, Section 13.5). Mild hypoxaemia, due presumably to microscopic fat embolism, is common after fractures of long bones,[41] and fat and bone marrow cell embolization can also produce hypoxaemia after hip arthroplasty.[42]

Functional abnormalities also occur after lymphangiography, due to microembolism of droplets of the oily medium. An injection of 20 mL of ethiodol in the pedal lymphatics produces an average reduction in D_LCO of about 30 per cent, with the nadir seen after 2–3 days.[43] In most subjects with otherwise healthy lungs there is no measurable change in blood gases, but those with preexisting lung disease are at greater risk of serious functional disturbance. D_LCO is useful as a screening test to identify those at risk, but the problem is rare nowadays as the technique is used so infrequently.

Pulmonary air embolism has been shown to produce transient perfusion scan defects similar to those seen with thrombotic PE, but the abnormalities typically resolve in a few hours.[44]

15.4 PULMONARY VENO-OCCLUSIVE DISEASE

Pulmonary function has been reported only in occasional cases of this rare condition. The features are generally similar to those found in primary or thromboembolic pulmonary arterial hypertension, with similar appearances on $\dot{V}/\dot{Q}$ scanning.[45] Lung volumes are usually normal but fall in the presence of radiographically evident pulmonary oedema. Reductions in PaO_2 and D_LCO can be profound.[46]

15.5 PULMONARY ARTERIOVENOUS MALFORMATIONS

15.5.1 Characteristics of hypoxaemia

Pulmonary arteriovenous malformations (AVMs) are abnormal communications between pulmonary arteries and pulmonary veins, usually congenital in nature. They result in anatomical shunts, which cause arterial hypoxaemia not corrected by breathing 100 per cent oxygen. Patients characteristically have a low PaO_2 and SaO_2 and also a low $PaCO_2$ with a respiratory alkalosis due to chronic hyperventilation.[47] The severity of the hypoxaemia is a function of blood flow through the AVMs and depends on their size and number. Characteristically, the hypoxaemia of AVMs varies with posture and also with the degree of lung inflation. Most patients show the phenomenon of orthodeoxia, in which PaO_2 and SaO_2 are lower in the upright than in the supine position. This occurs because most patients have AVMs that are predominantly basally situated, and it reflects the disproportionately large, gravity-dependent, basal blood flow in the upright posture.[48] Oxygenation therefore needs to be interpreted in light of the posture in which SaO_2 was measured or arterial blood was sampled. Apparent discrepancies in results can result from ignoring this simple observation.

Blood flowing through the shunt bypasses alveoli and is not exposed directly to alveolar pressure. At high lung volumes, therefore, where pulmonary vascular resistance normally increases, the fistula tends to 'steal' more blood and its vessels may be distended further by the surrounding inflated lung. The increased flow at high volumes may result in the well-recognized physical sign of a bruit, increasing in intensity on inspiration.

15.5.2 Measurements of anatomical shunt

Classically, the size of the anatomical shunt is quantified by measuring PaO_2 after the subject has breathed 100 per cent oxygen for 15–20 min, on the principle that, if hypoxaemia were due to mismatching of ventilation and perfusion, breathing pure oxygen would eventually result in normalization of arterial oxygenation, whereas if blood is

bypassing gas exchanging areas of the lung, normal oxygenation cannot be achieved (see Chapter 4, Section 4.4.2.4). In patients with pulmonary AVMs the percentage shunt calculated in this way shows an alinear relationship to resting arterial saturation (Fig. 15.4). An alternative method for calculating the shunt is by comparison of the number of isotopically labelled particles deposited systemically with that in the lungs following intravenous injection. Comparison of uptake by the kidneys with the lungs (on the assumption that the kidneys receive 10% of the cardiac output) gives values for anatomical shunt similar to those obtained by breathing 100 per cent oxygen.[50] With the more commonly used oxygen method, considerable care needs to be taken that the subject is indeed breathing pure oxygen, using an airtight mouthpiece and wearing a noseclip, and that the blood is sampled anaerobically and analysed rapidly. Due to the large PO_2 gradient in this situation between arterial blood and room air, introduction of even a tiny air bubble will cause serious underestimation of PaO_2 and consequent overestimation of the shunt.

15.5.3 Co-diffusing capacity and exercise performance

A mild or moderate reduction in both D_LCO and KCO is common in patients with pulmonary AVMs,[51,52] probably because most lesions are

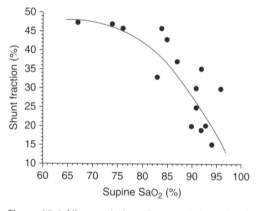

Figure 15.4 Alinear relation of per cent shunt fraction breathing 100 per cent oxygen and oxygen saturation in a group of patients with pulmonary arteriovenous malformations. Redrawn from ref. 49 with permission from the American Thoracic Society.

SaO_2, oxygen saturation.

multiple and smaller ones may not be visualized. Hyperventilation persists on exercise,[47] but exercise capacity is relatively well preserved.[49] The effect of exercise on oxygenation is variable; changes in oxygen saturation correlate with changes in the shunt fraction, which may either increase or decrease so that, on average in large groups of patients, oxygenation shows little change.[51]

15.5.4 Effects of therapeutic embolization

The standard treatment for pulmonary AVMs is by embolization, usually using small metal coils introduced into the vessels feeding the lesions. These decrease the shunt, increasing PaO_2 and SaO_2. Measurements of oxygenation and shunt fraction are key in monitoring progress and recognizing increasing size of the lesions or the development of new ones requiring further treatment. Successful embolization is often accompanied by a small increase in both D_LCO and KCO,[52,53] but some reduction often persists even after treating all the radiographically visible lesions, presumably because smaller vascular abnormalities remain. Objective evidence of improved exercise capacity has been demonstrated in a minority of patients after embolization.[53]

15.6 SYSTEMIC VASCULITIDES

Patients with the Churg–Strauss syndrome or 'allergic angiitis and granulomatosis' are characteristically asthmatic and therefore have evidence of variable airflow obstruction.[54] A combined obstructive and restrictive ventilatory defect may be seen as the condition is also associated with a variable degree of consolidation.

Wegener's granulomatosis (now categorized as 'anti-neutrophil cytoplasmic antibody (ANCA)-associated vasculitis') is characterized radiographically by one or more large, often cavitating opacities but sometimes more generalized shadowing is seen. Depending on the extent of the lung disease, reduced VC, TLC and D_LCO may be seen.[55] Airway obstruction is also common as a result of disease affecting either the central or peripheral airways. In one series, an obstructive defect on spirometry was seen more frequently than volume restriction.[55] Extensive narrowing of the central airway can produce the characteristic flow volume curve appearances of upper airway narrowing (see Chapter 12, Section 12.1.2). Maximum respiratory pressures are often impaired, even in subjects without overt respiratory involvement or corticosteroid treatment. Exercise capacity is reduced, as might be expected with a systemic illness associated with weakness.[56] Most data on D_LCO suggest that this is reduced approximately in proportion to the volume loss, such that KCO is normal or mildly impaired.[55,56]

REFERENCES

1 Santolicandro A, Prediletto R, Fornai E, et al. Mechanisms of hypoxemia and hypocapnia in pulmonary embolism. Am J Respir Crit Care Med 1995; 152: 336–47.
2 Harris B, Bailey D, Miles S, et al. Objective analysis of tomographic ventilation–perfusion scintigraphy in pulmonary embolism. Am J Respir Crit Care Med 2007; 175: 1173–80.
3 Manier G, Castaing Y. Influence of cardiac output on oxygen exchange in acute pulmonary embolism. Am Rev Respir Dis 1992; 145: 130–36.
4 Stein PD, Terrin ML, Hales CA, et al. Clinical, laboratory, roentgenographic, and electrocardiographic findings in patients with acute pulmonary embolism and no pre-existing cardiac or pulmonary disease. Chest 1991; 100: 598–603.
5 Stein PD, Goldhaber SZ, Henry JW. Alveolar–arterial oxygen gradient in the assessment of acute pulmonary embolism. Chest 1995; 107: 139–43.
6 Jones JS, Neff TL, Carlson SA. Use of the alveolar–arterial oxygen gradient in the assessment of acute pulmonary embolism. Am J Emerg Med 1998; 16: 333–7.
7 Rodger MA, Carrier M, Jones GN, et al. Diagnostic value of arterial blood gas measurement in suspected pulmonary embolism. Am J Respir Crit Care Med 2000; 162: 2105–8.
8 Kline JA, Hernandez-Nino J, Newgard CD, et al. Use of pulse oximetry to predict in-hospital complications in normotensive patients with pulmonary embolism. Am J Med 2003; 115: 203–8.
9 Kline JA, Kubin AK, Patel MM, Easton EJ, Seupal RA. Alveolar dead space as a predictor of severity of pulmonary embolism. Acad Emerg Med 2000; 7: 611–17.

10 Hogg K, Dawson D, Tabor T, Tabor B, Mackway-Jones K. Respiratory dead space measurement in the investigation of pulmonary embolism in outpatients with pleuritic chest pain. *Chest* 2005; **128**: 2195–202.

11 Wimalaratna HSK, Farrell J, Lee HY. Measurement of diffusing capacity in pulmonary embolism. *Respir Med* 1989; **83**: 481–6.

12 Fennerty AG, Gunawardena KA, Smith AP. The transfer factor and its subdivisions in patients with pulmonary emboli. *Eur Respir J* 1988; **1**: 98–101.

13 Hull RD, Raskob GE, Coates G, Panju AA. Clinical validity of a normal perfusion lung scan in patients with suspected pulmonary embolism. *Chest* 1990; **97**: 23–6.

14 PIOPED investigators. Value of the ventilation/perfusion scan in acute pulmonary embolism: results of the prospective investigation of pulmonary embolism diagnosis (PIOPED). *J Am Med Assoc* 1990; **263**: 2753–9.

15 Brandsbetter RD, Naccarato E, Sperber RJ, *et al.* Normal lung perfusion scan with extensive thromboembolic disease. *Chest* 1987; **92**: 565–6.

16 Holst H, Mare K, Jarund A, *et al.* An independent evaluation of a new method for automated interpretation of lung scintigrams using artificial neural networks. *Eur J Nucl Med* 2001; **28**: 33–8.

17 Frigyesi A. An automated method for the detection of pulmonary embolism in V/Q-scans. *Med Image Anal* 2003; **7**: 341–9.

18 Reinartz P, Kaiser HJ, Wildberger JE, *et al.* SPECT imaging in the diagnosis of pulmonary embolism: automated detection of match and mismatch defects by means of image-processing techniques. *J Nucl Med* 2006; **47**: 968–73.

19 Kapitan KS, Buchbinder M, Wagner PD, Moser KM. Mechanisms of hypoxaemia in chronic thromboembolic pulmonary hypertension. *Am Rev Respir Dis* 1989; **139**: 1149–54.

20 Kapitan KS, Clausen JL, Moser KM. Gas exchange in chronic thromboembolism after pulmonary thromboendarterectomy. *Chest* 1990; **98**: 14–19.

21 Williams MH, Adler JJ, Colp C. Pulmonary function studies as an aid in the differential diagnosis of pulmonary hypertension. *Am J Med* 1969; **47**: 378–83.

22 Rich S, Dantzker DR, Ayres SM, *et al.* Primary pulmonary hypertension: a national prospective study. *Ann Intern Med* 1987; **107**: 216–23.

23 Meyer FJ, Ewert R, Hoeper MM, *et al.* Peripheral airway obstruction in primary pulmonary hypertension. *Thorax* 2002; **57**: 473–6.

24 Meyer FJ, Lossnitzer D, Kristen AV, *et al.* Respiratory muscle dysfunction in idiopathic pulmonary arterial hypertension. *Eur Respir J* 2005; **25**: 125–30.

25 Burke CM, Glanville AR, Morris AJR, *et al.* Pulmonary function in advanced pulmonary hypertension. *Thorax* 1987; **42**: 131–5.

26 Sun XG, Hansen JE, Oudiz RJ, Wasserman K. Pulmonary function in primary pulmonary hypertension. *J Am Coll Cardiol* 2003; **41**: 1028–35.

27 Oppenheimer BW, Berger KI, Hadjiangelis NP, *et al.* Membrane diffusion in diseases of the pulmonary vasculature. *Respir Med* 2006; **100**: 1247–53.

28 Hoeper MM, Pietz MW, Golpon H, Welte T. Prognostic value of blood gas analyses in patients with idiopathic pulmonary arterial hypertension. *Eur Respir J* 2007; **29**: 944–50.

29 Dantzker DR, Bower JS. Mechanisms of gas exchange abnormality in patients with chronic obstructive pulmonary vascular disease. *J Clin Invest* 1979; **64**: 1050–55.

30 Chapman PJ, Bateman ED, Benatar SR. Primary pulmonary hypertension and thromboembolic pulmonary hypertension: similarities and differences. *Respir Med* 1990; **84**: 485–8.

31 D'Alonzo GE, Gianotti LA, Pohil RL, *et al.* Comparison of progressive exercise performance of normal subjects and patients with primary pulmonary hypertension. *Chest* 1987; **92**: 57–62.

32 Riley MS, Porszasz J, Engelen MP, Brundage BH, Wasserman K. Gas exchange responses to continuous incremental cycle ergometry exercise in primary pulmonary hypertension in humans. *Eur J Appl Physiol* 2000; **83**: 63–70.

33 Miyamoto S, Nagaya N, Satoh T, *et al.* Clinical correlates and prognostic significance of six-minute walk test in patients with primary pulmonary hypertension: comparison with cardiopulmonary exercise testing. *Am J Respir Crit Care Med* 2000; **161**: 487–92.

34 Provencher S, Chemia D, Herve P, *et al.* Heart rate responses during the 6-minute walk test in pulmonary arterial hypertension. *Eur Respir J* 2006; **27**: 114–20.

35 Barst RJ, Rubin LJ, Long WA, *et al.* A comparison of continuous intravenous epoprostenol (prostacyclin) with conventional therapy for primary pulmonary hypertension. The Primary Pulmonary Hypertension Study Group. *N Engl J Med* 1996; **334**: 296–302.

36 Reichenberger F, Mainwood A, Doughty N, *et al.* Effects of nebulised iloprost on pulmonary function and gas exchange in severe pulmonary hypertension. *Respir Med* 2007; **101**: 217–22.

37 Rafanan AL, Golish JA, Dinner DS, Hague LK, Arroliga AC. Nocturnal hypoxemia is common in primary pulmonary hypertension. *Chest* 2001; **120**: 894–9.

38 Minai OA, Pandya CM, Golish JA, *et al.* Predictors of nocturnal oxygen desaturation in pulmonary arterial hypertension. *Chest* 2007; **131**: 109–17.

39 Schulz R, Baseler G, Ghofrani HA, *et al.* 2002; Nocturnal periodic breathing in primary pulmonary hypertension. *Eur Respir J* **19**: 658–63.

40 Schulz R, Fegbeutel C, Olschewski H, *et al.* Reversal of nocturnal periodic breathing in primary pulmonary hypertension after lung transplantation. *Chest* 2004; **125**: 344–7.

41 Wong MW, Tsui HF, Yung SH, Chan KM, Cheng JC. Continuous pulse oximeter monitoring for inapparent hypoxemia after long bone fractures. *J Trauma* 2004; **56**: 356–62.

42 Kim YH, Oh SW, Kim JS. Prevalence of fat embolism following bilateral simultaneous and unilateral total hip arthroplasty performed with or without cement: a prospective, randomized clinical study. *J Bone Joint Surg* 2002; **84**: 1372–9.

43 Weg JG, Harkleroad LE. Aberrations in pulmonary function due to lymphangiography. *Dis Chest* 1968; **53**: 534–40.

44 Sessler CN, Kiser PE, Raval V. Transient pulmonary perfusion scintigraphic abnormalities in pulmonary air embolism. *Chest* 1989; **95**: 910–11.

45 Bailey CL, Channick RN, Auger WR, *et al.* 'High probability' perfusion lung scans in pulmonary venoocclusive disease. *Am J Respir Crit Care Med* 2000; **162**: 1974–8.

46 Elliott CG, Colby TV, Hill T, Crapo RO. Pulmonary veno-occlusive disease associated with severe reduction of single-breath carbon monoxide diffusing capacity. *Respiration* 1988; **53**: 262–6.

47 Terry PB, White RI, Barth KH, Kaufman SL, Mitchell SE. Pulmonary arteriovenous malformations: physiologic observations and results of therapeutic balloon embolization. *N Engl J Med* 1983; **308**: 1197–200.

48 Robin ED, Laman D, Horn BR, Theodore J. Platypnea related to orthodeoxia caused by true vascular lung shunts. *N Engl J Med* 1976; **294**: 941–3.

49 Chilvers ER, Whyte MKB, Jackson JE, Allison DJ, Hughes JMB. Effect of percutaneous transcatheter embolization on pulmonary function, right-to-left shunt and arterial oxygenation in patients with pulmonary arteriovenous malformations. *Am Rev Respir Dis* 1990; **142**: 420–25.

50 Whyte MKB, Peters AM, Hughes JMB, *et al.* Quantification of right to left shunt at rest and during exercise in patients with pulmonary arteriovenous malformations. *Thorax* 1992; **47**: 790–96.

51 Pennington DW, Gold WM, Gordon RL, *et al.* Treatment of pulmonary arteriovenous malformations by therapeutic embolization: rest and exercise physiology in eight patients. *Am Rev Respir Dis* 1992; **145**: 1047–51.

52 Dutton JA, Jackson JE, Hughes JM, *et al.* Pulmonary arteriovenous malformations: results of treatment with coil embolization in 53 patients. *Am J Roentgenol* 1995; **165**: 1119–25.

53 Gupta P, Mordin C, Curtis J, *et al.* Pulmonary arteriovenous malformations: effect of embolization on right-to-left shunt, hypoxemia, and exercise tolerance in 66 patients. *Am J Roentgenol* 2002; **179**: 347–55.

54 Chumbley LC, Harrison EG, DeRemee RA. Allergic granulomatosis and angiitis (Churg–Strauss syndrome). *Mayo Clin Proc* 1977; **52**: 477–84.

55 Rosenberg DM, Weinberger SE, Fulmer JD, *et al.* Functional correlates of lung involvement in Wegener's granulomatosis. *Am J Med* 1980; **69**: 387–94.

56 Newall C, Schinke S, Savage CO, Hill S, Harper L. Impairment of lung function, health status and functional capacity in patients with ANCA-associated vasculitis. *Rheumatology* 2005; **44**: 623–8.

16

Diseases of the Pleura and Chest Wall

16.1 EXTRAPULMONARY RESTRICTION

Disorders of the pleural space, thoracic skeleton or inspiratory muscles prevent full expansion of the lungs and produce a similar functional picture of extrapulmonary volume restriction. Respiratory muscle weakness is considered in Chapter 20, Section 20.2. In addition to failure to distend the lungs fully, there are secondary functional effects on the lungs themselves. The effects of lung compression by a distorted thoracic cage, of microatelectasis owing to lack of a periodic full inspiration, or of mismatching of ventilation and perfusion, therefore often contribute to the results of conventional tests. In general the integrity of the alveolar–capillary membrane is retained, but impairment of full expansion may reduce carbon monoxide diffusing capacity ($D_L CO$) to some extent, while $K CO$ is typically high normal or frankly increased due to mismatching of alveolar and pulmonary capillary blood volumes (see Chapter 3, Section 3.1.2).

16.2 PNEUMOTHORAX

In the days when artificial pneumothorax was induced for treatment of tuberculosis, several studies were reported of its functional effects, but less information is available in patients with spontaneous pneumothorax. Air in the pleural space 'uncouples' the lung from the chest wall, causing not only partial deflation of the lung but also expansion of the chest wall in accordance with their individual pressure–volume (PV) relationships (Fig. 16.1). The changes in volume of the two components depend on their relative compliances: since these are normally similar at functional residual capacity (FRC), the volume reduction of one and increase of the other should also be similar, a conclusion supported by measurements of the volume expired during refilling an artificial pneumothorax.[1] Consequently, in a patient with a pneumothorax, the VC is reduced, but the reduction is less than the volume of air in the pleural space.[2]

Large differences between plethysmographic and gas dilution estimates of TLC are seen, with the difference approximating the volume of pneumothorax. In theory, it might be expected that the plethysmographic 'total thoracic volume' (i.e. TLC + pneumothorax volume) at full inflation would be greater than the normal TLC. In practice, however, this appears not to be the case, possibly because at full inflation the tendency for the ipsilateral chest wall to exceed its normal capacity is countered by mediastinal shift impeding complete expansion of the contralateral unaffected lung.[2] The traditional radiological technique of taking an expiratory film detects air in the pleural space more readily because if lung collapse is incomplete its volume is less on expiration and the pleural air therefore represents a larger proportion of the hemithorax.

Provided that there is free communication around the lung, a pneumothorax equalizes the

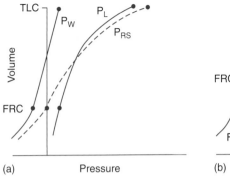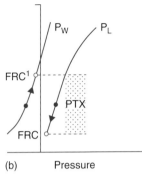

Figure 16.1 Theoretical effects of air in the pleural space on lung and chest wall in the affected hemithorax.
(a) Normal relations of chest wall (P_W) and lung recoil (P_L) to volume, with functional residual capacity (FRC) set by
the balance between P_L and P_W – i.e. recoil of the respiratory system (P_{RS}) is zero. (b) A pneumothorax (PTX)
uncouples the lung and chest wall so that each adopts a relaxation volume determined by the pleural pressure and
respective pressure–volume curve. FRC of the lung is reduced (● → ○), while the end expiratory volume of the chest
wall (FRC^1) increases. The volume of the pneumothorax equals (FRC^1 − FRC).

TLC, total lung capacity.

pleural pressure over the surface of the ipsilateral
lung. The consequent loss of the normal gradient of
pleural pressure abolishes gravity-dependent differences in regional lung volume[3] and might therefore
be expected to make the distribution of ventilation
more even. However, with moderate or large pneumothoraces, this is countered by a greater tendency
to airway closure in the partially collapsed lung.

Studies of gas exchange in animals during induc-
tion of a pneumothorax show an immediate fall in
arterial oxygenation, with a gradual return to normal levels over several hours. In patients with a persisting spontaneous pneumothorax (but otherwise
apparently normal lungs), a mild reduction in PaO_2
and an increase in alveolar–arterial PO_2 difference
($AaPO_2$) is common, even some days or weeks after
the acute event.[4] The effect is greater with larger
pneumothoraces, and measurement while breathing 100 per cent oxygen suggests an increased
'anatomical' shunt, compatible with continuing
perfusion of non-ventilated alveoli, presumably due
to areas of atelectasis. Immediately after aspiration
of a pneumothorax, the 'anatomical' shunt lessens
but the $AaPO_2$ and the dead space/tidal volume
ratio (V_D/V_T) may actually deteriorate initially due
to worsening ventilation/perfusion mismatching as
lung units open and the previously partly compensated relationships are disturbed.[4]

It is usually assumed that the lungs of the typical
young patient with spontaneous pneumothorax are
normal apart from the characteristic superficial apical 'blebs' that are evident at thorascopy. Follow-up
isotopic studies in such individuals may, however,
show more widespread changes, with reduction of
both ventilation and perfusion of the apical regions
of both the affected and (apparently) unaffected
lungs.[5] The functional features of generalized
emphysema with increased TLC and low K_{CO} are
seen in a significant proportion of patients,[6] especially in those presenting for the first time after the
age of 30 years. In younger patients long-term
effects of pneumothorax are minimal, although a
very mild restrictive defect may be seen years later,
especially if talc poudrage was used.[7]

16.3 PLEURAL EFFUSION

The relative paucity of data on pulmonary function
in patients with pleural effusion is mainly a result of
the difficulty in finding 'clean' cases, i.e. patients with
pleural fluid and no significant pulmonary disease. As
with pneumothorax, fluid between the visceral and
parietal pleural surfaces modifies the PV relations of
the lungs and chest wall, but the effects are less easy
to predict. When the pleural space contains a column of liquid, the gravitational effect on distribution
of pleural pressure is altered. In the normal situation
the pleural surface pressure and its vertical gradient
are determined by the recoil of lungs and chest wall

and by gravitational effects due to the weight of the lungs supported by the abdominal contents, but in the liquid column of a pleural effusion the gradient is determined by hydrostatic forces. If, in the presence of an effusion, the pleural liquid pressure is greater than normal, some expansion of the chest wall would be expected over the area of the effusion, while above the effusion normal pleural surface pressure relationships should apply. However, because the ribcage tends to move as a unit, there may still be a tendency to enlargement, although this will be resisted by the recoil of the lungs. Occasional patients are seen with 'tension' pleural effusion, where there is clinical and radiographic evidence of considerable expansion of the hemithorax: in this situation pleural pressure is markedly positive.[8] More often the pressure in the pleural effusion is below or only slightly above atmospheric. Its measurement is sometimes used as a clinical guide when large volumes of pleural fluid are aspirated, with the aim of avoiding a very negative pressure, which might precipitate pulmonary oedema.[9]

With pleural effusion, unlike pneumothorax, the reduction in TLC is seen equally with gas dilution and plethysmographic techniques – but both underestimate the total thoracic volume. Increases in gaseous lung volumes after aspiration are generally much smaller than the volume of fluid removed.[2,10–12] The increase in VC is related only approximately to the volume of fluid aspirated, and a greater increase is seen in subjects with markedly positive pleural fluid pressure.[11] Measurements of oesophageal pressure suggest that lung recoil pressure at TLC ($P_L$max) increases after removal of fluid. At first sight this may surprise as an increase in lung volume is normally associated with a reduced $P_L$max owing to less effective action of the inspiratory muscles at greater volumes. The explanation is that the efficacy of the respiratory muscles should be related not to the lung volume alone but to the chest wall volume: although lung volume at full inspiration is greater after aspiration, the chest wall volume decreases.[10]

In the presence of a pleural effusion, the arterial Po_2 is usually somewhat reduced and the $AaPo_2$ increased. The distribution of ventilation and perfusion is less well matched than normal, with broadening of the distribution of $\dot{V}_A/\dot{Q}$ ratios, but the main contributor to the hypoxaemia is a modest intrapulmonary shunt,[13] due presumably to areas of atelectasis. The immediate effect of aspiration of fluid on gas exchange is minor,[13] and relief of symptoms is probably due to improved mechanical function.[10]

Radioisotope studies of regional ventilation in the upright posture in patients with moderate-sized pleural effusion show a reduction at the affected lung base and delayed washout of inhaled xenon, implying reduced local ventilation.[14] Although overall $\dot{V}_A/\dot{Q}$ mismatching is increased, on a crude regional basis, reductions in local ventilation and perfusion usually appear well matched. Most pleural effusions develop more insidiously than pneumothorax, perhaps allowing more effective compensatory changes.

16.4 PLEURAL THICKENING

When 'pleural pressure' is used to partition the mechanical performance of the respiratory system into components due to the lungs and the chest wall, the two pleural layers are notionally separated, with the visceral pleura considered together with the lungs and the parietal pleura with the chest wall. In theory, therefore, if pathological changes of one or other pleural layer could be analysed separately, different functional consequences might result, but in practice the distinction is unimportant.

16.4.1 Localized pleural thickening

In the commonest form of pleural abnormality associated with asbestos exposure, hyaline or calcified plaques produce localized thickening of the parietal pleura, particularly over the lower half of the chest and diaphragm. Studies of large groups of asbestos workers with plaques diagnosed by plain chest radiography show minor reductions of VC and TLC.[15,16] However, distinction of plaques from lesser degrees of diffuse pleural thickening, and recognition of mild pulmonary fibrosis, may be difficult with plain radiography, and more recent computed tomography (CT)-based studies suggest that plaques alone are functionally irrelevant.[17,18]

16.4.2 Diffuse pleural thickening

Most cases of extensive bilateral pleural thickening result from asbestos exposure. The severity of the resulting restrictive ventilatory defect correlates with the extent and severity of the thickening, whether determined by plain radiography[17,18] or high-resolution CT (HRCT) scanning.[18] Of particular importance is radiographic obliteration of the costophrenic angles, which can have a disproportionately severe effect on lung volumes.[16,19] Functionally, this area is particularly important as it corresponds to the 'zone of apposition' between the visceral and parietal pleura, from which lung surface is 'recruited' as the lung expands during inspiration (see Chapter 1, Section 1.5.1). Loss of this surface reserve is the main mechanism of volume restriction due to pleural thickening, as limiting the separation of the diaphragm and ribcage during inspiration seriously impairs the motion of both.[20] Once established, the effects of asbestos-related diffuse pleural thickening on spirometric volumes remain relatively stable over time.[21]

Pathologically, both the visceral and parietal pleura are thickened in these patients so that the effects on respiratory mechanics are potentially complex. Also, some evidence of pulmonary fibrosis (asbestosis) is frequently found by HRCT, particularly in the adjacent subpleural lung. Attributing the contributions of intra- and extrapulmonary disease to the overall functional picture may be challenging. Because of secondary effects on lung distensibility, extrapulmonary as well as intrapulmonary, volume restriction is associated with a reduction of pulmonary compliance. With other extrapulmonary causes of volume restriction, such as respiratory muscle weakness, the maximum transpulmonary pressure ($P_L$max) is a useful distinguishing feature as it is increased in intrapulmonary restriction (e.g. pulmonary fibrosis) but reduced when full expansion is limited from without (see Fig. 1.7b in Chapter 1). Although a low $P_L$max was originally proposed as characteristic of pleural restriction,[22] a later study showed that an increased $P_L$max is more typical.[23] There has to be some doubt about the validity of oesophageal pressure as a guide to the true pleural pressure in such patients, but, in practice, the PV curve of the lungs does not distinguish between alveolar and diffuse pleural fibrosis. In clinical testing, the K_{CO} is a much more useful discriminator as, typically, it is raised with pleural disease but usually reduced with extensive alveolar fibrosis.

Increased dead space and total ventilation[24] and arterial oxygen desaturation[25] have been reported during exercise in patients with radiographically extensive bilateral pleural thickening, but it is unclear whether these result from pleural thickening per se or from coexistent asbestosis not detected by plain radiography. Maximal respiratory muscle pressures are generally normal in patients with extensive pleural thickening.[26]

16.4.3 Effects of surgical treatment of pleural disease

Surgical decortication of a lung is occasionally performed for breathless patients with extensive pleural thickening. With unilateral pleural thickening, this can produce worthwhile functional improvement, even after many years.[27] However, no information is available on the functional outcome of surgery in patients with bilateral diffuse pleural thickening.

During pleurectomy, which is sometimes performed for recurrent or persistent pneumothorax, a variable amount of the parietal pleura is removed. Since, however, spontaneous pneumothorax usually results from rupture of small blebs on the surface of the upper lobes, often only the inside of the upper ribcage is stripped, and this would be predicted to have little effect on expansion of the lung and chest wall on that side. Even with more extensive surgery, the diaphragmatic pleura is not removed, so that expansion of the chest wall by recruitment of surface from the zone of apposition is likely to be preserved. The long-term functional effects of surgical or chemical procedures for securing adhesion of the visceral and parietal pleura are generally minimal. Ultrasonography shows that unilateral chemical or surgical sclerosis results in reduced diaphragmatic excursion compared with the non-treated side; there is less effect with surgical sclerosis than chemical, presumably because the latter is likely to obliterate the surface reservoir provided by the zone of apposition.[28]

16.5 ANKYLOSING SPONDYLITIS

Ribcage expansion is diminished in ankylosing spondylitis but the chest wall is still able to expand via its abdominal pathway. Movement of the diaphragm is usually unimpeded and, unlike the situation in scoliosis, hypercapnic respiratory failure does not result from uncomplicated ankylosing spondylitis. A mild or moderate reduction in VC is common, but the TLC is often normal or reduced only slightly; residual volume and FRC are therefore often increased.[29–31] Chest wall compliance is reduced in proportion to the reduction of VC.[29] In patients with reduced TLC, reduction in pulmonary compliance is also seen, as with other extrapulmonary causes of volume restriction. A modest reduction in maximum respiratory pressures has been reported.[32,33]

Disturbances of gas exchange in ankylosing spondylitis are minor, but there may be mild hypoxaemia. In the absence of lung disease, $D_L CO$ is relatively well preserved and $K CO$ is high normal or mildly increased.[32] Regional studies have shown some reduction in ventilation at the lung apices, as might be expected with predominantly diaphragmatic breathing, but a normal distribution of perfusion.[30] Exercise performance has been reported as well preserved[34] or modestly impaired.[35,36]

16.6 SCOLIOSIS

Severe scoliosis or kyphoscoliosis is a well-recognized cause of respiratory disability that, when severe, can lead to respiratory failure and cor pulmonale. Most authorities prefer the term 'scoliosis' to 'kyphoscoliosis', as the former describes the primary abnormality. Rotation and lateral flexion of the spine restrict lung expansion,[37] and in most patients the 'kyphos' is due to prominence of the posterior angles of the ribs on the side of the convexity rather than to forward angulation of the spine. The severity of scoliosis is usually measured from radiographs by the method of Cobb: the higher the Cobb angle, the more severe the distortion and the more restricted are lung volumes.[38,39]

One problem in the assessment of lung function in scoliosis is uncertainty about the appropriate reference values, as the condition itself reduces body height. Other reference standards such as tibial length, arm span and height estimated from the angle and length of the spine have been proposed, but none is entirely satisfactory. Although span as the most appropriate surrogate has been questioned, in practice it is the most commonly used predictor and regression equations incorporating span instead of height have been developed.[40]

The typical pattern of lung volumes in scoliosis is reductions in VC, TLC and FRC, with a normal or proportionately less reduced RV. Even relatively mild curvature can be associated with significant volume restriction.[41] Calculation from the data of Kafer shows that a Cobb angle of 100° would be expected to give average mean values of VC and TLC of 53 per cent and 64 per cent of predicted respectively.[38] The simplest mechanical explanation for the reduction in lung volumes is abnormal stiffness (reduced compliance) of the chest wall.[38] However, measurements in children during anaesthesia and paralysis suggest that chest wall compliance is surprisingly normal, even when lung volumes are reduced,[42] suggesting that, at least in younger individuals, other factors may be important. Potential contributors include impaired mechanical advantage of the inspiratory muscles resulting from distortion of their normal points of skeletal attachment,[42] reduced respiratory muscle strength[43,44] and reduced lung compliance.[45,46]

Maldistribution of ventilation and perfusion is common and likely with any significant degree of scoliosis. The V_D/V_T and $AaPO_2$ both increase and PaO_2 falls.[47] The PaO_2 increases normally on breathing 100 per cent oxygen. With increasing severity of scoliosis the tidal volume decreases and, without a compensatory increase in total ventilation, alveolar ventilation will fall and $PaCO_2$ increase, leading to chronic ventilatory failure and cor pulmonale.

Radioisotope studies show more even gravity-dependent regional distribution of lung function than normal,[48] sometimes with a reversal of the normal vertical gradient. In the case of perfusion this is probably due to an increase in pulmonary artery pressure. On the concave side of the spinal curve, the volume of the lung is smaller, diaphragmatic excursion is less and the distribution of ventilation is more uneven.[49]

The $D_L CO$ is reduced approximately in proportion to lung volume, but $K CO$ is often high and is related inversely to the size of the lungs,[50] as would be expected with extrapulmonary volume restriction.

On exercise, the pulmonary artery pressure, which may already be elevated at rest, rises abnormally and in inverse proportion to the lung volume.[51] Measurements of cardiac output are, however, usually normal,[48] although the heart rate response is often excessive.[52] In severe scoliosis, exercise is limited by ventilatory factors and the maximum exercise ventilation is predictably reduced in proportion to the mechanical abnormality. In mild or moderate scoliosis exercise capacity is reduced even with relatively normal spirometric volumes when limitation by ventilatory factors would not be expected; the impairment may be due to unfitness and deconditioning.[52,53]

The ventilatory response to CO_2 is impaired in many patients, but this is a consequence of the mechanical abnormality and the slope of the response is reduced in proportion to the VC.[38] Respiratory drive during unstimulated tidal breathing, as assessed by measurement of the mouth occlusion pressure ($P_{0.1}$), is increased in proportion to the severity of the restrictive defect.[54] Although ventilatory failure with a raised $PaCO_2$ is often regarded as an ominous feature, this may be unduly pessimistic, as, even in the era before non-invasive ventilation, patients with scoliosis often survived for several years and the prognosis is appreciably better than for patients with chronic obstructive pulmonary disease (COPD) and a similar reduction of FEV_1.[55]

Hypoventilation and consequent arterial oxygen desaturation during sleep are common and most severe in those with daytime hypoxaemia or hypercapnia.[56] As in other conditions (see Fig. 6.3 in Chapter 6), desaturation is most severe in phasic rapid-eye-movement (REM) sleep when activity of inspiratory muscles other than the diaphragm is reduced. The situation may be exacerbated by the diaphragm operating at a mechanical disadvantage due to the anatomical distortions resulting from scoliosis.[57]

16.6.1 Effects of treatment of scoliosis

Braces are sometimes employed in adolescents in an attempt to reduce the scoliosis. The Milwaukee or Boston brace fits tightly around the abdomen and lower chest, reducing tidal expansion of the abdomen and lower ribcage and causing increased movement of the upper ribs;[58] as a result both VC and TLC are further reduced.[59]

The effects of orthopaedic surgery on lung function are generally disappointing and in younger subjects may be difficult to interpret because of growth during the interim. Lung volumes show a slight decline in the first few months, with subsequent recovery to preoperative values.[60,61] Exercise performance also fails to improve and may even decline postoperatively.[62] In general, the aim of improving respiratory function is not a valid indication for surgical intervention.[60]

Nocturnal non-invasive ventilation (NIV) is well established as the treatment of choice of patients with hypercapnic respiratory failure due to scoliosis. Marked improvements in daytime blood gases are seen.[63,64] It is presumed that correction of nocturnal hypercapnia by assisted ventilation leads to renal excretion of bicarbonate ions, thus 'resetting' the respiratory centres and increasing the ventilatory drive by day. Small improvements in VC and maximum respiratory pressures have also been reported,[63,64] but the mechanisms are unclear.

16.7 THORACOPLASTY

The deleterious functional effects of thoracoplasty have become increasingly evident many years after the procedure, with respiratory failure sometimes developing 30–40 years later. The operation, one of several forms of 'collapse' therapy, involved removal of a variable number of upper ribs usually overlying a tuberculous lung. A thoracoplasty violates the normal stability of the ribcage, effectively creating a flail segment, which moves paradoxically and which may also interfere with expansion of the lung on the normal side.[65] Scoliosis develops in many cases and contributes to the severity of the restrictive ventilatory defect.[66] A combined restrictive and obstructive defect is common with the latter due not only to previous smoking but probably also to the consequences of the previous tuberculosis.[67,68] The synergistic effects of airway narrowing and instability of the ribcage seem particularly to predispose to hypercapnic respiratory failure.[67] The $D_L CO$ and KCO are generally well preserved.[66] Exercise capacity is reduced in proportion to the reduced ventilatory capacity, as assessed by the FEV_1, which predicts performance more accurately than does the VC because of the frequent coexistence of airway narrowing.[69] Nocturnal hypoxaemia is commonly seen, related closely to the level of oxygenation when awake.[70]

16.8 PECTUS EXCAVATUM

Pectus deformities of the chest are usually regarded as of more cosmetic than physiological interest, but minor reductions in spirometric volumes are found[71,72] and exercise performance is impaired in individuals with more marked deformity. The exact mechanism is uncertain, but cardiovascular rather than ventilatory limitation is responsible,[73,74] and a reduction in stroke volume on exercise has been shown.[73] The impaired performance is not simply due to deconditioning.[74] Surgical repair improves cardiovascular[75] but not pulmonary[76] function, and there is often a modest deterioration of ventilatory function, with more marked restriction following surgery, despite improved exercise performance.[77,78]

REFERENCES

1 Heaf PJD, Prime FJ. Mechanical aspects of artificial pneumothorax. *Lancet* 1954; **2**: 468–70.

2 Gilmartin JJ, Wright AJ, Gibson GJ. Effects of pneumothorax or pleural effusion on pulmonary function. *Thorax* 1985; **40**: 60–65.

3 Anthonisen NR. Regional lung function in spontaneous pneumothorax. *Am Rev Respir Dis* 1977; **115**: 873–6.

4 Norris RM, Jones JG, Bishop JM. Respiratory gas exchange in patients with spontaneous pneumothorax. *Thorax* 1968; **23**: 427–33.

5 Bense L, Hedenstierna G, Lewander R, Wiman C, Thornstrom S. Regional lung function of non smokers with healed spontaneous pneumothorax. *Chest* 1986; **90**: 352–7.

6 Schramel FM, van Keimpema AR, Janssen JP, Golding RP, Postmus PE. Pulmonary function of patients with spontaneous pneumothorax in relation to the extent of emphysema-like changes. *Respir Med* 1996; **90**: 491–6.

7 Lange P, Mortensen J, Groth S. Lung function 22–35 years after treatment of idiopathic spontaneous pneumothorax with talc poudrage or simple drainage. *Thorax* 1988; **43**: 559–61.

8 Neff TA, Buchanan ED. Tension pleural effusion. *Am Rev Respir Dis* 1975; **111**: 543–8.

9 Feller-Kopman D, Walkey A, Berkowitz D, Ernst A. The relationship of pleural pressure to symptom development during therapeutic thoracentesis. *Chest* 2006; **129**: 1556–60.

10 Estenne M, Yernault J-C, De Troyer A. The mechanism of relief of dyspnoea after thoracocentesis in patients with large pleural effusions. *Am J Med* 1983; **74**: 813–19.

11 Light RW, Stansbury DW, Brown SE. The relationship between pleural pressures and changes in

12 Zerahn B, Jensen BV, Olsen F, Petersen JR, Kanstrup IL. The effect of thoracentesis on lung function and transthoracic electrical bioimpedance. *Respir Med* 1999; **93**: 196–201.

13 Agusti AG, Cardus J, Roca J, et al. Ventilation–perfusion mismatch in patients with pleural effusion: effects of thoracentesis. *Am J Respir Crit Care Med* 1997; **156**: 1205–9.

14 Anthonisen NR, Martin RR. Regional lung function in pleural effusion. *Am Rev Respir Dis* 1977; **116**: 201–7.

15 Schwartz DA, Fuortes LJ, Galvin JR, et al. Asbestos-induced pleural fibrosis and impaired lung function. *Am Rev Respir Dis* 1990; **141**: 321–6.

16 Lilis R, Miller A, Godbold J, Chan E, Selikoff IJ. Pulmonary function and pleural fibrosis: quantitative relationships with an integrative index of pleural abnormalities. *Am J Industr Med* 1991; **20**: 145–61.

17 Van Cleemput J, De Raeve H, Verschakelen JA, et al. Surface of localized pleural plaques quantitated by computed tomography scanning: no relation with cumulative asbestos exposure and no effect on lung function. *Am J Respir Crit Care Med* 2001; **163**: 705–10.

18 Copley SJ, Wells. AU, Rubens MB, et al. Functional consequences of pleural disease evaluated with chest radiography and CT. *Radiology* 2001; **220**: 237–43.

19 Ameille J, Matrat M, Paris C, et al. 2004; Asbestos-related pleural diseases: dimensional criteria are not appropriate to differentiate diffuse pleural thickening from pleural plaques. *Am J Industr Med* **45**: 289–96.

20 Singh B, Eastwood PR, Finucane KE, Panizza JA, Musk AW. Effect of asbestos-related pleural fibrosis on excursion of the lower chest wall and diaphragm. *Am J Respir Crit Care Med* 1999; **160**: 1507–15.

21 Yates DH, Browne K, Stidolph PN, Neville E. Asbestos-related bilateral diffuse pleural thickening: natural history of radiographic and lung function abnormalities. *Am J Respir Crit Care Med* 1996; **153**: 301–6.

22 Colp C, Reichel J, Park SS. Severe pleural restriction: the maximum static pulmonary recoil pressure as an aid in diagnosis. *Chest* 1975; **67**: 658–64.

23 Corris PA, Best JJK, Gibson GJ. Effects of diffuse pleural thickening on respiratory mechanics. *Eur Respir J* 1988; **1**: 248–52.

24 Miller A, Bhuptani AD, Sloane MF, Brown LK, Teirstein AS. Cardio-respiratory responses to incremental exercise in patients with asbestos related pleural thickening and normal or slightly abnormal lung function. *Chest* 1993; **103**: 1045–50.

25 Britton MG, Apps MCP, Maxwell DL, Hughes DTD, Hanson A. The value of earlobe oximetry in

the assessment of disability in asbestos-related disease. *Respir Med* 1989; **83**: 43–9.

26 Al Jarad N, Carroll MP, Laroche C, *et al.* Respiratory muscle function in patients with asbestos-related pleural disease. *Respir Med* 1994; **88**: 115–20.

27 Petty TL, Filley GF, Mitchell RS. Objective function improvement by decortication after 20 years of artificial pneumothorax for pulmonary tuberculosis. *Am Rev Respir Dis* 1961; **84**: 572–8.

28 Loring SH, Kurachak SC, Wohl MEB. Diaphragmatic excursion after pleural sclerosis. *Chest* 1989; **95**: 374–8.

29 Sharp JT, Sweany SK, Henry JP, *et al.* Lung and thoracic compliances in ankylosing spondylitis. *J Lab Clin Med* 1964; **63**: 254–63.

30 Stewart RM, Ridyard JB, Pearson JD. Regional lung function in ankylosing spondylitis. *Thorax* 1976; **31**: 433–7.

31 Aggarwal NA, Gupta D, Wanchu A, Tindal SK. Use of static lung mechanics to identify early pulmonary involvement in patients with ankylosing spondylitis. *J Postgrad Med* 2001; **47**: 89–94.

32 Vanderschueren D, Decramer M, Van den Daele P, Dequeker J. Pulmonary function and maximal transrespiratory pressures in ankylosing spondylitis. *Ann Rheumat Dis* 1989; **48**: 632–5.

33 Sahin G, Calikolu M, Ozge C, *et al.* Respiratory muscle strength but not BASFI score relates to diminished chest expansion in ankylosing spondylitis. *Clin Rhematol* 2004; **23**: 199–202.

34 Seckin U, Bolukbasi N, Gursel G, *et al.* Relationship between pulmonary function and exercise tolerance in patients with ankylosing spondylitis. *Clin Exp Rheumatol* 2000; **18**: 503–6.

35 Carter R, Riantawan P, Banhaus SW, Sturrock RD. An investigation of factors limiting aerobic capacity in patients with ankylosing spondylitis. *Respir Med* 1999; **93**: 700–708.

36 Seckin U, Bolukbasi N, Gursel G, *et al.* Relation between preliminary function and exercise tolerance in patients with ankylosing spondylitis. *Clin Exp Rheumatol* 2000; **18**: 503–6.

37 Leong JC, Lu WW, Luk KD, Karlberg EM. Kinematics of the chest cage and spine during breathing in healthy individuals and in patients with adolescent idiopathic scoliosis. *Spine* 1999; **24**: 1310–15.

38 Kafer ER. Idiopathic scoliosis: mechanical properties of the respiratory system and the ventilatory response to carbon dioxide. *J Clin Invest* 1975; **55**: 1153–63.

39 Kearon C, Viviani GR, Kirkley A, Killian KJ. Factors determining pulmonary function in adolescent idiopathic thoracic scoliosis. *Am Rev Respir Dis* 1993; **148**: 288–94.

40 Linderholm H, Lindgren U. Prediction of spirometric values in patients with scoliosis. *Acta Orthop Scand* 1978; **49**: 469–74.

41 Newton PO, Faro FD, Gollogly S, *et al.* Results of preoperative pulmonary function testing of adolescents with idiopathic scoliosis: a study of six hundred and thirty-one patients. *J Bone Joint Surg* 2005; **87**: 1937–46.

42 Caro CG, DuBois AB. Pulmonary function in kyphoscoliosis. *Thorax* 1961; **16**: 282–90.

43 Smyth RJ, Chapman KR, Wright TA, Crawford JS, Rebuck AS. Pulmonary function in adolescents with mild idiopathic scoliosis. *Thorax* 1984; **39**: 901–4.

44 Lisboa C, Moreno R, Fava M, Ferretti R, Cruz E. Inspiratory muscle function in patients with severe kyphoscoliosis. *Am Rev Respir Dis* 1985; **132**: 48–52.

45 Cooper DM, Rojas JV, Mellins RB, Keim HA, Mansell AL. Respiratory mechanics in adolescents with idiopathic scoliosis. *Am Rev Respir Dis* 1984; **130**: 16–22.

46 Conti G, Rocco M, Antonelli M, *et al.* Respiratory system mechanics in the early phase of acute respiratory failure due to severe kyphoscoliosis. *Intensive Care Med* 1997; **23**: 539–44.

47 Kafer ER. Idiopathic scoliosis: gas exchange and the age dependence of arterial blood gases. *J Clin Invest* 1976; **58**: 825–33.

48 Bergofsky EH. Respiratory failure in disorders of the thoracic cage. *Am Rev Respir Dis* 1979; **119**: 643–70.

49 Giordano A, Fuso L, Galli M, *et al.* Evaluation of pulmonary ventilation and diaphragmatic movement in idiopathic scoliosis using radioaerosol ventilation scintigraphy. *Nucl Med Commun* 1997; **18**: 105–11.

50 Siegler D, Zorab PA. The influence of lung volume on gas transfer in scoliosis. *Br J Dis Chest* 1982; **76**: 44–50.

51 Shneerson JM. Pulmonary artery pressure in thoracic scoliosis during and after exercise while breathing air and pure oxygen. *Thorax* 1978; **33**: 747–54.

52 Kearon C, Viviani G, Killian KJ. Factors influencing work capacity in adolescent idiopathic thoracic scoliosis. *Am Rev Respir Dis* 1993; **148**: 295–303.

53 Barrios C, Perez-Encinas C, Maruenda JI, Laguia M. Significant ventilatory functional restriction in adolescents with mild or moderate scoliosis during maximal exercise tolerance test. *Spine* 2005; **30**: 1610–15.

54 Ramonatxo M, Milic-Emili J, Prefaut C. Breathing pattern and load compensatory responses in young scoliotic patients. *Eur Respir J* 1988; **1**: 421–7.

55 Libby DB, Briscoe WA, Boyce B, Smith JP. Acute respiratory failure in scoliosis or kyphosis. *Am J Med* 1982; **73**: 532–8.

56 Midgren B, Petersson K, Hansson L, *et al.* Nocturnal hypoxaemia in severe scoliosis. *Br J Dis Chest* 1988; **82**: 226–36.

57 Sawicka EH, Branthwaite MA. Respiration during sleep in kyphoscoliosis. *Thorax* 1987; **42**: 801–8.

58 Kennedy JD, Robertson CF, Hudson I, Phelan PD. Effect of bracing on respiratory mechanics in mild idiopathic scoliosis. *Thorax* 1989; **44**: 548–53.

59 Kennedy JD, Robertson CF, Olinsky A, Dickens DRV, Phelan PD. Pulmonary restrictive effect of bracing in mild idiopathic scoliosis. *Thorax* 1987; **42**: 959–61.

60 Wong CA, Cole AA, Watson L, *et al.* Pulmonary function before and after anterior spinal surgery in adult idiopathic scoliosis. *Thorax* 1996; **51**: 534–6.

61 Graham EJ, Lenke LG, Lowe TG, *et al.* Prospective pulmonary function evaluation following open thoracotomy for anterior spinal fusion in adolescent idiopathic scoliosis. *Spine* 2000; **25**: 2319–25.

62 Lenke LG, White DK, Kemp JS, *et al.* Evaluation of ventilatory efficiency during exercise in patients with idiopathic scoliosis undergoing spinal fusion. *Spine* 2002; **27**: 2041–5.

63 Buyse B, Meersseman W, Demedts M. Treatment of chronic respiratory failure in kyphoscoliosis: oxygen or ventilation? *Eur Respir J* 2003; **22**: 525–8.

64 Gonzalez C, Ferris G, Diaz J, *et al.* Kyphoscoliotic ventilatory insufficiency: effects of long-term intermittent positive-pressure ventilation. *Chest* 2003; **124**: 857–62.

65 Hauge BN. Diaphragmatic movement and spirometric volume in patients with one functioning lung. *Scand J Respir Dis* 1971; **52**: 84–99.

66 Bredin CP. Pulmonary function in long-term survivors of thoracoplasty. *Chest* 1989; **95**: 18–19.

67 Phillips MS, Miller MR, Kinnear WJM, Gough SE, Shneerson JM. Importance of airflow obstruction after thoracoplasty. *Thorax* 1987; **42**: 348–52.

68 O'Connor TM, O'Riordan DM, Stack M, Bredin CP. Airways obstruction in survivors of thoracoplasty; reversibility is greater in non-smokers. *Respirology* 2004; **9**: 130–33.

69 Phillips MS, Kinnear WJM, Shaw D, Shneerson JM. Exercise responses in patients treated for pulmonary tuberculosis by thoracoplasty. *Thorax* 1989; **44**: 268–74.

70 Brander PE, Salmi T, Partinen M, Sovijarvi AR. Nocturnal oxygen saturation and sleep quality in long-term survivors of thoracoplasty. *Respiration* 1993; **60**: 325–31.

71 Castile RG, Staats BA, Westbrook PR. Symptomatic pectus deformities of the chest. *Am Rev Respir Dis* 1982; **126**: 564–8.

72 Kelly RE Jr, Shamberger RC, Mellins RB, *et al.* Prospective multicenter study of surgical correction of pectus excavatum: design, perioperative complications, pain, and baseline pulmonary function facilitated by internet-based data collection. *J Am Coll Surg* 2007; **205**: 205–16.

73 Beiser GD, Epstein SE, Stampfer M, *et al.* Impairment of cardiac function in patients with pectus excavatum with improvement after operative correction. *N Engl J Med* 1972; **287**: 267–72.

74 Malek MH, Fonkalsrud EW, Cooper CB. Ventilatory and cardiovascular responses to exercise in patients with pectus excavatum. *Chest* 2003; **124**: 870–82.

75 Malek MH, Berger DE, Housh TJ, *et al.* Cardiovascular function following surgical repair of pectus excavatum: a metaanalysis. *Chest* 2006; **130**: 506–16.

76 Malek MH, Berger DE, Marelich WD, *et al.* Pulmonary function following surgical repair of pectus excavatum: a meta-analysis. *Eur J Cardiothorac Surg* 2006; **30**: 637–43.

77 Morshuis W, Folgering H, Barentsz J, van Lier H, Lacquet L. Pulmonary function before surgery for pectus excavatum and at long-term follow-up. *Chest* 1994; **105**: 1646–52.

78 Lacquet LK, Morshuis WJ, Folgering HT. Long-term results after correction of anterior chest wall deformities. *J Cardiovasc Surg* 1998; **39**: 683–8.

17

Function of the Transplanted Lung

17.1 FACTORS INFLUENCING POST-TRANSPLANTATION FUNCTION

The increasing use of lung transplantation over the past 20 years has provided a major focus for evaluating respiratory function, both in pre-transplant assessment and in post-transplant monitoring. Among the many factors that influence the function of transplanted lungs are the following:

- *Nature of the pre-transplant disease*: the advanced stages of many diseases are accepted indications for transplantation. These include various types of interstitial lung disease, in which the native lungs are generally shrunken and fibrotic and a marked restrictive ventilatory defect is present; chronic airway disease, particularly chronic obstructive pulmonary disease (COPD) and cystic fibrosis, in which varying degrees of lung and chest wall hyperinflation are present; and pulmonary hypertension, both primary and secondary to congenital heart disease, in which mechanical abnormalities of the native lungs and chest wall are minor or absent.
- *Type of transplant*: most early success was with combined heart–lung transplantation (HLT). Subsequently, bilateral lung transplantation (BLT) and single lung transplantation (SLT) without transplantation of the heart have become much more common. Bilateral lung transplantation is now performed mainly for patients with chronic suppurative lung disease (cystic fibrosis or bronchiectasis), and sometimes for COPD and emphysema. Its use in the latter group has declined with increasing success of SLT, which is also the most common form of transplantation for patients with diffuse parenchymatous (interstitial) lung disease.
- *Time elapsed since transplantation*: respiratory function usually improves progressively over several weeks after uncomplicated transplantation, followed by stabilization with subsequent decline at very varying rates.
- *Development of complications*: these include pulmonary infections, acute and chronic organ rejection, obliterative bronchiolitis (OB) and stenoses at the sites of anastomoses.

17.2 HEART–LUNG AND BILATERAL LUNG TRANSPLANTATION

17.2.1 Lung volumes and elasticity

Once stability is reached 3–6 months after transplantation, lung volumes, including FEV_1, VC and TLC, are usually near normal in patients after BLT,[1] although a mild restrictive defect with VC averaging 70–80 per cent of predicted values usually persists after HLT.[2] In the absence of major complications there is often a further slight increase in VC and TLC over the subsequent 12–18 months, with average TLC still slightly less than the values predicted for the recipient.[3,4]

Patients receiving transplants for chronic airway disease, in whom preoperative TLC is usually greater than predicted, tend to show a reduction whereas those with the most restricted volumes preoperatively show an increase.[5,6] To some extent this pattern may be predetermined by matching of donor and recipient size, but a similar pattern is seen when lungs are used from a donor whose predicted TLC is appreciably larger than that of the recipient.[5] The ultimate value of TLC, therefore, depends mainly on the normal chest wall size of the recipient,[6] although a slightly lower value than predicted is seen in some patients.[7] Despite the near-normal TLC, RV and functional residual capacity (FRC) are increased, suggesting that at high lung volumes the chest wall adapts to the size of the transplanted lungs while at lower volumes distortions of the chest wall acquired before transplantation may persist, elevating FRC and RV and impeding complete expiration.[6]

Detailed study of the elastic behaviour of the transplanted lungs suggests relatively normal function after both HLT[8] and BLT.[6,7] Static lung compliance is mildly reduced in parallel with the smaller VC, and the exponential shape constant, K, is normal or mildly reduced.[6,8] A reduced maximum lung recoil pressure ($P_L$max) at full inflation in patients with small-volume lungs implies that the restriction is of extrapulmonary origin.

17.2.2 Airway function

In the absence of complications, airway function is generally normal and reductions in maximum expiratory flow are explicable in terms of lower lung volumes.[2] Abnormally high values of the FEV_1/VC ratio and/or specific airway conductance are seen in some patients in the early stages after HLT.[9] This is attributed to lower vagal tone of the airway smooth muscle due to the inevitable extrinsic denervation of the transplanted organ. These individuals may have an unusual pattern of flow limitation during forced expiration, with the maximum expiratory flow–volume (MEFV) curve showing a virtual plateau of flow at higher lung volumes and a marked 'shoulder' or 'knee' in the mid-VC, a pattern again

attributable to unusually low tone of bronchial smooth muscle (Fig. 17.1).[9] Very sensitive tests of function of the peripheral airways, such as the slope (phase III) of the single breath nitrogen washout test, may suggest peripheral dysfunction even without other evidence of early obliterative bronchiolitis (see Chapter 2, Section 2.1.9).[7]

Some data have suggested frequent bronchial hyperresponsiveness, but when care is taken to exclude patients with contemporary evidence of lung rejection or infection, as well as any recipients or donors who might have had asthma, bronchial responsiveness is not abnormal.[10]

17.2.3 Gas exchange function

A moderate reduction in carbon monoxide diffusing capacity (D_LCO) is common after both HLT[2] and BLT,[1] even in individuals with relatively normal lung volumes and no evidence of rejection or infection. Pulmonary gas exchange, however (which is of course usually grossly abnormal preoperatively), improves dramatically and arterial P_{O_2} returns to normal in most patients. A degree of hyperventilation is often present at rest, resulting in mild hypocapnia and respiratory alkalosis.[2]

17.2.4 Ventilatory responses

Studies of ventilatory responses to chemical stimuli have given somewhat conflicting results. One study of patients after HLT showed a reduced slope of the ventilatory response to CO_2,[11] but in a second study the ventilatory response was normal and the mouth occlusion pressure response was greater than normal.[12] Both studies showed that the ventilation was achieved with an unusually high tidal volume and low frequency response, a pattern that resembles the effects of vagotomy in animals or vagal blockade in humans. Ventilatory responses to hypoxia were similar to those in control subjects.

17.3 SINGLE LUNG TRANSPLANTATION

17.3.1 Single lung transplantation for interstitial lung disease

Marked improvements in lung volumes and D_LCO are seen once the patient has stabilized; TLC may

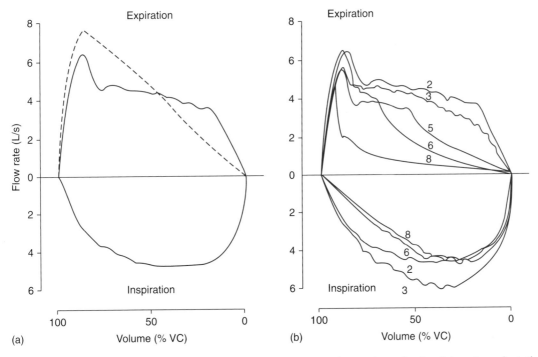

Figure 17.1 Maximum expiratory and inspiratory flow–volume curves in a patient after heart–lung transplantation (HLT). (a) Curves 2 months post-HLT compared with predicted (broken line), showing 'knee' appearance of maximum expiratory flow–volume (MEFV) curve with flows exceeding predicted in later expiration. (b) Sequential curves (numbers indicate months post-HLT), showing reduction in flow and change in shape of MEFV curves with increasing concavity as patient develops progressive airway obstruction due to obliterative bronchiolitis. Redrawn from ref. 9 with permission from the American Thoracic Society.

VC, vital capacity.

increase to normal,[13] or a mild restrictive defect may remain.[14] The VC is more consistently less than predicted and RV is increased.[13] Most of the increase in volumes occurs within 3 months of surgery, with a slight further increase over the first year.[14]

Lung scans show that the transplanted lung receives most of the perfusion almost immediately, relative perfusion of the transplant increasing from a mean of 63 per cent at 3 days to 77 per cent at 3 months in one series.[14] Similarly, ventilation is distributed preferentially to the transplanted lung, although the relative proportion is usually rather less than that of perfusion (Fig. 17.2).[13,15] Consequently, there may be minor degrees of ventilation/perfusion mismatching; oxygenation is usually close to normal but mild hypocapnia often persists.[14] The $D_L CO$ improves towards normal, although some reduction is common in proportion to the reduced volume[14] and K_{CO} is relatively normal.[13]

17.3.2 Single lung transplantation for chronic airway obstruction

Following successful SLT for chronic airway disease there is a temporal difference in the shifts of perfusion and ventilation, with redistribution of the former occurring within days while ventilation of the transplanted lung continues to increase for several weeks.[16] In the stable state the relative distribution of perfusion in patients undergoing SLT for emphysema is similar to that seen after SLT for pulmonary fibrosis (Fig. 17.2).[13] The eventual distribution of ventilation, however, is different in that single lungs transplanted for emphysema receive relatively more ventilation than perfusion and more than those transplanted for restrictive conditions.[13] The $D_L CO$ and K_{CO} also tend to be higher after transplantation for emphysema, and K_{CO} is often above the normal range,[13] presumably reflecting the generally better ventilation of the transplanted lung.

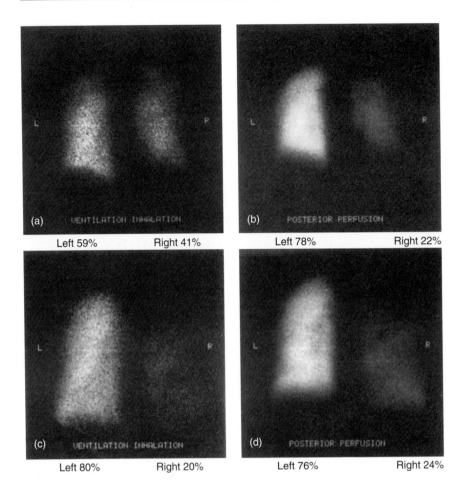

Figure 17.2 Posterior views of xenon ventilation (a,c) and perfusion (b, d) scans of (a,b) a patient following left single lung transplantation (SLT) for pulmonary fibrosis and (c,d) a patient following left SLT for chronic obstructive pulmonary disease (COPD). Figures indicate per cent total uptake of isotope with each scan. Note that the relative ventilation of the native lung in the patient with COPD is less than in pulmonary fibrosis, whereas the relative distribution of perfusion is similar in both. Reproduced from: Chacon RA *et al*. Comparison of the functional results of single lung transplantation for pulmonary fibrosis and chronic airway obstruction. *Thorax* 1998; **53**: 43–9, with permission from the BMJ Publishing Group.

The TLC and FRC of both lungs together (measured plethysmographically) are usually greater than predicted.[13,17] The post-transplantation value is related both to the predicted TLC of the recipient (as in HLT and BLT) and to the TLC pre-transplantation, reflecting continued hyperinflation of the native lung.[13] Computed tomography (CT) measurement of the volume of the two lungs individually suggests that, on average, the volume of the native lung is unchanged post-SLT, whereas the TLC of the transplanted lung is less than predicted; the FRC of the transplanted lung, however, is normal, i.e. the graft is relatively hyperinflated.[18]

The general introduction of SLT for patients with COPD and emphysema was delayed by fears that a hyperinflated native lung would seriously interfere with ventilation of the graft. The data (e.g. see Fig. 17.2) suggest that this is not a serious issue in the majority of patients, but hyperinflation is often demonstrable radiographically as mediastinal shift and flattening of the diaphragm on the side of the native lung. This is more likely to occur with very severe preoperative airway obstruction and a larger RV, and it is associated with a persistently higher RV and lower FEV_1 and FVC post-transplantation.[19]

Three-dimensional reconstruction of the area and shape of the diaphragm by spiral CT shows that its configuration returns to normal on the ipsilateral side after SLT, but the area of the dome of the ipsilateral diaphragm is smaller than in healthy subjects because the mediastinum is displaced towards the graft.[20]

The combination of a healthy transplanted lung and a lung with severe airway narrowing produces marked asynchrony of lung filling and emptying. This is apparent on the MEFV curve as a prolonged 'tail', which represents the delayed emptying of the native lung. This effect also impairs the value of single-breath tests for early recognition of airway obstruction (obliterative bronchiolitis – see below) post-transplant. However, if the nitrogen slope is measured with the subject in the lateral decubitus posture, the contributions of the graft and native lung can be distinguished; in particular, measurements obtained with the graft in the non-dependent position reflect the distribution of ventilation in that lung.[21]

Conventional criteria such as the FEV_1/VC ratio inevitably indicate overall airway obstruction due to the, albeit modest, persisting ventilation of the native lung.[13,17] The presence of the native lung with severe airway narrowing also predisposes to expiratory flow limitation (EFL) during tidal breathing. Although EFL is not usually present at rest,[22] it is more likely with increased ventilation on exercise, leading to increasing dynamic hyperinflation.[17,23] This phenomenon is much more likely to occur after SLT than BLT, and the overall improvement in spirometric volumes is inevitably less after SLT for COPD than after BLT.[24]

Comparison of right and left lungs transplanted for COPD shows no functional differences other than those attributable to the natural larger size of the right lung, so that right-sided grafts produce slightly greater FEV_1 and VC and receive relatively more perfusion and ventilation than do left-sided grafts.[25]

17.3.3 Single lung transplantation for pulmonary hypertension

Single lung transplantation for pulmonary vascular disease results in greater mismatching of ventilation and perfusion than other indications, as virtually all the perfusion is diverted immediately to the transplanted lung because of the considerable difference in pulmonary vascular resistance of the two lungs. Ventilation follows to a minor extent so that even after 3 months the graft is relatively underventilated in relation to its perfusion; this is accompanied by arterial hypoxaemia of varying severity, although usually appreciably less than in the preoperative state.[26]

17.4 RESPIRATORY MUSCLE FUNCTION AFTER LUNG TRANSPLANTATION

Several studies have shown evidence of reduced respiratory muscle strength and/or endurance after HLT,[11,27] BLT[28] and SLT.[29] Several factors are likely to contribute in different proportions in different populations: they include preoperative deconditioning, preoperative and/or postoperative steroid treatment[30,31] and other immunosuppressive agents.[32] Non-respiratory muscles may be similarly affected, and in some populations, e.g. people with cystic fibrosis, respiratory muscle function may be relatively better preserved than limb muscle function.[31] After SLT, asynchrony of action of the respiratory muscles on the two sides may be an additional factor impairing their function.[33] On the other hand, restoration of more normal thoracic geometry improves diaphragmatic function, at least on the side of the transplanted lung, in patients with severe COPD. In one study of diaphragmatic function after BLT for COPD,[34] maximum transdiaphragmatic pressure measured during a forceful voluntary sniff was found to increase postoperatively, as would be expected with the reduction in absolute lung volume and consequently more optimal muscle fibre length at FRC.

17.5 BREATHING DURING SLEEP AFTER TRANSPLANTATION

Two studies of breathing during sleep in patients post-HLT showed no clinically significant adverse effects on breathing or oxygenation.[35,36] Although weight gain and sleepiness are both common after lung transplantation, development of the obstructive sleep apnoea syndrome is unusual.[37]

17.6 EXERCISE AFTER LUNG TRANSPLANTATION

Improvements in exercise performance and capacity are readily demonstrable after successful lung transplantation.[38,39] Nevertheless, a marked reduction in capacity compared with healthy subjects has been reported in several studies, often with $\dot{V}o_2$max values averaging only 40–50 per cent of predicted.[38–41] The findings are generally similar, irrespective of the original diagnosis[23] and of the type of transplant performed.[42] Exercise ventilation has been reported as normal[40] or high[43] for the metabolic load; after HLT the increased ventilation is achieved with a larger tidal volume and lower frequency than normal.[44] The 'anaerobic threshold' is reached relatively early during progressive exercise testing.[38,41] Following HLT pulmonary gas exchange during exercise is usually relatively normal. After SLT the proportional distribution of ventilation and perfusion to the two lungs on exercise is similar to resting values,[45] but there may be mild arterial desaturation on maximal exercise, which has been attributed to possible limitation of diffusion in the native lung.[46] Grading of dyspnoea using the Borg scale shows normal values for a given exercise ventilation after HLT, implying (as would be expected) that the sensation is not significantly affected by, nor dependent upon, afferent information from the lungs or airways.[47]

Exercise performance after SLT for interstitial disease or COPD is generally similar, implying that the native lung does not usually impede the function of the transplant.[48] Although in many patients exercise pre-transplantation was limited by abnormal respiratory mechanics, this is not usually a major factor in patients after uncomplicated transplantation.[38,42]

Although cardiac dysfunction may contribute in a few cases,[49] peripheral circulatory and muscle function are likely to be the main determinants of exercise performance after lung transplantation. Clear relationships between exercise capacity and peripheral muscle strength have been demonstrated.[31,50] General deconditioning probably plays a major role, with impaired peripheral circulation leading to excessive anaerobic metabolism and lactate production.[51] Immunosuppressive treatment has also been invoked as a possible cause of impaired extraction and utilization of oxygen by the exercising muscles.[41]

The 6-min walk test (6 MWT) is often used in both pre-transplant assessment and post-transplant monitoring. In one large study of factors determining 6 MWT distance in patients with no complications 1 year after transplantation, the distance walked was less in those with shorter pre-transplant 6 MWT distances, while longer distances postoperatively were associated with BLT and a diagnosis of cystic fibrosis.[52]

17.7 COMPLICATIONS OF LUNG TRANSPLANTATION

17.7.1 Acute infection and rejection

The changes in pulmonary function seen with acute graft rejection and acute infection are generally similar, with reductions in FEV_1, FVC, maximum mid-expiratory flow (FEF_{25-75}), TLC and D_Lco.[53,54] Spirometric indices may be less sensitive for detecting complications after SLT for obstructive lung disease than in patients with SLT for fibrotic or pulmonary vascular disease[55] because of more frequent spirometric abnormality following uncomplicated transplantation in the former group. Sequential measurements showing a decline have a high positive predictive value, such that an apparent change should provoke further investigation, but the negative predictive value is less, implying that stable measurements cannot rule out allograft dysfunction.[54]

Following SLT, ventilation and perfusion scanning are sensitive to complications in the transplanted lung. In patients with grafts for fibrotic or obstructive lung disease, a reduction in ipsilateral perfusion is seen with acute rejection, presumably due to an increase in pulmonary vascular resistance in the graft. Improvements are demonstrable within a couple of days of effective treatment.[56] Changes in distribution of ventilation are usually less marked than perfusion.[57] With SLT for pulmonary vascular disease the picture is different, as perfusion is much less likely to be diverted to the native lung due to grossly increased vascular resistance. The pattern here is of a shift in ventilation with less, or no detectable, change in distribution of perfusion.[26,57]

17.7.2 Anastomotic complications

Localized stenoses can occur at the site of either airway or vascular anastomoses. Stenosis following SLT results in marked redistribution of ventilation or perfusion respectively. With bronchial stenosis, characteristic appearances of the maximum flow–volume curves and/or the forced expiratory spirogram may be detected (see Fig. 12.7 in Chapter 12).[58]

17.7.3 Obliterative bronchiolitis (bronchiolitis obliterans syndrome)

Obliterative bronchiolitis causes progressive and often severe airway obstruction and can occur following all types of lung transplantation. The condition, which is usually regarded as a manifestation of chronic rejection, is defined in functional terms as 'bronchiolitis obliterans syndrome' (BOS), as histopathological confirmation of obliteration of small airways is not always available. Its severity is graded in terms of the reduction in FEV_1 compared with baseline measurements (see Chapter 9, Section 9.17). Originally a fall in FEV_1 of 20 per cent or more was the criterion used for recognition of the syndrome, but latterly a category of 'potential BOS' has been defined as a reduction in FEV_1 greater than 10 per cent but less than 20 per cent.[59] As the condition worsens there is progressive reduction of FEV_1, FEV_1/VC and maximum expiratory flow.[3,9] The contour of the MEFV curve changes progressively with increasing concavity towards the volume axis in the later part of expiration (see Fig. 17.1).[9] The diagnosis of BOS is supported by finding a falling FEV_1 with little or no change in K_{CO} or, after SLT, in the distribution of perfusion.[60] In advanced disease TLC may increase but since in many patients TLC is less than predicted, its value in BOS is usually within the normal range.[61] The mechanical abnormalities are accompanied by deteriorating gas exchange and worsening hypoxaemia. $PaCO_2$ is usually reduced in mild or moderate disease[61] but inevitably rises if obstruction becomes severe.

The simple spirometric and flow volume indices that become abnormal earliest are FEV_1, FEV_1/VC, and maximum expiratory flow in the mid-VC range.[62] Detailed evaluation of forced expiratory tests using moments analysis is not demonstrably superior to simple spirometric measurements,[62] but indices of ventilation distribution using either single-breath[63] or multibreath washout[64] methods are more sensitive than spirometry in the earliest stages of the condition. Although measurements of FEF_{25-75} are applied widely in transplant populations, FEV_1 itself is a more accurate predictor of impending disease in the 'pre-BOS' category.[65]

Once the condition is established and FEV_1 has shown a clear decline, the single-breath nitrogen test offers no further advantage over FEV_1 as the nitrogen slope and FEV_1 are then closely correlated.[7] Function tends to decline more rapidly in females, in those with more rapid onset of the condition and with preoperative idiopathic pulmonary fibrosis.[66]

References

1 Cooper JD, Patterson GA, Grossman R, *et al*. Double-lung transplant for advanced chronic obstructive lung disease. *Am Rev Respir Dis* 1989; **139**: 303–7.

2 Theodore J, Jamieson SW, Burke CM, *et al*. Physiologic aspects of human heart–lung transplantation: pulmonary function status of the post-transplanted lung. *Chest* 1984; **86**: 349–57.

3 Theodore J, Marshall S, Kramer M, *et al*. The 'natural history' of the transplanted lung: rates of pulmonary functional changes in long-term survivors of heart lung transplantation. *Transplant Proc* 1991; **23**: 1165–6.

4 Lloyd KS, Barnard P, Holland VA, Noon GP, Lawrence EC. Pulmonary function after heart–lung transplantation using larger donor organs. *Am Rev Respir Dis* 1990; **142**: 1026–9.

5 Tamm M, Higenbottam TW, Dennis CM, Sharples LD, Wallwork J. Donor and recipient predicted lung volume and lung size after heart–lung transplantation. *Am J Respir Crit Care Med* 1994; **150**: 403–7.

6 Chacon RA, Corris PA, Dark JH, Gibson GJ. Respiratory mechanics after heart–lung and bilateral lung transplantation. *Thorax* 1997; **52**: 718–22.

7 Arens R, McDonough JM, Zhao H, *et al*. Altered lung mechanics after double-lung transplantation. *Am J Respir Crit Care Med* 1998; **158**: 1403–9.

8   Glanville AR, Theodore J, Harvey J, Robin ED. Elastic behaviour of the transplanted lung: exponential analysis of static pressure–volume relationships. *Am Rev Respir Dis* 1988; **137**: 308–12.

9   Estenne M, Ketelbout P, Primo G, Yernault J-C. Human heart–lung transplantation: physiological aspects of the denervated lung and post transplant obliterative bronchiolitis. *Am Rev Respir Dis* 1987; **135**: 976–8.

10 Herve P, Picard N, Ladurie M le R, *et al*. Lack of bronchial hyperresponsiveness to methacholine and to isocapnic dry air hyperventilation in heart/lung and double lung transplant recipients with normal lung histology. *Am Rev Respir Dis* 1992; **145**: 1503–5.

11 Sanders MH, Owens GR, Sciurba FC, *et al*. Ventilation and breathing pattern during progressive hypercapnia and hypoxia after human heart–lung transplantation. *Am Rev Respir Dis* 1989; **140**: 38–44.

12 Duncan SR, Kagawa FT, Stames VA, Theodore J. Hypercarbic ventilatory responses of human heart–lung transplant recipients. *Am Rev Respir Dis* 1991; **144**: 126–30.

13 Chacon RA, Corris PA, Dark JH, Gibson GJ. Comparison of the functional results of single lung transplantation for pulmonary fibrosis and chronic airway obstruction. *Thorax* 1998; **53**: 43–9.

14 Grossman RF, Frost A, Zamel N, *et al*. Results of single lung transplantation for bilateral pulmonary fibrosis. *N Engl J Med* 1990; **322**: 727–33.

15 Markstaller K, Kauczor HU, Puderbach M, *et al*. ^{3}He-MRI-based vs. conventional determination of lung volumes in patients after unilateral lung transplantation: a new approach to regional spirometry. *Acta Anaesthesiol Scand* 2002; **46**: 845–52.

16 Kaiser LR, Cooper JD, Trulock EP, *et al*. The evolution of single lung transplantation for emphysema. *J Thorac Cardiovasc Surg* 1991; **102**: 333–41.

17 Murciano D, Ferretti A, Boczkowski J, *et al*. Flow limitation and dynamic hyperinflation during exercise in COPD patients after single lung transplantation. *Chest* 2000; **118**: 1248–54.

18 Estenne M, Cassart M, Poncelet P, Gevenois PA. Volume of graft and native lung after single-lung transplantation for emphysema. *Am J Respir Crit Care Med* 1999; **159**: 641–5.

19 Yonan NA, el-Gamel A, Egan J, *et al*. Single lung transplantation for emphysema: predictors for native lung hyperinflation. *J Heart Lung Transplant* 1998; **17**: 192–201.

20 Cassart M, Verbandt Y, de Francquen P, Gevenois PA, Estenne M. Diaphragm dimensions after single-lung transplantation for emphysema. *Am J Respir Crit Care Med* 1999; **159**: 1992–7.

21 Van Muylem A, Scillia P, Knoop C, Paiva M, Estenne M. Single-breath test in lateral decubitus reflects function of single lungs grafted for emphysema. *J Appl Physiol* 2006; **100**: 834–8.

22 Murciano D, Pichot MH, Boczkowski J, *et al*. Expiratory flow limitation in COPD patients after single lung transplantation. *Am J Respir Crit Care Med* 1997; **155**: 1036–41.

23 Martinez FJ, Orens JB, Whyte RI, *et al*. Lung mechanics and dyspnea after lung transplantation for chronic airflow obstruction. *Am J Respir Crit Care Med* 1996; **153**: 1536–43.

24 Pochetinno A, Kotloff RM, Rosengard BR, *et al*. Bilateral versus single lung transplantation for chronic obstructive pulmonary disease: intermediate-term results. *Ann Thorac Surg* 2000; **70**: 1813–18.

25 Levine SM, Anzueto A, Gibbons WJ, *et al*. Graft position and pulmonary function after single lung transplantation for obstructive lung disease. *Chest* 1993; **103**: 444–8.

26 Kramer MR, Marshall SE, McDougall IR, *et al*. The distribution of ventilation and perfusion after single-lung transplantation in patients with pulmonary fibrosis and pulmonary hypertension. *Transplant Proc* 1991; **23**: 1215–16.

27 Ambrosino N, Bruschi C, Callegari G, *et al*. Time course of exercise capacity, skeletal and respiratory muscle performance after heart–lung transplantation. *Eur Respir J* 1996; **9**: 1508–14.

28 Brath H, Lahrmann H, Wanke T, *et al*. The effect of lung transplantation on the neural drive to the diaphragm in patients with severe COPD. *Eur Respir J* 1997; **10**: 424–9.

29 Ratnovsky A, Elad D, Izbicki G, Kramer MR. Mechanics of respiratory muscles in single-lung transplant recipients. *Respiration* 2006; **73**: 642–50.

30 Nava S, Fracchia C, Callegari, G, *et al*. Weakness of respiratory and skeletal muscles after a short course of steroids in patients with acute lung rejection. *Eur Respir J* 2002; **20**: 497–9.

31 Pinet C, Scillia P, Cassart M, *et al*. Preferential reduction of quadriceps over respiratory muscle strength and bulk after lung transplantation for cystic fibrosis. *Thorax* 2004; **59**: 783–9.

32 Williams TJ, Snell GI. Early and long-term functional outcomes in unilateral, bilateral, and living-related transplant recipients. *Clin Chest Med* 1997; **18**: 245–57.

33 Ratnovsky A, Kramer MR, Elad D. Breathing power of respiratory muscles in single-lung transplanted emphysematic patients. *Respir Physiol Neurobiol* 2005; **148**: 263–73.

34 Wanke T, Merkle M, Formanek D, *et al*. Effect of lung transplantation on diaphragmatic function in

patients with chronic obstructive pulmonary disease. *Thorax* 1994; **49**: 459–64.

35 Sanders MH, Costantino JP, Owens GR, *et al.* Breathing during wakefulness and sleep after human heart–lung transplantation. *Am Rev Respir Dis* 1989; **140**: 45–51.

36 Shea SA, Horner RL, Banner NR, *et al.* The effect of human heart–lung transplantation upon breathing at rest and during sleep. *Respir Physiol* 1988; **72**: 131–50.

37 Dhar R, Corris PA, Lordan J, Fisher A, Gibson GJ. Weight gain and sleepiness after lung transplantation. *Am J Respir Crit Care Med* 2007; **175** (suppl.): A376.

38 Oelberg DA, Systrom DM, Markowotz DH, *et al.* Exercise performance in cystic fibrosis before and after bilateral lung transplantation. *J Heart Lung Transplant* 1998; **17**: 1104–12.

39 Systrom DM, Pappagionopoulos P, Fishman RS, Wain JC, Ginns LC. Determinants of abnormal maximum oxygen uptake after lung transplantation for chronic obstructive pulmonary disease. *J Heart Lung Transplant* 1998; **17**: 1220–30.

40 Pelligrino R, Rodarte JR, Frost AE, Reid MB. Breathing by double lung recipients during exercise: response to expiratory threshold loading. *Am J Respir Crit Care Med* 1998; **157**: 106–10.

41 Tirdel GB, Girgis R, Fishman RS, Theodore J. Metabolic myopathy as a cause of the exercise limitation in lung transplant recipients. *J Heart Lung Transplant* 1998; **17**: 1231–7.

42 Schwaiblmair M, Reichenspurner H, Muller C, *et al.* Cardiopulmonary exercise testing before and after lung and heart–lung transplantation. *Am J Respir Crit Care Med* 1999; **159**: 1277–83.

43 Estenne M, Primo G, Yernault J-C. Cardiorespiratory responses to dynamic exercise after human heart–lung transplantation. *Thorax* 1987; **42**: 629–30.

44 Sciurba F, Owens G, Sanders M, *et al.* Exercise response in heart–lung transplant recipients: evidence for an altered breathing pattern. *N Engl J Med* 1988; **319**: 1186–93.

45 Ross DJ, Waters PF, Waxman AD, Koerner SK, Mohsenifar Z. Regional distribution of lung perfusion and ventilation at rest and during steady-state exercise after unilateral lung transplantation. *Chest* 1993; **104**: 130–35.

46 Miyoshi S, Trulock EP, Schaefers H-J, *et al.* Cardiopulmonary exercise testing after single and double lung transplantation. *Chest* 1990; **97**: 1130–36.

47 Tapper DP, Duncan SR, Kraft S, *et al.* Detection of inspiratory resistive loads by heart–lung transplant recipients. *Am Rev Respir Dis* 1992; **145**: 458–60.

48 Gibbons WJ, Levine SM, Bryan CL, *et al.* Cardiopulmonary exercise responses after single lung transplantation for severe obstructive lung disease. *Chest* 1991; **100**: 106–11.

49 Vachiery JL, Niset G, Antoine M, *et al.* Haemodynamic response to dynamic exercise after heart–lung transplantation. *Eur Respir J* 1999; **14**: 1131–5.

50 Reinsma GD, ten Hacken NH, Grevink RG, *et al.* Limiting factors of exercise performance 1 year after lung transplantation. *J Heart Lung Transpl* 2006; **25**: 1310–16.

51 Ross DJ, Waters PF, Mohsenifar Z, *et al.* Haemodynamic responses to exercise after lung transplantation. *Chest* 1993; **103**: 46–53.

52 Sager JS, Kotloff RM, Ahya VN, *et al.* Association of clinical risk factors with functional status following lung transplantation. *Am J Transplant* 2006; **6**: 2191–201.

53 Otulana BA, Higenbottam T, Scott J, *et al.* Lung function associated with histologically diagnosed acute lung rejection and pulmonary infection in heart–lung transplant patients. *Am Rev Respir Dis* 1990; **142**: 329–32.

54 Van Muylem A, Melot C, Antoine M, Knoop C, Estenne M. Role of pulmonary function in the detection of allograft dysfunction after heart–lung transplantation. *Thorax* 1997; **52**: 643–7.

55 Becker FS, Martinez FJ, Brunsting LA, *et al.* Limitations of spirometry in detecting rejection after single lung transplantation. *Am J Respir Crit Care Med* 1994; **150**: 159–66.

56 Toronto Lung Transplant Group. Unilateral lung transplantation for pulmonary fibrosis. *N Engl J Med* 1986; **314**: 1140–45.

57 Levine SM, Jenkinson SG, Bryan CL, *et al.* Ventilation–perfusion inequalities during graft rejection in patients undergoing single lung transplantation for primary pulmonary hypertension. *Chest* 1992; **101**: 401–5.

58 Gascoigne AD, Corris PA, Dark JH, Gibson GJ. The biphasic spirogram: a clue to unilateral narrowing of a mainstem bronchus. *Thorax* 1990; **45**: 637–8.

59 Estenne M, Maurer JR, Boehler A, *et al.* Bronchiolitis obliterans syndrome 2001: an update of the diagnostic criteria. *J Heart Lung Transplant* 2002; **21**: 297–310.

60 Bjortuft A, Geiran OR, Fjeld J, *et al.* Single lung transplantation for chronic obstructive pulmonary disease: pulmonary function and impact of bronchiolitis obliterans syndrome. *Respir Med* 1996; **90**: 553–9.

61 Burke CM, Theodore J, Dawkins KD, *et al.* Post-transplant obliterative bronchiolitis and other late

sequelae in human heart–lung transplantation. *Chest* 1984; **84**: 824–9.

62 Chacon RA, Corris PA, Dark JH, Gibson GJ. Tests of airway function in detecting and monitoring treatment of obliterative bronchiolitis after lung transplantation. *J Heart Lung Transplant* 2000; **19**: 263–9.

63 Estenne M, Van Muylem A, Knoop C, Antoine M. Detection of obliterative bronchiolitis after lung transplantation by indexes of ventilation distribution. *Am J Respir Crit Care Med* 2000; **162**, 1047–51.

64 Van Muylem A, Verbanck S, Estenne M. Monitoring the lung periphery of transplanted lungs. *Respir Physiol Neurobiol* 2005; **148**: 141–51.

65 Hachem RR, Chakinala MM, Yusen RD, *et al.* The predictive value of bronchiolitis obliterans syndrome stage 0-p. *Am J Respir Crit Care Med* 2004; **169**: 468–72.

66 Lama VN, Murray S, Lonigro RJ, *et al.* Course of FEV_1 after onset of bronchiolitis obliterans syndrome in lung transplant recipients. *Am J Respir Crit Care Med* 2007; **175**: 1192–8.

18

Sleep Apnoea Syndromes

18.1 BACKGROUND AND DEFINITIONS

The first definitive investigation of patients with obstructive sleep apnoea, reported only 40 years ago, was in patients with the obesity hypoventilation syndrome (OHS, previously known as the Pickwickian syndrome).[1] Patients with OHS have chronic hypercapnia and are usually very obese (see Chapter 24, Section 24.2), but subsequently, with the wider availability of sleep investigations, it became apparent that patients with OHS were only a small minority of the total population with the obstructive sleep apnoea syndrome (OSAS) and that most individuals with OSAS have normal daytime blood gases.

Based on the pattern of airflow and movements of the ribcage and abdomen, Gastaut *et al.* described three types of apnoea: 'obstructive', 'central' and 'mixed' (see Chapter 6, Section 6.4.1).[1] Most mixed apnoeas are essentially obstructive, with the respiratory efforts undetected in the earlier part of the apnoea.

Central sleep apnoea syndromes are much less common than OSAS. They are seen particularly in infants with an immature respiratory control system, while in adults central sleep apnoea occurs most commonly in cardiac disease as a manifestation of Cheyne–Stokes breathing. It is also seen in some patients with central nervous or neuromuscular disease and occasionally, in the absence of other pathology, as an idiopathic syndrome (see Section 18.3).

18.2 OBSTRUCTIVE SLEEP APNOEA

18.2.1 Pathophysiology of obstructive sleep apnoea

Sleep-disordered breathing results from an interaction between, on the one hand, the structure and function of the upper airway and, on the other hand, the stability of the ventilatory control system during sleep. Obstructive sleep apnoea (OSA) is essentially a disorder of the former but instability of respiratory control may also exert an important influence.[2] The level of ventilatory drive determines the activity of both the respiratory 'pump' muscles and the muscles that support the upper airway; the latter have a major influence on the collapsibility or compliance of the pharynx.

Any control system involving a feedback loop is potentially unstable due to the inevitable delay between sensing the input signal and effecting the response. Since the output from the medullary respiratory control neurons drives the upper airway muscles, the stability of respiratory control influences the calibre of the upper airway. Thus, it has, for example, been shown that obstruction of the upper airway in OSA occurs at the nadir of fluctuating respiratory drive.[3]

Table 18.1 Factors predisposing to obstructive sleep apnoea

Male sex
Obesity (especially central, neck)
Retroplaced mandible (overbite)
Small maxilla
Large tonsils
Large tongue

18.2.1.1 Factors contributing to obstructive sleep apnoea

See Table 18.1.

The pharyngeal airway has little effective bony support and consequently it is unusually subject to dynamic forces that narrow or dilate it. This is advantageous for swallowing but, potentially, is a serious disadvantage for breathing, especially if the airway calibre is also compromised. The upper airway narrows during sleep, even in healthy subjects, due to the overall reduction in ventilatory drive and the loss of tonic activity of the pharyngeal muscles. In individuals with OSAS, the pharyngeal airway is not only smaller than normal but also more collapsible, i.e. its compliance is increased.[4] In addition to inadequate or ineffectual support by the pharyngeal dilator muscles (see below), other factors may contribute to increased pharyngeal compliance. These include long-term effects of vibration injury due to snoring, which frequently precedes OSAS, and the consequent oedema and inflammatory changes increasing tissue volume and possibly damaging the sensory nerve endings responsible for pharyngeal reflexes (see below).[5] Airway size and compliance interact in that, the smaller the airway when awake, the more likely are dynamic changes during sleep to cause complete occlusion. Also, the higher resistance of a small airway exaggerates the swings in pharyngeal pressure and consequently increases the dynamic forces acting on an abnormally compliant airway. Exaggerated tidal pressure swings may also result from high nasal airway resistance upstream from the site of obstruction, although this does not appear to be a major factor in most individuals with OSAS.[6]

Increased compliance of the upper airway with greater respiratory variation in size during sleep has been demonstrated in patients with OSAS using ultrafast magnetic resonance imaging (MRI).[7] The same phenomenon is demonstrable under general anaesthesia, with the tendency of the airway to collapse correlating with the severity of OSAS.[8] The site of periodic collapse or narrowing during sleep is usually the velopharynx (behind the soft palate) or oropharynx (between the tip of the soft palate and the epiglottis). Lung volume has a major effect on pharyngeal compliance, as breathing at higher volumes stretches the airway in the craniocaudal dimension, thereby stiffening it and reducing the likelihood of closure.[9] Posture is also an important determinant of pharyngeal size, which is less in the supine position due to the effects of gravity on the lower jaw and tongue. Posture has a major effect on the severity of OSAS in some individuals; the frequency of apnoeas and consequent severity of desaturation is often greater in the supine posture, although most patients with moderate or severe symptoms have apnoeas and hypopnoeas in all sleep postures. However, some patients, particularly those with milder disease, have positional sleep apnoea, with apnoeas and hypopnoeas effectively confined to the supine posture.[10]

Gender differences are well recognized in OSAS, with two to three times as many men as women affected. Male patients with OSAS[11] and even healthy men[12] have a more collapsible upper airway (less negative critical closing pressure (P_{crit}); see below) than women of equivalent body mass index (BMI). The difference is probably related to the different distribution of adipose tissue in the two sexes.[13] For a given BMI, women in general have a lower apnoea/hypopnoea index (AHI) than men; alternatively, for a given AHI, women tend to be heavier than men. In women the prevalence of OSAS is much less before than after the menopause; although prevalence of OSAS increases after the menopause, it remains somewhat lower than in men after controlling for age and BMI.[14] Hormone replacement therapy with oestrogens is accompanied by less nocturnal desaturation for a given BMI, presumably due to less frequent sleep apnoea.[15]

Data on the effects of age are somewhat conflicting. In general population studies, the frequency of sleep-disordered breathing increases progressively with age, but the age distribution of patients diagnosed with OSAS usually shows peak values in the fifties and sixties and lower rates in older individuals.[16] Whether this reflects reduced awareness among older individuals or a 'survivor effect' related to the adverse consequences of untreated OSAS is unclear.

Various abnormalities of the soft tissues may contribute to pharyngeal narrowing. Obesity, which is the most common risk factor for OSAS in adults, is associated with greater deposition of adipose tissue as fat pads around the airway.[17] Other potential contributors include enlargement of the tongue and soft palate,[18] while enlargement or persistence of the tonsils is also important, particularly in children and some younger adults. A difference in airway shape has been described, with a relatively greater anteroposterior (AP) diameter than lateral (the converse of the normal situation), which may impair the efficacy of the pharyngeal dilator muscles.[19]

The position and orientation of the facial bones and mandible is particularly important, as even a slightly retroplaced mandible is associated with a more vertical orientation and appreciable reduction in pharyngeal dimensions compared with the average.[20] In some ethnic groups, particularly those of Chinese and South East Asian origin, BMI appears to be relatively less important and variations in craniofacial bony stricture more so. Consequently, among these races many individuals have severe OSAS with relatively normal or only mildly increased bodyweight.[21,22]

18.2.1.2 Critical closing pressure

Throughout inspiration the intra-airway pressure resulting from contraction of the inspiratory 'pump' muscles is always subatmospheric. Normally, the tendency to narrow and close is opposed by a combination of the passive recoil of the airway wall and the action of the pharyngeal dilating muscles. If intra-airway pressure is lowered progressively, a critical value will be reached at which the airway closes completely. This critical closing pressure (P_{crit}) can be measured during assisted ventilation via a tight-fitting mask by abrupt reduction of the nasal pressure. The reduction in airflow at different nasal pressures is measured and P_{crit} estimated by plotting flow against pressure (Fig. 18.1).[23,24] This gives a quantitative index of the net effects of narrowing and dilating forces on the pharyngeal lumen. In non-apnoeic, non-snoring healthy individuals, P_{crit} is markedly negative (i.e. the pharynx resists collapse), while during sleep in those with OSAS it is much less negative or even positive,[25] implying that continuous activity of the

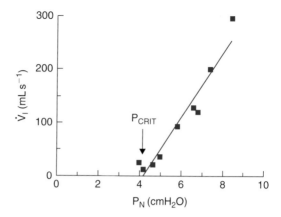

Figure. 18.1 Estimation of critical closing pressure of pharynx (P_{CRIT}) by abrupt reductions of nasal pressure during application of positive airway pressure in a sleeping individual with obstructive sleep apnoea. Each point represents the nasal pressure (P_N) and resulting inspiratory flow; in this example, flow ceases at an abnormally high P_{CRIT} of approximately $+4\,cmH_2O$. Modified from ref. 23, with permission from the American Thoracic Society.

$\dot{V}_I$, inspiratory flow.

pharyngeal dilator muscles is required to maintain patency of the airway.

18.2.1.3 Pharyngeal dilator muscles

Several muscles are involved in stabilizing the pharynx during inspiration. They include muscles that influence the position of the hyoid bone (geniohyoid, sternohyoid) and those attached to the tongue (e.g. genioglossus) and to the palate (e.g. tensor palatini). Some show background tonic activity and most are activated during inspiration, with their activity regulated by both reflex mechanisms and central respiratory drive. Subatmospheric pressure in the airway stimulates mechanoreceptors located mainly in the larynx, resulting in increased output to the genioglossus and other muscles via a reflex arc.[26] In addition, the medullary respiratory control neurons drive the pharyngeal dilator muscles almost synchronously with the respiratory pump muscles. In fact, activation of genioglossus with each breath occurs marginally before each breath and before activation of the pump muscles, which has the effect of 'priming' the upper airway in advance of development of a negative intra-airway pressure.[27] In individuals with OSAS, even though the more

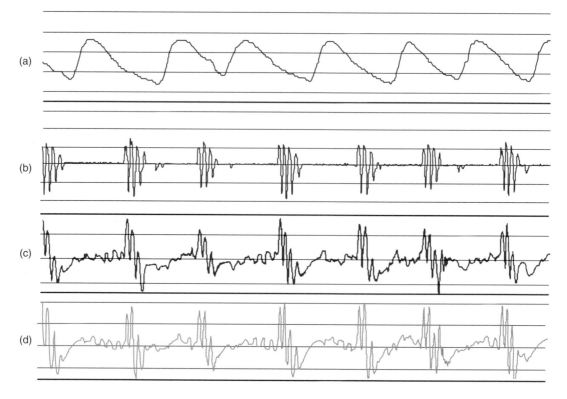

Figure. 18.2 Recognition of obstructive sleep apnoea using limited sleep study. Signals are **(a)** oxygen saturation (oximeter), **(b)** nasal airflow (nasal cannulae), **(c)** ribcage motion and **(d)** abdominal motion (inductance bands). Note that, during each period of apnoea (zero airflow), ribcage and abdominal motion continue but are out of phase with each other.

collapsible upper airway results in increased activity of the pharyngeal dilator muscles, this is insufficient to maintain airway patency.[28]

18.2.1.4 Influence of respiratory control instability

Although more important in the genesis of central than obstructive apnoeas, instability of the respiratory control system can also impact on the latter. The overall stability of the control system can be described in terms of the 'loop gain', which has two components, 'controller gain' and 'plant gain' (see Chapter 6, Section 6.2.1). The respiratory controller gain depends on the ventilatory responses to hypoxia or hypercapnia, while the plant gain describes the effectiveness of carbon dioxide (CO_2) elimination for a given level of ventilation. If the overall loop gain is high, the response is disproportionate to the stimulus and the underdamped

system causes oscillation of ventilation, which may then set up a self-perpetuating cycle of periodic breathing. This is likely to become more obvious during sleep when the stabilizing effect of the wakefulness drive is lost. The contribution of such a mechanism to the pathogenesis of obstructive sleep apnoeas is uncertain, but greater instability is demonstrable in patients with more severe OSA.[2]

18.2.1.5 Chest wall motion

During an obstructive as opposed to central apnoea, respiratory efforts continue and are associated with movements of the ribcage and abdomen that are out of phase with each other (Fig. 18.2). The inspiratory paradox can occur (i.e. volume diminishing) in either the ribcage or the abdominal compartment, with the pattern varying between individuals.[29,30] If the diaphragm predominates, ribcage paradox is seen due to the lowered pleural pressure as the diaphragm contracts; if the ribcage muscles are dominant, paradoxical motion of the abdomen occurs. Abdominal paradox tends to be seen in more obese subjects and recruitment of the abdominal muscles may contribute to this pattern in some subjects.[29]

18.2.1.6 Termination of apnoea

As the apnoea progresses, the activity of the 'pump' muscles gradually increases, presumably due to the increasing chemical drive to breathe consequent on hypoxaemia and increasing $PaCO_2$, although the latter develops much more slowly than the former. These stimuli also result in increased activity of the upper airway muscles.[31] The importance of hypoxaemia is demonstrable by administration of oxygen, which reduces muscle activity and prolongs apnoea.[31] The termination of an obstructive apnoea depends on partial arousal, which is accompanied by a considerable increase in activity of the upper airway dilator muscles and consequent de-occlusion of the airway. The stimulus to arousal is probably mediated mechanically rather than chemically, as in healthy subjects arousals are seen with increasing efforts at similar intrathoracic pressures regardless of the stimulus, whether hypoxia, hypercapnia or an added external resistance.[32] It has been suggested that a stimulus to arousal may also be fatigue developing in the diaphragm as it contracts forcefully and repeatedly against an occluded airway, but the evidence for this is inconclusive.

18.2.1.7 Effect of sleep state

Obstructive apnoeas and the consequent oxygen desaturation are generally more severe in rapid-eye-movement (REM) sleep, presumably due to the greater suppression of inspiratory (including upper airway) muscle activity. Obstructive apnoeas tend to become more prolonged as the night progresses, probably due to the greater proportion of REM sleep later in the night.

18.2.1.8 'Central' apnoeas in obstructive sleep apnoea syndrome

Many patients with OSAS have some events that appear to be 'central' in nature, while other patients have mixed apnoeas, and in a few snoring patients apparently central apnoeas dominate.[33] In some patients, the apparent nature of the apnoea varies with posture, with central or mixed apnoeas when supine becoming clearly obstructive when the subject assumes the lateral position.[34] In such individuals conventional treatment for OSAS with nasal continuous positive airway pressure (CPAP) is usually effective. Higher pressures may, however, be required than for typical OSAS, and lower pressures may appear to convert central apnoeas to mixed or obstructive events.[34] These observations suggest that, in many individuals with apparently central sleep apnoea, the cessation of effort is a reflex response to occlusion of the airway. As discussed above, the termination of an obstructive apnoea is accompanied by greatly increased muscle activity with consequent hyperventilation and hypocapnia. Potentially this can destabilize the respiratory control and in some individuals it may result in cessation of respiratory effort at the onset of the next apnoea,[35] so that an obstructive apnoea may then appear to be 'central' or 'mixed'.

18.2.1.9 Effects on nocturnal blood gases

The most obvious functional consequence of apnoea or hypopnoea is arterial oxygen desaturation. The recorded fall in SaO_2 commences about 10 s after the onset of apnoea, a delay that is due in part to the response time of the oximeter and in part to the circulation time. The rate at which SaO_2 falls is a function of the oxygen 'stores' in the lungs and blood and of the rate at which oxygen is consumed during apnoea. The overall magnitude of the fall depends on the rate of fall and its duration. The nadir SaO_2 depends importantly on the pre-apnoeic value, so that, inevitably, anyone with awake desaturation is likely to show more marked dips for a given duration of apnoea. Conversely, younger subjects with healthy lungs may show only minor falls in SaO_2 in the face of quite severe OSAS.

The rate of fall of SaO_2 is related more closely to the mixed venous oxygen saturation than to the arterial value, as the venous blood 'pool' of oxygen is greater than the arterial 'pool'.[36] Desaturation is usually more severe in REM than non-REM sleep because of the longer duration of apnoeas.[37] In occasional patients with OSAS, unusually severe desaturation is related to the presence of a patent foramen ovale that allows interatrial right-to-left shunting during the vigorous respiratory efforts of the obstructive apnoeas.[38]

Transient rises in $PaCO_2$ during apnoeas are more difficult to detect than reductions in oxygen saturation, partly because transcutaneous PCO_2 electrodes respond much more slowly than oximeters and partly because the increase in $PaCO_2$ during an apnoea is very much less than the falls in PaO_2 and saturation, due to the large difference in relative body 'stores'. Small overall increases in both transcutaneous[39] and end tidal[40] PCO_2 have been reported overnight in patients with OSAS. Measurements of daytime blood gases are discussed below (see Section 18.2.4.1).

18.2.2 Obstructive sleep apnoea and obstructive sleep apnoea syndrome

Several epidemiological studies have shown that the prevalence of sleep-disordered breathing in apparently healthy individuals is surprisingly large, with only a minority developing relevant symptoms. Hence, it is important to distinguish OSA, the phenomenon, from OSAS, the syndrome, which implies attributable symptoms in addition. Depending on the definitions used, only about 20–30 per cent of individuals with OSA have OSAS.

As discussed in Chapter 6, Section 6.4.1, an apnoea is defined conventionally as cessation of breathing for more than 10 s, but, like most other definitions in this field, this is purely arbitrary. Initially OSAS was defined in terms of the apnoea index (AI), i.e. the average number of apnoeas per 1 h of sleep; one popular definition still used sometimes in North America is an AI of more than 5. However, with greater experience it has become clear that this is a gross oversimplification and of little practical value. Not only do many asymptomatic and apparently healthy subjects have an AI greater than 5, but also the full-blown syndrome with all the typical symptoms can be seen in patients with periodic hypopnoea rather than complete apnoea.[41] This realization led to introduction of the apnoea/hypopnoea index (AHI), which is now the most commonly used index of severity. It should, however, be noted that the distribution of AHI in the general population is continuous

Table 18.2 Severity of obstructive sleep apnoea syndrome

Classification	Apnoea/hypopnoea index (events/h)*
Mild	5–15
Moderate	15–30
Severe	>30

*Plus daytime sleepiness.
Reproduced from ref. 42 with permission from the American Academy of Sleep Medicine.

rather than bimodal and that it increases with age.[16] One commonly used definition of OSAS specifies an AHI of more than 15 per hour,[41] although more than 10 per hour is also used. The AHI together with the presence of attributable symptoms is used to classify the severity of OSAS as mild, moderate or severe (Table 18.2).[42] Again, however, it should be emphasized that such cut-off values are arbitrary as, in effect, there is a continuum from normality through 'sleepy snorers' to patients with severe OSAS who may have many hundreds of apnoeas per night. There are, for example, some snoring individuals with severe daytime sleepiness in whom measurements during sleep do not fit any of the criteria for OSAS. These are sometimes referred to as having the 'upper airway resistance syndrome',[43] which can be recognized by inspiratory flow limitation on the airflow signal (see Chapter 6, Section 6.3.3). It is likely that the mechanism of daytime sleepiness in such individuals is similar to that in full blown OSAS, i.e. sleep disruption with recurrent transient arousal during sleep associated with the increased effort of breathing through a partially obstructed upper airway.

It is a reasonable assumption that daytime sleepiness is in some way related to impaired sleep quality, sleep deprivation or sleep disruption. Consequently, many studies have examined whether the electroencephalogram (EEG) structure of sleep, e.g. the frequency of awakening or transient partial arousal, relates better to daytime sleepiness than the rather crude AHI, but the results have been disappointing. In community surveys of OSA, the AHI shows no correlation with daytime sleepiness, which is hardly surprising in light of the high prevalence of sleepiness in the population and the numerous other everyday causes (e.g. sleep deprivation, shift work, insomnia). On the other hand, in populations of patients presenting to sleep clinics there usually is a relationship, albeit weak, between AHI and the severity of daytime sleepiness. Despite several attempts to refine the prediction of symptoms by using more specific measurements of sleep, none has been shown to be superior to the AHI, although detailed studies have shown that the severity of nocturnal hypoxaemia and indices of sleep disruption correlate independently with the severity of daytime sleepiness.[44,45]

18.2.3 Investigation and measurement

Historically, patients with suspected sleep apnoea were investigated by detailed polysomnography (PSG) in hospital. Although still regarded as the definitive investigation in some centres, this is both impracticable and unnecessary in most patients in whom OSAS is suspected. Full PSG still has an important role in the investigation of sleepiness when other conditions enter the differential diagnosis and also in patients with important comorbidity such as chronic airway disease, cardiac failure or neuromuscular disease. At the other extreme, oximetry alone using a pulse oximeter allows recognition of more severe OSAS but suffers from a lack of both specificity and sensitivity. Between the extremes of detailed PSG and oximetry alone are various limited sleep study systems ('respiratory polysomnography'), which are increasingly used in domiciliary investigation (Fig. 18.2). These are discussed in detail in Chapter 6, Section 6.5.3.

18.2.4 Awake measurements of respiratory function in obstructive sleep apnoea syndrome

18.2.4.1 Arterial blood gases

When awake, the majority of patients with OSAS have arterial blood gases within normal limits, but a minority have hypercapnia and hypoxaemia. Many of these patients have coexistent chronic obstructive pulmonary disease (COPD), while others have extreme obesity and fit the criteria for the obesity hypoventilation syndrome (see Chapter 24, Section 24.2). However, the overall prevalence of daytime blood gas abnormalities in OSAS may have been underestimated in earlier studies and in most economically advanced countries probably is

increasing pari passu the severity of obesity. In general, daytime blood gases become more abnormal as BMI increases[46,47] and as lung volumes become more restricted.[48,49] Two studies of patients without airway obstruction showed hypercapnia in 20–30 per cent of patients with BMI above 40[47,48] and even in 7 per cent of those with BMI below 30.[47]

Patients with diurnal respiratory failure are likely to develop polycythaemia, pulmonary hypertension and cor pulmonale.[50] Nocturnal hypoxaemia alone, however, is rarely sufficient to cause polycythaemia. A decreased affinity of haemoglobin for oxygen, with an increase in the P_{50} value, has been demonstrated in OSAS, with the P_{50} related inversely to the mean nocturnal SaO_2. This shift to the right of the oxyhaemoglobin dissociation curve may have a protective effect against the development of polycythaemia and cor pulmonale.[51]

18.2.4.2 Ventilatory responses

Studies of the ventilatory responses to CO_2 and hypoxia in OSAS have produced somewhat conflicting results. Most show average values in the normal range.[52–54] Reduced responses are sometimes reported in patients with daytime hypercapnia,[52] but this is likely in any condition associated with a raised $PaCO_2$ (see Chapter 5, Section 5.2.1). Sleep deprivation may also be relevant as it reduces the ventilatory response of healthy subjects.[55] One study comparing measurements before and after a night's sleep in patients with untreated OSAS showed a lower response in the morning, with shifts of the response curves to the right and a lower ventilation for a given saturation or end tidal PCO_2 but no change in the slope of the responses.[56]

18.2.4.3 Maximum and tidal airflow

Some patients with OSAS show abnormal maximum flow–volume curves related to narrowing and/or instability of the upper airway. Sometimes a 'sawtooth' pattern, with irregular oscillations of maximum expiratory and/or inspiratory flow (see Fig. 1.36 in Chapter 1) is seen,[57] while in other patients there may be disproportionate reduction of maximum inspiratory flow,[58] as is found with structural narrowing of the extrathoracic airway (see Chapter 12, Section 12.1.2.2). Flow oscillations occur particularly in patients with more severe

OSAS.[59] The sensitivity of abnormal maximum flow–volume curves for recognition of OSAS improves if measurements are made in the supine posture,[60] but it is still too low for the measurement to be reliable as a general screening test.[59,60]

Use of the negative expiratory pressure technique (see Chapter 1, Section 1.6.5.8) may show evidence of abnormal collapsibility of the upper airway during awake tidal breathing, with flow limitation demonstrable particularly in the supine posture.[61,62] In one study, a correlation was found between the proportion of the tidal volume over which flow limitation was detectable awake and the frequency of apnoeas when asleep.[61]

18.2.4.4 Lung volumes, diffusing capacity and exercise

Conventional measurements of lung volumes and carbon monoxide diffusing capacity ($D_L CO$) are normal in patients with uncomplicated OSAS after allowing for the effects of obesity.[63] Reduced exercise capacity, expressed as weight-corrected $\dot{V}O_2max$, has been reported in patients with OSAS, but whether this reflects abnormal physiological function or lack of fitness and/or motivation is not clear.[64]

18.2.5 Effects of treatment of obstructive sleep apnoea syndrome

18.2.5.1 Continuous positive airway pressure (CPAP)

The treatment of OSAS was revolutionized by the introduction in 1981 of nasal CPAP,[65] which rapidly became the treatment of choice for the great majority of patients with significant symptoms. The principle is very simple: by applying a positive pressure via the nose (sometimes via the nose and mouth), any tendency to narrowing and collapse of the airway can be overcome, the airway wall is stabilized, and sleep quality and daytime symptoms are improved. The pressure required to overcome the apnoeas and hypopnoeas varies between individuals and, within an individual, may also vary depending on several factors including posture and sleep stage. Usually, treatment is initiated after a simple 'titration' study over a single night or half a night, with the pressure adjusted either manually during continuous monitoring or automatically using an auto-setting device. The aim is usually to eliminate 90 per cent or 95 per cent of the sleep-related events (Fig. 18.3). Most patients then continue with a fixed-pressure device set at the titrated level and sleep investigations are repeated only if justified by continuing or recurrent symptoms. Major changes in weight or other therapeutic manoeuvres may also justify a repeat study in order to retitrate the pressure or determine whether continued treatment is required. Regular use of auto-titrating machines is recommended by some. These deliver a variable pressure that increases if obstructive events or flow limitation are detected, with the applied pressure decreasing automatically during periods when no obstructive events or flow limitation are occurring. Different machines vary in their algorithms for recognizing sleep breathing events: they may sense, variously, vibration due to snoring, evidence of flow limitation or changing impedance detected by

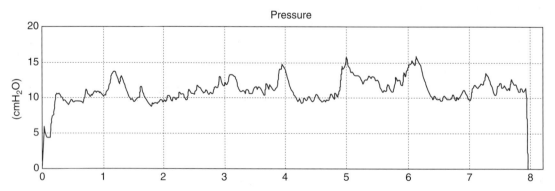

Figure. 18.3 Titration of optimum continuous positive airway pressure using auto-setting positive pressure equipment during sleep. Vertical lines represent 1-h intervals. The pressure required to overcome apnoeas and hypopnoeas varies between $8.5\,cmH_2O$ and $16\,cmH_2O$, and the estimated ninety-fifth percentile pressure for the whole night is $14\,cmH_2O$.

forced oscillation. Compared with conventional CPAP, auto-titrating machines are associated with a slight reduction in the average overall pressure but, in practice, most patients are treated satisfactorily with a fixed-pressure device.[66]

Subtle changes in awake respiratory function have been reported after a period of regular CPAP treatment. Even though most patients with OSAS have normal awake blood gases and normal conventional respiratory function, small increases in PaO_2 occur,[67] as well as minor increases in ventilatory and mouth occlusion pressure responses to CO_2.[54] In patients with more definite daytime hypercapnia and hypoxaemia, long-term treatment with CPAP improves daytime and night-time blood gases.[68] Improved performance in progressive exercise has also been reported.[69]

18.2.5.2 Mandibular advancement devices

Intra-oral mandibular advancement devices represent an alternative to CPAP for some patients with OSAS,[70] although they are less predictably effective at reducing the AHI and the severity of oxygen desaturation.[71] One study suggested that maximum flow–volume curves might have a role in predicting those patients likely to respond better to this approach: one of the factors associated with a greater likelihood of benefit was a higher ratio of $\dot{V}_E max_{50}/\dot{V}_I max_{50}$.[72]

18.2.5.3 Effects of weight loss

Weight loss is a logical treatment for obese patients with OSAS and is achieved most effectively by various forms of bariatric surgery. In morbidly obese patients with OSAS, this has been shown to result in increased pharyngeal dimensions,[73] with concomitant marked decreases in AHI and the severity of nocturnal desaturation.[74,75]

18.3 CENTRAL SLEEP APNOEA

18.3.1 Causes of central sleep apnoea

See Table 18.3.

The prevalence of clinically significant central sleep apnoea is much less than OSAS, but the range of conditions in which central apnoea can occur is broader. Although, in principle, the pathophysiology underlying obstructive and central apnoeas and the resulting patterns of abnormality are distinct, some overlap is seen due to interactions between the stability of the upper airway and the overall respiratory control system (see Chapter 6, Section 6.2). As mentioned above, it has been shown in some individuals with OSAS that airway closure occurs at the nadir of varying drive and, conversely, central apnoea can occur as a reflex response to airway closure. In some patients with otherwise typical OSAS, central apnoea due to instability of respiratory control may be unmasked by treatment with CPAP (see Section 18.3.3).

Central sleep apnoea results ultimately from failure of respiratory drive. This may be low continuously due to inadequate or ineffectual central output, or intermittently, if the stimulus to the respiratory centres is varying. In the former case, persistent hypoventilation and hypercapnia are present (see Table 18.3). Neuromuscular causes and the obesity hypoventilation syndrome are covered in Chapter 20, Section 20.2.1.7 and Chapter 24, Section 24.2 respectively. The effects of heavy acute sedation on breathing are well recognized, but it has also become apparent that individuals receiving long-term opiate therapy can develop frequent central sleep apnoea.[76,77] The apnoeas occur particularly in non-REM sleep and their frequency is dose-dependent. The prevalence of this problem is unclear but it may be more common than appreciated.[77]

Table 18.3 Causes of central sleep apnoea in adults

Cause	Section
With raised $Paco_2$	
Central hypoventilation	20.1.2
Severe respiratory muscle weakness	20.2.1.7
Obesity–hypoventilation syndrome	24.2
Chronic opiate use	
With low/normal $Paco_2$	
Normal subjects: sleep onset, altitude	
Congestive heart failure	19.2.4
Stroke	20.3.1.3
Idiopathic	
CPAP-induced/'complex'	

CPAP, continuous positive airway pressure.

Central sleep apnoea with a normal or, more commonly, reduced $PaCO_2$ occurs with the development of unstable breathing during sleep due to the uncovering of the 'apnoeic threshold' in the face of an overall increase in loop gain (see Chapter 6, Section 6.2.1). It may occur transiently in normal subjects at sleep onset due to the fluctuating awake/asleep state and consequent variation in the 'wakefulness drive'.[78] It is common and more persistent in healthy individuals sleeping at altitude, when the frequency of central sleep apnoea is related closely to the severity of hypocapnia.[79] Frequent arousal from sleep at altitude tends to exacerbate the instability of control and is likely to perpetuate the periodic breathing and central apnoeas.[80] The commonest pathological setting associated with periodic central sleep apnoea in adults is in association with Cheyne–Stokes breathing in patients with congestive cardiac failure (see Chapter 19, Section 19.2.4). Central apnoeas may also be seen along with other sleep breathing disorders in patients after stroke (see Chapter 20, Section 20.3.1.3).

18.3.2 Idiopathic central sleep apnoea syndrome

Patients with periodic central apnoea and no apparent underlying cause are categorized as having idiopathic central sleep apnoea syndrome. They represent only a small minority of patients attending sleep clinics. The breathing typically shows a cyclical pattern during sleep for at least part of the night, sometimes with a superficial resemblance to Cheyne–Stokes breathing, but typically the cycle duration is appreciably shorter and oxygen desaturation tends to be less marked.[81,82] The apnoeas are usually more common in non-REM than REM sleep. Patients with these features have a mildly reduced arterial PCO_2 awake and measurements of end tidal or transcutaneous PCO_2 suggest that low values are maintained during sleep. Awake ventilatory responses are characteristically high. The consequent high loop gain of the ventilatory control system leads to exaggerated responses that perpetuate the fluctuating stimulus and response. Reducing the overall stimulus to breathe by adding supplementary oxygen overnight has been shown to reduce the frequency of central apnoeas.[83]

18.3.3 'Complex sleep apnoea syndrome'

In some patients with apparently typical OSAS, initiation of treatment with CPAP appears to unmask a potentially unstable respiratory control system, with the development of central apnoeas. Such individuals have both upper airway obstruction and periodic breathing, a combination that has been labelled the 'complex sleep apnoea syndrome'.[84] This is sometimes recognized during initial CPAP titration and may improve with suppression of the apnoeas during continuing CPAP therapy.[85] However, in some individuals the problem can persist and be manifest as poor control of symptoms despite resolution of the obstructive events. As in the idiopathic central sleep apnoea syndrome, such individuals have persistent, albeit mild, sleep hypocapnia. Also as in the idiopathic central sleep apnoea syndrome, the abnormalities are more marked in non-REM than in REM sleep. It is assumed that the CPAP treatment, in addition to overcoming the obstructive events, induces mild hyperventilation and a consequently lower $PaCO_2$, which unmasks the effect of periodic respiratory drive.[86] The central apnoeas can be suppressed by restoring end tidal PCO_2 close to waking levels with the addition of a very low concentration of CO_2 into the CPAP mask.[87] More practicable is use of 'adaptive servoventilation', which stabilizes breathing in some individuals,[88] as it does with Cheyne–Stokes breathing (see Chapter 19, Section 19.2.4.6).

REFERENCES

1 Gastaut H, Tassinari CA, Duron B. Polygraphic study of the episodic diurnal and nocturnal (hypnic and respiratory) manifestations of the Pickwick syndrome. *Brain Res* 1966; **1**: 167–86.

2 Younes M, Ostrowski M, Thompson W, Leslie C, Shewchuk W. Chemical control stability in patients with obstructive sleep apnea. *Am J Respir Crit Care Med* 2001; **163**: 1181–90.

3 Onal E, Lopata M. Periodic breathing and the pathogenesis of occlusive sleep apnoea. *Am Rev Respir Dis* 1982; **126**: 676–80.

4 Gleadhill I, Schwartz A, Wise R, *et al.* Upper airway collapsibility in snorers and in patients with obstructive hypopnoea and apnoea. *Am Rev Respir Dis* 1991; **143**: 1300–303.

5 Boyd JH, Petrof BJ, Hamid O, Fraser R, Kimoft RJ. Upper airway muscle inflammation and denervation changes in obstructive sleep apnoea. *Am J Respir Crit Care Med* 2004; **170**: 541–6.

6 Atkins M, Taskar V, Clayton N, Stone P, Woodcock AA. Nasal resistance in obstructive sleep apnoea. *Chest* 1994; **105**: 1133–5.

7 Ciscar MA, Juan G, Martinez V, *et al.* Magnetic resonance imaging of the pharynx in OSA patients and healthy subjects. *Eur Respir J* 2001; **17**: 79–86.

8 Eastwood PR, Szollosi I, Platt PR, Hillman DR. Comparison of upper airway collapse during general anaesthesia and sleep. *Lancet* 2002; **359**: 1207–9.

9 Heinzer RC, Stanchina ML, Malhotra A, *et al.* Effect of increased lung volume on sleep disordered breathing in patients with sleep apnoea. *Thorax* 2006; **61**: 435–9.

10 Mador MJ, Kufel TJ, Magalang UJ, *et al.* Prevalence of positional sleep apnea in patients undergoing polysomnography. *Chest* 2005; **128**: 2130–37.

11 Jordan AS, Wellman A, Edwards JK, *et al.* Respiratory control stability and upper airway collapsibility in men and women with obstructive sleep apnea. *J Appl Physiol* 2005; **99**: 2020–27.

12 Pillar G, Malhotra A, Fogel R, *et al.* Airway mechanics and ventilation in response to resistive loading during sleep: influence of gender. *Am J Respir Crit Care Med* 2000; **162**: 1627–32.

13 O'Donnell CP, Schwartz AR, Smith PL. Upper airway collapsibility. *Am J Respir Crit Care Med* 2000; **162**: 1606–7.

14 Bixler EO, Vgontzas AN, Lin HM, *et al.* Prevalence of sleep-disordered breathing in women: effects of gender. *Am J Respir Crit Care Med* 2001; **163**: 608–13.

15 Saaresranta T, Polo-Kantola P, Virtanen I, *et al.* Menopausal estrogen therapy predicts better nocturnal oxyhemoglobin saturation. *Maturitas* 2006; **55**: 255–63.

16 Young T, Peppard PE, Gottlieb DJ. Epidemiology of obstructive sleep apnoea: a population health perspective. *Am J Respir Crit Care Med* 2002; **165**: 1217–39.

17 Watanabe T, Isono S, Tanaka A, Tansawa H, Nishimo T. Contribution of body habitus and craniofacial characteristics to segmental closing pressures of the passive pharynx in patients with sleep-disordered breathing. *Am J Respir Crit Care Med* 2002; **165**: 260–65.

18 Schwab RJ, Gupta KB, Gefter WB, *et al.* Upper airway and soft tissue anatomy in normal subjects and patients with sleep-disordered breathing: significance of the lateral pharyngeal walls. *Am J Respir Crit Care Med* 1995; **152**: 1673–89.

19 Leiter JC. Upper airway shape: is it important in the pathogenesis of obstructive sleep apnoea? *Am J Respir Crit Care Med* 1996; **153**: 894–8.

20 Fleetham JA. Upper airway imaging in relation to obstructive sleep apnoea. *Clin Chest Med* 1992; **13**: 399–416.

21 Li KK, Kushida C, Powell NB, Riley RW, Guilleminault C. Obstructive sleep apnea syndrome: a comparison between Far-East Asian and white men. *Laryngoscope* 2000; **110**: 1689–93.

22 Ip MS, Lam B, Lauder IJ, *et al.* A community study of sleep-disordered breathing in middle-aged Chinese men in Hong Kong. *Chest* 2001; **119**: 62–9.

23 Schwartz AR, O'Donnell CP, Baron J, *et al.* The hypotonic upper airway in obstructive sleep apnea. *Am J Respir Crit Care Med* 1998; **157**: 1051–7.

24 Patil SP, Punjabi NM, Schneider H, *et al.* A simplified method for measuring critical pressures during sleep in the clinical setting. *Am J Respir Crit Care Med* 2004; **170**: 86–93.

25 Gold AR, Marcus CL, Dipalo F, Gold MS. Upper airway collapsibility during sleep in upper airway resistance syndrome. *Chest* 2002; **121**: 1531–40.

26 Fogel R, Malhotra A, Pillar G, *et al.* Genioglossal activation in patients with obstructive sleep apnoea versus control subjects: mechanisms of muscle control. *Am J Respir Crit Care Med* 2001; **164**: 2025–30.

27 Horner RL. Impact of brainstem sleep mechanisms on pharyngeal motor control. *Respir Physiol* 2000; **119**: 113–21.

28 Pierce R, White D, Malhotra A, *et al.* Upper airway collapsibility, dilator muscle activation and resistance in sleep apnoea. *Eur Respir J* 2007; **30**: 345–53.

29 Staats BA, Bonekat HW, Harris CD, Offord KP. Chest wall motion in sleep apnoea. *Am Rev Respir Dis* 1984; **130**: 59–63.

30 Kimoff RJ, Cheong TH, Olha AE, *et al.* Mechanisms of apnoea termination in obstructive sleep apnoea: role of chemoreceptor and mechanoreceptor stimuli. *Am J Respir Crit Care Med* 1994; **149**: 707–14.

31 Hudgel DW, Hendricks C, Dadley A. Alteration in obstructive apnea pattern induced by changes in oxygen and carbon dioxide inspired concentrations. *Am Rev Respir Dis* 1988; **138**: 16–19.

32 Gleeson K, Zwillich CW, White DP. The influence of increasing ventilatory effort on arousal from sleep. *Am Rev Respir Dis* 1990; **142**: 296–300.

33 Bradley TD, McNicholas WT, Rutherford R, *et al.* Clinical and physiologic heterogeneity of the central sleep apnea syndrome. *Am Rev Respir Dis* 1986; **134**: 217–21.

34 Issa FG, Sullivan CE. Reversal of central sleep apnea using nasal CPAP. *Chest* 1986; **90**: 165–71.

35 Iber C, Davies SF, Chapman RC, Mahowald MM. A possible mechanism for mixed apnea in obstructive sleep apnea. *Chest* 1986; **89**: 800–805.

36 Fletcher EC, Costarangos C, Miller T. The rate of fall of arterial oxyhaemoglobin saturation in obstructive sleep apnea. *Chest* 1989; **96**: 717–22.

37 Series F, Cormier Y, LaForge J. Influence of apnea type and sleep stage on nocturnal postapneic desaturation. *Am Rev Respir Dis* 1990; **141**: 1522–6.

38 Johannson MC, Eriksson P, Peker Y, *et al.* The influence of patent foramen ovale on oxygen desaturation in obstructive sleep apnoea. *Eur Respir J* 2007; **29**: 149–55.

39 Chin K, Hirai M, Kuriyama T, *et al.* Changes in the arterial P_{CO_2} during a single night sleep in patients with obstructive sleep apnoea. *Intern Med* 1997; **36**: 454–60.

40 Fuse K, Satoh M, Yokata T, *et al.* Regulation of ventilation before and after sleep in patients with obstructive sleep apnoea. *Respirology* 1999; **4**: 125–30.

41 Gould CA, Whyte KF, Rhind GB, *et al.* The sleep hypopnea syndrome. *Am Rev Respir Dis* 1988; **137**: 895–8.

42 American Academy of Sleep Medicine. Sleep related breathing disorders in adults: recommendations for syndrome definition and measurement techniques in clinical research. *Sleep* 1999; **22**: 667–89.

43 Guilleminault C, Stoohs R, Clerk A, Cetel M, Maistros P. A cause of excessive daytime sleepiness: the upper airway resistance syndrome. *Chest* 1993; **104**: 781–7.

44 Punjabi NM, O'Hearn DJ, Neubauer DN, *et al.* Modeling hypersomnolence in sleep-disordered breathing: a novel approach using survival analysis. *Am J Respir Crit Care Med* 1999; **159**: 1703–9.

45 Mediano E, Barcelo A, de la Pena M, *et al.* Daytime sleepiness and polysomnographic variables in sleep apnoea patients. *Eur Respir J* 2007; **30**: 110–13.

46 Verin E, Tardif C, Pasquis P. Prevalence of daytime hypercapnia or hypoxia in patients with OSAS and normal lung function. *Respir Med* 2001; **95**: 693–6.

47 Laaban J-P, Chailleus E. Daytime hypercapnia in adult patients with obstructive sleep apnea syndrome in France, before initiating nocturnal nasal continuous positive airway pressure therapy. *Chest* 2005; **127**: 710–15.

48 Resta O, Foschino-Barbaro MP, Bonfitto P, *et al.* Prevalence and mechanisms of diurnal hypercapnia in a sample of morbidly obese subjects with obstructive sleep apnoea. *Respir Med* 2000; **94**: 240–46.

49 Akashiba T, Kawahara S, Kosaka N, *et al.* Determinants of chronic hypercapnia in Japanese men with obstructive sleep apnea syndrome. *Chest* 2002; **121**: 415–21.

50 Krieger J, Sforza E, Apprill M. Pulmonary hypertension, hypoxaemia and hypercapnia in obstructive sleep apnea patients. *Chest* 1989; **96**: 729–37.

51 Maillard D, Fleury B, Housset B, *et al.* Decreased oxyhaemoglobin affinity in patients with sleep apnoea syndrome. *Am Rev Respir Dis* 1991; **143**: 486–9.

52 Sin DD, Jones RL, Man GC. Hypercapnic ventilatory response in patients with and without obstructive sleep apnea: do age, gender, obesity, and daytime Pa_{CO_2} matter? *Chest* 2000; **117**: 454–9.

53 Verbraecken J, Willemen M, De Cock W, *et al.* Influence of longterm CPAP therapy on CO_2 drive in patients with obstructive sleep apnea. *Respir Physiol* 2000; **123**: 121–30.

54 Moura SM, Bittencourt LR, Bagnato MC, *et al.* Acute effect of nasal continuous positive air pressure on the ventilatory control of patients with obstructive sleep apnea. *Respiration* 2001; **68**: 243–9.

55 White DP, Douglas NJ, Pickett CK, Zwillich CW, Weil JV. Sleep deprivation and control of ventilation. *Am Rev Respir Dis* 1983; **128**: 984–6.

56 Fuse K, Satoh M, Yokota T, *et al.* Regulation of ventilation before and after sleep in patients with obstructive sleep apnea. *Respirology* 1999; **4**: 125–30.

57 Sanders MH, Martin RJ, Pennock BE, Rogers RM. The detection of sleep apnoea in the awake patient. *J Am Med Assoc* 1981; **245**: 2414–18.

58 Haponik EF, Bleecker ER, Allen RP, *et al.* Abnormal inspiratory flow–volume curves in patients with sleep-disordered breathing. *Am Rev Respir Dis* 1981; **124**: 571–4.

59 Katz I, Zamel N, Slutsky AS, Rebuck AS, Hoffstein V. An evaluation of flow–volume curves as a screening test for obstructive sleep apnoea. *Chest* 1990; **98**: 337–40.

60 Shore ET, Millman RP. Abnormalities in the flow–volume loop in obstructive sleep apnoea sitting and supine. *Thorax* 1984; **39**: 775–9.

61 Liistro G, Veriter C, Drury M, Aubert G, Stanescu D. Expiratory flow limitation in awake sleep-disordered breathing subjects. *Eur RespirJ* 1999; **14**: 185–90.

62 Verin E, Tardif C, Portier F, *et al.* Evidence for expiratory flow limitation of extrathoracic origin in patients with obstructive sleep apnea. *Thorax* 2002; **57**: 423–8.

63 Hoffstein V, Oliver Z. Pulmonary function and sleep apnea. *Sleep Breath* 2003; **7**: 159–65.

64 Lin CC, Hsieh WY, Chou CS, Liaw SF. Cardiopulmonary exercise testing in obstructive sleep apnea syndrome. *Respir Physiol Neurobiol* 2006; **150**: 27–34.

65 Sullivan CE, Issa FG, Berthon-Jones M, Eves L. Reversal of obstructive sleep apnoea by continuous positive airway pressure applied through the nares. *Lancet* 1981; **1**: 862–5.

66 Ayas NT, Patel SR, Malhotra A, *et al*. Auto-titrating versus standard continuous positive airway pressure for the treatment of obstructive sleep apnea: results of a meta-analysis. *Sleep* 2004; **27**: 249–53.

67 Verbraecken J, Willemen M, De Cock W, Van de Heyning P, De Backer WA. Continuous positive airway pressure and lung inflation in sleep apnea patients. *Respiration* 2001; **68**: 357–64.

68 Sforza E, Krieger J, Weizenblum E, *et al*. Long-term effects of treatment with nasal continuous positive airway pressure on daytime lung function and pulmonary hemodynamics in patients with obstructive sleep apnea. *Am Rev Respir Dis* 1990; **141**: 866–70.

69 Lin CC, Lin CK, Wu KM, Chou CS. Effect of treatment by nasal CPAP on cardiopulmonary exercise test in obstructive sleep apnea syndrome. *Lung* 2004; **182**: 199–212.

70 Kushida CA, Morgenthaler TI, Littner MR, *et al*. Practice parameters for the treatment of snoring and obstructive sleep apnoea with oral appliances: an update for 2005. *Sleep* 2006; **29**: 240–43.

71 Ferguson KA, Cartwright R, Rogers R, Schmidt-Nowara W. Oral appliances for snoring and obstructive sleep apnoea: a review. *Sleep* 2006; **29**: 244–62.

72 Zeng B, Ng AT, Darendeliler MA, Petocz P, Cistulli PA. Use of flow–volume curves to predict oral appliance treatment outcome in obstructive sleep apnea. *Am J Respir Crit Care Med* 2007; **175**: 726–30.

73 Busetto L, Enzi G, Inelmen EM, *et al*. Obstructive sleep apnea syndrome in morbid obesity: effects of intragastric balloon. *Chest* 2005; **128**: 618–23.

74 Scheuller M, Weider D. Bariatric surgery for treatment of sleep apnea syndrome in 15 morbidly obese patients: long-term results. *Otolaryngol Head Neck Surg* 2001; **125**: 299–302.

75 Dixon JB, Schachter LM, O'Brien PE. Polysomnography before and after weight loss in obese patients with severe sleep apnea. *Int J Obes* 2005; **29**: 1048–54.

76 Wang D, Teichtahl H, Drummer O, *et al*. Central sleep apnea in stable methadone maintenance treatment patients. *Chest* 2005; **128**: 1348–56.

77 Walker JM, Farney RJ, Rhondeau SM, *et al*. Chronic opioid use is a risk factor for the development of central sleep apnea and ataxic breathing. *J Clin Sleep Med* 2007; **3**: 455–61.

78 Dunai J, Kleiman J, Trinder J. Ventilatory instability during sleep onset in individuals with high peripheral chemosensitivity. *J Appl Physiol* 1999; **87**: 661–72.

79 Burgess KR, Johnson PL, Edwards N. Central and obstructive sleep apnoea during ascent to high altitude. *Respirology* 2004; **9**: 222–9.

80 Khoo MC, Anholm JD, Ko SW, *et al*. Dynamics of periodic breathing and arousal during sleep at extreme altitude. *Respir Physiol* 1996; **103**: 33–43.

81 Xie A, Rutherford R, Rankin F, Wong B, Bradley TD. Hypocapnia and increased ventilatory responsiveness in patients with idiopathic central sleep apnea. *Am J Respir Crit Care Med* 1995; **152**: 1950–55.

82 Eckert DJ, Jordan AS, Merchia P, Malhotra A. Central sleep apnoea: pathophysiology and treatment. *Chest* 2007; **131**: 595–607.

83 Franklin KA, Eriksson P, Sahlin C, Lundgren R. Reversal of central sleep apnea with oxygen. *Chest* 1997; **111**: 163–9.

84 Morgenthaler TI, Kagramanov V, Hanak V, Decker PA. Complex sleep apnea syndrome: is it a unique clinical syndrome? *Sleep* 2006; **29**: 1203–9.

85 Dernaika T, Tawk M, Nazir S, Younis W, Kinasewitz GT. The significance and outcome of continuous positive airway pressure-related central sleep apnea during split-night sleep studies. *Chest* 2007; **132**: 81–7.

86 Thomas RJ, Terzano MG, Parrino L, Weiss W. Obstructive sleep-disordered breathing with a dominant cyclic alternating pattern: a recognisable polysomnographic variant with practical clinical implications. *Sleep* 2004; **27**: 229–34.

87 Thomas RJ, Daly RW, Weiss JW. Low-concentration carbon dioxide is an effective adjunct to positive airway pressure in the treatment of refractory mixed central and obstructive sleep-disordered breathing. *Sleep* 2005; **28**: 69–77.

88 Allam JS, Olson EJ, Gay PC, Morgenthaler TI. Efficacy of adaptive servoventilation in treatment of complex and central sleep apnoea syndromes. *Chest* 2007; **132**: 1839–46.

PART C

RESPIRATORY FUNCTION IN SYSTEMIC DISEASES

19

Cardiac Disease

Study of the respiratory function of patients with cardiac disease has a venerable history, dating back to the observations in the nineteenth century by John Cheyne and William Stokes of the characteristic pattern of waxing and waning tidal breathing to which their names are eponymously attached. The first description by Cheyne was of a patient following a severe stroke, but he also had advanced cardiac disease. For most of the twentieth century, studies concentrated largely on the respiratory function of patients with valvular heart disease. Latterly there has been considerable growth of interest in patients with chronic congestive heart failure (CHF), particularly in relation to its effects on exercise performance and breathing during sleep.

Another important link between cardiac disease and respiratory function is evident in epidemiological studies of risk factors for developing ischaemic heart disease. Several studies, including the large Framingham Study in the USA,[1] have shown that reduction in VC and/or FEV_1 is related strongly to subsequent mortality from ischaemic heart disease. Various possible explanations have been proposed, but the precise nature of the relationship is uncertain: one obvious link is smoking, but this is not the sole explanation as the correlation is strong also in non-smokers.[2] Another possible mechanism is that lower-than-average lung function reflects poor overall fitness and obesity.[2,3]

Heart disease can affect the function of the lungs directly, e.g. by reducing their distensibility, or indirectly by a poor cardiac output increasing anaerobic metabolism and, consequently, ventilation. Many individuals have to cope with both heightened ventilatory demand and impaired pulmonary performance. Individuals with exertional breathlessness often present a diagnostic dilemma, and attribution of the symptom to cardiac or lung disease (or both) can present a difficult challenge.

19.1 ACUTE CARDIAC FAILURE

19.1.1 Effects on respiratory mechanics

When oedema is confined to the pulmonary interstitium only mild reductions of lung volumes are likely, but once alveolar 'flooding' occurs the effect is more profound. In one study of acute left ventricular failure (LVF) due to hypertension, for example, a mean VC of only 45 per cent of predicted was reported.[4] Even in the absence of radiographic evidence, pulmonary congestion produces a measurable reduction in VC, which may take several weeks to return to normal.[5] 'Cardiac asthma' implies narrowing of the airways. Although usually attributed to peribronchial oedema, there is little evidence that this is the mechanism; alternative explanations include mucosal swelling and reflex effects.[6] Wheezing, orthopnoea and paroxysmal nocturnal dyspnoea are common to both bronchial asthma and LVF and clinically the distinction can be difficult. Simple measurements of spirometry or peak expiratory flow (PEF) can be very helpful as 'cardiac asthma' is associated with only mild or moderate impairment of airway function.[5] In one study the average PEF of patients admitted to hospital with LVF was 224 L min^{-1} compared with a mean of 108 L min^{-1} in a comparable group with an acute exacerbation of bronchial asthma.[7] Although not completely specific, values of PEF exceeding 200 L min^{-1} in this situation favour LVF as the cause of acute shortness of breath and wheezing.

19.1.2 Effects on pulmonary gas exchange

Abnormal pulmonary gas exchange occurs even in apparently uncomplicated myocardial infarction. Its consequences are seen as reduced PaO_2 and SaO_2,[8] with widening of the alveolar–arterial PO_2 ($AaPO_2$) gradient. The arterial desaturation is due in part to basal airway closure and mismatching of ventilation and perfusion within lung regions. The severity of hypoxaemia may be amplified by the effect of a low cardiac output and consequent greater desaturation of mixed venous blood.[9] Moreover, the PaO_2 may not correct completely on 100 per cent oxygen,[10] implying a degree of 'anatomical' shunt. This would be expected with continued perfusion of 'flooded' alveoli, but its presence in less florid, and presumably interstitial, oedema is not explained fully.

The standard textbook account of blood gases in patients with acute LVF describes hypoxaemia with a normal or low $PaCO_2$. The literature, however, records many instances of hypercapnia,[11,12] at least transiently. A metabolic (lactic) acidosis is also not uncommon and, if combined with a respiratory acidosis, may result in extremely low values of pH.[11] In one series of 101 mainly elderly patients with cardiogenic pulmonary oedema, no fewer than 55 had a combined acidosis and 12 others had a respiratory acidosis alone.[12] It may be relevant that many of the patients had received opiates or oxygen before the blood gases were measured. Nevertheless, the figures cast serious doubt on the received wisdom that acute pulmonary oedema is typically associated with hypocapnia. Abnormal blood gases usually improve rapidly with appropriate medical management, including oxygen treatment.[8] Continuous positive airway pressure (CPAP) or pressure support ventilation is beneficial in more severe cases,[13] improving gas exchange by raising lung volume and reducing cardiac preload.

19.2 CHRONIC CARDIAC FAILURE

19.2.1 Resting ventilation and gas exchange

Patients with chronic CHF have increased resting oxygen consumption due mainly to the increased ventilation,[14] which in turn results from a combination of increased ventilatory drive, an inefficient pattern of breathing with rapid frequency and small tidal volume, and impaired gas exchange. The regional distribution of ventilation may be abnormal, particularly in patients with cardiomegaly who, in the supine position, have reduced ventilation of the left lower lobe due to mechanical compression.[15] Regional redistribution of perfusion may also be seen with more uniform distribution or even a reversal of the normal gradient, particularly in patients with a markedly raised left atrial pressure. Airway closure during tidal breathing is common and results from a low functional residual capacity (FRC) rather than an increase in closing capacity.[16] This increases $AaPO_2$ and contributes to a varying degree of hypoxaemia, while $PaCO_2$ is typically low with a respiratory alkalosis.[16,17]

19.2.2 Respiratory mechanics

A restrictive ventilatory defect of variable severity is typical, with cardiomegaly per se contributing to the reduced volumes in many patients.[18] Static lung compliance is reduced, due to the effects of vascular congestion and oedema, but the reduction is not clearly related to the severity as assessed by symptoms and exercise capacity.[19]

Patients with chronic heart failure commonly have reduced muscle bulk and associated weakness, which also affects the respiratory muscles.[17,20] In some individuals this contributes to the restriction of lung volumes. Reduction of maximum static inspiratory pressure correlates with the severity of CHF[21] and of breathlessness during daily activities.[16,20]

Patients with end-stage CHF show little spirometric evidence of airway obstruction,[22] although a mildly reduced FEV_1/VC is seen in some patients with advanced disease.[21] The reported abnormalities of residual volume in CHF are divergent, probably owing to varying combinations of opposing trends. On the one hand, stiffening of alveolar walls opposes full deflation by holding the alveoli open, as in mitral stenosis (see below), and airway narrowing or closure are also associated with a raised RV; on the other hand, with frank alveolar oedema the number of air containing alveoli is reduced, so that the RV (gas volume) falls, even though the total volume of the thoracic contents (gas + fluid + heart) may not be reduced. Non-specific bronchial hyperrespon-siveness is demonstrable in some patients with chronic cardiac failure.[6] It is attributed to airway oedema and may lessen after treatment with diuretics.[23]

Patients with acute or chronic heart failure characteristically complain of orthopnoea. Expiratory flow limitation in the upright posture may occur with pulmonary oedema,[24] but it is not usually found in CHF.[16] However, when the patient assumes the recumbent posture it is much more frequent and is an important contributor to orthopnoea.[24,25] It results from a posture-related increase in respiratory resistance, which is demonstrable within 5 min of assuming the supine posture.[26]

Following successful heart transplantation, lung volumes usually increase and may normalize.[27,28] Much of the increase in VC is attributable simply to a smaller heart size.[29]

19.2.3 Carbon monoxide diffusing capacity

A moderate reduction in carbon monoxide diffusing capacity (D_LCO) is characteristic of CHF,[27,28,30] with lower values in patients with more severe disease.[30] The KCO has been reported to be either normal[31] or mildly reduced.[32] In the latter series,[32] patients were studied before and after appropriate medical treatment, which resulted in an increase in KCO to normal values.

Detailed study of the membrane (D_m) and capillary blood volume (V_c) components of diffusing capacity shows consistently low values of the former[33,34] and a close inverse correlation between D_m and pulmonary vascular resistance.[34] As might be expected, the V_c component is increased, especially in more severe heart failure,[35] and it correlates with the pulmonary capillary wedge pressure.[34] Any increase in V_c, however, is insufficient to counter the reduction in D_m, which accounts for the overall reduction in D_LCO.

Unlike lung volumes, D_LCO does not usually increase after heart transplantation. Indeed, some series have shown a small further reduction.[27,36] This may be due to a lower V_c consequent on less pulmonary congestion, with unchanged function of the alveolar–capillary membrane due to non-reversible damage.[31]

19.2.4 Cheyne–Stokes breathing and sleep breathing disorders

19.2.4.1 Cheyne–Stokes breathing awake

Cheyne–Stokes breathing (Cheyne–Stokes respiration, CSR) is common in patients with chronic heart failure. Although more easily recognized during sleep, it is also present in many individuals while awake and was recorded in 30 per cent of patients with stable CHF in one study.[37] It may also be detectable during exercise testing,[38,39] particularly in patients with more severely impaired cardiac function and lower $\dot{V}O_2max$.[38]

19.2.4.2 Prevalence of sleep-disordered breathing in congestive heart failure

Estimates of the prevalence of sleep-disordered breathing have varied between 24 per cent and 82 per cent in different populations of patients with CHF.[40–45] The proportions with predominantly central and obstructive apnoea have also varied markedly. The prevalence is higher in those with more severe cardiac disease,[44] in whom central sleep apnoea (CSA) as a feature of Cheyne–Stokes breathing tends to dominate.[40–42] Across populations with a broad range of severity, obstructive apnoea may be relatively more common.[43,45] The highest prevalence of sleep apnoea was reported in a series of patients investigated only 1 month after being treated for an episode of acute cardiac failure.[42] Sleep apnoea is more likely in patients with atrial fibrillation or other dysrhythmias.[40,41] As might be expected, patients with dominant obstructive apnoea tend to be heavier and more likely to snore.[40]

19.2.4.3 Pathophysiology of Cheyne–Stokes respiration and central sleep apnoea in chronic heart failure

The physiological consequences of CHF provide the ideal background for destabilization of respiratory control and consequent development of CSR/CSA. Congestive heart failure is associated with hyperventilation, probably due to stimulation of pulmonary vagal receptors, resulting in a chronically low arterial P_{CO_2} that is therefore closer to the apnoeic threshold. The circulation of the blood is slowed in cardiac failure, increasing the delay between stimulus and ventilatory response, which encourages the control system to overshoot. The underlying instability is exaggerated during sleep by transient arousal causing hyperventilation and a further fall in Pa_{CO_2} below the apnoeic threshold (see Chapter 6, Section 6.2.1).

Patients with CSR/CSA have a lower Pa_{CO_2} awake than those with CHF without sleep-disordered breathing.[46] The stimulus to hyperventilation is likely to be pulmonary vascular congestion stimulating vagal receptors, as the awake Pa_{CO_2} correlates inversely with pulmonary wedge pressure.[47] An increased ventilatory response to CO_2 when awake is also characteristic[48,49] and contributes to the control instability. A direct correlation has been shown between awake ventilatory responses to CO_2 and the apnoea/hypopnoea

index (AHI) asleep.[49,50] The circulation time is an important determinant of the cycle length of the oscillations of respiratory drive,[46] with the cycle duration inversely proportional to the cardiac output.[51] Consequently, the cycle length of CSR/CSA in patients with CHF is appreciably longer than in other forms of central sleep apnoea and may exceed 1 min.[50] The longer ventilatory periods typically show more gradual increase and decline.[51] Arterial P_{CO_2} normally rises a little during sleep, but patients with CSR/CSA fail to show this rise.[52] The periodic hypopnoea and apnoea is followed by a fall in Sa_{O_2} (Fig. 19.1). In principle the waxing and waning breathing pattern should be mirrored by symmetrical decreases and increases in Sa_{O_2}, rather than the 'sawtooth' pattern sometimes described in obstructive sleep apnoea due to the more rapid recovery of Sa_{O_2} following each apnoea. In practice, however, the pattern of oximetry alone is not sufficiently specific

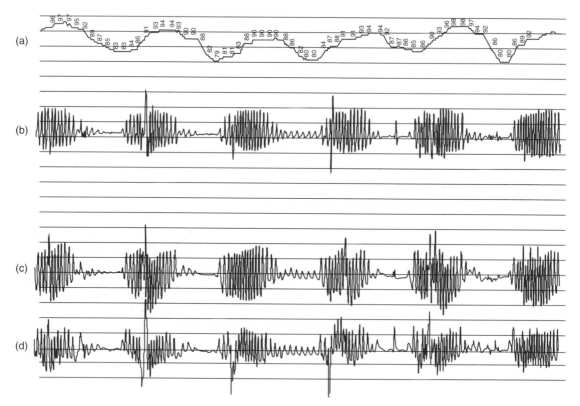

Figure 19.1 Cheyne–Stokes breathing with central sleep apnoea in a patient with congestive heart failure. Signals are (a) oxygen saturation (oximeter), (b) flow (nasal cannulae), (c) ribcage movement and (d) abdominal movement (inductance bands). Note waxing and waning of ventilation with periods of hypopnoea or apnoea, but the ribcage and abdomen move in phase.

for accurate distinction.[53] The severity of CSA/CSR is affected by posture, with less frequent apnoea and better oxygenation in the lateral than the supine position. This effect is independent of changes in size of the upper airway; the explanation is unclear but may relate to differences in lung volume and lung oxygen 'stores' in the two postures.[54] Cheyne–Stokes breathing characteristically is usually more apparent during non-rapid-eye-movement (REM) sleep, when behavioural influences on breathing are less than in REM sleep. Frequent arousal is a common consequence of the waxing and waning of breathing. However, unlike the obstructive sleep apnoea syndrome (OSAS), in which arousal occurs at the termination of apnoea, with CSR arousal tends to occur close to the peak of ventilation.[55] As with OSAS, recurrent arousal is accompanied by increased catecholamine secretion and increases in systemic blood pressure, which may be relevant to the adverse prognosis associated with CSR.[54] Daytime sleepiness may result from the sleep disturbance associated with CSR,[56] but, for reasons that are unclear, this appears to be less common than in patients with OSAS.

19.2.4.4 Pathophysiology of obstructive sleep apnoea in congestive heart failure

The potential mechanisms of OSA in CHF have not been elucidated fully and may vary between individuals. Clearly, the presence of significant obesity is likely to predispose to OSA, as it would in individuals with no heart disease, and the high prevalence of OSA in the otherwise healthy community means that it will occur coincidentally in some people.

The distinction between CSA/CSR and OSA in CHF is not always clear-cut, as many individuals show features of both and the 'diagnosis' reflects the dominant pattern. With CSR, the periodic waning of respiratory drive affects the muscles supporting the upper airway as well as the 'respiratory pump' muscles. Reduction of drive to the pharyngeal dilators is likely to predispose the airway to narrowing or closure,[57] potentially producing the picture of obstructive hypopnoea or apnoea. A further possible contributor is oedema of the airway wall with reduction in its lumen and an increase in

its compliance, particularly in the supine position.[58] The cycle duration in individuals with OSA associated with heart failure is typically longer than in those without heart disease.[59] Within an individual the pattern of sleep apnoea can change over a night's sleep and between nights.[60,61] In some the proportion of obstructive events declines while central events increase later in the night.[60] This is accompanied by a reduction in $PaCO_2$ and increasing cycle length, suggesting deteriorating cardiac function as the night progresses, which presumably further destabilizes the respiratory control system. As with CSR/CSA, OSA in patients with CHF is often not accompanied by excessive daytime sleepiness. Remarkably, in one study, the level of sleepiness of patients with OSA and CHF was lower than in community controls matched for severity of sleep-disordered breathing.[62]

19.2.4.5 Prognostic importance of Cheyne–Stokes breathing in congestive heart failure

Several studies have shown that CSR is associated with a poor prognosis and increased mortality in CHF. Although a large proportion of this association is due to more severe cardiac disease in people with CSR, there is probably also a true independent adverse risk associated with CSR/CSA.[63,64] Recognition of CSR while awake may be particularly important, as in one study this accounted for the adverse prognosis[65] and in another study the presence of CSR during both sleep and exercise carried a particularly poor prognosis.[66] A positive prognostic factor in the latter study was use of β-blockers, which were associated with better survival.[66] Since β-blockers were not used widely for heart failure until recently, it is possible that the adverse prognosis associated with CSR/CSA may now be less relevant.

19.2.4.6 Effects of treatment of sleep-disordered breathing in congestive heart failure

Patients with symptomatic obstructive sleep apnoea associated with CHF are usually treated with CPAP in similar fashion to individuals without heart disease. A small randomized controlled trial (RCT) showed that suppression of obstructive apnoeas by CPAP was accompanied by a significant increase in left ventricular ejection fraction (LVEF).[67]

Many different forms of treatment have been tried in patients with CSR/CSA (Table 19.1). Treating the underlying heart failure itself may improve the breathing pattern. A period of intensive treatment reduces both pulmonary capillary wedge pressure and the frequency of central apnoeas,[68] while acute infusion of a vasodilator at cardiac catheterization reduces the amplitude of oscillations of ventilation and shortens the cycle duration in patients with awake CSR.[69] An alternative approach to improving myocardial function in patients with heart failure is by cardiac resynchronization therapy; in an uncontrolled study of patients with CSR/CSA this significantly reduced the frequency of sleep apnoeas and improved nocturnal oxygenation.[70] Similarly, following cardiac transplantation, CSR/CSA improves, although it may not resolve completely.[71] However, following transplantation, a significant proportion of patients develop obstructive sleep apnoea,[71,72] which is mainly due to gaining weight.[72]

Supplementary oxygen has been used for many years as a means of suppressing CSR, which it does quite effectively, thereby improving both oxygenation and sleep quality.[73-75] Nocturnal oxygen also reduces sympathetic activation and catecholamine levels and improves daytime exercise performance.[76] Whether this influences long-term outcome has not been studied adequately.[77] An alternative method of stabilizing nocturnal breathing is by inspiring a low concentration of CO_2 as only a small increase in the prevailing low $PaCO_2$ is effective in restoring regular respiration.[78] This approach has, however, been reported to increase catecholamine levels[79] and is not currently a viable method of treatment. The carbonic anhydrase inhibitor acetazolamide is used widely to treat periodic breathing at altitude. It works by producing a metabolic acidosis and increasing the difference between $PaCO_2$ and the apnoeic threshold. In a recent small RCT it was shown to reduce the frequency of central apnoeas and improve oxygenation in CHF.[80]

In patients with central as opposed to obstructive sleep apnoea, CPAP increases intrathoracic pressure and lung volume. In principle the latter should be advantageous for oxygenation and the former for left ventricular function, as left ventricular (LV) transmural pressure and afterload are reduced, while cardiac preload will also be lower due to a smaller end diastolic volume.[81] However, it has a possible adverse effect on cardiac output in patients with a low LV filling pressure, such as occurs with atrial fibrillation.[82] Early reports of the effectiveness of CPAP for treating CSR/CSA were encouraging, with improvements in the nocturnal breathing disturbance, oxygenation, LV ejection fraction and symptoms.[82,83] However, in the large multicentre Canadian Continuous Positive Airway Pressure for Patients with Central Sleep Apnea and Heart Failure (CANPAP) trial, these effects did not translate into an overall improvement in survival.[84] In a subsequent post hoc analysis it appeared that those patients on CPAP treatment in whom CSR/CSA was most effectively suppressed showed a greater improvement of LVEF and significantly longer survival.[85]

Other modes of ventilatory support have also been evaluated. Non-invasive ventilation (NIV) by bilevel pressure support was shown in one small randomized study to be as effective as CPAP at improving nocturnal ventilation and circulation time,[86] but in another retrospective study it proved more likely to worsen then to improve CSR.[87] A novel non-invasive ventilator has been developed specifically to stabilize breathing during sleep by varying the amount of ventilatory support from breath to breath in order to stabilize the tidal volume to a long-term running average value.[88] An RCT of this technique of 'adaptive servoventilation' (ASV) showed effective control of

Table 19.1 Therapeutic modalities influencing Cheyne–Stokes breathing (CSR) and central sleep apnoea (CSA) in congestive heart failure

Treatment of heart failure	Drugs
	Cardiac resynchronization therapy
	Heart transplantation
Treatment of CSR/CSA	CO_2
oxygen	Acetazolamide
	CPAP
	Adaptive servoventilation

CPAP, continuous positive airway pressure.

nocturnal ventilation, a reduction in daytime hyperventilation and an increase in $PaCO_2$ with an objective improvement in alertness.[89] A longer-term comparison with CPAP showed better compliance and a greater improvement in LVEF with ASV.[90]

19.2.5 Exercise testing in chronic heart failure

19.2.5.1 Pattern of exercise response

Maximum exercise performance and maximum (peak) oxygen consumption ($\dot{V}O_2max$) are limited to an extent dependent on the severity of CHF. The ventilatory response to exercise of patients with CHF is greater than normal for the metabolic rate. Ventilation is inefficient due to the characteristic pattern of relatively increased breathing frequency and small tidal volume, which results in a high dead space/tidal volume (V_D/V_T) ratio and excessive dead space ventilation.[91] The pattern of rapid shallow breathing is a consequence of the reduced pulmonary compliance,[92] and tidal volume reaches a maximal value at relatively low work rates during progressive exercise, with further increases in ventilation dependent on increasing frequency only.[93] Ventilation is also constrained in some individuals by the development of increasing expiratory flow limitation.[94,95]

In addition to the excessive dead space ventilation, alveolar ventilation is abnormally high and $PaCO_2$ low.[96] The increased drive to breathe may result partly from mechanical stimulation of pulmonary receptors due to pulmonary congestion and partly from early anaerobic metabolism. The 'anaerobic threshold' is typically low, after which there is a disproportionate increase in CO_2 output compared with $\dot{V}O_2$ and consequently a high respiratory exchange ratio.[91] Increased anaerobic metabolism is supported by a higher blood lactate concentration for a given $\dot{V}O_2$,[97] but the lactate concentration is not related clearly to the excessive ventilation.[96] Arterial oxygenation usually remains relatively normal, even in patients with severe heart failure.[91] Measurements of D_LCO on exercise in CHF show values less than normal and D_LCO may fall near peak exercise, consistent with development of interstitial oedema.[98] The 6-min walk test is commonly used in overall assessment of patients with CHF and has been shown to have adequate reproducibility and responsiveness in this population.[99]

19.2.5.2 Prognostic value of progressive exercise testing in congestive heart failure

Progressive exercise tests have been shown in several studies to give powerful prognostic information in patients with chronic heart failure (Table 19.2).[100–116] These observations have become of considerable importance in clinical decision-making about the optimal timing of cardiac transplantation for advanced heart failure. Of the specific indices, two have been shown consistently to relate strongly to 'survival' (which usually implies 'transplant-free survival'):

- the symptom-limited maximum or peak oxygen consumption ($\dot{V}O_2max$) corrected for body weight;
- the slope of the relationship between ventilation and CO_2 production ($\dot{V}_E/\dot{V}CO_2$).

Some studies have suggested that correction of $\dot{V}O_2max$ by estimated lean body mass (LBM) rather than overall weight improves the prediction, while others focused on the peak 'oxygen pulse' (i.e. $\dot{V}O_2max$ divided by maximum heart rate) corrected for LBM. Several studies include estimates of optimal cut-off values for dichotomizing the population into those with greater or lesser risk of mortality, but increasing experience has shown that this approach is somewhat simplistic as the likelihood of mortality varies across a range of values.

It should be noted that, as with the prognostic data on Cheyne–Stokes breathing discussed above (see Section 19.2.4.5), many of these data were collected in the era before widespread use of β-blockers for treating CHF, which have significantly changed the prognosis. As β-blockers have been shown to reduce mortality without influencing $\dot{V}O_2max$, some of the earlier conclusions may now be less valid. In particular, the threshold value of $\dot{V}O_2max$ of $14 \, mL \, min^{-1} kg^{-1}$, which is used widely as a guide for referral for heart transplantation, requires re-evaluation as a lower threshold may now be more appropriate.[110,113]

Table 19.2 Optimal exercise-related predictors of 'survival' in congestive heart failure (CHF)

Reference	Indices	Cut-off for better survival
100	$\dot{V}O_2$max (mL min^{-1} kg^{-1})	>14
101	$\dot{V}O_2$max (% predicted)	>50
102	$\dot{V}O_2$max (mL min^{-1} kg^{-1})	>15
	$\dot{V}_E/\dot{V}CO_2$ at AT	<50
103	$\dot{V}_E/\dot{V}CO_2$ slope	–
	$\dot{V}O_2$max (mL min^{-1} kg^{-1})	–
104	$\dot{V}_E/\dot{V}CO_2$ slope	–
105	$\dot{V}O_2$max (mL min^{-1} kg^{-1})	Continuous variable 10–20
	$\dot{V}_E/\dot{V}CO_2$ slope	Continuous variable 30–55
106	$\dot{V}_E/\dot{V}CO_2$ slope	≤130% predicted
107	$\dot{V}O_2$max (mL min^{-1} kg LBM^{-1})	>19
108	$\dot{V}O_2$max	Continuous variable
109	Periodic breathing on exercise	–
110	No β-blocker: $\dot{V}_E/\dot{V}CO_2$ slope	<33
	$\dot{V}O_2$max (mL min^{-1} kg^{-1})	Continuous variable 10–18
	With β-blocker: $\dot{V}O_2$max (mL min^{-1} kg^{-1})	>10
111	$\dot{V}O_2$max (mL min^{-1} kg LBM^{-1})	–
112	Peak 'oxygen pulse lean'	≥14 mL/beat
113	$\dot{V}O_2$max (mL min^{-1} kg^{-1})	Continuous variable
114	$\dot{V}O_2$max (mL min^{-1} kg^{-1})	>14
	$\dot{V}_E/\dot{V}CO_2$ slope	<34
115	$\dot{V}O_2$max	–
	$\Delta\dot{V}O_2$max	–
116	$\dot{V}_E/\dot{V}CO_2$ slope	–

LBM, lean body mass; $\Delta\dot{V}O_2$max, change in $\dot{V}O_2$max over time.

'Peak oxygen pulse lean' = $\dot{V}O_2$max /peak heart rate corrected for LBM. AT, anaerobic threshold.

19.3 VALVULAR HEART DISEASE

19.3.1 Mitral valve disease

19.3.1.1 Effects on pulmonary mechanics and lung volumes

Many of the functional features seen with mitral valve disease resemble those of chronic heart failure. Patients with mitral disease characteristically have a reduced VC and increased RV, with a TLC close to normal.[17] The static pressure–volume (PV) curve of the lungs shows a reduced compliance but a reduction in maximum lung recoil pressure ($P_L$max) at full inflation, which may be due in part to inspiratory muscle weakness.[118] The likely increase in non-gaseous thoracic contents (heart, blood, tissue) may also contribute to the reduction in $P_L$max since their volumes are ignored in the PV curve of the lungs as plotted conventionally; the total thoracic volume is therefore underestimated and the apparently reduced $P_L$max may be appropriate for the larger volume. The reduced VC is probably due to a combination of factors, including muscle weakness, stiffening of the lungs by vascular congestion and fibrosis, and cardiomegaly. An inverse relation is seen between the VC or TLC and the radiographically measured cardiothoracic ratio (Fig. 19.2).[117]

Elevation of RV is the rule with mitral valve disease. It has been attributed to the effect of congested vessels in alveolar walls impeding their deflation. Wheezing is frequent in patients with mitral disease and evidence of mild airflow obstruction is often present. Distinction of the effects of mitral disease from those of primary airway disease is sometimes difficult. However, in non-smoking patients the FEV_1/VC ratio is at most only mildly reduced.[117,119] A further distinguishing feature is the absence of an increase in TLC in patients with mitral disease alone, whereas it is usually high in patients with primary airway disease. Non-specific bronchial hyperresponsiveness is present in many patients with mitral valve disease.[6,120] The severity of hyperresponsiveness relates to the degree of pulmonary venous congestion, as judged by the pulmonary capillary wedge pressure,[120] and also to indices of airway narrowing.[121] In the latter respect the hyperresponsiveness of mitral valve disease

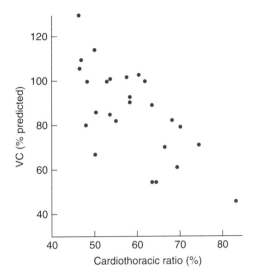

Figure 19.2 Relation between vital capacity (VC) and cardiac size (assessed by the cardiothoracic ratio on a posteroanterior chest radiograph) in 26 patients with mitral valve disease and no radiographic evidence of cardiac failure. $r = 0.69$, $P < 0.001$. Modified from: Rhodes KM *et al*. Relation between severity of mitral valve disease and routine lung function tests in non-smokers. *Thorax* 1982; **37**: 751–5, with permission from the BMJ Publishing Group.

resembles that seen in chronic obstructive pulmonary disease (COPD) rather than asthma.

19.3.1.2 Effects on carbon monoxide uptake

An increased pulmonary capillary blood volume resulting from a high left atrial pressure would be expected to increase the D_LCO, and this has been reported occasionally in mild disease. More commonly, this tendency is outweighed by impaired diffusion across the alveolar–capillary membrane so that the D_LCO is less than normal. The effective alveolar volume is also usually reduced so that KCO is generally little affected and within the normal range in most patients.[117,122]

19.3.1.3 Relation of respiratory function to severity of mitral disease

With all the measurements discussed above there are trends to increasing abnormality with increasing haemodynamic disturbance.[48,56] For instance, patients with an increased pulmonary capillary wedge pressure have more abnormal function that those with normal wedge pressures,[122] and significant inverse correlations have been shown between FEV_1, VC, D_LCO and K_{CO} and various indices of the severity of mitral valve narrowing or pulmonary hypertension assessed by cardiac catheterization.[117]

19.3.1.4 Isotope scans

A raised left atrial pressure gives a characteristic appearance to the perfusion lung scan (Fig. 19.3), with increased apical perfusion and reduced perfusion of the lung bases.[123] The findings are compatible with elevated pulmonary vascular pressures and interstitial oedema at the lung bases so that 'zone 4' (see Chapter 2, Section 2.2.1) is

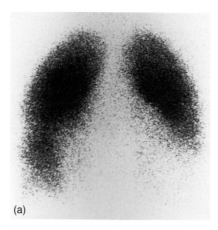

(a)

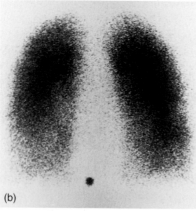

(b)

Figure 19.3 Perfusion lung scan in a patient with mitral stenosis, showing preferential distribution to upper zones. (a) Anterior; (b) posterior.

exaggerated. Chronic pulmonary congestion of whatever aetiology can produce this pattern, but the effect is seen most obviously in mitral stenosis. Ventilation is also shifted away from the lung bases so that overall regional matching of ventilation and perfusion is retained.[123]

19.3.1.5 Effects on exercise performance

Exercise in patients with mitral valve disease is usually limited by the restricted cardiac output, and tachycardia is common, especially when the rhythm is atrial fibrillation. As with chronic heart failure (see Section 19.2.5.1), ventilation is greater than normal for a given oxygen consumption and patients with mitral disease characteristically breathe with a small tidal volume and rapid frequency. The tidal volume on exercise as a proportion of the VC is similar to normal.[124]

19.3.1.6 Effects of mitral valve surgery

After surgical correction of mitral valve disease, changes in both static function and exercise performance correlate with improvement in symptoms but are often modest.[125] Increases in FEV_1 and VC are small but there is a more marked fall in RV.[125,126] Bronchial hyperreactivity declines significantly consistent with reduced pulmonary congestion, even without any change in spirometric volumes.[120]

The D_LCO may show a small initial fall, compatible with a reduction in pulmonary congestion,[127] but after a few months values are similar to preoperative values.[125,127] The characteristic regional distribution of pulmonary perfusion becomes more normal but the change is less in patients with more severe disease preoperatively.[128]

Measurements of exercise performance postoperatively confirm increased work capacity.[125,127] Because of an increased stroke volume the relation between heart rate and workload is less steep after surgery, which allows a greater maximum workload before the heart rate becomes limiting.[125] Ventilation at a standard submaximal work load may be less after surgery,[124] but the maximum ventilation at maximum exercise is greater than preoperatively because the workload is greater. The tidal volume for a given ventilation is larger after surgery, presumably because of relief of pulmonary congestion.[124]

19.3.2 Aortic valve disease

The effects of aortic valve disease on pulmonary function have been less studied than those of mitral disease. Since the lesion is one stage further removed from the pulmonary vascular bed, the effects are generally less marked. Mechanical function and diffusing capacity are normal provided that pulmonary wedge pressure is normal, but in patients with a raised wedge pressure mild reductions of VC, TLC and $D_L CO$ are seen, with RV remaining normal.[129] There is no evidence of significant airflow obstruction. Aortic valve replacement improves exercise capacity and leads to reduction of exercise ventilation.[130] Unlike mitral disease, exercise in aortic valve disease is often limited by angina so that relief of this may allow greater exercise tolerance, with little or no change in submaximal indices.

19.4 CONGENITAL HEART DISEASE

19.4.1 Left-to-right shunts

Most interest in the respiratory function of patients with left-to-right shunts has centred on the $D_L CO$ and its derivatives. In patients with increased pulmonary blood flow due to atrial or ventricular septal defects (ASD, VSD), raised values of both $D_L CO$ and KCO are commonly found due to an increased pulmonary capillary blood volume. The abnormality is usually more marked with ASD than with VSD. If pulmonary hypertension develops, the increase in $D_L CO$ is less obvious, owing to a fall in the effective alveolar volume, but the elevation of KCO may persist.[131]

The effects on mechanical performance of the lungs resemble those of mitral stenosis: in patients with normal resting vascular pressures the abnormalities are subtle and may be evident only as a slightly increased residual volume. In middle age a restrictive defect is common, and in some patients there is reduction of VC and TLC, and there is evidence of mild airway narrowing with a slightly raised airway resistance and minor reduction of FEV_1/VC ratio.[131,132]

There may be evidence of abnormal gas exchange, with mild hypoxaemia and an increased $AaPO_2$. Even if oxygen desaturation is only mild,

this may represent significant ventilation/perfusion mismatching as the unusually high saturation of pulmonary arterial blood in patients with a left-to-right shunt should normally result in a very small $AaPO_2$. Studies of regional perfusion in patients with left-to-right shunts show the expected increased perfusion of the upper zones, so that the overall impression is of more even distribution. This pattern occurs with either an increased flow at normal pressure or a normal flow at high pressure. Inversion of the normal vertical gradient, such as occurs with mitral stenosis, is not usually seen as this pattern probably reflects an actual reduction of basal flow due to increased interstitial pressure accompanying raised pulmonary venous pressure.[133]

In adults with ASD, exercise performance is frequently abnormal, even in asymptomatic individuals. The $\dot{V}O_2 max$ is reduced and the slope of the relationship of ventilation to $\dot{V}CO_2$ increased; both abnormalities correlate with the severity of left-to-right shunting.[134,135] Closure of the ASD results in an improvement in exercise capacity irrespective of the severity of symptoms.[134]

19.4.2 Right-to-left shunts

The most obvious abnormality of respiratory function in patients with Fallot's tetralogy or the Eisenmenger syndrome is the reduction of arterial oxygenation, which is often gross. The reduced oxygen content is partially compensated by an increase in haemoglobin concentration. The primary effect of polycythaemia is an increase in oxygen content (concentration) and not in percentage saturation or partial pressure. An important feature of the arterial hypoxaemia of right-to-left shunts is its failure to correct on breathing 100 per cent oxygen – but some rise of PaO_2 is to be expected because the effect of any ventilation/perfusion imbalance in the lungs is removed. Patients with right-to-left shunts have many similarities to healthy subjects who live at high altitude and, like them, they show a blunted ventilatory response to hypoxia. In patients with cyanotic congenital heart disease this appears to be an effect of acclimatization, as the hypoxic response is restored after correction of the circulatory abnormality.[136]

The failure of oxygenation in these patients is readily apparent but the problem of carbon dioxide elimination is less well recognized.

The shunted blood contains CO_2 at mixed venous tension, and therefore maintenance of a normal arterial P_{CO_2} demands an increased ventilation. This is usually achieved at rest so that most patients have a Pa_{CO_2} that is normal or slightly low (the reduction may be due in part to a mild metabolic acidosis). However, on exercise, despite abnormally high ventilation, the compensatory changes are inadequate and a marked rise in Pa_{CO_2} along with a fall in Pa_{O_2} is typical.[137]

The lung perfusion scan of a patient with right-to-left shunt shows a characteristic pattern because of the loss of some isotope into the systemic circulation before it reaches the lungs; as a result, activity is seen in other organs, in particular kidneys, liver or spleen (Fig. 19.4). After palliative surgery to create a systemic-to-pulmonary (left-to-right) shunt, a reduction in distribution of the isotope to the side of the anastomosis is seen because of the diluting effect of blood shunted from the systemic circulation.

In patients with the Eisenmenger syndrome, the $D_{L}CO$ and K_{CO} are typically reduced.[138] The abnormality may be underestimated in polycythaemic patients if the standard correction factor for haemoglobin concentration is applied (see Chapter 21, Section 21.2). Lung volumes are often mildly reduced, and many patients have mild airway obstruction with slight reductions of FEV_1/VC and of maximum expiratory flows at low lung volumes.[138]

On progressive exercise testing, a severe reduction in $\dot{V}_{O_2}max$ is likely, particularly in patients with the Eisenmenger syndrome.[139] In adult congenital heart disease in general the slope of ventilation against CO_2 production during progressive exercise is a good predictor of mortality, but it is less useful in patients with cyanotic heart disease.[140]

Occasionally, right-to-left shunting via a patent foramen ovale (PFO) causes hypoxaemia, which can present difficulty in diagnosis. This can occur when distortion of atrial anatomy leads to preferential direction of deoxygenated venous blood, usually from the inferior vena cava, through a PFO or ASD. The effect may be greater in the upright than the supine position and this situation is one of the causes of the 'platypnoea orthodeoxia' syndrome. It has also been described in patients with distorted anatomy due to pneumonectomy[141] or dilatation of the aortic root[142] as well as transiently and repeatedly during the frustrated inspiratory efforts of obstructive sleep apnoea.[143]

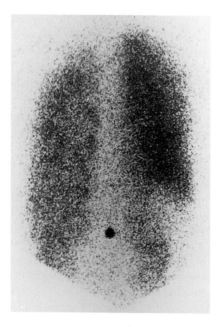

Figure 19.4 Perfusion lung scan in a patient with right-to-left shunt (ventricular septal defect, VSD), showing abnormal activity in the kidneys.

REFFERENCES

1 Kannel WB, Hubert H, Lew EA. Vital capacity as a predictor of cardiovascular disease: the Framingham study. *Am Heart J* 1983; **105**: 311–15.

2 Lange R, Nyboe J, Jensen G, Schnohr P, Appleyard M. Ventilatory function impairment and risk of cardiovascular death and of fatal or non-fatal myocardial infarction. *Eur Respir J* 1991; **4**: 1080–87.

3 Weiss ST. Pulmonary function as a phenotype physiologic marker of cardiovascular morbidity and mortality. *Chest* 1991; **99**: 265–6.

4 Cosby RS, Stowell EC, Hartwig WR, Mayo M. Pulmonary function in left ventricular failure, including cardiac asthma. *Circulation* 1957; **15**: 492–501.

5 Light RW, George RB. Serial pulmonary function in patients with acute heart failure. *Arch Intern Med* 1983; **143**: 429–33.

6 Snashall PD, Chung KF. Airway obstruction and bronchial hyperresponsiveness in left ventricular failure and mitral stenosis. *Am Rev Respir Dis* 1991; **144**: 945–56.

7   McNamara RM, Cionni DJ. Utility of the peak expiratory flow rate in the differentiation of acute dyspnoea: cardiac vs. pulmonary origin. *Chest* 1992; **101**: 129–32.

8   Wilson AT, Channer KS. Hypoxaemia and supplemental oxygen therapy in the first 24 hours after myocardial infarction: the role of pulse oximetry. *J R Coll Physicians Lond* 1997; **31**: 657–61.

9   West JB. Ventilation–perfusion relationships. *Am Rev Respir Dis* 1977; **116**: 919–43.

10 Al Bazzaz FJ, Kazemi H. Arterial hypoxemia and distribution of pulmonary perfusion after uncomplicated myocardial infarction. *Am Rev Respir Dis* 1972; **106**: 721–8.

11 Anthonisen NR, Smith HJ. Respiratory acidosis as a consequence of pulmonary oedema. *Ann Intern Med* 1965; **62**: 991–9.

12 Avery WG, Samet P, Sackner MA. The acidosis of pulmonary oedema. *Am J Med* 1970; **48**: 320–24.

13 Park M, Sangean MC, Volpe M de S, *et al.* Randomised, prospective trial of oxygen, continuous positive airway pressure, and bilevel positive airway pressure by face mask in acute cardiogenic pulmonary edema. *Crit Care Med* 2004; **32**: 2407–15.

14 Riley M, Elborn JS, McKane WR, *et al.* Resting energy expenditure in chronic cardiac failure. *Clin Sci* 1991; **80**: 633–9.

15 Alexander MSM, Peters AM, Cleland JP, Lavender JP. Impaired left lower lobe ventilation in patients with cardiomegaly: an isotope study of mechanics. *Chest* 1992; **101**: 1189–93.

16 Torchio R, Gulotta C, Greco-Lucchina P, *et al.* Closing capacity and gas exchange in chronic heart failure. *Chest* 2007; **129**: 1330–36.

17 Ambrosino N, Opasich C, Crotti, P, *et al.* Breathing pattern, ventilatory drive and respiratory muscle strength in patients with chronic heart failure. *Eur Respir J* 1994; **7**: 17–22.

18 Olson TP, Beck KC, Johnson JB, Johnson BD. Competition for intrathoracic space reduces lung capacity in patients with chronic heart failure: a radiographic study. *Chest* 2006; **130**: 164–71.

19 Evans SA, Watson L, Cowley AJ, Johnston ID, Kinnear WJ. Static lung compliance in chronic heart failure: relation with dyspnoea and exercise capacity. *Thorax* 1995; **50**: 245–8.

20 McParland C, Krishnan B, Wang Y, Gallagher CG. Inspiratory muscle weakness and dyspnoea in chronic heart failure. *Am Rev Respir Dis* 1992; **146**: 467–72.

21 Dimopoulou I, Daganou M, Tsintzas OK, Tzelepis GE. Effects of severity of long-standing congestive heart failure on pulmonary function. *Respir Med* 1998; **92**: 1321–5.

22 Naum CC, Sciurba FC, Rogers RM. Pulmonary function abnormalities in chronic severe cardiomyopathy preceding cardiac transplantation. *Am Rev Respir Dis* 1992; **145**: 1334–8.

23 Pison C, Malo J-L, Rouleau J-L, *et al.* Bronchial hyperresponsiveness to inhaled methacholine in subjects with chronic left heart failure at a time of exacerbation and after increasing diuretic therapy. *Chest* 1989; **96**: 230–35.

24 Boni E, Bezzi M, Carminati L, *et al.* Expiratory flow limitation is associated with orthopnea and reversed by vasodilators and diuretics in left heart failure. *Chest* 2005; **128**: 1050–57.

25 Torchio R, Gulotta C, Greco-Lucchina P, *et al.* Orthopnea and tidal expiratory flow limitation in chronic heart failure. *Chest* 2006; **130**: 472–9.

26 Yap JC, Moore DM, Cleland JG, Pride NB. Effect of supine posture on respiratory mechanics in chronic left ventricular failure. *Am J Respir Crit Care Med* 2000; **162**: 1285–91.

27 Ravenscraft SA, Gross CR, Kubo SH, *et al.* Pulmonary function after successful heart transplantation: one year follow-up. *Chest* 1993; **103**: 54–8.

28 Niset G, Ninane V, Antoine M, Yernault JC. Respiratory dysfunction in congestive heart failure: correction after heart transplantation. *Eur Respir J* 1993; **6**: 1197–201.

29 Hosenpud JD, Stibolt TA, Atwal K, *et al.* Abnormal pulmonary function specifically related to congestive heart failure: comparison of patients before and after cardiac transplantation. *Am J Med* 1990; **88**: 493–6.

30 Agostoni P, Bussotti M, Cattadori G, *et al.* Gas diffusion and alveolar–capillary unit in chronic heart failure. *Eur Heart J* 2006; **27**: 2538–43.

31 Mettauer B, Lampert E, Charloux A, *et al.* Lung membrane diffusing capacity, heart failure, and heart transplantation. *Am J Cardiol* 1999; **83**: 62–7.

32 Petersen CL, Kjaer A. Impact of medical treatment on lung diffusion capacity in elderly patients with heart failure: baseline characteristics and 1-year follow up after medical treatment. *Int J Cardiol* 2005; **98**: 453–7.

33 Puri S, Baker BL, Dutka DP, *et al.* Reduced alveolar–capillary membrane diffusing capacity in chronic heart failure: its pathophysiological relevance and relationship to exercise performance. *Circulation* 1995; **91**: 2769–74.

34 Assayag P, Benamer H, Aubry P, *et al.* Alteration of the alveolar–capillary membrane diffusing capacity in chronic left heart disease. *Am J Cardiol* 1998; **82**: 459–64.

35 Puri S, Baker BL, Oakley CM, Hughes JM, Cleland JG. Increased alveolar/capillary membrane resistance to gas transfer in patients with chronic heart failure. *Br Heart J* 1994; **72**: 140–44.

36 Al-Rawas OA, Carter R, Stevenson RD, Naik SK, Wheatley DJ. Exercise intolerance following heart transplantation: the role of pulmonary diffusing capacity impairment. *Chest* 2000; **118**: 1661–70.

37 Ponikowski P, Anker SD, Chua TP, *et al.* Oscillatory breathing patterns during wakefulness in patients with chronic heart failure: clinical implications and role of augmented peripheral chemosensitivity. *Circulation* 1999; **100**: 2418–24.

38 Corra U, Giordano A, Bosimini E, *et al.* Oscillatory ventilation during exercise in patients with chronic heart failure: clinical correlates and prognostic implications. *Chest* 2002; **121**: 1572–80.

39 Leite JJ, Mansur AJ, de Freitas HF, *et al.* Periodic breathing during incremental exercise predicts mortality in patients with chronic heart failure evaluated for cardiac transplantation. *J Am Coll Cardiol* 2003; **41**: 2175–81.

40 Javaheri S, Parker TJ, Liming JD, *et al.* Sleep apnea in 81 ambulatory male patients with stable heart failure: types and their prevalences, consequences, and presentations. *Circulation* 1998; **97**: 2154–9.

41 Sin DD, Fitzgerald F, Parker JD, *et al.* Risk factors for central and obstructive sleep apnea in 450 men and women with congestive heart failure. *Am J Respir Crit Care Med* 1999; **160**: 1101–6.

42 Tremel F, Pepin JL, Veale D, *et al.* High prevalence and persistence of sleep apnoea in patients referred for acute left ventricular failure and medically treated over 2 months. *Eur Heart J* 1999; **20**: 1201–9.

43 Ferrier K, Campbell A, Yee B, *et al.* Sleep-disordered breathing occurs frequently in stable outpatients with congestive heart failure. *Chest* 2005; **128**: 2116–22.

44 Rao A, Georgiadou P, Francis DP, *et al.* Sleep-disordered breathing in a general heart failure population: relationships to neurohumoral activation and subjective symptoms. *J Sleep Res* 2006; **15**: 81–8.

45 Schulz R, Blau A, Borgel J, *et al.* Sleep apnoea in heart failure. *Eur Respir J* 2007; **29**: 1201–5.

46 Naughton M, Benard D, Tam A, Rutherford R, Bradley TD. Role of hyperventilation in the pathogenesis of central sleep apneas in patients with congestive heart failure. *Am Rev Respir Dis* 1993; **148**: 330–38.

47 Lorenzi-Filho G, Azevedo ER, Parker JD, Bradley TD. Relationship of carbon dioxide tension in arterial blood to pulmonary wedge pressure in heart failure. *Eur Respir J* 2002; **19**: 37–40.

48 Wilcox I, McNamara SG, Dodd MJ, Sullivan CE. Ventilatory control in patients with sleep apnoea and left ventricular dysfunction: comparison of obstructive and central sleep apnoea. *Eur Respir J* 1998; **11**: 7–13.

49 Javaheri S. A mechanism of central sleep apnea in patients with heart failure. *N Engl J Med* 1999; **341**: 949–54.

50 Solin P, Roebuck T, Johns DP, Walters EH, Naughton MT. Peripheral and central ventilatory responses in central sleep apnea with and without congestive heart failure. *Am J Respir Crit Care Med* 2000; **162**: 2194–200.

51 Ha. MJ, Xie A, Rutherford L, *et al.* Cycle length of periodic breathing in patients with and without heart failure. *Am J Respir Crit Care Med* 1996; **154**: 376–81.

52 Xie A, Skatrud JB, Puleo DS, Rahko PS, Dempsey JA. Apnea–hypopnea threshold for CO_2 in patients with congestive heart failure. *Am J Respir Crit Care Med* 2002; **165**: 1245–50.

53 Series F, Kimoff RJ, Morrison D, *et al.* Prospective evaluation of nocturnal oximetry for detection of sleep-related breathing disturbances in patients with chronic heart failure. *Chest* 2005; **127**: 1507–14.

54 Szollosi I, Roebuck T, Thompson B, Naughton MT. Lateral sleeping position reduces severity of central sleep apnea/Cheyne–Stokes respiration. *Sleep* 2006; **29**: 1045–51.

55 Trinder J, Merson R, Rosenberg JI, *et al.* Pathophysiological interactions of ventilation, arousals and blood pressure oscillations during Cheyne–Stokes respiration in patients with heart failure. *Am J Respir Crit Care Med* 2000; **162**: 808–13.

56 Hanly P, Zuberi-Khokhar N. Daytime sleepiness in patients with congestive heart failure and Cheyne–Stokes respiration. *Chest* 1995; **107**: 952–8.

57 Alex CG, Onal E, Lopata M. Upper airway occlusion during sleep in patients with Cheyne–Stokes respiration. *Am Rev Respir Dis* 1986; **133**: 42–5.

58 Shepard J, Pevernogie D, Stanson A, *et al.* Effects of changes in central venous pressure on upper airway size in patients with obstructive sleep apnoea. *Am J Respir Crit Care Med* 1996; **153**: 250–54.

59 Ryan CM, Bradley TD. Periodicity of obstructive sleep apnea in patients with and without heart failure. *Chest* 2005; **127**: 536–42.

60 Tkacova R, Niroumand M, Lorenzi-Filho G, Bradley TD. Overnight shift from obstructive to central apneas in patients with heart failure: role of P_{CO_2} and circulatory delay. *Circulation* 2001; **103**: 238–43.

61 Tkacova R, Wang H, Bradley TD. Night-to-night alterations in sleep apnea type in patients with heart failure. *J Sleep Res* 2006; **15**: 321–8.

62 Arzt M, Young T, Finn L, *et al.* Sleepiness and sleep in patients with both systolic heart failure and obstructive sleep apnea. *Arch Intern Med* 2006; **166**: 1716–22.

63 Lanfranchi PA, Braghiroli A, Bosimini E, *et al.* Prognostic value of nocturnal Cheyne–Stokes respiration in chronic heart failure. *Circulation* 1999; **99**: 1435–40.

64 Javaheri S, Shukla R, Zeigler H, Wexler L. Central sleep apnea, right ventricular dysfunction, and low diastolic blood pressure are predictors of mortality in systolic heart failure. *J Am Coll Cardiol* 2007; **49**: 2028–34.

65 Andreas S, Hagenah G, Moller C, Werner GS, Kreuzer H. Cheyne–Stokes respiration and prognosis in congestive heart failure. *Am J Cardiol* 1996; **78**: 1260–64.

66 Corrà U, Pistano M, Mezzani A, *et al.* Sleep and exertional periodic breathing in chronic heart failure: prognostic importance and interdependence. *Circulation* 2006; **113**: 44–50.

67 Kaneko Y, Floras JS, Usui K, *et al.* Cardiovascular effects of continuous positive airway pressure in patients with heart failure and obstructive sleep apnea. *N Engl J Med* 2003; **348**: 1233–41.

68 Solin P, Bergin P, Richardson M, *et al.* Influence of pulmonary capillary wedge pressure on central apnea in heart failure. *Circulation* 1999; **99**: 1574–9.

69 Olson TP, Frantz RP, Snyder EM, *et al.* Effects of acute changes in pulmonary wedge pressure on periodic breathing at rest in heart failure patients. *Am Heart J* 2007; **153**: 104.e1–7.

70 Sinha A-M, Skobel EC, Breithardt OA, *et al.* Cardiac resynchronization therapy improves central sleep apnea and Cheyne–Stokes respiration in patients with chronic heart failure. *J Am Coll Cardiol* 2004; **44**: 68–71.

71 Mansfield DR, Solin P, Roebuck T, *et al.* The effect of successful heart transplant treatment of heart failure on central sleep apnea. *Chest* 2003; **124**: 1675–81.

72 Javaheri S, Abraham WT, Brown C, *et al.* Prevalence of obstructive sleep apnoea and periodic limb movement in 45 subjects with heart transplantation. *Eur Heart J* 2004; **25**: 260–66.

73 Hanly PJ, Millar TW, Steljes DG, *et al.* The effect of oxygen on respiration and sleep in patients with congestive heart failure. *Ann Intern Med* 1989; **111**: 777–82.

74 Staniforth AD, Kinnear WJ, Starling R, Hetmanski DJ, Cowley AJ. Effect of oxygen on sleep quality, cognitive function and sympathetic activity in patients with chronic heart failure and Cheyne–Stokes respiration. *Eur Heart J* 1998; **19**: 922–8.

75 Javaheri S, Ahmed M, Parker TJ, Brown CR. Effects of nasal O_2 on sleep-related disordered breathing in ambulatory patients with stable heart failure. *Sleep* 1999; **22**: 1101–6.

76 Andreas S, Clemens C, Sandholzer H, Figulla HR, Kreuzer H. Improvement of exercise capacity with treatment of Cheyne–Stokes respiration in patients with congestive heart failure. *J Am Coll Cardiol* 1996; **27**: 1486–90.

77 Javaheri S. Pembrey's dream: the time has come for a long-term trial of nocturnal supplemental nasal oxygen to treat central sleep apnea in congestive heart failure. *Chest* 2003; **123**: 322–5.

78 Lorenzi-Filho G, Rankin F, Bies I, Bradley TD. Effects of inhaled carbon dioxide and oxygen on Cheyne–Stokes respiration in patients with heart failure. *Am J Respir Crit Care Med* 1999; **159**: 1490–98.

79 Andreas S, Weidel K, Hagenah G, Heindl S. Treatment of Cheyne–Stokes respiration with nasal oxygen and carbon dioxide. *Eur Respir J* 1998; **12**: 414–19.

80 Javaheri S. Acetazolamide improves central sleep apnea in heart failure: a double-blind, prospective study. *Am J Respir Crit Care Med* 2006; **173**: 234–7.

81 Arzt M, Bradley TD. Treatment of sleep apnea in heart failure. *Am J Respir Crit Care Med* 2006; **173**: 1300–308.

82 Kiely JL, Deegan P, Buckley A, *et al.* Efficacy of nasal continuous positive airway pressure therapy in chronic heart failure: importance of underlying cardiac rhythm. *Thorax* 1998; **53**: 957–62.

83 Naughton MT, Liu PP, Bernard DC, Goldstein RS, Bradley TD. Treatment of congestive heart failure and Cheyne–Stokes respiration during sleep by continuous positive airway pressure. *Am J Respir Crit Care Med* 1995; **151**: 92–7.

84 Bradley TD, Logan AG, Kimoff RJ, *et al.* Continuous positive airway pressure for central sleep apnea and heart failure. *N Engl J Med* 2005; **353**: 2025–33.

85 Arzt M, Floras JA, Logan AG, *et al.* Suppression of central sleep apnea by continuous positive airway pressure and transplant-free survival in heart failure: a post hoc analysis of the Canadian Continuous Positive Airway Pressure for Patients with Central Sleep Apnea and Heart Failure Trial (CANPAP). *Circulation* 2007; **115**: 3173–80.

86 Kohnlein T, Welte T, Tan LB, Elliott MW. Assisted ventilation for heart failure patients with Cheyne–Stokes respiration. *Eur Respir J* 2002; **20**: 934–41.

87 Johnson KG, Johnson DC. Bilevel positive airway pressure worsens central apneas during sleep. *Chest* 2005; **128**: 2141–50.

88 Teschler H, Dohring J, Wang Y-M, Berthon-Jones M. Adaptive pressure support servo-ventilation: a novel treatment for Cheyne–Stokes respiration in heart failure. *Am J Respir Crit Care Med* 2001; **164**: 614–19.

89 Pepperell JCT, Maskell NA, Jones DR, *et al.* A randomized controlled trial of adaptive ventilation for Cheyne–Stokes breathing in heart failure. *Am J Respir Crit Care Med* 2003; **168**: 1109–14.

90 Philippe C, Stoica-Herman M, Drouot X, *et al.* Compliance with and effectiveness of adaptive servoventilation versus continuous positive airway pressure in the treatment of Cheyne–Stokes respiration in heart failure over a six month period. *Heart* 2006; **92**: 337–42.

91 Wasserman K, Zhang YY, Gitt A, *et al.* Lung function and exercise gas exchange in chronic heart failure. *Circulation* 1997; **96**: 2221–7.

92 Agostoni P, Pelligrino R, Conca C, Rodarte JR, Brusasco V. Exercise hyperpnea in chronic heart failure: relationships to lung stiffness and expiratory flow limitation. *J Appl Physiol* 2002; **92**: 1409–16.

93 Witte KK, Thackray SD, Nikitin NP, Clelend JG, Clark AL. Pattern of ventilation during exercise in chronic heart failure. *Heart* 2003; **89**: 610–14.

94 Johnson BD, Beck KC, Olson LJ, *et al.* Ventilatory constraints during exercise in patients with chronic heart failure. *Chest* 2000; **117**: 321–32.

95 Schroeder CA, Balfe DL, Khan SS, Mohsenifar Z. Airflow limitation and breathing strategy in congestive heart failure patients during exercise. *Respiration* 2003; **70**: 137–42.

96 Wensel R, Francis DP, Georgiadou P, *et al.* Exercise hyperventilation in chronic heart failure is not caused by systemic lactic acidosis. *Eur J Heart Failure* 2005; **7**: 1105–11.

97 Steele IC, Moore A, Nugent AM, *et al.* Non-invasive measurement of cardiac output and ventricular ejection fractions in chronic cardiac failure: relationship to impaired exercise tolerance. *Clin Sci* 1997; **93**: 195–203.

98 Olson LJ, Snyder EM, Beck KC, Johnson BD. Reduced rate of alveolar–capillary recruitment and fall of pulmonary diffusing capacity during exercise in patients with heart failure. *J. Cardiac Failure* 2006; **12**: 299–306.

99 O'Keefe ST, Lye M, Donnellan C, Carmichael DN. Reproducibility and responsiveness of quality of life assessment and six minute walk test in elderly heart failure patients. *Heart* 1998; **80**: 377–82.

100 Mancini DM, Eisen H, Kussmaul W, *et al.* Value of peak exercise oxygen consumption for optimal timing of cardiac transplantation in ambulatory patients with heart failure. *Circulation* 1991; **83**: 778–786.

101 Stelken AM, Younis LT, Jennison SH, *et al.* Prognostic value of cardiopulmonary exercise testing using percent achieved of predicted peak oxygen uptake for patients with ischemic and dilated cardiomyopathy. *J Am Coll Cardiol* 1996; **27**: 345–52.

102 MacGowan GA, Janosko K, Cecchetti A, Murali S. Exercise-related ventilatory abnormalities and survival in congestive heart failure. *Am J Cardiol* 1997; **79**: 1264–6.

103 Chua TP, Ponikowski P, Harrington D, *et al.* Clinical correlates and prognostic significance of the ventilatory response to exercise in chronic heart failure. *J Am Coll Cardiol* 1997; **29**: 1585–90.

104 Robbins M, Francis G, Pashkow FJ, *et al.* Ventilatory and heart rate responses to exercise: better predictors of heart failure mortality than peak oxygen consumption. *Circulation* 1999; **100**: 2411–17.

105 Francis DP, Shamim W, Davies LC, *et al.* Cardiopulmonary exercise testing for prognosis in chronic heart failure: continuous and independent prognostic value from V_E/Vco_2 slope and peak Vo_2. *Eur Heart J* 2000; **21**: 154–61.

106 Kleber F, Vietzke G, Wernecke KD, *et al.* Impairment of ventilatory efficiency in heart failure: prognostic impact. *Circulation* 2000; **101**: 2803–9.

107 Osman AF, Mehra MR, Lavie CJ, Nunez E, Milani RV. The incremental prognostic importance of body fat adjusted peak oxygen consumption in chronic heart failure. *J Am Coll Cardiol* 2000; **36**: 2126–31.

108 Myers J, Gullestad L, Vagelos R, *et al.* Cardiopulmonary exercise testing and prognosis in severe heart failure: 14 mL/kg/min revisited. *Am Heart J* 2000; **139**: 78–84.

109 Leite JJ, Mansur AJ, de Freitas HF, *et al.* Periodic breathing during incremental exercise predicts mortality in patients with chronic heart failure evaluated for cardiac transplantation. *J Am Coll Cardiol* 2003; **41**: 2175–81.

110 Corrà U, Mezzani A, Bosimini E, *et al.* Limited predictive value of cardiopulmonary exercise indices in patients with moderate chronic heart failure treated with carvedilol. *Am Heart J* 2004; **147**: 553–60.

111 Cicoira M, Davos CH, Francis DP, *et al.* Prediction of mortality in chronic heart failure from peak oxygen consumption adjusted for either body weight or lean tissue. *J Card Fail* 2004; **10**: 421–6.

112 Lavie CJ, Milani RV, Mehra MR. Peak exercise oxygen pulse and prognosis in chronic heart failure. *Am J Cardiol* 2004; **93**: 588–93.

113 O'Neill JO, Young JB, Pothier CE, Lauer MS. Peak oxygen consumption as a predictor of death in patients with heart failure receiving beta-blockers. *Circulation* 2005; **111**: 2313–18.

114 Arena R, Myers J, Abella J, Peberdy MA. Influence of heart failure etiology on the prognostic value of peak oxygen consumption and minute ventilation/carbon dioxide production slope. *Chest* 2005; **128**: 2812–17.

115 Corrà U, Mezzani A, Bosimini E, Giannuzzi P. Prognostic value of time-related changes of cardiopulmonary exercise testing indices in stable chronic heart failure: a pragmatic and operative scheme. *Eur J Cardiovasc Prev Rehabil* 2006; **13**: 186–92.

116 Bard RL, Gillespie BW, Clarke NS, Egan TG, Nicklas JM. Determining the best ventilatory efficiency measure to predict mortality in patients with heart failure. *J Heart Lung Transplant* 2006; **25**: 589–95.

117 Rhodes KM, Evemy K, Nariman S, Gibson GJ. Relation between severity of mitral valve disease and routine lung function tests in non-smokers. *Thorax* 1982; **37**: 751–5.

118 De Troyer A, Estenne M, Yernault J-C. Disturbance of respiratory muscle function in patients with mitral valve disease. *Am J Med* 1980; **69**: 867–73.

119 Chatterji RS, Panda BN, Tewari SC, Rao KS. Lung function in mitral stenosis. *J Assoc Physicians India* 2000; **48**: 976–80.

120 Gulec S, Ertas F, Tutar E, *et al*. Bronchial hyperreactivity in patients with mitral stenosis before and after successful percutaneous mitral balloon valvulotomy. *Chest* 1999; **116**: 1582–6.

121 Rolla G, Bucca C, Brussino L, *et al*. Bronchial responsiveness, oscillations of peak flow rate and symptoms in patients with mitral stenosis. *Eur Respir J* 1992; **5**: 213–18.

122 Yernault L-C, Englert M, De Troyer A. Mechanical and diffusing lung properties in patients with rheumatic valve disease, in *Cardiac Lung* (eds C Giuntini and P Panuccio), Piccin, Padua, 1979, pp. 35–47.

123 Dawson A, Rocamora JM, Morgan JR. Regional lung function in chronic pulmonary congestion with and without mitral stenosis. *Am Rev Respir Dis* 1976; **113**: 51–9.

124 Reed JW, Ablett M, Cotes JE. Ventilatory responses to exercise and to carbon dioxide in mitral stenosis before and after valvotomy: causes of tachypnoea. *Clin Sci* 1978; **54**: 9–16.

125 Rhodes KM, Evemy K, Nariman S, Gibson GJ. Effects of mitral valve surgery on static lung function and exercise performance. *Thorax* 1985; **40**: 107–12.

126 Yoshioka T, Nakanishi N, Okubo S, *et al*. Improvement in pulmonary function in mitral stenosis after percutaneous transvenous mitral commissurotomy. *Chest* 1990; **89**: 290–94.

127 Gomez-Hospital JA, Cequier A, Romero PV, *et al*. Persistence of lung function abnormalities despite sustained success of percutaneous mitral valvotomy: the need for an early indication. *Chest* 2005; **127**: 40–46.

128 Ohno K, Nakahara K, Hirose H, Nahano S, Kawashima Y. Effects of valvular surgery on overall and regional lung function in patients with mitral stenosis. *Chest* 1987; **92**: 224–8.

129 Yernault J-C, De Troyer A. Mechanics of breathing in patients with aortic valve disease. *Bull Eur Physiopathol Respir* 1980; **16**: 491–500.

130 Gilmour DG, Spiro SG, Raphael MJ, Freedman S. Exercise tests before and after heart valve replacement. *Br J Dis Chest* 1976; **70**: 185–94.

131 De Troyer A, Yernault J-C, Englert M. Mechanics of breathing in patients with atrial septal defect. *Am Rev Respir Dis* 1977; **115**: 413–21.

132 Hamano K, Gohra H, Katoh T, *et al*. Late postoperative respiratory function in adults after surgical correction of atrial septal defects: analysis of respiratory dysfunction patterns. *Scand Cardiovasc J* 1998; **32**: 135–6.

133 Dollery CT, West JB, Wilcken DEL, *et al*. Regional pulmonary blood flow in patients with circulatory shunts. *Br Heart J* 1961; **23**: 225–35.

134 Brochu MC, Baril JF, Dore A, *et al*. Improvement in exercise capacity in asymptomatic and mildly symptomatic adults after atrial septal defect percutaneous closure. *Circulation* 2002; **106**: 1821–6.

135 Tronjnarska O, Szyszka A, Gwizdale A, *et al*. Evaluation of exercise capacity with cardiopulmonary exercise testing and type B natriuretic peptide concentrations in adult patients with patient atrial septal defect. *Cardiology* 2006; **106**: 154–60.

136 Edelman NH, Lahiri S, Braudo L, *et al*. The blunted ventilatory response to hypoxia in cyanotic congenital heart disease. *N Engl J Med* 1970; **282**: 405–11.

137 Davies H, Gazetopoulos N. Dyspnoea in cyanotic congenital heart disease. *Br Heart J* 1965; **27**: 28–41.

138 MacArthur CGC, Hunter D, Gibson GJ. Ventilatory function in the Eisenmenger syndrome. *Thorax* 1979; **34**: 348–53.

139 Diller GP, Dimopoulos K Okonko D, *et al*. Exercise intolerance in adult congenital heart disease: comparative severity, correlates, and prognostic implication. *Circulation* 2005; **112**: 828–35.

140 Dimopoulos K, Okonko DO, Diller GP, *et al*. Abnormal ventilatory response to exercise in adults with congenital heart disease relates to cyanosis and predicts survival. *Circulation* 2006; **113**: 2796–802.

141 Marini C, Miniati M, Ambrosino N, *et al*. Dyspnoea and hypoxaemia after lung surgery: the role of interatrial right-to-left shunt. *Eur Respir J* 2006; **28**: 174–81.

142 Pemberton J, Irvine T, Stewart MJ, Antunes G, Gibson GJ. Platypnoea orthodeoxia in a patient with aortic root dilatation and a patent foramen ovale. *Eur J Echocardiogr* 2007; **8**: 151–62.

143 Johansson MC, Eriksson P, Peker Y, *et al*. The influence of patent foramen ovale on oxygen desaturation in obstructive sleep apnoea. *Eur Respir J* 2007; **29**: 149–55.

20

Neuromuscular Disease

The central nervous system (CNS) provides both the rhythm generator and the neural pathways controlling respiration, and the respiratory muscles are the effector organs for breathing; consequently, neuromuscular diseases can interfere with respiratory function at several levels. Lesions in the brain may affect the respiratory drive or motor control of the respiratory muscles, while a wide range of conditions affecting the spinal cord, peripheral nerves and skeletal muscles can result in respiratory muscle dysfunction or weakness.

20.1 ABNORMALITIES OF RESPIRATORY CONTROL

In some diseases, such as poliomyelitis, both central control and peripheral respiratory function may be disturbed; in others, such as certain myopathies, an additional central abnormality is sometimes suspected when disturbance of respiratory function appears out of proportion to the muscle weakness. Analysis of abnormal ventilatory control is, however, bedevilled by the dependence of conventional tests of respiratory sensitivity, such as the responses to hypercapnia or hypoxia, on the integrity of the effector system, i.e. the respiratory muscles. Furthermore, once hypercapnia has developed, the ventilatory response to carbon dioxide (CO_2) is likely to be reduced because the accompanying elevation of bicarbonate

concentration results in attenuation of the respiratory stimulus (see Chapter 5, Section 5.2.1).

20.1.1 Patterns of breathing with central nervous system lesions

The neurons responsible for generating the fundamental respiratory rhythm are in the medulla (see Chapter 5, Section 5.1). Their output via the metabolic (automatic) respiratory control pathway is modulated by chemical and neural afferent information from both peripheral and central sites and is transmitted to the respiratory muscles via the reticulospinal tract. In addition, however, the pattern of tidal breathing is influenced by the behavioural (volitional) control pathway via the corticospinal tract (see Fig. 5.1 in Chapter 5). The latter is relevant particularly when awake and in rapid-eye-movement (REM) sleep but much less so during non-REM sleep.

Various abnormal breathing patterns may be seen in patients with chronic CNS diseases, and these have been related to particular sites of disease (Fig. 20.1),[1] but with acute brain injury their localizing value is less specific.[2,3] The most familiar is Cheyne–Stokes breathing, in which the tidal volume waxes and wanes smoothly with a characteristic periodicity interspersed by brief periods of apnoea, most evident during sleep. The various mechanisms contributing to Cheyne–Stokes breathing are discussed in Chapter 6, Section 6.2.1. It is

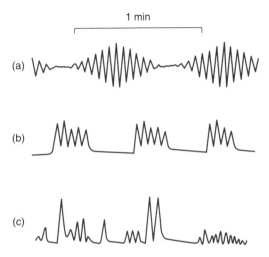

1 min

(a)

(b)

(c)

Figure 20.1 Schematic diagram of breathing patterns seen in neurological diseases. (a) Classic Cheyne–Stokes respiration, showing smooth waxing and waning of the tidal volume punctuated by brief periods of apnoea. (b) Periodic breathing with brief clusters of breaths and without the symmetry of Cheyne–Stokes respiration. (c) Grossly irregular or 'ataxic' respiration.

seen in its most developed form in chronic heart failure (see Chapter 19, Section 19.2.4), while among neurological conditions it has been associated particularly with disease (usually vascular) affecting both cerebral hemispheres. In some patients both cerebrovascular and cardiac disease may be contributory, as in the original case described by John Cheyne.[4]

Periodic or 'cluster' breathing with a shorter cycle and a less symmetrical and regular contour than Cheyne–Stokes respiration has less localizing value but is often seen with disease affecting the brainstem. Grossly irregular or 'ataxic' breathing with no obvious periodicity is also more characteristic of medullary lesions (Fig. 20.1). Pontine lesions are occasionally associated with 'apneustic' breathing with prolonged inspiratory pauses.[5]

Gross hyperventilation is seen occasionally with lesions of the midbrain and upper pons, but the precise mechanism of the increased drive to breathe is often uncertain.[1] Hyperventilation in CNS disease is very rare in the absence of coexisting cardiopulmonary disease, particularly pulmonary congestion or oedema. Because of impaired pulmonary function, the low $PaCO_2$ resulting from the hyperventilation is usually

accompanied by a low PaO_2 and a widened alveolar–arterial PO_2 ($AaPO_2$) gradient. Although the CNS lesion itself may be responsible for the associated pulmonary oedema, the hyperventilation usually results from stimulation of pulmonary receptors. True 'central' or 'neurogenic' hyperventilation can be inferred with confidence only in patients with no cardiopulmonary dysfunction and a normal $AaPO_2$. This picture is very rare but has been described particularly with diffuse cerebral lymphoma.[6,7]

The observations of Plum and colleagues on which most of the above conclusions are based were mainly in patients with chronic lesions in a stable state.[1,5,8] Patients presenting acutely show less clear correlations between breathing patterns and lesions at specific sites. In one large study of patients admitted to a neurosurgical unit with head injury, tumour or subarachnoid haemorrhage, there was a strong association between medullary lesions and grossly irregular breathing, but other patterns were of no localizing value, presumably because, in acutely ill patients, widespread metabolic brain dysfunction limits their specificity.[2]

20.1.2 Disorders of automatic (metabolic) respiratory control

20.1.2.1 Congenital central hypoventilation syndrome

The rare syndrome of congenital central hypoventilation ('Ondine's curse') is characterized by chronic hypoventilation, often most evident during non-REM sleep (when ventilation is driven primarily by the metabolic control system). Although most cases are recognized shortly after birth, patients may also present in later childhood or adult life.[9] The cause has been identified as a mutation of the PHOX2B gene, which is also an important determinant of function of the autonomic nervous system. The condition shows an autosomal dominant inheritance pattern. Conventionally, congenital central hypoventilation syndrome is diagnosed only in the absence of an identifiable brainstem lesion,[10] but PHOX2B mutations have also been described in patients with central hypoventilation and structural abnormalities in the brainstem.[11]

20.1.2.2 Acquired central hypoventilation

When poliomyelitis was common, ataxic breathing was recognized in many patients with bulbar disease as the lesions of bulbar poliomyelitis correspond closely to the site of the ventral group of respiratory neurons in the upper medulla.[12] Similar disruption of the automatic control pathway can occur acutely with a variety of pathological conditions, including trauma, encephalitis, stroke and tumours;[8,13] these may affect the medulla either directly or by causing raised intracranial pressure, resulting in depression of ventilation with hypercapnia and hypoxaemia. A similar syndrome with central sleep apnoea sometimes occurs after bilateral cervical cordotomy for relief of intractable pain. In this procedure, not only are the ascending spinoreticular tracts interrupted but also the adjacent descending reticulospinal tracts of the 'metabolic' respiratory control system may be damaged. Unexpected death during sleep, due presumably to central apnoea, is a well-recognized complication of this procedure.[14,15]

20.1.2.3 Functional picture of central hypoventilation syndromes

Patients with central hypoventilation syndromes have normal mechanical ventilatory function. A blood gas picture of 'pure' hypoventilation would be expected, i.e. a normal $AaPo_2$ gradient, but any coexisting pulmonary abnormality, such as infection, may result in disproportionate hypoxaemia and increased $AaPo_2$. Hypercapnia is likely to be exacerbated if opioid or other sedative drugs are used. When awake, some individuals may be able to maintain normal blood gases, but responses to CO_2 or hypoxia are greatly diminished or absent.[16] Despite the absent chemical responses, ventilation increases on exercise, but the increase is less than normal so that $PaCO_2$ tends to rise and PaO_2 to fall.[17]

20.1.2.4 Treatment of central hypoventilation

One approach to treatment of central hypoventilation is pacing of the diaphragm by repetitive stimulation of the phrenic nerve. This has been used successfully in some patients but, since the upper airway muscles are not being driven normally, it can precipitate obstructive sleep apnoea.[18] Nocturnal non-invasive ventilation (NIV) is the more commonly used, and frequently successful, therapeutic approach.

20.1.3 Disorders of volitional respiratory control

Bilateral lesions of the pyramidal (corticospinal) tracts are seen occasionally with infarcts in the mid-pontine region. This results in the so-called 'locked-in syndrome' with almost complete loss of voluntary movement, including the ability to override the automatic drive to breathe. Automatic breathing is preserved because the medulla continues to function normally, but patients cannot influence the monotonously regular ventilatory pattern.[19] The ventilatory response to CO_2 is preserved,[20] but supramedullary volitional influences on breathing are lost.

Volitional control of breathing may also be impaired by strokes and other lesions that affect the cerebral hemispheres, and by Parkinson's disease and other extrapyramidal disorders.

20.2 CONSEQUENCES OF RESPIRATORY MUSCLE WEAKNESS

Most patients with respiratory muscle weakness, whether due to primary muscle diseases, peripheral neuropathies or motor neuron disease, have global weakness affecting all inspiratory and expiratory muscles. Isolated unilateral diaphragmatic paralysis due to localized phrenic nerve damage is commonly seen and, much more rarely, bilateral diaphragmatic paralysis occurs and results in a characteristic functional picture. Selective paralysis of other respiratory muscle groups is seen with localized spinal cord lesions and is discussed later (see Section 20.3.4).

20.2.1 Global respiratory muscle weakness

20.2.1.1 Direct measurements of respiratory muscle function

Respiratory muscle function can be assessed simply and directly by measuring the pressure developed during maximum voluntary inspiratory and expiratory efforts. Values of maximal inspiratory and expiratory static alveolar pressures obtained by recording at the mouth during sustained efforts against a closed airway are reasonably reproducible, provided that certain precautions are taken (see Chapter 1, Section 1.5.2.1). For the inspiratory muscles, an alternative is to measure the sniff nasal inspiratory pressure (SNIP), a dynamic measurement obtained via the occluded nostril during a forceful sniff. Some patients find this a more natural manoeuvre, but in more severe weakness the static inspiratory pressure may be more reliable.[21] Many laboratories perform both tests and use the numerically greater as the 'true' measurement. The expiratory equivalent of the SNIP is a measurement of intrathoracic or abdominal pressure during coughing, but since this requires oesophageal intubation it is impracticable for routine testing.

Measurements of maximum respiratory pressures are sensitive to respiratory muscle weakness and may be markedly impaired before significant volume loss is recognizable.[22] All volitional tests of respiratory muscle weakness are, however, open to the objection of effort dependence. Their value is also compromised in some individuals by inadequate technique and in some conditions where weakness of bulbar muscles or upper motor neuron lesions impair the ability to generate the necessary effort. In such situations assessment of respiratory muscle function by various non-volitional techniques of electrical or magnetic stimulation is preferable (see Chapter 1, Section 1.5.3.1). However, the availability of such methodology is restricted to a small number of laboratories with a major interest in this area.

20.2.1.2 Lung volumes

The most frequently detected abnormality of lung volumes in patients with respiratory muscle weakness is a reduction in the VC. This is often 'pruned' at both its upper and lower limits due to weakness of the inspiratory muscles limiting full inflation and weakness of the expiratory muscles preventing full expiration and thus increasing residual volume. The VC is reduced further by the abnormally low compliance of both the lungs[23] and the chest wall.[24] Indeed, in patients with severe weakness,

the VC is related more closely to the reduced pulmonary compliance than to the direct effect of loss of distending force.[25,26] The mechanism of the reduced distensibility of the lungs is not clear: it is probably not due simply to widespread microatelectasis,[27] but it may reflect altered behaviour of surfactant resulting from inability to inflate the lungs fully.

Impaired expiratory muscle strength directly increases RV, but any reduction in lung compliance may counter this effect, such that in some patients RV is normal. In healthy older individuals, RV is determined by progressive narrowing and closure of airways rather than by expiratory muscle force (see Chapter 8, Section 8.5.2.1). However, when weakness develops, RV may become more effort-dependent, so that forceful expiration can no longer be sustained sufficiently for airway narrowing to become the limiting factor. With severe expiratory weakness this gives a characteristic appearance to the tail of the maximum expiratory flow–volume (MEFV) curve, with flow ceasing abruptly so that it appears to 'fall off' the curve (Fig. 20.2).[28]

Measurements of functional residual capacity (FRC) in patients with muscle weakness are variable, with both reduced and increased values reported in different series. Any reduction of lung distensibility will encourage a reduction of FRC, and a greater-than-normal value of lung recoil pressure (P_L) of FRC would then be expected. In practice, P_L at FRC is usually reduced,[23,26] probably due to altered passive pressure–volume characteristics of the chest wall (Fig. 20.3). In some patients with muscle weakness, however, FRC is increased; this is usually associated with a marked rise in RV and is commonly seen, for example, in motor neuron disease.[28,29] Patients with this condition are generally older than most others with severe respiratory muscle disease, and the difference may be related to age.

20.2.1.3 Airway function

A reduction in the forced expiratory ratio (FEV_1/VC) is theoretically possible with severe expiratory muscle weakness but in practice is not seen. FEV_1/VC and specific airway conductance are typically normal or increased,[23] and resistance measured by forced oscillation is also normal.[30]

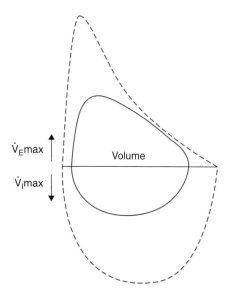

Figure 20.2 Schematic diagram of maximum flow–volume curves in a patient with severe muscle weakness (solid line) compared with normal (broken line). The volume axis represents change in absolute lung volume. The forced vital capacity (FVC) of the patient is reduced by inability both to inspire and to expire fully. Peak expiratory flow is reduced and at the end of expiration flow 'falls off' the expected curve because of expiratory muscle weakness. Maximum inspiratory flow $\dot{V}_I$max, is impaired at all lung volumes.

$\dot{V}_E$max, maximum expiratory flow.

However, peak expiratory flow (which is strictly effort-dependent) is impaired, as are maximum inspiratory flows at all lung volumes (see Fig. 20.2). Consequently, the maximum flow–volume curve in patients with respiratory muscle weakness may resemble that of upper (extrathoracic) airway obstruction – but the characteristic plateau of expiratory flow (see Fig. 12.2 in Chapter 12) is not seen. Oscillations of maximum expiratory and/or inspiratory flow ('sawtooth' appearance; see Fig. 1.36 in Chapter 1) may be present, particularly when the upper airway muscles are also weak.

A major clinical effect of expiratory weakness is reduced efficacy of coughing. This normally requires a markedly positive intrathoracic pressure, which compresses the intrathoracic airways and mobilizes secretions by the resulting shearing forces. The effect of coughing can be visualized on the MEFV curve as a transient of flow that exceeds the maximum value generated at the same thoracic volume during continuous forced expiration. The absence of such expiratory flow transients during coughing implies severe expiratory weakness.[31]

20.2.1.4 Measurements of ventilation

The maximum voluntary ventilation is typically reduced and the early literature suggested this was

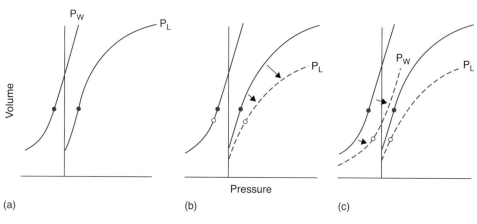

(a)   (b)   (c)

Figure 20.3 Determinants of functional residual capacity (FRC) illustrated by static pressure–volume (PV) curves. (a) In the normal subject FRC (solid circles) is determined by the balance of recoil pressure of the lungs (P_L) and chest wall (P_W). (b) With severe muscle weakness, the compliance of the lungs is reduced (broken line) and, if there were no change in the static PV curve of the chest wall, the balance of recoil pressures would produce a greater-than-normal value of P_L at the smaller FRC (open circles). (c) In practice, P_L at FRC is less than normal because the static PV curve of the chest wall is also altered and chest wall compliance (slope over tidal breathing range) is reduced.

the most sensitive test of respiratory muscle weakness. Its sensitivity has, however, been overrated and it is usually reduced in approximate proportion to VC.[29,32]

The pattern of resting breathing in patients with muscle weakness typically shows a rapid frequency and reduced tidal volume. This is inefficient in terms of gas exchange but may be mechanically imposed by increased stiffness (low compliance) of the lungs.

20.2.1.5 Pulmonary gas exchange

In acute neuromuscular illnesses the PaO_2 may be appreciably reduced, but the picture is often complicated by respiratory infection.[33] In chronic disease, the $AaPO_2$ is normal or only slightly increased, even with quite severe weakness.[23] In patients with mild weakness, the arterial PCO_2 is frequently below normal,[32] but hypercapnia supervenes when the bellows function of the chest wall is no longer adequate to maintain normal ventilation (Fig. 20.4). The tendency to alveolar hypoventilation is exacerbated by the typical breathing pattern of respiratory muscle weakness with a small tidal volume, which implies that an abnormally large proportion of the total ventilation is wasted on the irreducible anatomical dead space. Consequently, the $PaCO_2$ at rest is related inversely to the tidal volume.[34]

Patients with hypercapnia due to respiratory muscle weakness are at risk of worsening hypercapnia if treated with uncontrolled oxygen. Even with low oxygen flows, the inspired oxygen concentration increases unpredictably and can result in life-threatening hypercapnia.[35]

The single-breath carbon monoxide diffusing capacity (D_LCO) in patients with muscle weakness is usually normal or reduced only mildly. A slight reduction is likely because of inability fully to distend the lungs and therefore to expose all the alveolar surface to carbon monoxide. As with other causes of extrapulmonary restriction, KCO is often greater than normal.

20.2.1.6 Ventilatory control and exercise

Abnormal central control of ventilation may contribute to hypercapnia in some conditions, but its relevance has been overestimated. In many earlier studies, weakness of the respiratory muscles was not assessed directly and no account was taken of the effect of weakness on ventilatory responses. In most instances hypercapnia and/or a reduced ventilatory response slope are attributable simply to weakness.[29] Furthermore, the mouth occlusion

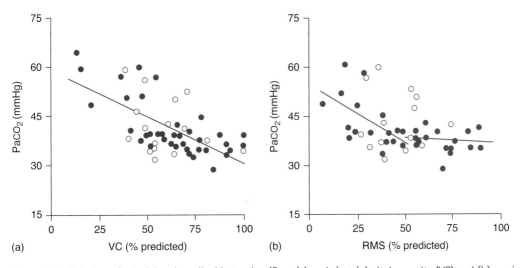

Figure 20.4 Relation of arterial carbon dioxide tension ($PaCO_2$) (awake) to (a) vital capacity (VC) and (b) respiratory muscle strength (RMS – arithmetic average of maximum static expiratory and inspiratory alveolar pressures ($P_E$max, $P_I$max)), each as per cent predicted in a population of patients with generalized muscle weakness. Open circles represent patients with coexisting chronic airway obstruction. Modified from: Braun NMT et al. Respiratory muscle and pulmonary function in polymyositis and other proximal myopathies. *Thorax* 1983; **38**: 616–23, with permission from the BMJ Publishing Group.

pressure ($P_{0.1}$) during tidal breathing at rest is typically greater than normal in patients with respiratory muscle weakness,[36] and in less weak patients $PaCO_2$ is less than normal (Fig. 20.4). Both of these observations imply increased, rather than decreased, ventilatory drive. Substitution of $P_{0.1}$ for ventilation when assessing the response to chemical stimulation has given variable results. In many patients with chronic respiratory muscle weakness the slope of the $P_{0.1}/PCO_2$ response is less than normal,[37,38] but since generation of $P_{0.1}$ is inevitably dependent on inspiratory muscle contraction its use in this situation does not circumvent the problem of impaired effector function being an inadequate index of respiratory drive. This conclusion is also supported by the interesting 'model' offered by patients with myasthenia gravis studied before and after administration of an anticholinesterase drug. In this situation improvements in maximum respiratory pressures are accompanied by an increase in slopes of both the ventilatory and $P_{0.1}$ responses to CO_2.[38]

Exercise and the maximum oxygen consumption achievable by patients with respiratory muscle weakness are usually limited by generalized weakness affecting the limbs rather than by cardiorespiratory factors. The limited data available suggest that the relation of workload to PO_2 is usually normal and that indices of submaximal exercise performance are also normal.[39]

20.2.1.7 Breathing during sleep

In slowly progressive respiratory muscle weakness, hypercapnia develops first during sleep, when ventilation is inevitably reduced compared with the awake state, and only later does $PaCO_2$ become persistently elevated by day.[40] Gradual retention of bicarbonate ions in response to respiratory acidosis during sleep probably contributes to the subsequent development of diurnal hypercapnia. The various patterns of abnormality of breathing during sleep reported in individuals with respiratory muscle weakness include hypopnoeas and apnoeas, which may be central, 'pseudo-central' or obstructive, and more prolonged periods of hypoventilation.[41] Pseudo-central events are actually obstructive but superficially appear to be central as the inspiratory effort is too weak to be identified by conventional external sensors, although oesophageal pressure

monitoring or electromyographic (EMG) studies show that efforts are continuing.[42] The most commonly seen discrete sleep-breathing events are central hypopnoeas with associated dips in oxygen saturation; these are more frequent and prolonged in REM sleep, particularly phasic REM sleep.[41] During REM sleep the overall activity of skeletal muscles is greatly suppressed, although activation of the diaphragm is normally relatively better preserved. In patients with respiratory muscle weakness, particularly those with diaphragmatic weakness, REM hypopnoea and hypoventilation result from inadequate diaphragmatic recruitment. Predominantly obstructive apnoeas or hypopnoeas have been reported in some studies. Obstructive events are more likely in individuals with a high body mass index (BMI) and in those who snore or who have other predisposing characteristics such as macroglossia.[41,43] With milder respiratory muscle weakness, sleep-related hypopnoeas tend to predominate with more sustained hypoventilation seen as respiratory muscle weakness progresses.[44] Because the pattern of abnormality varies and, at least in more severely affected individuals, persistent hypoventilation is frequent, the apnoea hypopnoea index (AHI) is an inadequate descriptor of the severity of sleep disordered breathing in this population.

Nocturnal hypoxaemia can result from any or all of the above breathing abnormalities and, in addition, may be due to ventilation/perfusion mismatching, particularly in the supine posture. Desaturation is characteristically most marked during phasic REM sleep and is also more marked in older subjects and those with higher BMI.[41]

Several studies have investigated the relations of breathing and oxygenation during sleep to daytime respiratory function in patients with respiratory muscle weakness. As would be expected, nocturnal saturation correlates with daytime PaO_2 and $PaCO_2$ (inversely); in general, any desaturation while awake is likely to amplify breathing related falls in SaO_2 when asleep.[41] Since nocturnal desaturation and hypercapnia are likely to precede daytime respiratory failure, potentially more sensitive predictors of abnormal nocturnal gas exchange have been sought. Broadly, the more severe the mechanical abnormality, as assessed by maximum pressures and VC, the more severe the nocturnal hypercapnia and desaturation, although correlations

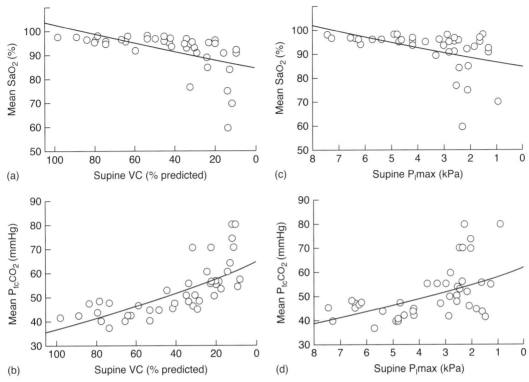

Figure 20.5 Relations of mean nocturnal oxygen saturation (Sao$_2$) (a,c) and mean transcutaneous Pco$_2$ (P$_{tc}$co$_2$) (b,d) to supine vital capacity (VC) (a,b) and maximum inspiratory alveolar pressure (P$_I$max) (c,d) in a population of patients with generalized muscle weakness. Modified from: Ragette R *et al.* Patterns and predictors of sleep disordered breathing in primary myopathies. *Thorax* 2002; **57**: 724–8, with permission from the BMJ Publishing Group.

are not close[41,44] and relationships are alinear (Fig. 20.5). Whether sleep studies should be part of routine monitoring of patients with respiratory muscle weakness is controversial, as the value of early detection of nocturnal breathing abnormalities has not been established. Studies of the influence of respiratory function on survival have consistently shown that simple daytime measurements such as VC or maximum static inspiratory alveolar pressure (P$_I$max) are better predictors of survival than nocturnal oxygen saturation.[45,46] Similarly, the combination of daytime respiratory function with symptoms, particularly orthopnoea and daytime sleepiness, is better than nocturnal measurements as a predictor of benefit from treatment with NIV.[47]

Non-invasive nocturnal ventilatory support via a facemask or other interface is used widely in patients with hypercapnic respiratory failure due to chronic respiratory muscle weakness. It also has a role in some patients with sleep-related symptoms,

even in the absence of daytime hypercapnia.[40,48,49] In patients with ventilatory failure, considerable improvement is seen in both nocturnal oxygenation and daytime blood gases (Fig. 20.6). Most studies show no significant change in mechanical function of the lungs and thorax after a period of treatment.[48] The improvement in daytime PaCO$_2$ is probably related to the reduction in bicarbonate concentration that accompanies better nocturnal ventilation. Consequently, the ventilatory response to hypercapnia increases following a period of nocturnal treatment, as the lower bicarbonate concentration implies a greater stimulus to the respiratory centres when breathing a hypercapnic gas mixture.

20.2.2 Bilateral diaphragmatic paralysis

Most cases of bilateral paralysis of the diaphragm are seen in the context of generalized weakness of the respiratory muscles, but occasional patients are encountered with selective weakness or paralysis.

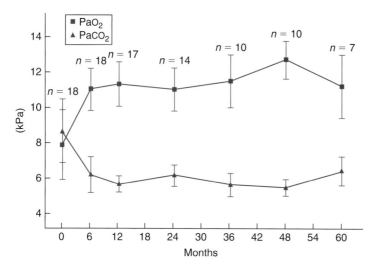

Figure 20.6 Evolution of awake Pa_{O_2} and Pa_{CO_2} in patients with Duchenne muscular dystrophy treated for up to 5 years with non-invasive ventilation. Modified from: Simonds AK *et al.* Impact of nasal ventilation on survival in hypercapnic Duchenne muscular dystrophy. *Thorax* 1998; 53: 949–52, with permission from the BMJ Publishing Group.

20.2.2.1 Effects on maximum pressures and lung volumes

Bilateral diaphragmatic paralysis (BDP) is characterized functionally by an absent, or virtually absent, transdiaphragmatic pressure on maximal inspiratory efforts or during bilateral phrenic or cervical electrical or magnetic stimulation. The VC typically shows a marked fall (often greater than 50%) in the supine posture compared with the erect, which corresponds to the patient's common complaint of extreme orthopnoea and to the observation of inspiratory paradox of the abdominal wall in the supine position.[50] In the upright posture, maintenance of a more normal VC is aided by gravity and abdominal paradox is less likely to be apparent, as patients adapt to the adverse mechanics by expiratory contraction of the muscles of the abdominal wall followed by relaxation and consequent forward abdominal motion at the onset of inspiration.[51] A history of difficulty swimming or lower body immersion in water is also characteristic and is due to the effects of hydrostatic forces on the abdomen and diaphragm. Measurement of VC in subjects in water shows a marked reduction, with ventilation nevertheless preserved by an augmented drive to breathe and increase in respiratory rate.[52]

20.2.2.2 Effects on tidal breathing

During tidal breathing with complete BDP, the changes in pleural surface pressure (P_{pl}) and sub-diaphragmatic abdominal pressure (P_{ab}) are identical, as the increasingly negative P_{pl} during inspiration is transmitted via the paralysed diaphragm. Consequently, the ratio $\Delta P_{ab}/\Delta P_{pl}$ is +1, whereas in healthy subjects during tidal breathing P_{pl} and P_{ab} change in the opposite sense to each other with a ratio on average (seated) of about -2.[53] This ratio has been shown to be proportional to maximum transdiaphragmatic pressure (P_{di}max) recorded during maximum voluntary efforts, and its measurement may be helpful in patients unable to perform such manoeuvres adequately.[53]

20.2.2.3 Effects on gas exchange

The effects of isolated BDP on gas exchange are generally less severe than suggested by some earlier reports,[51] probably because several of the patients reported with BDP also had generalized weakness.[54] With isolated BDP, increased activity of other respiratory muscles is apparently sufficient to maintain virtually normal blood gases in most patients while awake both at rest and on exercise,[54] although exercise capacity is moderately reduced with lower maximum ventilation than normal.[55] Regional ventilation and perfusion show the expected reductions at the lung bases.[56]

20.2.2.4 Effects on breathing during sleep

The results of investigation during sleep are variable, with some reporting no abnormal rise in transcutaneous P_{CO_2}[54] and others finding hypercapnia.[57] Arterial desaturation during sleep is more consistently detectable. As would be expected, desaturation is seen particularly during REM sleep,[58] as this is when, in healthy subjects, ventilation is particularly dependent on diaphragmatic function. Some studies have suggested that patients with severe diaphragmatic weakness adapt by suppressing REM sleep,[58] but others appear able to maintain a normal duration of REM sleep.[59] In patients with BDP, the severity of REM desaturation is proportional to the postural fall in VC when awake, emphasizing the importance of diaphragmatic function for maintaining oxygenation, especially during REM sleep.[58,60]

20.2.2.5 Effects of treatment of bilateral diaphragmatic paralysis

Some patients improve symptomatically with NIV, even when daytime blood gases are not particularly abnormal. The improvement may be due to restoring the ability of sleep in the supine posture when ventilation is assisted, whereas adopting this posture without ventilatory support is likely to seriously disrupt sleep. The surgical procedure of diaphragmatic plication is reserved mainly for patients with unilateral diaphragmatic paralysis (see below) but has also been reported to improve VC and pulmonary gas exchange in selected patients with isolated BDP.[61]

20.2.3 Unilateral diaphragmatic paralysis

Unilateral diaphragmatic palsy (UDP) is frequently a solitary neuromuscular abnormality resulting from localized damage to the ipsilateral phrenic nerve by tumour, trauma or infection. In the face of normal function of the other respiratory muscles,

conventional tests of respiratory function may remain within normal limits, but values of VC and TLC in the upright posture of 70–80 per cent predicted are commonly found.[62–64] In many patients with UDP the phrenic palsy results from malignant infiltration and the underlying cause may then dominate the functional pattern. In general, the functional abnormalities of UDP are intermediate between those of BDP and normality. As with bilateral paralysis, many patients show a marked reduction of VC in the supine position.[63,64] The postural effect is greater with right-sided paralysis, due to the effect of gravity on the liver.[64]

Maximum inspiratory pressure and sniff P_{di} show moderate reductions.[65,66] The ratio $\Delta P_{ab}/\Delta P_{pl}$ during upright tidal breathing is more positive than normal and intermediate between normality and BDP, in proportion to the reduction in P_{di}max.[53,62]

Studies of regional gas exchange show diminished function at the lung base overlying the paralysed muscle, with relatively more reduction of ventilation than perfusion.[63,67] A small fall in Pa_{O_2} occurs on assuming the supine position, possibly reflecting an increased tendency to airway closure.[64] The D_LCO is usually normal but K_{CO} may be modestly increased.[64] Exercise capacity is somewhat reduced.[55]

Surgical plication results in significant improvement in lung volumes[68] and P_{di}max,[69] with restoration of a more normal $\Delta P_{ab}/\Delta P_{pl}$ ratio during tidal breathing.[53]

20.3 SPECIFIC CONDITIONS OF THE CENTRAL NERVOUS SYSTEM

20.3.1 Stroke

20.3.1.1 Effect of site of stroke

The effect of a stroke on respiratory function is critically dependent on the site and extent of the neurological damage. Because of the large area of the cerebral cortex involved with volitional muscle control, a localized cortical infarct has little or no effect on respiratory function. By contrast, as with motor control elsewhere in the body, even a small infarct affecting the internal capsule has a much greater effect. Electromyographic studies in patients with hemiplegia show marked reduction in activity of both the inspiratory intercostal muscles and the diaphragm on the ipsilateral side. The reduction is relatively greater for the intercostal muscles than for the diaphragm,[70] presumably reflecting greater bilateral innervation of the latter. As would be expected, voluntary manoeuvres under the control of the behavioural pathway are more affected than functions dependent on metabolic control. For example, both ultrasonic measurements of diaphragmatic motion[71] and optoelectronic plethysmography of chest movements[72] show symmetrical movement during quiet resting breathing but reduced movement on the hemiplegic side during voluntary deep breathing.

Strokes affecting the midbrain and medulla are likely to have more profound effects on breathing in the acute stages than are lesions at higher levels. The various abnormalities of resting breathing pattern associated with lesions at various levels are discussed above (see Section 20.1.1) in relation to differential involvement of the corticospinal or reticulospinal pathways of ventilatory control.

20.3.1.2 Acute effects on oxygenation

Awake hypoxaemia is very common in the first few days after stroke. In some patients this is related to periodic breathing of Cheyne–Stokes pattern, which may be detectable even in conscious patients.[73] In one study this pattern was found in half the conscious patients studied and its occurrence was unrelated to the location of the recent infarct.[74] Hypoxaemia is common even in patients in whom periodic breathing has been excluded.[74,75] The severity of oxygen desaturation is greater in older subjects and in those with more severe strokes.[75] Some data suggest that the effect is particularly marked when patients are nursed supine,[74] but this may be due to associated respiratory comorbidity rather than to the stroke per se.[76] Although, in principle, hypoxaemia is likely to be deleterious for some patients, hyperoxia may also be harmful and routine administration of oxygen after stroke does not improve survival.[77]

20.3.1.3 Sleep-disordered breathing after stroke

Several studies have shown a high frequency of sleep-disordered breathing after stroke,[78–81] with a high prevalence of both central and obstructive apnoeas and hypopnoeas. Analysis of cause and effect is complicated by evidence that pre-existing obstructive sleep apnoea probably increases the risk of developing a stroke.[78] However, sequential sleep studies after stroke[79,81] show evidence of improvement over several weeks. Irrespective of whether sleep-disordered breathing antedates or follows the stroke, several studies have shown that its presence has a significant effect on the long-term outcome. It is associated with longer hospitalization, greater long-term functional impairment and an increased likelihood of death and dependency.[82–84] The severity of sleep-disordered breathing post-stroke is not related clearly to the site or extent of the stroke, but it is more common in patients with evidence of pre-existing cerebrovascular disease.[82,85]

In patients with central sleep apnoea or Cheyne–Stokes breathing post-stroke there is no relation to the location or type of stroke, but such individuals tend to have lower nocturnal transcutaneous P_{CO_2} and a greater prevalence of left ventricular systolic dysfunction.[86]

20.3.1.4 Findings in convalescent patients

Asymmetrical chest movement during volitional manoeuvres persists in patients with a significant hemiparesis.[72] Many patients convalescing from a stroke have demonstrable weakness of both inspiratory and expiratory muscles, as shown by impaired maximum respiratory pressures.[87]

20.3.2 Parkinson's disease and related conditions

20.3.2.1 Parkinson's disease

Parkinson's disease is characterized by bradykinesia, rigidity and tremor of skeletal muscles, abnormalities that particularly affect the performance of repetitive movements. Consequently, unlike in other neuromuscular diseases, maximum voluntary ventilation may be impaired disproportionately and therefore may be more sensitive than other tests of respiratory muscle function in Parkinson's disease.[88] Dyscoordinate activity during tidal breathing is demonstrable by electromyography.[89]

A restrictive ventilatory defect is frequently present.[90] Maximum inspiratory pressures are commonly reduced even in mild disease,[91,92] and respiratory muscle endurance is also decreased.[91] Contrary to earlier reports, there is no evidence of generalized airway narrowing,[93,94] but abnormalities suggesting upper airway dysfunction are frequently found, with a reduction in effort-dependent maximum flows on inspiration and expiration, often with oscillation of flow giving a 'sawtooth' appearance (Fig. 20.7).[94–96] The oscillations have been shown to correspond to rhythmic or irregular movements of glottic and supraglottic structures consistent with dyscoordination of the upper airway muscles.[94,95]

Muscle dysfunction sufficient to cause hypercapnia is very rare, but the combination of central alveolar hypoventilation and parkinsonism has been reported as sequelae of encephalitis lethargica.[97] Exercise performance may be reasonably well preserved in patients with only mild disease,[98] but otherwise maximum exercise capacity and $\dot{V}O_2$max are reduced in proportion to maximum respiratory pressures.[92] Studies during sleep show an increased prevalence of snoring and obstructive sleep apnoea, particularly in patients with more advanced disease.[99] Treatment with

levodopa (L-dopa) has been shown to improve respiratory muscle function, with demonstrable effects on maximum flow–volume curves (Fig. 20.7).[96]

20.3.2.2 Multisystem atrophy

In multisystem atrophy (e.g. Shy–Drager syndrome) extrapyramidal features are accompanied by degenerative changes affecting the autonomic nervous system. There may be severe upper airway narrowing (accompanied by stridor) due to laryngeal dysfunction.[100] This may be due to either paralysis of the laryngeal abductor muscles[101] or active contraction of the laryngeal adductor muscles during inspiration.[102] Abnormalities persist during sleep, with hypoventilation and oxygen desaturation.[101,103] Tidal breathing is often notably irregular even during slow-wave sleep, consistent with a defect in the metabolic pathway of respiratory control, probably related to degeneration of brainstem autonomic systems.[104] Consequently, periodic breathing of Cheyne–Stokes type is sometimes seen during sleep,[101] and periods of central apnoea may persist even after tracheostomy to relieve the laryngeal obstruction.[105]

20.3.3 Arnold–Chiari malformation and syringomyelia

The Arnold–Chiari malformation results in caudal displacement of the cerebellum and sometimes the medulla through the foramen magnum, and is frequently associated with syringomyelia and/or syringobulbia. Reported abnormalities of respiratory function include central alveolar hypoventilation, sleep apnoea and the consequences of vocal cord paralysis. Occasionally, otherwise unexplained ventilatory failure is a presenting feature of Arnold–Chiari malformation with syringomyelia.[106] Various mechanisms may be relevant, including insensitivity of the peripheral chemoreceptors resulting from impaired glossopharyngeal nerve function,[107] compression of the medulla by herniation through the foramen magnum and a syrinx interrupting the reticulospinal pathways that mediate automatic respiratory control. Some patients present with hypercapnic respiratory failure,[106] while others may have relatively normal daytime blood gases but severe sleep apnoea, which can appear to be either central[108] or

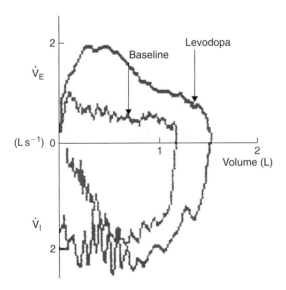

Figure 20.7 Maximum expiratory and inspiratory flow volume curves from a patient with Parkinson's disease before and after a single dose of levodopa. Modified from ref. 96 with permission from the American College of Chest Physicians.

obstructive.[109] Cervical decompression can produce considerable improvement in the sleep-disordered breathing.[108]

20.3.4 Spinal cord lesions

20.3.4.1 Effects of cervical cord injury

Most measurements of respiratory function have been reported in patients with traumatic spinal cord injury, but similar abnormalities are seen with vascular or neoplastic conditions. The effects on respiratory function depend critically on the level of the damage. Lesions above the phrenic nerve outflow, i.e. at C1 or C2, result in paralysis of all the main respiratory muscles due to interruption of the descending pathways, with apnoea followed rapidly by death unless ventilatory support is instituted.[110] Lesions of the lower cervical cord leave the diaphragm and inspiratory accessory muscles intact, but inspiratory intercostal and most expiratory action is lost as the latter depends mainly on the integrity of the abdominal wall muscles. Loss of expiratory muscle function has little relevance for normal tidal expiration but greatly reduces the efficacy of coughing. Patients with low cervical tetraplegia retain the function of pectoralis major, which has sufficient expiratory action to cause some dynamic airway compression, a phenomenon that is essential for the efficacy of coughing.[111]

In contrast to patients with bilateral diaphragmatic paralysis, who are severely orthopnoeic, paralysis of the other inspiratory muscles with retention of normal diaphragmatic function has a more profound effect in the upright position. Measurements of chest wall motion show that diaphragmatic contraction unsupported by activity of the other inspiratory muscles produces paradoxical movement of the upper ribcage, while the lower ribs expand normally.[112] In some patients the stability of the ribcage is maintained by reflex EMG activity in the parasternal intercostal muscles[113] or by activity of the scalene muscles.[114] For the same reason, supine values of VC and FEV_1 are typically larger than those measured seated, at least with injury at levels down to T1.[115,116] In general, the lower the level of injury, the less effect on spirometric volumes. The TLC is reduced proportionally less than VC, and RV may be increased. However, in some patients RV remains normal, perhaps because of decreased

lung and/or chest wall distensibility.[117] If expiratory muscle function were lost completely, FRC would be identical to RV, but a small expiratory reserve volume is found even with high cervical injuries,[116] due to the action of muscles of the neck and upper chest wall. The maximum inspiratory pressure that patients with tetraplegia can generate is about half the normal value.[113] Some improvement can be achieved by training the residually functional respiratory muscles by resistance breathing, particularly with only partial spinal cord transection: the benefit is seen more in terms of endurance than respiratory muscle strength.[118]

Maximum expiratory flow is inevitably reduced, but the forced expiratory ratio remains normal.[119] Bronchial hyperresponsiveness to inhaled methacholine is demonstrable in patients with tetraplegia using measurements of either FEV_1[120] or specific airway conductance.[121] Also, a large bronchodilator effect and reduced airway responsiveness are seen with use of the anticholinergic bronchodilator ipratropium.[121] Bronchial responsiveness in patients with tetraplegia has been attributed to loss of the sympathetic innervation of the lung, leaving bronchoconstrictor cholinergic activity unopposed; loss of the ability to stretch airway smooth muscle by deep breathing may also play a role.[120]

Sequential studies after cervical cord injury show that more profound disturbances are present in the first few weeks, following which FEV_1 and VC can increase appreciably. In the first few days many patients show significant arterial hypoxaemia. In general, the higher the lesion, the more severe the gas exchange abnormality, and, with lesions at the level of C4, hypercapnia is often present initially.[119] A high prevalence of sleep-disordered breathing has been reported a few weeks after cervical cord injury.[122]

20.3.4.2 Effects of thoracic cord injury

Transection of the thoracic spinal cord and consequent paraplegia is accompanied by less severe reduction in VC than is seen in tetraplegia. The postural effect on VC is less consistent than in patients with cervical cord injury, sometimes with greater values in the supine position.[116,123] The most important respiratory consequence of paraplegia due to thoracic cord injury is the reduced force of coughing due to paralysis or weakness of the abdominal muscles.

The rate of decline of FEV_1 and VC several years after injury is probably more rapid then normal in both tetraplegia[115,124] and paraplegia.[125]

20.3.5 Multiple sclerosis

As the neurological sites of demyelination vary in multiple sclerosis, so do the resulting effects on respiratory function. A variety of abnormalities has been described, with reduced respiratory muscle pressures the commonest;[126,127] lung volume restriction,[128] impaired exercise capacity,[129] acute hypercapnic respiratory failure,[130] sleep apnoea,[131] impaired ventilatory response to CO_2[132] and paroxysmal hyperventilation[131] have all been reported singly or in combination.

Respiratory problems are unusual as the presenting feature of the disease but are common with relapses. Occasionally an acute relapse is associated with respiratory arrest. Respiratory failure can be accompanied by irregular respiration while awake, and by central sleep apnoea due to a lesion affecting the metabolic pathway of ventilatory control in the medulla[133] or weakness of the diaphragm and other respiratory muscles due to demyelination of the cervical spinal cord.[131] Nocturnal hypoxaemia is commonly found when overnight measurements are made.[128]

In general, patients more disabled by multiple sclerosis have worse respiratory function.[128] In ambulant individuals with little involvement of the upper limbs, function is usually relatively well preserved, while those confined to a wheelchair due to weakness of the legs have more marked reductions in VC and maximum respiratory pressures. Exercise capacity can be related directly to respiratory muscle strength,[129] and the respiratory muscle weakness may be improved by resistance training.[134]

20.3.6 Poliomyelitis

In the first half of the twentieth century the high prevalence of poliomyelitis and the consequent use of ventilatory support with the 'iron lung' was a major stimulus to the clinical assessment of respiratory function. Indeed, the 'iron lung' itself was a precursor of the whole-body plethysmograph. It was noted in early studies that polio could affect

breathing by involving either the spinal cord or the brainstem, and it was among the earliest recognized causes of central alveolar hypoventilation. In a classic study, Plum and Swanson distinguished the grossly ataxic breathing pattern of patients with acute bulbar poliomyelitis and apnoea during drowsiness and sleep from the less severe abnormality shown by those in whom disease was confined to the spinal cord.[8] Careful pathological studies of the brainstem of patients dying from bulbar polio showed that the lesions were located in the upper medulla close to the ventral respiratory group of neurons controlling the automatic respiratory pathway.[9] In patients who recovered from the acute illness, the evidence of abnormal ventilatory control usually disappeared.

In recent years it has been appreciated that late respiratory complications of poliomyelitis can develop. This effect corresponds to the delayed increase in weakness in other muscles that can appear up to 30 years after the original illness. Weakness develops mainly in those muscles that were affected acutely and is apparently due to late degeneration and loss of the relevant motor neurons. It has been shown that individuals currently requiring no ventilatory support, but who had been ventilated during the acute illness, have significantly weaker inspiratory muscles than those who were never ventilated,[135] and patients are seen with gradually increasing respiratory muscle weakness leading to chronic respiratory failure. This 'post-polio' syndrome tends to occur in those who had evidence of respiratory muscle weakness during their original illness and/or those who develop a marked scoliosis. Spirometric volumes are lower in individuals who were ventilated acutely and in those who contracted polio after the age of 10 years;[136] nocturnal hypoventilation is a common consequence, with apnoeas that may be either central or obstructive.[137] Not surprisingly, patients with evidence of bulbar involvement are more likely to have central apnoeas, which occur particularly during non-REM sleep.[138] Treatment with nocturnal NIV is frequently used in this population.

20.3.7 Motor neuron disease (amyotrophic lateral sclerosis)

Amyotrophic lateral sclerosis (ALS) shares with poliomyelitis the propensity to affect both medullary and spinal motor neurons. Respiratory infections and failure are common terminal events and, even in less symptomatic patients, respiratory muscle weakness is the rule.[29,139] Occasionally, severe respiratory weakness develops early when there is little limb weakness; such patients can present with breathlessness and cause diagnostic difficulty.[140] In most individuals severe diaphragmatic weakness or paralysis mirrors severe weakness of the other respiratory muscles.[29]

A reduced VC is often accompanied by an increased RV and sometimes an increased FRC. Consequently, TLC is often surprisingly normal despite fairly severe weakness.[28,29] In patients with severe expiratory weakness the MEFV curve shows abrupt termination of flow (see Fig. 20.2). This appearance is exaggerated by the addition of only a small external resistance, emphasizing the vulnerability of such patients to minor respiratory illnesses that are likely to have a similar functional effect.[28]

The ventilatory response to CO_2 is reduced in proportion to the impairment of maximum respiratory pressures and of VC; elevation of $PaCO_2$ usually implies severe weakness and a poor prognosis. Hypercapnia is related closely to the severity of inspiratory muscle weakness measured either as nasal inspiratory pressure during a forceful sniff (SNIP) or transdiaphragmatic pressure during the same manoeuvre (sniff P_{di}) (Fig. 20.8).[141] However, no clear relationship holds in patients with more

severe bulbar weakness, probably because assessment of respiratory muscle strength by volitional tests is then much less reliable.[141]

Sleep studies in ALS frequently show abnormalities, with patterns of REM-related hypopnoea and desaturation and/or overall hypoventilation.[45,142] Although obstructive events have been described in some patients,[45] they are less common. The AHI is an insensitive index of the severity of sleep-disordered breathing[45] and relates less well to overall quality of life than do measurements of respiratory muscle function awake.[143] Patients with more severe weakness are particularly vulnerable during REM sleep; one study showed reduced or absent REM sleep in individuals with more severe diaphragmatic dysfunction,[144] which may represent an adaptation to the vulnerability of their breathing during sleep.

The prognosis for survival in ALS has been shown in several studies to relate to the severity of respiratory muscle weakness in preference to all other features of the disease. The indices most closely correlated with survival have varied in different studies and include maximum inspiratory pressure, VC,[45] SNIP,[145] and the rate of decline of VC estimated either from a single measurement and assuming a value of 100 per cent predicted at presentation[146] or from sequential measurements.[147] Despite the frequent finding of abnormal breathing during sleep, this does not add usefully to awake measurements when estimating likely survival.[45]

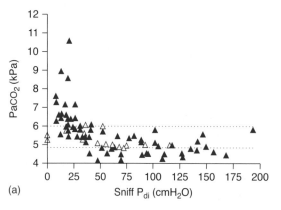 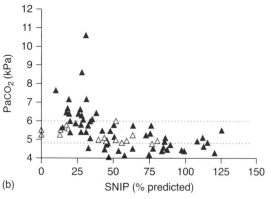

(a) Sniff P_{di} (cmH$_2$O)

(b) SNIP (% predicted)

Figure 20.8 Relations between arterial PCO_2 ($PaCO_2$) and (a) sniff transdiaphragmatic pressure (P_{di}) and (b) sniff nasal inspiratory pressure (SNIP) in patients with motor neuron disease (amyotrophic lateral sclerosis, ALS). Open triangles indicate patients with predominant bulbar features; dotted lines indicate normal range of $PaCO_2$. Note hyperbolic relationships and general similarity to relation between $PaCO_2$ and respiratory muscle weakness in patients with other forms of respiratory muscle weakness (cf. Fig. 20.4b). Modified with permission from ref. 141.

The value of NIV in ALS has been more controversial than in other causes of advanced respiratory muscle weakness, mainly because the prognosis is more limited than that of most muscular dystrophies and myopathies. One standard guideline recommends offering NIV for symptomatic chronic hypercapnia,[148] but the presence of orthopnoea with demonstrable respiratory muscle weakness may be more sensitive.[47] A randomized controlled trial using one or other of these criteria as the indication to initiate treatment with NIV confirmed improved survival and quality of life in patients without severe bulbar dysfunction.[49] In addition, use of NIV may slow the rate of decline of VC.[47] Patients with more severe bulbar impairment, however, show less good tolerance of NIV, and its benefit is then less certain.[49]

Chronic spinal muscular atrophy of adults (Kugelberg–Welander syndrome) involves only the lower motor neurons and has a much better prognosis than ALS, but occasionally it causes diaphragmatic paralysis and ventilatory failure.[51,149]

20.4 SPECIFIC CONDITIONS OF PERIPHERAL NERVE AND MUSCLE

20.4.1 Neuropathies

20.4.1.1 Guillain–Barré syndrome

In polyneuritis of the Guillain–Barré type, generalized weakness progresses rapidly over weeks or days and about 30 per cent of patients develop sufficient respiratory weakness to require mechanical ventilation.[150,151] Blood gases are relatively insensitive as a guide to the likely need for ventilatory support, as hypercapnia is a late event. However, sequential measurements of VC and/or maximum respiratory pressures have been shown to be useful in several studies.[150–152] The various thresholds predicting the likely need for intervention include a VC of 15–20 mL/kg bodyweight[150,152] or less than 60 per cent predicted,[151] or a decline in VC exceeding 30 per cent.[152] With measurements of maximum pressures, $P_I$max <30 cmH$_2$O or $P_E$max <40 cmH$_2$O is similarly predictive.[152] Follow-up data on respiratory function are sparse but recovery is often slow and some patients do not regain completely normal muscle function.

20.4.1.2 Other peripheral neuropathies

Respiratory muscle weakness undoubtedly occurs in many other generalized neuropathies but, in most, little or no direct information on respiratory function is available. In hereditary motor and sensory neuropathy (Charcot–Marie–Tooth disease) diaphragmatic weakness has been reported,[153,154] as also has generalized weakness sufficient to cause hypercapnic respiratory failure.[155]

20.4.1.3 Phrenic nerve lesions

Localized phrenic nerve lesions causing unilateral diaphragmatic paralysis are seen most commonly with infiltration by tumour. Injury to one[156] or, less commonly, both[157] phrenic nerves is also a well-recognized consequence of cardiac surgery, particularly when an ice-cold solution is used to produce cardioplegia (so called 'frostbitten phrenic syndrome'). This used to be a relatively common consequence of cardiac surgery when topical cardiac cooling with ice 'slush' was used, but it is much less likely if this is avoided.[158] In most cases recovery occurs over a few weeks, but prolonged ventilatory assistance may be required.[159]

The phrenic nerves are sometimes involved in neuralgic amyotrophy (brachial neuritis), which affects the nerves of the brachial plexus. Diaphragmatic paralysis may be unilateral or simultaneously or sequentially bilateral.[160] Sequential measurements of diaphragmatic function usually show some evidence of recovery, but this can take several months and is often incomplete.[161]

20.4.2 Myasthenic disorders

20.4.2.1 Myasthenia gravis

Patients with generalized myasthenia gravis typically show a chronic reduction in global respiratory muscle strength and endurance.[162] A reduction in P_{di} during voluntary manoeuvres such as a forceful sniff is demonstrable more readily than any impairment on phrenic nerve stimulation at a frequency of 1 Hz (twitch P_{di}), so that the ratio twitch P_{di}/sniff P_{di} is unusually high. The discrepancy is attributable to varying neural activation with different frequencies of stimulation, since voluntary manoeuvres are associated with a frequency of 3–5 Hz at which fatigue is more likely to be seen[163] and fatiguability is demonstrable by phrenic stimulation if similar higher frequencies are used.[164] Maximum flow–volume curves in myasthenia have been reported to show evidence of functional upper airway obstruction related to weakness of upper airway muscles.[165]

During sleep, REM-related oxygen desaturation may be seen,[166] as in other causes of generalized respiratory muscle weakness. Obstructive sleep apnoea has also been reported in some patients[167,168] and may be related to weakness of the upper airway muscles. Following acute administration of an anticholinesterase drug (e.g. neostigmine), increases are demonstrable in lung volumes[169] and maximum respiratory pressures,[162,163] but in one study there was no improvement in respiratory muscle endurance.[162] The improved strength is accompanied by an increase in both ventilatory and mouth occlusion pressure responses to CO_2.[38] Some individuals show an increase in airway resistance after being given an anticholinesterase. This has been attributed to increased parasympathetic tone in the airways, but it is not seen in all subjects and may be relevant only to those with pre-existing airway obstruction or bronchial hyperresponsiveness.

Occasionally, patients develop severe respiratory muscle weakness due to decompensated myasthenia gravis ('myasthenic crisis'), with consequent acute respiratory failure requiring ventilatory support. Data on the value of monitoring respiratory function in this situation are variable: one study showed that sequential VC measurement was a poor predictor of the need for ventilatory support,[170] whereas others have reported that VC and maximum respiratory pressures (using thresholds similar to those described above in patients with Guillain–Barré syndrome) are helpful in predicting the likely need for intubation and ventilatory support.[171]

20.4.2.2 Lambert–Eaton syndrome

In the myasthenic (Lambert–Eaton) syndrome, respiratory muscle weakness is common and its severity is generally proportional to the degree of limb muscle weakness.[172] In this condition repetitive muscle contraction has the converse effect to that seen in myasthenia gravis, i.e. increasing rather than decreasing force, a phenomenon that has been demonstrated by repeated measurements

of P_Imax.[173] Weakness sufficient to cause hypercapnic respiratory failure occurs occasionally.[174]

20.4.3 Muscular dystrophies

20.4.3.1 Duchenne muscular dystrophy

In Duchenne muscular dystrophy, the severity of respiratory muscle weakness usually parallels the level of general disability.[175] Affected boys usually show a normal increase in VC until around the age of 10 years, after which it plateaus and subsequently declines.[176] The average rate of subsequent decline of VC is about 8 per cent predicted per year.[177] A complicating scoliosis is often a contributory factor. Maximum respiratory pressures are more sensitive and show weakness from an earlier stage,[175] but, overall, VC is a reliable predictor of mortality.[177] The residual volume is increased in more severely affected patients.

Gas exchange while awake is usually only mildly impaired except in the most disabled patients.[175] As expected, gas exchange is more frequently abnormal during sleep, with an overall reduction in ventilation compared with normal in both REM and non-REM sleep,[178] together with REM-related desaturation associated with periods of hypopnoea and/or apnoea; these are usually central but may also be obstructive.[179,180]

Hypercapnia while awake was associated historically with a poor prognosis, but nocturnal NIV increases survival appreciably and greatly improves daytime blood gases (see Fig. 20.6),[181] even though VC continues to deteriorate.

20.4.3.2 Late-onset muscular dystrophies

In the late-onset dystrophies such as facioscapulohumeral, limb-girdle and Becker muscular dystrophy, evidence of mild or moderate respiratory muscle weakness may be found.[182–184] Occasionally the weakness is sufficiently severe to cause hypercapnic respiratory failure.[185]

20.4.4 Myotonic dystrophy (dystrophia myotonica, Steinert's disease)

The abnormal respiratory function of patients with myotonic dystrophy has been the subject of many

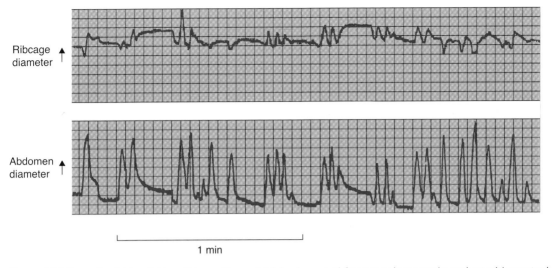

Figure 20.9 Example of 'chaotic' breathing pattern of tidal volume and frequency in an awake patient with myotonic dystrophy; recording made with pairs of magnetometers measuring anteroposterior diameters of ribcage and abdomen. Modified with permission from ref. 29.

studies over the past 50 years. Chronic hypercapnia is well recognized, and this, together with somnolence, increased sensitivity to sedatives, an abnormal resting breathing pattern (Fig. 20.9) and reduced ventilatory response to CO_2, led early authors to infer an abnormality of central respiratory control.

20.4.4.1 Respiratory muscle function

It is now appreciated that some of the above features are attributable to dysfunction of the respiratory muscles, as the severity of weakness was often underestimated in earlier studies. Reduced maximum respiratory pressures are demonstrable in most patients at the time of presentation. Characteristically, $P_E$max is numerically more impaired than $P_I$max.[29] The severity of respiratory muscle weakness is easily underestimated on clinical grounds if it is inferred from weakness of other muscles.

20.4.4.2 Hypercapnia and ventilatory responses

Hypercapnia correlates with the severity of respiratory muscle weakness in myotonic dystrophy in a similar fashion to other muscle diseases (Fig. 20.10).[37,186] The reduced ventilatory response to CO_2 is also related to the degree of weakness and

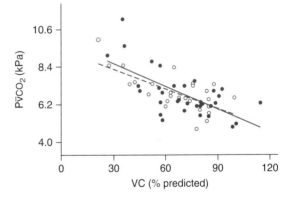

Figure 20.10 Relations between mixed venous P_{CO_2} $P\bar{v}_{CO_2}$ (measured by rebreathing) and vital capacity (VC) in groups of patients with myotonic dystrophy (open circles, broken line) and non-myotonic respiratory muscle weakness (solid circles, solid line). The lines represent linear regressions and are similar in the two groups. Modified with permission from ref. 37.

to the consequent restrictive ventilatory defect.[29] Data on the mouth occlusion pressure $(P_{0.1})$ response to CO_2 show, variously, increased,[187] normal[188] and reduced[37] values. In weak individuals, however, even a low value need not imply reduced central respiratory drive, since $P_{0.1}$ is dependent on muscle function and the slope increases if strength improves.[38]

20.4.4.3 Awake tidal breathing

Some patients with myotonic dystrophy have a bizarre pattern of resting tidal volume and frequency[34,142] that resembles the 'ataxic' breathing associated with brainstem lesions (see Fig. 20.9). The cause is uncertain: it is not related clearly to the severity of weakness or to the presence of chronic hypercapnia.[189] It is unlikely that myotonia per se is relevant, as EMG recordings show little evidence of myotonic discharges from the respiratory muscles during quiet breathing.[190] Myotonic activity becomes more evident with voluntary or chemically induced hyperventilation,[190] but it has no obvious clinical effect as maximum voluntary ventilation over 15 s is impaired to a similar relative degree as the VC.[29] Moreover, in the benign condition of myotonia congenita, there is no evidence of impaired lung or respiratory muscle function at rest.[191] It seems likely, therefore, that irregular tidal breathing in myotonic dystrophy does result from abnormal CNS function. However, if it were due to a defect in the metabolic pathway of ventilatory control, abnormal breathing would be expected to be most evident in deep non-REM sleep, since this is when the metabolic control pathway is considered to be dominant. The converse is actually the case, with breathing most irregular when awake or in light sleep.[192,193] It is, therefore, unlikely that irregular breathing in myotonic dystrophy originates in the brainstem and its origin is unclear.

20.4.4.4 Breathing during sleep in myotonic dystrophy

Several detailed studies of breathing during sleep have been reported in myotonic dystrophy. Episodes of apnoea and hypopnoea are relatively common and may be either central or obstructive.[194–196] However, the frequency of events is usually less than that seen in subjects with sleepiness due to obstructive sleep apnoea syndrome. Obesity is commoner in patients with myotonic dystrophy than in most other conditions associated with respiratory muscle weakness, and the frequency of obstructive events during sleep correlates with BMI.[196] Daytime somnolence is a major feature of patients with myotonic dystrophy and, although either hypercapnia or sleep-disordered breathing may contribute in occasional individuals, it appears that these are not the main cause in the majority[195,197,198] and a central cause of daytime sleepiness is more likely.

20.4.4.5 Summary of respiratory features of myotonic dystrophy

The respiratory function of patients with myotonic dystrophy is potentially confusing and can be summarized as follows:

- Respiratory muscle weakness is very common and easily overlooked clinically.
- Neither the ventilatory nor the $P_{0.1}$ response is helpful in distinguishing central from peripheral causes of CO_2 insensitivity, as both are dependent on respiratory muscle function.
- Hypercapnia is common and related closely to the severity of respiratory muscle weakness as in other conditions causing muscle weakness.
- Both central and obstructive sleep apnoeas are often present but are not responsible for daytime sleepiness in most individuals.
- The mechanisms of both disordered resting ventilation and sleepiness remain uncertain but are probably neurogenically determined.

Nocturnal ventilatory support may be helpful in some patients with myotonic dystrophy and hypercapnia, but the acceptability and benefit of this form of treatment is generally much less than in other conditions associated with severe respiratory muscle weakness.[199]

20.4.5 Miscellaneous myopathies and polymyositis

Many forms of congenital and acquired muscle disease can affect the respiratory muscles causing a restrictive ventilatory defect and, eventually, hypercapnic respiratory failure (Table 20.1). Among the commoner acquired conditions are polymyositis,[200] alcohol myopathy[32] and steroid myopathy.[201]

The classification of the large number of congenital syndromes that affect skeletal muscle is evolving rapidly as the specific gene abnormalities causing them are identified. Many of the congenital muscle conditions cause early mortality, and only those presenting in adults or with conditions associated with prolonged survival are considered

Table 20.1 Myopathies associated with respiratory muscle weakness in adults

	Reference
Acquired disorders	
Inflammatory myopathies	
Polymyositis and inclusion body myositis	200
Drugs/toxins	
Steroids	201
Alcohol	32
Genetic disorders	
Metabolic myopathies	
Acid maltase deficiency (Pompe's disease)	202, 203
Mitochondrial myopathies	204–206
Miscellaneous disorders	
Bethlem myopathy	207
Nemaline myopathy	208, 209
Distal myopathies	210, 211
Multicore myopathy	212

here. Respiratory muscle weakness and other functional abnormalities are common in several of the large range of metabolic myopathies. These disorders of muscle energy metabolism are grouped into three broad categories: impaired carbohydrate utilization, abnormal lipid metabolism and the mitochondrial diseases.

One of the commoner disorders of carbohydrate metabolism that can present in adult life is acid maltase deficiency (glycogenosis type II, Pompe disease).[202,203] This results from a deficiency of the lysosomal enzyme α-glucosidase, which is involved in the metabolism of glycogen. Unusually among neuromuscular diseases, the respiratory muscles often appear to be disproportionately affected and patients can present with severe respiratory weakness while still ambulant.[203] Severe diaphragmatic weakness or paralysis is relatively common and is associated closely with sleep-disordered breathing (mainly REM-related hypopnoeas) and chronic hypercapnia.[202]

The mitochondrial myopathies include syndromes with various pathological, biochemical and clinical features. They are multisystem disorders and result from impaired energy production due to a reduced capacity to generate mitochondrial adenosine triphosphate (ATP). They include conditions previously categorized as ragged red fibre disease, oculocraniosomatic neuromuscular disease and Kearns–Sayre syndrome. Respiratory muscle weakness can be sufficiently severe to cause hypercapnic respiratory failure.[204] A major symptom is exercise limitation, which may be due to either breathlessness or fatigue and myalgia in the exercising muscles. This may be seen in patients with relatively normal lung function, although some reduction in maximum respiratory pressures is usual.[205] Exercise performance is characterized by an abnormal relationship between $\dot{V}O_2$ and workload, such that oxygen consumption tends to flatten off at higher work levels causing an overall reduction in capacity. During submaximal exercise both heart rate and ventilation are markedly increased in relation to $\dot{V}O_2$ (Fig. 20.11).

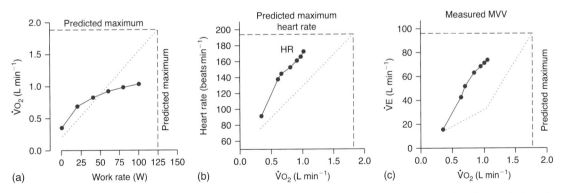

Figure 20.11 Examples of progressive exercise in a patient with mitochondrial myopathy. Note the alinear relation of $\dot{V}O_2$ to work rate with marked flattening off of $\dot{V}O_2$ at higher work rates (a), and excessive heart rate (b) and ventilatory (c) responses during submaximal exercise. Modified from ref. 205, with permission from the American Thoracic Society.

REFERENCES

1 Plum F, Posner JB. *The Diagnosis of Stupor and Coma*, 3rd edn, FA Davis, Philadelphia, PA, 1980.

2 North JB, Jennett S. Abnormal breathing patterns associated with acute brain damage. *Arch Neurol* 1974; **31**: 338–44.

3 Lee MC, Klassen AC, Resch JA. Respiratory pattern disturbances in ischaemic cerebral vascular disease. *Stroke* 1974; **5**: 612–16.

4 Cheyne J. A case of apoplexy in which the fleshy part of the heart was converted into fat. *Dublin Hospital Reports* 1818; **2**: 216–23.

5 Plum F, Alvord EC. Apneustic breathing in man. *Arch Neurol* 1964; **10**: 101–12.

6 Bateman DE, Gibson GJ, Hudgson P, Tomlinson BE. Central neurogenic hyperventilation in a conscious patient with a primary cerebral lymphoma. *Ann Neurol* 1985; **17**: 402–5.

7 Laigle-Donadey F, Iraqi W, Strauss C, *et al.* Primary central nervous system lymphoma presenting with central neurogenic hyperventilation: a case report and review of the literature. *Rev Neurol (Paris)* 2005; **161**: 940–48.

8 Plum F, Swanson AG. Abnormalities in central regulation of respiration in acute and convalescent poliomyelitis. *Arch Neurol Psychiatry* 1958; **80**: 267–85.

9 Bolton CF, Chen R, Wijdicks EFM, Zifko UA. *Neurology of Breathing*, Butterworth, Philadelphia, PA, 2004.

10 Antic NA, Malow BA, Lange N, *et al.* PHOX2B mutation-confirmed congenital central hypoventilation syndrome: presentation in adulthood. *Am J Respir Crit Care Med* 2006; **174**: 923–7.

11 Weese-Mayer DE, Shannon CD, Keens GT, Silvestri JM. Idiopathic congenital hypoventilation syndrome: diagnosis and management. *Am J Respir Crit Care Med* 1999; **160**: 368–73.

12 Bachetti T, Robbiano A, Parodi S, *et al.* Brainstem anomalies in two patients affected by congenital central hypoventilation syndrome. *Am J Respir Crit Care Med* 2006; **174**: 706–9.

13 Farmer WC, Glenn WWL, Gee JBL. Alveolar hypoventilation syndrome. *Am J Med* 1978; **64**: 39–49.

14 Tranmer BI, Tucker WS, Bilbao JM. Sleep apnea following percutaneous cervical cordotomy. *Can J Neurol Sci* 1987; **14**: 262–7.

15 Lahuerta J, Buxton P, Lipton S, Bowsher D. The location and function of respiratory fibres in the second cervical spinal cord segment: respiratory dysfunction syndrome after cervical cordotomy. *J Neurol Neurosurg Psychiatry* 1992; **55**: 1142–5.

16 Paton JY, Swaminathan S, Sargent CW, Keens TG. Hypoxic and hypercapnic ventilatory responses in awake children with congenital central hypoventilation syndrome. *Am Rev Respir Dis* 1989; **140**: 368–72.

17 Paton JY, Swaninathan S, Sargent CW, Hawksworth A, Keens TG. Ventilatory response to exercise in children with congenital central hypoventilation syndrome. *Am Rev Respir Dis* 1993; **147**: 1185–91.

18 Glenn WWL, Gee JBL, Cole DR, *et al.* Combined central alveolar hypoventilation and upper airway obstruction. *Am J Med* 1978; **64**: 50–60.

19 Nordgren RE, Markesbery WR, Fukuda K, Reeves AG. Seven cases of cerebromedullospinal disconnection: the 'locked-in' syndrome. *Neurology* 1971; **21**: 1140–48.

20 Heywood P, Murphy K, Corfield DR, *et al.* Control of breathing in man; insights from the 'locked-in' syndrome. *Respir Physiol* 1996; **106**: 13–20.

21 Hart N, Polkey MI, Sharshar T, *et al.* Limitations of sniff nasal pressure in patients with severe neuromuscular weakness. *J Neurol Neurosurg Psychiatry* 2003; **74**: 1685–7.

22 Black LF, Hyatt RE. Maximal static respiratory pressures in generalized neuromuscular disease. *Am Rev Respir Dis* 1971; **103**: 641–50.

23 Gibson GJ, Pride NB, Newsom Davis J, Loh LC. Pulmonary mechanics in patients with respiratory muscle weakness. *Am Rev Respir Dis* 1977; **115**: 389–95.

24 Estenne M, Heilporn A, Delhez L, Yernault J-C, De Troyer A. Chest wall stiffness in patients with chronic respiratory muscle weakness. *Am Rev Respir Dis* 1983; **128**: 1002–7.

25 Gibson GJ, Pride NB. Lung mechanics in diaphragmatic paralysis. *Am Rev Respir Dis* 1979; **119** (suppl.): 119–20.

26 De Troyer A, Borenstein S, Cordier R. Analysis of lung volume restriction in patients with respiratory muscle weakness. *Thorax* 1980; **35**: 603–10.

27 Estenne M, Gevenois PA, Kinnear W, *et al.* Lung volume restriction in patients with chronic respiratory muscle weakness: the role of microatelectasis. *Thorax* 1993; **48**: 698–701.

28 Kreitzer SM, Saunders NA, Tyler HR, Ingram RH. Respiratory muscle function in amyotrophic lateral sclerosis. *Am Rev Respir Dis* 1978; **117**: 437–47.

29 Serisier DE, Mastaglia FL, Gibson GJ. Respiratory muscle function and ventilatory control. I in patients with motor neurone disease. II in patients with myotonic dystrophy. *Q J Med* 1982; **51**: 205–26.

30 Wesseling G, Quaedvlieg FCM, Wouters EFM. Oscillatory mechanics of the respiratory system in neuromuscular disease. *Chest* 1992; **102**: 1752–7.

31 Szeinberg A, Tabachnik E, Rashed N, *et al.* Cough capacity in patients with muscular dystrophy. *Chest* 1988; **94**: 1232–5.

32 Braun NMT, Arora NS, Rochester DF. Respiratory muscle and pulmonary function in polymyositis and other proximal myopathies. *Thorax* 1983; **38**: 616–23.

33 Harrison BDW, Collins JV, Brown KGE, Clark TJH. Respiratory failure in neuromuscular diseases. *Thorax* 1971; **26**: 579–84.

34 Misuri G, Lanini B, Gigliotti F, *et al.* Mechanism of CO_2 retention in patients with neuromuscular disease. *Chest* 2006; **117**: 447–53.

35 Gay PC, Edmonds LC. Severe hypercapnia after low-flow oxygen therapy in patients with neuromuscular disease and diaphragmatic dysfunction. *Mayo Clin Proc* 1995; **70**: 327–30.

36 Baydur A. Respiratory muscle strength and control of ventilation in patients with neuromuscular disease. *Chest* 1991; **99**: 330–38.

37 Gibson GJ, Gilmartin JJ, Veale D, Walls TJ, Serisier DE. Respiratory muscle function in neuromuscular disease, in *Breathlessness* (eds NL Jones and KJ Killian), CME, Hamilton, Canada, 1992, pp. 66–71.

38 Spinelli A, Marconi G, Gorini M, Pizzi A, Scano G. Control of breathing in patients with myasthenia gravis. *Am Rev Respir Dis* 1992; **145**: 1359–66.

39 Carroll JE, Hagberg JM, Brooke MH, Shumate JB. Bicycle ergometry and gas exchange measurements in neuromuscular diseases. *Arch Neurol* 1979; **36**: 457–61.

40 Ward S, Chatwin M, Heather S, Simonds AK. Randomised controlled trial of non-invasive ventilation (NIV) for nocturnal hypoventilation in neuromuscular and chest wall disease patients with daytime normocapnia. *Thorax* 2005; **60**: 1019–24.

41 Bourke SC, Gibson GJ. Sleep and breathing in neuromuscular disease. *Eur Respir J* 2002; **19**: 1194–201.

42 Smith PE, Calverley PMA, Edwards RHT. Hypoxaemia during sleep in Duchenne muscular dystrophy. *Am Rev Respir Dis* 1988; **137**: 884–8.

43 Barbé F, Quera-Salva MA, McCann C, *et al.* Sleep-related respiratory disturbances in patients with Duchenne muscular dystrophy. *Eur Respir J* 1994; **7**: 1403–8.

44 Ragette R, Mellies U, Schwake C, Volt T, Teschler H. Patterns and predictors of sleep disordered breathing in primary myopathies. *Thorax* 2002; **57**: 724–8.

45 Gay PC, Westbrook PR, Daube JR, *et al.* Effects of alterations in pulmonary function and sleep variables on survival in patients with amyotrophic lateral sclerosis. *Mayo Clin Proc* 1991; **66**: 686–94.

46 Phillips MF, Smith PE, Carroll N, Edmonds RHT, Calverley PMA. Nocturnal oxygenation and prognosis in Duchenne muscular dystrophy. *Am J Respir Crit Care Med* 1999; **160**: 198–202.

47 Bourke SC, Bullock RE, Williams TL, Shaw PJ, Gibson GJ. Noninvasive ventilation in ALS: indications and effect on quality of life. *Neurology* 2003; **61**: 171–7.

48 Barbé F, Quera-Salva MA, de Lattre J, Gajdos P, Agusti AG. Long-term effects of nasal intermittent positive ventilation on pulmonary function and sleep architecture in patients with neuromuscular diseases. *Chest* 1996; **110**: 1179–83.

49 Bourke SC, Tomlinson M, Williams TL, *et al.* Effects on non-invasive ventilation on survival and quality of life in patients with amyotrophic lateral sclerosis: a randomised controlled trial. *Lancet Neurol* 2006; **5**: 140–47.

50 Mier-Jedrzejowicz A, Brophy C, Moxham J, Green M. Assessment of diaphragm weakness. *Am Rev Respir Dis* 1988; **137**: 877–83.

51 Newsom Davis J, Goldman M, Joh L, Casson M. Diaphragm function and alveolar hypoventilation. *Q J Med* 1976; **45**: 87–100.

52 Schoenhofer B, Koehler D, Polkey MI. Influence of immersion in water on muscle function and breathing pattern in patients with severe diaphragm weakness. *Chest* 2004; **125**: 2069–74.

53 Hillman DR, Finucane KE. Respiratory pressure partitioning during quiet inspiration in unilateral and bilateral diaphragmatic weakness. *Am Rev Respir Dis* 1988; **137**: 1401–5.

54 Laroche CM, Carroll N, Moxham J, Green M. Clinical significance of severe isolated diaphragm weakness. *Am Rev Respir Dis* 1988; **138**: 862–6.

55 Hart N, Nickol AH, Cramer D, *et al.* Effect of severe isolated unilateral and bilateral diaphragm weakness on exercise performance. *Am J Respir Crit Care Med* 2002; **165**: 1265–70.

56 Amis TC, Ciofetta G, Hughes JMB, Loh L. Regional lung function in bilateral diaphragmatic paralysis. *Clin Sci* 1980; **59**: 485–92.

57 Stradling JR. Bilateral diaphragm paralysis and sleep apnoea without diurnal respiratory failure. *Thorax* 1988; **43**: 75–7.

58 White JES, Drinnan MJ, Smithson AJ, Griffiths CJ, Gibson GJ. Respiratory muscle activity and oxygenation during sleep in patients with muscle weakness. *Eur Respir J* 1995; **8**: 807–14.

59 Bennett JR, Dunroy HM, Corfield DR, *et al.* Respiratory muscle activity during REM sleep in patients with diaphragm paralysis. *Neurology* 2004; **62**: 134–7.

60 Bye PTP, Ellis ER, Issa FG, Donnelly PM, Sullivan CE. Respiratory failure and sleep in neuromuscular disease. *Thorax* 1990; **45**: 241–7.

61 Stolk J, Versteegh MIM. Long-term effect of bilateral plication of the diaphragm. *Chest* 2000; **117**: 786–9.

62 Lisboa C, Paré PD, Pertuze J, *et al.* Inspiratory muscle function in unilateral diaphragmatic paralysis. *Am Rev Respir Dis* 1986; **134**: 488–92.

63 Ridyard JB, Stewart RM. Regional lung function in unilateral diaphragmatic paralysis. *Thorax* 1976; **31**: 438–42.

64 Clague HW, Hall DR. Effect of posture on lung volume: airway closure and gas exchange in hemidiaphragmatic paralysis. *Thorax* 1979; **34**: 523–6.

65 Laroche C, Mier AK, Moxham J, Green M. Diaphragm strength in patients with recent hemidiaphragmatic paralysis. *Thorax* 1988; **43**: 170–74.

66 Verin E, Marie JP, Tardif C, Denis P. Spontaneous recovery of diaphragmatic strength in unilateral diaphragmatic paralysis. *Respir Med* 2006; **100**: 1944–51.

67 Easton PA, Fleetham JA, De la Rocha A, Anthonisen NR. Respiratory function after paralysis of the right hemi-diaphragm. *Am Rev Respir Dis* 1983; **127**: 125–8.

68 Freeman RK, Wozniak TC, Fitzgerald EB. Functional and physiologic results of video-assisted thoracoscopic diaphragm plication in adult patients with unilateral diaphragm paralysis. *Ann Thorac Surg* 2006; **81**: 1853–7.

69 Ciccolella DE, Daly BDT, Celli BR. Improved diaphragmatic function after surgical application for unilateral diaphragmatic paralysis. *Am Rev Respir Dis* 1992; **146**: 797–9.

70 De Troyer A, Zegers de Beyl D, Thirion M. Function of the respiratory muscles in acute hemiplegia. *Am Rev Respir Dis* 1981; **123**: 631–2.

71 Cohen E, Mier A, Heywood P, *et al.* Diaphragmatic movement in hemiplegic patients measured by ultrasonography. *Thorax* 1994; **49**: 890–95.

72 Lanini B, Bianchi R, Romagnoli I, *et al.* Chest wall kinematics in patients with hemiplegia. *Am J Respir Crit Care Med* 2003; **168**: 109–13.

73 Nachtmann A, Siebler M, Rose G, Sitzer M, Steinmetz H. Cheyne–Stokes respiration in ischemic stroke. *Neurology* 1995; **45**: 820–21.

74 Elizabeth J, Singarayar J, Ellul J, Barer D, Lye M. Arterial oxygen saturation and posture in acute stroke. *Age Ageing* 1993; **22**: 269–72.

75 Sulter G, Elting JW, Stewart R, den Arend A, De Keyser J. Continuous pulse oximetry in acute hemiparetic stroke. *J Neurolog Sci* 2000; **179**: 65–9.

76 Rowat AM, Wardlaw JM, Dennis MS, Warlow CP. Patient positioning influences oxygen saturation in the acute phase of stroke. *Cerebrovasc Dis* 2001; **12**: 66–72.

77 Ronning OM, Guldvog B. Should stroke victims routinely receive supplemental oxygen? A quasi-randomized controlled trial. *Stroke* 1999; **30**: 2033–7.

78 Harbison JA, Gibson GJ. Snoring, sleep apnoea and stroke: chicken or scrambled egg? *Q J Med* 2000; **93**: 647–54.

79 Harbison J, Ford GA, James OFW, Gibson GJ. Sleep-disordered breathing following acute stroke. *Q J Med* 2002; **95**: 741–7.

80 Turkington PM, Bamford J, Wanklyn P, *et al.* Prevalence and clinical importance of upper airway obstruction in the first 24 hours after acute stroke. *Stroke* 2002; **33**: 2037–42.

81 Parra O, Arboix A, Bechich L, *et al.* Time course of sleep-related breathing disorders in first-ever stroke or transient ischemic attack. *Am J Respir Crit Care Med* 2000; **161**: 375–80.

82 Kaneko Y, Hajek VE, Zivanovic V, Raboud J, Bradley D. Relationship of sleep apnea to functional capacity and length of hospitalization following stroke. *Sleep* 2003; **26**: 293–7.

83 Parra O, Arboix A, Montserrat JM, *et al.* Sleep-related breathing disorders: impact on mortality of cerebrovascular disease. *Eur Respir J* 2004; **24**: 267–72.

84 Turkington PM, Allgar V, Bamford J, Wanklyn P, Elliott MW. Effect of upper airway obstruction in acute stroke on functional outcome at 6 months. *Thorax* 2004; **59**: 367–71.

85 Harbison J, Gibson GJ, Birchall D, Zammit-Maempel I, Ford GA. White matter disease and sleep-disordered breathing after acute stroke. *Neurology* 2003; **61**: 1–5.

86 Nopmaneejumruslers C, Kaneko Y, Hajek V, Zivanovic V, Bradley TD. Cheyne–Stokes respiration in stroke: relationship to hypocapnia and occult cardiac dysfunction. *Am J Respir Crit Care Med* 2005; **171**: 1048–52.

87 Teixeira-Salmela LF, Parreira VF, Britto RR, *et al.* Respiratory pressures and thoracoabdominal motion in community-dwelling chronic stroke survivors. *Arch Phys Med Rehab* 2005; **86**: 1974–8.

88 Polatli M, Akyol A, Cildag O, Bayulkem K. Pulmonary function tests in Parkinson's disease. *Eur J Neurol* 2001; **8**: 341–5.

89 Estenne M, Hubert M, de Troyer A. Respiratory muscle involvement in Parkinson's Disease. *N Engl J Med* 1984; **311**: 1516–17.

90 Shill H, Stacy M. Respiratory function in Parkinson's disease. *Clin Neurosci* 1998; **5**: 131–5.

91 Weiner P, Inzelberg R, Davidovich A, *et al.* Respiratory muscle performance and the perception of dyspnea in Parkinson's disease. *Can J Neurol Sci* 2002; **29**: 68–72.

92 Haas BM, Trew M, Castle PC. Effects of respiratory muscle weakness on daily living function, quality of life, activity levels, and exercise capacity in mild to moderate Parkinson's disease. *Am J Phys Med Rehab* 2004; **83**: 601–7.

93 Bogaard JM, Hovestadt A, Meerwaldt J, van der Meché A, Stigt J. Maximal expiratory and inspiratory flow–volume curves in Parkinson's disease. *Am Rev Respir Dis* 1989; **139**: 610–14.

94 De Bruin PFC, De Bruin VMS, Lees AJ, Pride NB. Effects of treatment on airway dynamics and respiratory muscle strength in Parkinson's disease. *Am Rev Respir Dis* 1993; **148**: 1576–80.

95 Vincken WG, Gauthier SG, Dollfuss RE, et al. Involvement of upper airway muscles in extrapyramidal disorders. *N Engl J Med* 1984; **311**: 438–42.

96 Herer B, Amulfi I, Housset B. Effects of levodopa on pulmonary function in Parkinson's disease. *Chest* 2001; **119**: 387–93.

97 Apps MCP, Sheaf PC, Ingram DA, Kennard C, Empey DW. Respiration and sleep in Parkinson's disease. *J Neurol Neurosurg Psychiatry* 1985; **48**: 1240–45.

98 Canning CG, Alison JA, Allen NE, Groeller H. Parkinson's disease: an investigation of exercise capacity, respiratory function, and gait. *Arch Phys Med Rehabil* 1997; **78**: 199–207.

99 Maria B, Sophia S, Michalis M, et al. Sleep breathing disorders in patients with idiopathic Parkinson's disease. *Respir Med* 2003; **97**: 1151–7.

100 Gilmartin JJ, Wright AJ, Cartlidge NEF, Gibson GJ. Upper airway obstruction complicating the Shy–Drager syndrome. *Thorax* 1984; **39**: 313–14.

101 Shimohata T, Shinoda Y, Nakayama H, et al. Daytime hypoxemia, sleep-disordered breathing, and laryngopharyngeal findings in multiple system atrophy. *Arch Neurol* 2007; **64**: 856–61.

102 Isono S, Shiba K, Yamaguchi M, et al. Pathogenesis of laryngeal narrowing in patients with multiple system atrophy. *J Physiol* 2001; **536**: 237–49.

103 Vetrugno R, Provini F, Cortelli P, et al. Sleep disorders in multiple system atrophy: a correlative videopolysomnographic study. *Sleep Med* 2004; **5**: 21–30.

104 McNicholas WT, Rutherford R, Grossman R, et al. Abnormal respiratory pattern generation during sleep in patients with autonomic dysfunction. *Am Rev Respir Dis* 1983; **128**: 429–33.

105 Jin K, Okabe S, Chida K, et al. Tracheostomy can fatally exacerbate sleep-disordered breathing in multiple system atrophy. *Neurology* 2007; **68**: 1618–21.

106 Alvarez D, Requena I, Arias M, et al. Acute respiratory failure as the first sign of Arnold–Chiari malformation associated with syringomyelia. *Eur Respir J* 1995; **8**: 661–3.

107 Bokinski GE, Hudson LD, Weil JV. Impaired chemosensitivity and acute respiratory failure in Arnold–Chiari malformation and syringomyelia. *N Engl J Med* 1973; **288**: 947–8.

108 Balk RA, Hiller FC, Lucas EA, et al. Sleep apnoea and the Arnold–Chiari malformation. *Am Rev Respir Dis* 1985; **132**: 929–30.

109 Tsara V, Serasli E, Kimiskidis V, et al. Acute respiratory failure and sleep-disordered breathing in Arnold–Chiari malformation. *Clin Neurol Neurosurg* 2005; **107**: 521–4.

110 Howard RS, Thorpe J, Barker R, et al. Respiratory insufficiency due to high anterior cervical cord infarction. *J Neurol Neurosurg Psychiatry* 1998; **64**: 358–61.

111 Estenne M, Van Muylem A, Gorini M, et al. Evidence of dynamic airway compression during cough in tetraplegic patients. *Am J Respir Crit Care Med* 1994; **150**: 1081–5.

112 Mortola JP, Sant'Ambrogio G. Motion of the rib cage and the abdomen in tetraplegic patients. *Clin Sci* 1978; **54**: 25–32.

113 De Troyer A, Heilporn A. Respiratory mechanics in quadriplegia: the respiratory function of the intercostal muscles. *Am Rev Respir Dis* 1980; **122**: 591–600.

114 Estenne M, De Troyer A. Relationship between respiratory muscle electromyogram and rib cage motion in tetraplegia. *Am Rev Respir Dis* 1985; **132**: 53–9.

115 Linn WS, Adkins RH, Gong H, Waters RL. Pulmonary function in chronic spinal cord injury: a cross-sectional survey of 222 southern California adult outpatients. *Arch Phys Med Rehab* 2000; **81**: 757–63.

116 Baydur A, Adkins RH, Milic-Emili J. Lung mechanics in individuals with spinal cord injury: effects of injury level and posture. *J Appl Physiol* 2001; **90**: 405–11.

117 Scanlon PD, Loring SH, Pichurko BM, et al. Respiratory mechanics in acute quadriplegia: lung and chest wall compliance and dimensional changes during respiratory manoeuvres. *Am Rev Respir Dis* 1989; **139**: 615–20.

118 Uiji SG, Houtman S, Folgering HT, Hopman MT. Training of the respiratory muscles in individuals with tetraplegia. *Spinal Cord* 1999; **37**: 575–9.

119 Ledsome JR, Sharp JM. Pulmonary function in acute cervical cord injury. *Am Rev Respir Dis* 1981; **124**: 41–4.

120 Singas E, Lesser M, Spungen AM, Bauman WA, Almenoff PL. Airway hyperresponsiveness to methacholine in subjects with spinal cord injury. *Chest* 1996; **110**: 911–15.

121 Mateus SRM, Beraldo PSS, Horan TA. Cholinergic bronchomotor tone and airway calibre in tetraplegic patients. *Spinal Cord* 2006; **44**: 269–74.

122 Berlowitz DJ, Brown DJ, Campbell DA, Pierce RJ. A longitudinal evaluation of sleep and breathing in the first year after cervical spinal cord injury. *Arch Phys Med Rehabil* 2005; **86**: 1193–9.

123 Estenne M, De Troyer A. Mechanism of the postural dependence of vital capacity in tetraplegic subjects. *Am Rev Respir Dis* 1987; **135**: 367–71.

124 Tow AM, Graves DE, Carter RE. Vital capacity in tetraplegics twenty years and beyond. *Spinal Cord* 2001; **39**: 139–44.

125 Linn SW, Spungen AM, Gong H, *et al*. Forced vital capacity in two large outpatient populations with chronic spinal cord injury. *Spinal Cord* 2001; **39**: 263–8.

126 Gosselink R, Kovacs L, Decramer M. Respiratory muscle involvement in multiple sclerosis. *Eur Respir J* 1999; **13**: 449–54.

127 Mutluay FK, Gurses HN, Saip S. Effects of multiple sclerosis on respiratory functions. *Clin Rehabil* 2005; **19**: 426–32.

128 Buyse B, Demedts M, Meekers J, *et al*. Respiratory dysfunction in multiple sclerosis: a prospective analysis of 60 patients. *Eur Respir J* 1997; **10**: 139–45.

129 Koseoglu BF, Gokkaya NKO, Ergun U, Inan L, Yesiltepe E. Cardiopulmonary and metabolic functions, aerobic capacity, fatigue and quality of life in patients with multiple sclerosis. *Acta Neurol Scand* 2006; **114**: 261–7.

130 Kuwahira I, Kondo T, Ohta Y, Yamagayashi H. Acute respiratory failure in multiple sclerosis. *Chest* 1990; **97**: 246–7.

131 Howard RS, Wiles CM, Hirsch NP, *et al*. Respiratory involvement in multiple sclerosis. *Brain* 1992; **115**: 479–94.

132 Tantucci C, Massucci M, Pipero R, *et al*. Control of breathing and respiratory muscle strength in patients with multiple sclerosis. *Chest* 1994; **105**: 1163–70.

133 Boor JW, Johnson RJ, Canales L, Dunn DP. Reversible paralysis of automatic respiration in multiple sclerosis. *Arch Neurol* 1977; **34**: 686–9.

134 Gosselink R, Kovacs L, Ketelaer P, Carton H, Decramer M. Respiratory muscle weakness and respiratory muscle training in severely disabled multiple sclerosis patients. *Arch Phys Med Rehab* 2000; **81**: 747–51.

135 Soliman MG, Higgins SE, El-Kabir DR, *et al*. Non-invasive assessment of respiratory muscle strength in patients with previous poliomyelitis. *Respir Med* 2005; **99**: 1217–22.

136 Dean E, Ross J, Road JD, Courtenay L, Madill KJ. Pulmonary function in individuals with a history of poliomyelitis. *Chest* 1991; **100**: 118–23.

137 Steljes DG, Kryger MH, Kirk BW, Millar TW. Sleep in postpolio syndrome. *Chest* 1990; **98**: 133–40.

138 Dean AC, Graham BA, Dalakas M, Sato S. Sleep apnea in patients with postpolio syndrome. *Ann Neurol* 1998; **43**: 661–4.

139 Schiffman PL, Belsh JM. Pulmonary function at diagnosis of amyotrophic lateral sclerosis: rate of deterioration. *Chest* 1993; **103**: 508–13.

140 Nightingale S, Bates D, Bateman DE, *et al*. Enigmatic dyspnoea: an unusual presentation of motor neurone disease. *Lancet* 1982; **1**: 933–5.

141 Lyall RA, Donaldson N, Polkey MI, Leigh PN, Moxham J. Respiratory muscle strength and ventilatory failure in amyotrophic lateral sclerosis. *Brain* 2001; **124**: 2000–2013.

142 Ferguson KA, Strong MJ, Ahmad D, George CFP. Sleep-disordered breathing in amyotrophic lateral sclerosis. *Chest* 1996; **110**: 664–9.

143 Bourke SC, Shaw PJ, Gibson GJ. Respiratory function vs. sleep-disordered breathing as predictors of QOL in ALS. *Neurology* 2001; **57**: 2040–44.

144 Arnulf I, Similowski T, Salachas F, *et al*. Sleep disorders and diaphragmatic function in patients with amyotrophic lateral sclerosis. *Am J Respir Crit Care Med* 2000; **161**: 849–56.

145 Morgan RK, McNally S, Alexander M, *et al*. Use of Sniff nasal-inspiratory force to predict survival in amyotrophic lateral sclerosis. *Am J Respir Crit Care Med* 2005; **171**: 269–74.

146 Armon C, Graves MC, Moses D, *et al*. Linear estimates of disease progression predict survival in patients with amyotrophic lateral sclerosis. *Muscle Nerve* 2000; **23**: 874–82.

147 Vender RL, Mauger D, Walsh S, Alam S, Simmons Z. Respiratory system abnormalities and clinical milestones for patients with amyotrophic lateral sclerosis with emphasis upon survival. *Amyotroph Lateral Scler* 2007; **8**: 36–41.

148 Miller RG, Rosenberg JA, Gelinas DF, *et al*. Practice parameter: the care of the patient with amyotrophic lateral sclerosis (an evidence-based review). *Neurology* 1999; **52**: 1311–23.

149 Haas H, Johnson LR, Gill TH, Armentrout TS. Diaphragm paralysis and ventilatory failure in chronic proximal spinal muscular atrophy. *Am Rev Respir Dis* 1981; **123**: 465–76.

150 Chevrolet J-C, Deléamont P. Repeated vital capacity measurement as predictive parameters for mechanical ventilation need and weaning success in Guillain–Barré syndrome. *Am Rev Respir Dis* 1991; **144**: 814–18.

151 Sharshar T, Chevret S, Bourdain F, *et al*. Early predictors of mechanical ventilation in Guillain–Barre syndrome. *Crit Care Med* 2003; **31**: 278–83.

152 Lawn ND, Fletcher DD, Henderson RD, Wolter TD, Wijdicks EF. Anticipating mechanical ventilation in

Guillain–Barre syndrome. *Arch Neurol* 2001; **58**: 893–8.

153 Chan CK, Mohensin V, Loke J, *et al.* Diaphragmatic dysfunction with hereditary motor and sensory neuropathy (Charcot–Marie–Tooth disease). *Chest* 1987; **91**: 567–70.

154 Laroche CM, Carroll N, Moxham J, *et al.* Diaphragm weakness in Charcot–Marie–Tooth disease. *Thorax* 1988; **43**: 478–9.

155 White J, Bullock RE, Hudgson P, Gibson GJ. Neuromuscular disease, respiratory failure and cor pulmonale. *Postgrad Med J* 1992; **68**: 820–23.

156 Dureuil B, Vires N, Pariente R, Desmonts JM, Aubier M. Effects of phrenic nerve cooling on diaphragmatic function. *J Appl Physiol* 1987; **63**: 1763–9.

157 Efthimiou J, Butler J, Benson MK, Westaby S. Bilateral diaphragm paralysis after cardiac surgery with topical hypothermia. *Thorax* 1991; **46**: 351–4.

158 Dimopoulou I, Daganou M, Dafni U, *et al.* Phrenic nerve dysfunction after cardiac operations: electrophysiologic evaluation of risk factors. *Chest* 1998; **113**: 8–14.

159 Diehl JL, Lofaso F, Deleuze P, *et al.* Clinically relevant diaphragmatic dysfunction after cardiac operations. *J Thorac Cardiovasc Surg* 1994; **107**: 487–98.

160 Lahrmann H, Grisold W, Authier FJ, Zifko UA. Neuralgic amyotrophy with phrenic nerve involvement. *Muscle Nerve* 1999; **22**: 437–42.

161 Hughes PD, Polkey MI, Moxham J, Green M. Long-term recovery of diaphragm strength in neuralgic amyotrophy. *Eur Respir J* 1999; **13**: 379–84.

162 Keenan SP, Alexander D, Road JD, *et al.* Ventilatory muscle strength and endurance in myasthenia gravis. *Eur Respir J* 1995; **8**: 1130–35.

163 Mier-Jedrzejowicz A, Brophy C, Green M. Respiratory muscle function in myasthenia gravis. *Am Rev Respir Dis* 1988; **138**: 867–73.

164 Mier A, Brophy C, Moxham J, Green M. Repetitive stimulation of phrenic nerves in myasthenia gravis. *Thorax* 1992; **47**: 640–44.

165 Putman MT, Wise RA. Myasthenia gravis and upper airway obstruction. *Chest* 1996; **109**: 400–404.

166 Quera-Salva MA, Guilleminault C, Chevret S, *et al.* Breathing disorders during sleep in myasthenia gravis. *Ann Neurol* 1992; **31**: 86–92.

167 Nicolle MW, Rask S, Koopman WJ, *et al.* Sleep apnea in patients with myasthenia gravis. *Neurology* 2006; **67**: 140–42.

168 Prudio J, Koenig J, Ermert S, Juhasz J. Sleep disordered breathing in medically stable patients with myasthenia gravis. *Eur J Neurol* 2007; **14**: 321–6.

169 De Troyer A, Borenstein S. Acute changes in respiratory mechanics after pyridostigmine injection in patients with myasthenia gravis. *Am Rev Respir Dis* 1980; **121**: 629–38.

170 Rieder P, Louis M, Jolliet P, Chevrolet JC. The repeated measurement of vital capacity is a poor predictor of the need for mechanical ventilation in myasthenia gravis. *Intensive Care Med* 1995; **21**: 663–8.

171 Thieben MJ, Blacker DJ, Liu PY, Harper CM Jr, Wijdicks EF. Pulmonary function tests and blood gases in worsening myasthenia gravis. *Muscle Nerve* 2005; **32**: 664–7.

172 Laroche CM, Mier AK, Spiro SG, *et al.* Respiratory muscle weakness in the Lambert–Eaton myasthenic syndrome. *Thorax* 1989; **44**: 913–18.

173 Wilcox PG, Morrison NJ, Anzarut ARA, Pardy RL. Lambert–Eaton myasthenic syndrome involving the diaphragm. *Chest* 1988; **93**: 604–6.

174 Nicolle MW, Stewart DJ, Remtulla H, Chen R, Bolton CF. Lambert–Eaton myasthenic syndrome presenting with severe respiratory failure. *Muscle Nerve* 1996; **19**: 1328–33.

175 Inkley SR, Oldenburg FC, Vignos PJ. Pulmonary function in Duchenne muscular dystrophy related to stage of disease. *Am J Med* 1974; **56**: 297–306.

176 Baydur A, Gilgoff I, Prentice W, Carlson M, Fischer DA. Decline in respiratory function and experience with long-term assisted ventilation in advanced Duchenne's muscular dystrophy. *Chest* 1990; **97**: 884–9.

177 Phillips MF, Quinlivan RC, Edwards RH, Calverley PM. Changes in spirometry over time as a prognostic marker in patients with Duchenne muscular dystrophy. *Am J Respir Crit Care Med* 2001; **164**: 2191–4.

178 Smith PEM, Edwards RHT, Calverley PMA. Ventilation and breathing pattern during sleep in Duchenne muscular dystrophy. *Chest* 1989; **96**: 1346–51.

179 Smith PEM, Calverley PMA, Edwards RHT. Hypoxaemia during sleep in Duchenne muscular dystrophy. *Am Rev Respir Dis* 1988; **137**: 884–8.

180 Khan Y, Heckmatt JZ. Obstructive apnoeas in Duchenne muscular dystrophy. *Thorax* 1994; **49**: 157–61.

181 Simonds AK, Muntoni F, Heather S, Fielding S. Impact of nasal ventilation on survival in hypercapnic Duchenne muscular dystrophy. *Thorax* 1998; **53**: 949–52.

182 Rideau Y, Jankowski LW, Grellet J. Respiratory function in the muscular dystrophies. *Muscle Nerve* 1981; **4**: 155–64.

183 Politano L, Nigro V, Passamano L, *et al.* Evaluation of cardiac and respiratory involvement in sarcoglycanopathies. *Neuromusc Disord* 2001; **11**: 178–85.

184 Poppe M, Bourke J, Eagle M, *et al.* Cardiac and respiratory failure in limb-girdle muscular dystrophy 2I. *Ann Neurol* 2004; **56**: 738–41.

185 Wohlgemuth M, van der Kooi EL, van Kesteren RG, van der Maarei SM, Padberg GW. Ventilatory support in facioscapulohumeral muscular dystrophy. *Neurology* 2004; **63**: 176–8.

186 Begin P, Mathieu J, Almirall J, Grassino A. Relationship between chronic hypercapnia and inspiratory-muscle weakness in myotonic dystrophy. *Am J Respir Crit Care Med* 1997; **156**: 133–9.

187 Bégin R, Bureau MA, Lupien L, *et al*. Pathogenesis of respiratory insufficiency in myotonic dystrophy. *Am Rev Respir Dis* 1982; **125**: 312–18.

188 Bégin R, Bureau MA, Lupien L, Lemieux B. Control and modulation of respiration in Steinert's myotonic dystrophy. *Am Rev Respir Dis* 1980; **121**: 281–9.

189 Bogaard JM, van der Meché FGA, Hendriks I, Ververs C. Pulmonary function and resting breathing pattern in myotonic dystrophy. *Lung* 1992; **170**: 143–54.

190 Rimmer KP, Golar SD, Lee MA, Whitelaw WA. Myotonia of the respiratory muscles in myotonic dystrophy. *Am Rev Respir Dis* 1993; **148**: 1018–22.

191 Estenne M, Borenstein S, De Troyer A. Respiratory muscle dysfunction in myotonia congenita. *Am Rev Respir Dis* 1984; **130**: 681–4.

192 Veale D, Cooper BG, Gilmartin JJ, *et al*. Breathing pattern awake and asleep in patients with myotonic dystrophy. *Eur Respir J* 1995; **8**: 815–18.

193 Ververs CC, Van der Meché FG, Verbraak AF, van der Sluys HC, Bogaard JM. Breathing pattern awake and asleep in myotonic dystrophy. *Respiration* 1996; **63**: 1–7.

194 Cirignotta F, Mondini S, Zucconi M, *et al*. Sleep related breathing impairment in myotonic dystrophy. *J Neurol* 1987; **235**: 80–85.

195 Gilmartin JJ, Cooper BG, Griffiths CJ, *et al*. Breathing during sleep in patients with myotonic dystrophy and non-myotonic muscle weakness. *Q J Med* 1991; **78**: 21–31.

196 Finnimore AJ, Jackson RV, Morton A, Lynch E. Sleep hypoxia in myotonic dystrophy and its correlation with awake respiratory function. *Thorax* 1994; **49**: 66–70.

197 Van der Meché FGA, Bogaard JM, van der Sluys JCM, *et al*. Daytime sleep in myotonic dystrophy is not caused by sleep apnoea. *J Neurol Neurosurg Psychiatry* 1994; **57**: 626–8.

198 Giubilei F, Antonini G, Bastianello S, *et al*. Excessive daytime sleepiness in myotonic dystrophy. *J Neurol Sci* 1999; **164**: 60–63.

199 Nugent AM, Smith IE, Shneerson JM. Domiciliary-assisted ventilation in patients with myotonic dystrophy. *Chest* **121**: 459–64.

200 Teixeira A, Cherin P, Demoule A, *et al*. 2005; Diaphragmatic dysfunction in patients with idiopathic inflammatory myopathies. *Neuromusc Disord* 2005; **15**: 32–9.

201 Weiner P, Azgad Y, Weiner M. The effect of corticosteroids on inspiratory muscle performance in humans. *Chest* 1993; **104**: 1788–91.

202 Mellies U, Ragette R, Schwake C, *et al*. Sleep-disordered breathing and respiratory failure in acid maltase deficiency. *Neurology* 2001; **57**: 1290–95.

203 Pellegrini N, Laforet P, Orlikowski D, *et al*. Respiratory insufficiency and limb muscle weakness in adults with Pompe's disease. *Eur Respir J* 2005; **26**: 1024–31.

204 Cros D, Palliyath S, Dimauro S, *et al*. Respiratory failure revealing mitochondrial myopathy in adults. *Chest* 1992; **102**: 824–8.

205 Flaherty KR, Wald J, Weisman IM, *et al*. Unexplained exertional limitation: characterization of patients with a mitochondrial myopathy. *Am J Respir Crit Care Med* 2001; **164**: 425–32.

206 Sanaker PS, Husebye ES, Fondenes O, Bindoff LA. Clinical evolution of Kearns–Sayre syndrome with polyendocrinopathy and respiratory failure. *Acta Neurol Scand* 2007; **187**: 64–7.

207 Van der Kooi AJ, de Voogt WG, Bertini E, *et al*. Cardiac and pulmonary investigations in Bethlem myopathy. *Arch Neurol* 2006; **63**: 1617–21.

208 Riley DJ, Santiago TV, Daniele RP, *et al*. Blunted respiratory drive in congenital myopathy. *Am J Med* 1977; **63**: 459–65.

209 Falga-Tirado C, Perez-Peman P, Ordi-Ros J, Bofill JM, Balcells E. Adult onset of nemaline myopathy presenting as respiratory insufficiency. *Respiration* 1995; **62**: 353–4.

210 Horowitz SH, Schmalbruch H. Autosomal dominant distal myopathy with desmin storage: a clinicopathologic and electrophysiologic study of a large kinship. *Muscle Nerve* 1994; **17**: 151–60.

211 Chinnery PF, Johnson MA, Walls TJ, *et al*. A novel autosomal dominant distal myopathy with early respiratory failure: clinico-pathologic characteristics and exclusion of linkage to candidate genetic loci. *Ann Neurol* 2001; **49**: 443–52.

212 Rimmer KP, Whitelaw WA. The respiratory muscles in multicore myopathy. *Am Rev Respir Dis* 1993; **148**: 227–31.

21

Blood Disorders

Effective transport of oxygen from the atmosphere to the metabolizing tissues depends on three main factors – pulmonary gas exchange, the circulation and the carriage of oxygen by the blood. In addition to its role in transport of physiological gases, the concentration of haemoglobin (Hb) in the blood influences tests of respiratory function by its effect on the diffusing capacity for carbon monoxide ($D_L CO$). Abnormal respiratory function can also occur with haemoglobins of abnormal molecular structure.

21.1 ANAEMIA

21.1.1 Effect on oxygenation

The capacity of anaemic blood to carry oxygen is reduced in proportion to the haemoglobin concentration. If the oxygen dissociation curve is constructed with oxygen content (concentration) plotted against partial pressure (Fig. 21.1a), it is contracted on the y axis compared with the normal

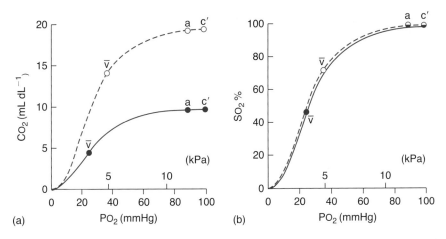

Figure 21.1 Haemoglobin–oxygen dissociation curve in anaemia (haemoglobin concentration 50% of normal–solid lines) compared with normal (broken lines). (a) Oxygen content (C_{O_2}) plotted against P_{O_2} to show the marked reduction in oxygen carriage by anaemic blood (the effect of oxygen in solution is ignored). (b) Per cent saturation (S_{O_2}) plotted against P_{O_2} shows identical curves. Also identified are the pressure, content and per cent saturation in end pulmonary capillary (c′), arterial (a) and mixed venous v̄ blood in the normal subject (open circles) and the patient with anaemia (solid circles). In the anaemic patient the mixed venous blood has a reduced oxygen content, saturation and pressure; the arterial blood has a greatly reduced oxygen content but per cent saturation and Pa_{O_2} are a little affected (see text for explanation).

curve; but with the alternative display in terms of percentage saturation, the curve appears normal (Fig. 21.1b). Anaemia does not affect tissue oxygen consumption so that, if the cardiac output is normal, the difference in oxygen content between arterial and mixed venous blood is also normal (Fick principle; see Equation 2.2 in Chapter 2), but the difference in percentage saturation is increased. Anaemic mixed venous blood is therefore abnormally low in both oxygen content (because the arterial oxygen content is low) and percentage saturation (because the tissues extract a normal amount of oxygen but the total available is less). Consequently, the Po_2 of anaemic mixed venous blood, $(P\bar{v}o_2)$ is also less than normal (Fig. 21.1).

Although anaemia reduces the oxygen content (concentration) of arterial blood in direct proportion to the concentration of haemoglobin, it has an insignificant effect on either the percentage saturation (Sao_2) or the partial pressure (Pao_2) of arterial blood. In theory, the likely reduction in mixed venous saturation and Po_2 would tend to lower Pao_2 a little due to the effect of the normal irreducible anatomical shunt, but other factors may counter this. In particular, the high cardiac output that accompanies anaemia tends to maintain mixed venous oxygenation, thereby reducing any effect of admixture of desaturated blood. Furthermore, in experimental animals subjected to isovolaemic anaemia, the overall matching of ventilation to perfusion improves and consequently Pao_2 actually shows a small increase.[1] Data in humans are very limited: in one study of patients with iron deficiency anaemia the mean alveolar–arterial Po_2 difference ($Aapo_2$) breathing air remained within the normal range – but it fell, and Pao_2 increased by an average of 4 mmHg, after correction of the anaemia.[2] However, in another study of eight patients with severe chronic iron deficiency there was a more important reduction of Pao_2 and a mean rise from 64 mmgHg to 76 mmHg after treatment.[3]

21.1.2 Effect on carbon monoxide diffusing capacity

Simple chronic anaemia has no direct effect on pulmonary mechanics, but the possibility of cardiac failure with a severely reduced haemoglobin should be borne in mind. More relevant to everyday practice is the effect of anaemia on the $D_L co$.

In a classic study, Roughton and Forster analysed the overall $D_L co$ in terms of diffusion across the alveolar–capillary membrane, the rate of reaction of CO with haemoglobin and the volume of blood in the pulmonary capillaries, developing the equation (see Chapter 3, Section 3.2):[4]

$$\frac{1}{D_L co} = \frac{1}{D_m} + \frac{1}{\theta\, V_c} \qquad (21.1)$$

where θ is the rate at which 1 mL of blood combines with CO (mL CO $min^{-1} mmHg^{-1}$). Therefore θ equals the product of the haemoglobin concentration and the uptake of CO per gram of haemoglobin.

Equation 21.1 can be rewritten as:

$$\frac{1}{D_L co} = \frac{1}{D_m} + \frac{1}{\theta' \times \dfrac{[Hb]}{14.6} \times V_c} \qquad (21.2)$$

where θ' is the rate of combination of CO at a standard haemoglobin concentration of $14.6\, g\, dL^{-1}$ and [Hb] is the actual concentration. Rearranging Equation 21.2 allows standardization of the measured $D_L co$ to a normal haemoglobin concentration.[5] The standardized value is that which would be obtained at the standard haemoglobin concentration of $14.6\, g\, dL^{-1}$ and is given by:

$$D_L co\ standardized = D_L co\ measured \times \frac{14.6a + [Hb]}{(1 + a) \times [Hb]} \qquad (21.3)$$

where 'a' can be shown to equal the ratio D_m/V_c. If a normal value of 0.7 is assumed for this ratio, Equation 21.3 simplifies to:

$$D_L co\ standardized = D_L co\ measured \times \frac{10.2 + [Hb]}{1.7 \times [Hb]} \qquad (21.4)$$

The effect of haemoglobin concentration on the measured $D_L co$, predicted by Equation 21.4, is shown in Fig. 21.2; a similar relationship holds for Kco. When correcting for the effects of anaemia, an assumed value for D_m/V_c of 0.7 may not always be justified. If this ratio is greater than 0.7, then so is the correction factor, but of course if D_m or V_c is abnormal, this will affect the measured total

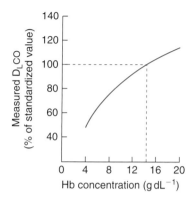

Figure 21.2 The predicted effect of haemoglobin concentration ([Hb]) on single-breath carbon monoxide diffusing capacity (D_Lco), expressed as a percentage of the value at a standard [Hb] of 14.6 g dL^{-1}. (D_Lco calculated using Equation 21.4.)

diffusing capacity in accordance with Equation 21.1. For example, with the development of heart failure in an anaemic patient, an increase in V_c might be expected, together with a reduction both in D_m and in the D_m/V_c ratio – so exact prediction of the effect on the D_Lco would then become very difficult. However, in uncomplicated anaemia, this method of correction generally works well. It has, for example, been shown to account satisfactorily for the reduced D_Lco in iron deficiency anaemia and for the increase after gradual correction of the iron deficiency,[5] and it also fits the results when anaemia is corrected more rapidly by blood transfusion.[6] Some authors have found that a simple proportional adjustment for haemoglobin concentration gives more accurate results,[7] but in practice Equation 21.4 is the most widely used method for correcting both D_Lco and Kco for anaemia.

21.1.3 Effects of anaemia on exercise performance

The increased cardiac output associated with chronic anaemia is maintained during exercise and results mainly from a rapid heart rate with some increase in stroke volume in more anaemic individuals.[8,9] Ventilation is also high for a given level of exercise.[10] In individuals with simple iron deficiency anaemia and normal cardiac and respiratory function, significant incapacity due to breathlessness is unlikely as long as the haemoglobin concentration exceeds 8 g dL^{-1}.[5]

In polycythaemia the total red cell mass is increased and a frequently encountered clinical problem is to decide whether this is the cause or the effect of abnormal respiratory function. Not only do chronically hypoxic patients develop polycythaemia, but also patients with primary polycythaemia (polycythaemia rubra vera) often have abnormal respiratory function, including a degree of hypoxaemia. The reduction in PaO_2 attributable to polycythaemia alone is usually mild, and a normal value is usually taken as excluding a cardiorespiratory cause. An absolute distinction may not always be possible, however; the most useful cut-off value is a PaO_2 of about 60 mmHg (8 kPa) with the subject awake and breathing air at sea level. Values less than 60 mmHg are unusual in uncomplicated primary polycythaemia, while the great majority of patients with secondary polycythaemia due to cardiac or pulmonary disease have a PaO_2 less than this value (which is approximately equivalent to an arterial oxygen saturation of 90%). The stimulus to red cell production may be underestimated by reliance on daytime measurements of oxygenation alone. In obstructive sleep apnoea, polycythaemia is usually seen only in patients who show daytime hypoxaemia, but occasionally it occurs as a consequence of nocturnal desaturation alone.[11]

In primary polycythaemia the 'anatomical' shunt is usually normal or increased only minimally, and the usually mild hypoxaemia is presumed to be due to $\dot{V}_A/\dot{Q}$ mismatching.[12,13] A natural model of the effects of polycythaemia is offered by high-altitude dwellers; those who develop a disproportionately increased red cell mass have greater $AaPO_2$ than average-altitude dwellers. Detailed analysis of pulmonary gas exchange using the multiple inert gas elimination technique (MIGET) suggests that this is due to the combined effects of lung units with very low $\dot{V}/\dot{Q}$ ratios and lower mixed venous oxygenation consequent on a reduced cardiac output due, presumably, to the greatly increased blood viscosity.[14] Some patients with primary polycythaemia have an increased physiological dead space; this is attributed to small vascular thromboses, which are well-recognized in patients with this condition.

Typically, D_Lco and Kco are greater than normal in primary polycythaemia,[15] and the increase

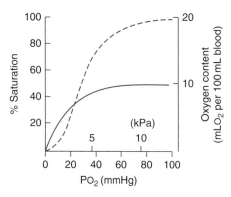

Figure 21.3 Effect of carboxyhaemoglobin on the haemoglobin–oxygen dissociation curve. The solid line shows the curve with a very high carboxyhaemoglobin concentration of 50 per cent, compared with the normal curve (broken line). The oxygen-carrying capacity of haemoglobin is reduced by 50 per cent and oxygen content (concentration) is therefore halved at a given Po_2. The true oxygen saturation, measured in vitro by spectrophotometry, is reduced in proportion (but saturation using an oximeter is likely to appear normal). In addition, the presence of a high carboxyhaemoglobin concentration alters the shape of the oxygen dissociation curve.

is often greater than predicted if the haemoglobin correction applied in anaemia (Equation 21.4) is used. The likeliest explanation is an increase in pulmonary capillary blood volume accompanying the expansion of the total blood volume,[15] which would render this correction inadequate.

21.3 CARBOXYHAEMOGLOBINAEMIA

Carbon monoxide (CO) competes with oxygen for binding sites on the Hb molecule. Since Hb has a much greater affinity for CO than for oxygen, a large proportion of its binding sites will be occupied by CO molecules at a relatively low partial pressure of CO. In addition, the presence of excess CO changes the shape of the haemoglobin–oxygen dissociation curve, shifting it to the left (Fig. 21.3) and thus inhibiting the release of oxygen to the metabolizing tissues, further compounding the problem of oxygen availability.

It is important to note that conventional indices of oxygenation are deceptively normal in patients with CO poisoning. The PaO_2 is essentially un-affected as it is a measurement of partial pressure

and not of oxygen concentration. Furthermore, oxygen saturation, as measured conventionally by a pulse oximeter, is also likely to be normal since carboxy-haemoglobin is measured along with oxygenated haemoglobin.[16] Although pulse oximeters fail to distinguish the two, direct spectrophotometry of blood in vitro measures oxygen saturation accurately.

Although the affinity of Hb is much greater (about 240 times) for CO than for oxygen, combination with Hb is competitive. Consequently, increasing the inspired oxygen concentration hastens the dissociation of carboxyhaemoglobin and its elimination; this is the rationale for treating CO poisoning with 100 per cent oxygen.[17]

21.4 HAEMOGLOBINOPATHIES

21.4.1 Sickle cell anaemia

Abnormal respiratory function is often found in individuals with sickle cell anaemia but inter-pretation is complicated by two main factors – uncertainty about the most appropriate reference values to use for lung volumes and uncertainty about the validity of measurements of oxygena-tion, especially when using a pulse oximeter.

21.4.1.1 Respiratory mechanics

A mild restrictive ventilatory defect is widely rec-ognized, with average reductions of VC and TLC of 10–15 per cent, even in comparison with appro-priate ethnically matched control subjects.[18–20] One reason may be that the usual method of stan-dardization for height is inappropriate, as individ-uals with sickle cell anaemia have different body proportions, with a shorter upper body relative to total stature and narrower lateral chest diameter than healthy subjects of the same ethnicity.[21] In addition to the restrictive ventilatory pattern, some data suggest that a significant minority of individuals with sickle cell disease have airway obstruction, with bronchial hyperresponsiveness[22] and an unusually brisk bronchodilator response.[23]

21.4.1.2 Measurements of pulmonary gas exchange

The oxygen dissociation curve of haemoglobin S is shifted to the right (i.e. its oxygen affinity is reduced compared with normal HbA), so that, for a given PaO_2, the saturation is less than normal. Studies of the validity of measuring oxygen saturation by pulse oximetry have given very variable results, with some suggesting underestimation[24-26] and others overestimation[27] of the true value. Majority opinion favours underestimation, but the extent of the discrepancy is probably not significant clinically.[26]

In the 'acute chest syndrome' associated with sickle cell disease, patients present with respiratory symptoms accompanied by hypoxaemia; the precise cause is often unclear, but contributory factors may include infection, intrapulmonary 'sickling' and fat embolism.[23] This, and other forms of sickle cell crisis, may be preceded by hypoxaemia. Nocturnal desaturation is a frequent finding[28] and may predispose to such crises.[29] Its cause is uncertain as it is not clearly attributable to episodic upper airway obstruction.[28]

Measurements of D_LCO in sickle cell disease show consistently low values, even after correction for anaemia;[18-20,22] on average, KCO is greater than normal, at least in children.[30]

21.4.1.3 Exercise performance

Maximum exercise capacity and $\dot{V}O_2$max are typically reduced. Exercise is accompanied by abnormally high ventilation, due largely to an increased physiological dead space probably resulting from the effects of intrapulmonary sickling and consequent vascular damage.[31] The reduction in exercise capacity is proportional to the reduced D_LCO,[19] consistent with pulmonary vascular disease and pulmonary hypertension.[19,32]

21.4.2 Thalassaemia

A mild restrictive ventilatory defect is common in thalassaemia major, with the reduction of lung volumes tending to become more marked with age.[33-36] Iron overload due to repeated transfusion has been suggested as a contributory factor, but the data are conflicting: one study showed more severe restriction with increasing cumulative iron 'burden',[33] but subsequent studies failed to confirm this.[34,35] D_LCO is more consistently reduced (even after correction for anaemia).[34,36] A mild reduction in PaO_2 is common,[34] but clinically significant

hypoxaemia at rest is unusual.[33] Exercise capacity and $\dot{V}O_2$ are reduced and cardiac output and heart rate are increased for a given $\dot{V}O_2$, as in chronic anaemia of other causes.[37] Oxygen desaturation on exercise is relatively common,[34] but the mechanism is uncertain.

21.4.3 Haemoglobins with altered oxygen affinity

A number of other, rare, genetically determined abnormal haemoglobins associated with alterations in affinity for oxygen have been described. These affect the position of the haemoglobin–oxygen dissociation curve and are usefully classified as haemoglobins with high and low oxygen affinity, depending on whether the P_{50} (see Chapter 4, Section 4.1) is, respectively, reduced or increased. High-affinity haemoglobins are more varied than low-affinity molecules and in most cases the abnormal haemoglobin comprises 40–50 per cent of the total.[38] With few exceptions, saturation of haemoglobin with oxygen at the high tensions that prevail in the lungs is virtually complete, and the main effect of abnormal affinity is on delivery of oxygen to the tissues rather than uptake in the lung. With low-affinity molecules oxygen delivery is enhanced, while with high-affinity molecules it is impaired, but the effects are usually mitigated by changes in haemoglobin concentration and therefore in oxygen content (Fig. 21.4). Thus, patients with high-affinity haemoglobins characteristically have polycythaemia, while those with low-affinity molecules are often anaemic.

Altered haemoglobin oxygen affinity disturbs the normal tight relation between oxygen partial pressure and saturation. As discussed in Chapter 5, Section 5.2.2, the normal response of ventilation to falling PaO_2 is hyperbolic, but the relation becomes rectilinear if ventilation is plotted against arterial oxygen saturation. It is not clear whether this is a coincidence resulting from similarities in the shapes of the ventilatory response to hypoxia and the oxygen dissociation curve, or whether it has a physiological basis related to the nature of the stimulus to the chemoreceptors in the carotid body. Use has been made of the 'natural experiment' in which the normal relation of SaO_2 to PaO_2 is uncoupled in patients with abnormal-affinity haemoglobins to investigate these two possibilities. The results show

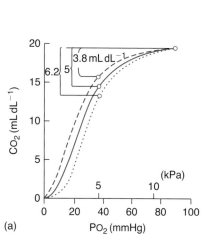
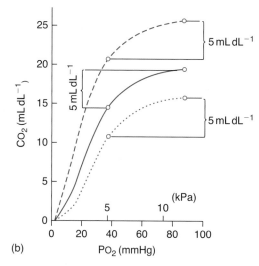

(a)   (b)

Figure 21.4 Effects of low- and high-affinity haemoglobins on oxygen carriage. Oxygen content (Co_2) is plotted against Po_2 and the effect of an increase (dotted line) and reduction (broken line) of P_{50} of 5 mmHg is illustrated. (a) Haemoglobin concentration [Hb] and oxygen-carrying capacity of the blood are unchanged. For given arterial and mixed venous pressures (open circles), a shift to the left (high-affinity haemoglobin) leads to reduced oxygen delivery to the tissues, with the arteriovenous oxygen content difference reduced from a normal value of 5 mL/100 mL blood to 3.8 mL/100 mL blood. Conversely, a shift to the right (low oxygen affinity) improves tissue oxygen availability ($a - \bar{v}$ content difference 6.2 mL dL^{-1}). The compensatory effect of an increased [Hb] with the high-affinity molecule and a reduced [Hb] with the low-affinity molecule is illustrated in (b), where values of [Hb] (and therefore oxygen-carrying capacity) have been chosen that maintain a normal $a - \bar{v}$ content difference of 5 mL dL^{-1}.

that, with a high-affinity haemoglobin, the relation of ventilation to oxygen tension remains normal, supporting the 'coincidence' hypothesis.[39]

21.5 MISCELLANEOUS CONDITIONS

21.5.1 Bone marrow transplantation

Obliterative bronchiolitis with progressive airway obstruction is a well-recognized complication of bone marrow and stem cell transplantation and is regarded as a manifestation of chronic graft versus host disease. Its prevalence appears to have declined in recent years.[40] Compromised respiratory function pre-transplantation increases the risk of post-transplant respiratory failure.[41] The functional pattern resembles obliterative bronchiolitis seen in other contexts (see Chapter 9, Section 9.17).

21.5.2 Acute leukaemia

An abnormality that occasionally caused misinterpretation is seen in some patients with acute

leukaemia and a very high white cell count; the phenomenon, colourfully termed 'leukocyte larceny',[42] results in a spuriously low value of arterial Po_2 due to the white cells consuming oxygen in the blood during the interval between sampling and analysis. Precursor white blood cells (blasts) are particularly active metabolically and the error increases with delay in analysis or failing to keep the blood cooled by ice.[43] Since the consumption of oxygen occurs in vitro, measurements of oxygen saturation by pulse oximetry are unaffected, a pattern of abnormality that may give the clue to the cause of the low measured Po_2.

REFERENCES

1   Deem S, Hedges RG, McKinney S, et al. Mechanisms of improvement in pulmonary gas exchange during isovolemic hemodilution. J Appl Physiol 1999; 87: 132–41.

2   Housley E. Respiratory gas exchange in chronic anaemia. Clin Sci 1967; 32: 19–26.

3 Guleria JS, Pande JN, Markose MM, *et al.* Pulmonary function in chronic severe anaemia. *Clin Sci* 1971; **40**: 317–25.

4 Roughton FJW, Forster RE. Relative importance of diffusion and chemical reaction rates in determining rate of exchange of gases in the human lung, with special reference to true diffusing capacity of pulmonary membrane and volume of blood in the lung capillaries. *J Appl Physiol* 1957; **11**: 290–302.

5 Cotes JE, Dabbs JM, Elwood PC, *et al.* Iron-deficiency anaemia: its effect on transfer factor for the lung (diffusing capacity) and ventilatory and cardiac frequency during sub-maximal exercise. *Clin Sci* 1972; **42**: 325–35.

6 Clark EH, Woods RL, Hughes JMB. Effect of blood transfusion on the carbon monoxide transfer factor of the lung in man. *Clin Sci* 1978; **54**: 627–31.

7 Marrades RM, Diaz O, Roca J, *et al.* Adjustment of $D_L CO$ for haemoglobin concentration. *Am J Respir Crit Care Med* 1997; **155**: 236–41.

8 Davies CTM, Chukweumeka AC, van Haaren JPM. Iron-deficiency anaemia: its effect on maximum aerobic power and responses to exercise in African males aged 17–40 years. *Clin Sci* 1973; **44**: 555–62.

9 Woodson RD, Wills RE, Lefant C. Effect of acute and established anaemia on O_2 tranport at rest, sub-maximal and maximal work. *J Appl Physiol* 1978; **44**: 36–43.

10 Sproule BJ, Mitchell JH, Miller WF. Cardiopulmonary physiological response to heavy exercise in patients with anaemia. *J Clin Invest* 1960; **39**: 378–88.

11 Moore-Gillon J, Treacher DF, Gaminara EJ, Pearson TC, Cameron IC. Intermittent hypoxia in patients with unexplained polycythaemia. *Br Med J* 1986; **293**: 588–90.

12 Lertzmann M, Frome BM, Israel LG, Cherniack RM. Hypoxia in polycythaemia vera. *Ann Intern Med* 1964; **60**: 409–17.

13 Murray JF. Arterial studies in primary and secondary polycythaemic disorders. *Am Rev Respir Dis* 1965; **92**: 435–49.

14 Manier G, Guenard H, Castaing Y, Varene N, Vargas E. Pulmonary gas exchange in Andean natives with excessive polycythaemia: effect of hemodilution. *J Appl Physiol* 1988; **65**: 2107–17.

15 Greening AP, Patel K, Goolden AWG, *et al.* Carbon monoxide diffusing capacity in polycythaemia rubra vera. *Thorax* 1982; **37**: 528–31.

16 Bozeman WP, Myers RA, Barish RA. Confirmation of the pulse oximetry gap in carbon monoxide poisoning. *Ann Emerg Med* 1997; **30**: 608–11.

17 Weaver LK, Howe S, Hopkins R, Chan KJ. Carboxy-hemoglobin half-life in carbon monoxide-poisoned patients treated with 100% oxygen at atmospheric pressure. *Chest* 2000; **117**: 801–8.

18 Miller GJ, Sergeant GR. An assessment of lung volumes and gas transfer in sickle-cell anaemia. *Thorax* 1971; **26**: 309–15.

19 Delclaux C, Zerah-Lancner F, Bachir D, *et al.* Factors associated with dyspnea in adult patients with sickle cell disease. *Chest* 2005; **128**: 3336–44.

20 Klings ES, Wyszynski DF, Nolan VG, Steinberg MH. Abnormal pulmonary function in adults with sickle cell anemia. *Am J Respir Crit Care Med* 2006; **173**: 1264–9.

21 Miller GJ, Sergeant GR, Saunders MJ, *et al.* Interpretation of lung function tests in the sickle-cell haemoglobinopathies. *Thorax* 1978; **33**: 85–8.

22 Vendramini EC, Vianna EO, De Lucena AI, *et al.* Lung function and airway hyperresponsiveness in adult patients with sickle cell disease. *Am J Med Sci* 2006; **332**: 68–72.

23 Vichinsky EP, Neumayr LD, Earles AN, *et al.* Causes and outcomes of the acute chest syndrome in sickle cell disease. National Acute Chest Syndrome Study Group. *N Engl J Med* 2000; **342**: 1855–65.

24 Needleman JP, Franco ME, Varlotta L, *et al.* Mechanisms of nocturnal oxyhemoglobin desaturation in children and adolescents with sickle cell disease. *Pediatr Pulmonol* 1999; **28**: 418–22.

25 Hargrave DR, Wade A, Evans JP, Hewes DK, Kirkham FJ. Nocturnal oxygen saturation and painful sickle cell crises in children. *Blood* 2003; **101**: 846–8.

26 Fitzgerald RK, Johnson A. Pulse oximetry in sickle cell anemia. *Crit Care Med* 2001; **29**: 1803–6.

27 Needleman JP, Setty BN, Varlotta L, Dampier C, Allen JL. Measurement of hemoglobin saturation by oxygen in children and adolescents with sickle cell disease. *Pediatr Pulmonol* 1999; **28**: 423–8.

28 Comber JT, Lopez BL. Evaluation of pulse oximetry in sickle cell anemia patients presenting to the emergency department in acute vasoocclusive crisis. *Am J Emerg Med* 1996; **14**: 16–18.

29 Homi J, Levee L, Higgs D, Thomas P, Sergeant G. Pulse oximetry in a cohort study of sickle cell disease. *Clin Lab Haematol* 1997; **19**: 17–22.

30 Sylvester KP, Patey RA, Kassim Z, *et al.* Lung gas transfer in children with sickle cell anaemia. *Respir Physiol Neurobiol* 2007; **158**: 70–74.

31 Pianosi P, D'Sousa SLA, Esseltine DW, Charge TD, Coster AJ. Ventilation and gas exchange during exercise in sickle cell anaemia. *Am Rev Respir Dis* 1991; **143**: 226–30.

32 Anthi A, Machado RF, Jison ML, *et al.* Hemodynamic and functional assessment of patients with sickle cell disease and pulmonary

hypertension. *Am J Respir Crit Care Med* 2007; **175**: 1272–9.

33 Factor JM, Pottipati SR, Rappaport I, *et al.* Pulmonary function abnormalities in thalassaemia major and the role of iron overload. *Am J Respir Crit Care Med* 1994; **149**: 1570–74.

34 Tai DY, Wang YT, Lou J, *et al.* Lungs in thalassaemia major patients receiving regular transfusion. *Eur Respir J* 1996; **9**: 1389–94.

35 Dimopoulou I, Kremastinos DT, Maris TG, Mavrogeni S, Tzelepis GE. Respiratory function in patients with thalassaemia and iron overload. *Eur Respir J* 1999; **13**: 602–5.

36 Kanj N, Shamseddine A, Gharzeddine W, *et al.* Relation of ferritin levels to pulmonary function in patients with thalassemia major and the acute effects of transfusion. *Eur J Haematol* 2000; **64**: 396–400.

37 Grant GP, Graziano JH, Seaman C, Mansell AL. Cardiorespiratory response to exercise in patients with thalassaemia major. *Am Rev Respir Dis* 1987; **136**: 92–7.

38 Bellingham AJ. Haemoglobins with altered oxygen affinity. *Br Med Bull* 1976; **32**: 234–8.

39 Rossoff LJ, Rebuck AS, Aberman A. The hypoxic ventilatory response in patients with high affinity hemoglobin. *Am Rev Respir Dis* 1980; **121**: 170–72.

40 Marras TK, Chan CK, Lipton JH, *et al.* Long-term pulmonary function abnormalities and survival after allogeneic marrow transplantation. *Bone Marrow Transplant* 2004; **33**: 509–17.

41 Parimon T, Madtes DK, Au DH, Clark JG, Chien JW. Pretransplant lung function, respiratory failure, and mortality after stem cell transplantation. *Am J Respir Crit Care Med* 2005; **172**: 384–90.

42 Fox MJ, Brody JS, Weintraub LR. Leukocyte larceny: a cause of spurious hypoxemia. *Am J Med* 1979; **67**: 742–6.

43 Charoenratanakul S, Loasuthi K. Pseudohypoxaemia in a patient with acute leukaemia. *Thorax* 1997; **52**: 394–5.

22

Renal Diseases

The kidneys and lungs share responsibility for maintaining acid–base homeostasis, and the effects of primary disturbances in the function of one system are often compensated by the other. Many patients with renal failure have abnormal respiratory function, with most interest centring on the phenomenon of hypoxaemia during haemodialysis and on the high prevalence of disordered breathing during sleep of patients with chronic renal failure. In addition, renal disease can affect respiratory function indirectly via its complications such as fluid retention and anaemia.

22.1 CHRONIC RENAL FAILURE

22.1.1 Effects on lung volumes

Many patients with chronic uraemia have 'waterlogged' lungs, which may produce a restrictive ventilatory defect. However, in the absence of pulmonary oedema or cardiomegaly, lung volumes are usually normal or near-normal,[1–4] although residual volume is sometimes increased.[3]

22.1.2 Effects on pulmonary gas exchange

Even in the absence of overt pulmonary oedema, studies using radioactive xenon may show reduced ventilation at the lung bases and an increased closing capacity, consistent with premature closure of small airways, possibly due to gravity-dependent subclinical peribronchial oedema.[5] In the absence of frank fluid retention such effects are of little clinical importance, and the consequent ventilation/perfusion mismatching usually produces only a minor increase in alveolar–arterial P_{O_2} difference $(A a P_{O_2})$, with Pa_{O_2} low normal or slightly reduced.[6]

The Pa_{CO_2} is often below normal, as would be expected with the metabolic acidosis that accompanies renal failure, but chronic hypocapnia often persists after correction of acidaemia. Suggested explanations include a persisting intracellular acidosis,[7] an unidentified metabolic stimulus to breathe[8] or heightened central chemosensitivity.[9]

22.1.3 Effects on carbon monoxide diffusing capacity

A frequent finding in chronic renal failure is a reduction in the carbon monoxide diffusing capacity $(D_L CO)$, which is seen irrespective of the aetiology of the renal failure.[2,5,6,10,11] The abnormality persists after correction for anaemia and is also reflected in a low $K CO$.[10,11] Partitioning of the single-breath measurement into its membrane (D_m) and pulmonary capillary (V_c) components shows that the reduction is due to a low D_m.[6,10] The reduction in $D_L CO$ (haemoglobin-corrected) is proportional to the severity[6] and duration[11] of renal failure. It does not improve acutely after dialysis[5] or in the longer term after transplantation.[2] It has been suggested that this apparently irreversible effect might be due to deposition of fibrin in alveolar walls following episodes of pulmonary oedema.[2,6] Another possible contributor is the development of pulmonary vascular disease, as pulmonary hypertension is common in patients with longstanding renal failure receiving haemodialysis.[12]

22.1.4 Effects on respiratory muscle function and exercise performance

Uraemia is accompanied by weakness of skeletal muscles, and impaired respiratory muscle strength has been demonstrated in some[13] but not all[14] studies. Such weakness is hardly surprising in view of the known effects of acidosis and alterations in the concentrations of electrolytes such as calcium, magnesium, potassium and phosphate, all of which may accompany uraemia.

Exercise capacity is markedly impaired by chronic renal failure; the reduction correlates with both the severity of anaemia[15] and the reduction in serum phosphorus concentration.[16] Treatment of anaemic patients with erythropoietin improves exercise capacity,[17,18] but it remains subnormal even after restoring haemoglobin concentration ([Hb]) to normal.[18]

22.2 ACUTE EFFECTS OF HAEMODIALYSIS

During each period of haemodialysis, the patient is subjected to rapid changes in acid–base status, with correction of a metabolic acidosis or the development of a frank alkalosis, although the arterial P_{CO_2} shows little or no change.[19,20] An observation that has evoked considerable interest and some controversy is the fall in arterial P_{O_2}, which is found consistently to accompany haemodialysis. The Pa_{O_2} usually falls within a few minutes of starting dialysis, reaching a nadir at about 2 h followed by some recovery by the end of the session.[4,21] Several possible explanations have been suggested (Table 22.1). A shift in the oxygen dissociation curve associated with the increasing pH during dialysis would lower Pa_{O_2} for a given oxygen saturation or content. Alternatively, increasing alkalosis may cause hypoxaemia by depressing central respiratory output and therefore reducing ventilation. Third, if

acetate is used as the dialysate, its metabolism will increase oxygen consumption. However, the two most likely mechanisms of hypoxaemia are ventilation/perfusion mismatching due to complement activation causing stasis of white blood cells in small pulmonary vessels,[22] and reduced ventilation due to CO_2 excretion via the dialysate, especially if this is an acetate solution.[19,23] Craddock et al. pointed out the temporal relation between the onset of hypoxaemia and the fall in blood leukocyte count during haemodialysis: in experimental animals they demonstrated stasis of white cells in small pulmonary vessels, apparently mediated by activation of complement induced by contact with the dialyser membrane.[22] The hypothesis of dialysis induced hypoxaemia due to leukostasis in small pulmonary vessels is supported by a consistent fall in $D_L CO$ with a similar time course to the drop in Pa_{O_2}. There are, however, several objections to this as the sole mechanism: first, hypoxaemia is seen during dialysis using membranes that do not cause leukopoenia;[24] second, if haemofiltration precedes dialysis, leukopoenia occurs during the former procedure without hypoxaemia, but a fall in Pa_{O_2} develops during the subsequent dialysis despite resolution of leukopoenia;[24] third, when dialysis is performed against a bicarbonate-buffered solution, the fall in Pa_{O_2} is less or absent, despite the development of leukopoenia.[21,25] These last findings emphasize the important point that CO_2 is normally excreted into the dialysis fluid, and this probably underlies the most important mechanism of the hypoxaemia. Loss of CO_2 by this route implies a relatively lower than normal CO_2 output at the mouth. Consequently, both the minute ventilation and the respiratory exchange ratio fall during dialysis. In one study, measurement of gas exchange at the mouth showed an average value of R of only 0.62 compared with a mean

Table 22.1 Potential mechanisms of haemodialysis-induced hypoxaemia

Shift of oxygen dissociation curve
Hypoventilation due to alkalosis
Increased oxygen consumption due to metabolism of dialysate
$\dot{V}/\dot{Q}$ mismatching due to leukostasis
Hypoventilation due to CO_2 unloading

predialysis value of 0.81.[23] The implication of this non-respiratory removal of CO_2 is clear if the simplified alveolar air equation (see Equation 2.4 in Chapter 2) is considered:

$$P_{A}O_2 = P_{I}O_2 - \frac{P_{A}CO_2}{R}$$

The alveolar PO_2 ($P_{A}O_2$) is calculated by using the arterial PCO_2 as the 'effective' alveolar PCO_2 ($P_{A}CO_2$) (see Fig. 2.13 in Chapter 2). The arithmetic dictates that, with a reduction of R, $P_{A}O_2$ must fall, inevitably also causing a fall in the arterial PO_2. Comparison of the measured reductions in PaO_2 during haemodialysis with the effects predicted from the rate of loss of CO_2 and corresponding fall in R suggest that this mechanism is quantitatively the most important contributor to dialysis-induced hypoxaemia.[19,23] The early fall in PaO_2 is probably due to leukostasis, but the overall effect of haemodialysis on ventilation/perfusion matching is towards a slight improvement.[26] A consequence of CO_2 'unloading' is to destabilize resting ventilation, and the reduced overall ventilation may be accompanied by irregular or periodic breathing and sometimes apnoeas, particularly if dialysing against an acetate solution.[20]

The extent of oxygen desaturation accompanying haemodialysis is unlikely to be important in subjects with normal cardiopulmonary function or in those with a mildly reduced predialysis PaO_2,[27] but it may be clinically relevant in those with more markedly impaired respiratory function.[28]

22.3 EFFECTS OF PERITONEAL DIALYSIS

During continuous ambulatory peritoneal dialysis (CAPD) the large volume of peritoneal fluid can restrict lung volumes and impair pulmonary gas exchange. In a study of serial changes in lung volumes, the initially reduced spirometric volumes were shown to revert to predialysis values over the first 2 weeks of treatment.[29] In patients established on treatment the only apparent effect on lung mechanics is a modest reduction in functional residual capacity (FRC), particularly in the supine posture.[30,31] Introduction of fluid into the abdomen increases the length of the diaphragm

acutely, and this results in an increase in maximum inspiratory and transdiaphragmatic pressures at the smaller FRC.[31] No acute changes are seen in CO uptake.[30] Unlike haemodialysis, CAPD is not associated with deceases in PaO_2.[29]

22.4 CHRONIC RENAL FAILURE AND SLEEP-DISORDERED BREATHING

Uraemia is commonly associated with daytime sleepiness, disturbed sleep, reduced sleep efficiency, sleep fragmentation and decreased slow-wave sleep.[32] There is also a high prevalence of sleep-disordered breathing (SDB) in end-stage renal disease, but the strength of any cause and effect relationship is uncertain. Estimates of the prevalence of SDB vary considerably in different studies, with values between 30 per cent and 70 per cent of patients quoted,[4] the prevalence depending on case selection and the criteria used for recognition of SDB. A study of unselected patients with end-stage renal disease suggested that about 16 per cent had both SDB and attributable symptoms.[33] Comparison with community controls matched for body mass index (BMI) and age has confirmed that the high prevalence is not artefactual.[34] Most reports have been in patients undergoing haemodialysis, but SDB is also common in patients with chronic renal failure who are not receiving replacement therapy.[35,36] Most studies show mainly obstructive apnoea,[4,36,37] although predominantly central apnoea has also been reported,[32] as well as an approximately even distribution of obstructive, central and 'mixed' events.[38]

Various potential mechanisms for the high prevalence of SDB in chronic renal failure have been suggested. Some may predispose to obstructive events, others to central events and some potentially to both (Table 22.2). As discussed in Chapter 18, Section 18.2.1.4, the factors predisposing to both obstructive and central events are sometimes related, as fluctuating central respiratory drive influences the activity of the upper airway dilator muscles and consequently the propensity to airway narrowing or collapse. The compliance of the upper airway is likely to be increased (i.e. the airway to be more 'floppy') in the presence of fluid retention and oedema, while the function of the airway dilator muscles

Table 22.2 Potential contributors to sleep-disordered breathing in chronic renal failure

Promoting central apnoea
↑ Ventilatory responses (high 'loop gain')
Low Pa_{CO_2}
Promoting obstructive apnoea
Upper airway oedema
Uraemic myopathy
Promoting central and obstructive apnoea
Autonomic neuropathy
Coexistent cardiac disease

themselves might be impaired by uraemia, which is known to affect skeletal muscle function elsewhere. Some, though not all, data suggest that respiratory chemosensitivity is heightened in chronic renal failure.[39] The consequent high 'loop gain' (see Chapter 6, Section 6.2.1) would tend to increase ventilatory instability, especially in the face of a low Pa_{CO_2}. The frequency of obstructive apnoeas correlates, albeit weakly, with deteriorating renal function,[36,37] while central apnoeas are more likely with lower Pa_{CO_2},[37] as might be expected as the prevailing arterial P_{CO_2} approaches the 'apnoea threshold' (see Chapter 6, Section 6.2.1).

Sleep-disordered breathing improves with nocturnal haemodialysis but is little affected by diurnal dialysis;[38] it also resolves after successful renal transplantation.[40]

22.5 GOODPASTURE'S SYNDROME

Serial estimation of D_LCO and K_{CO} to detect pulmonary haemorrhage has proved of clinical value in Goodpasture's (antiglomerular basement membrane) syndrome.[41] Increased CO uptake, however, is not specific for Goodpasture's syndrome as it also occurs in other conditions associated with lung haemorrhage.[42] The normal clearance mechanism for red blood cells shed in alveolar spaces is engulfment by alveolar macrophages, and only when this route is saturated does haemoptysis occur. Considerable alveolar haemorrhage may therefore occur without frank haemoptysis (unlike bronchial bleeding, where the ciliary 'escalator' operates and allows recognition of much smaller bleeds). Peripheral bleeding can be detected by finding haemosiderin-laden macrophages in the sputum or

in alveolar lavage fluid,[43] while overt haemoptysis is less sensitive than other indices, such as radiographic shadowing, a fall in [Hb] or a rise in K_{CO}. By simultaneously measuring the uptake and clearance of radioactively labelled $C^{15}O$, Ewan et al. showed that rises in K_{CO} in Goodpasture's syndrome were due to stagnant blood.[41] The clearance of CO from the lungs, estimated by external counting, was delayed, while uptake was increased due to the extravasated red cells that remained within the counting area. Sequential measurements with the standard single-breath technique alone have proved useful indicators of bleeding episodes without the need for isotopic measurements. Major episodes of alveolar haemorrhage are accompanied by a restrictive ventilatory defect and worsening hypoxaemia.[43] The K_{CO} is more sensitive to haemorrhage than is the total D_LCO because the reduction in alveolar volume caused by haemorrhage will counter any tendency for D_LCO to rise. It is important to correct the measurements for haemoglobin concentration – a simultaneous estimate is desirable because of rapid changes in [Hb] when haemorrhage occurs. Many patients with Goodpasture's syndrome have chronic uraemia, with the result that the baseline CO uptake may be low and, consequently, a significant rise in K_{CO} (e.g. 50%) may still result in a value in the normal range. Consequently a rise and fall of K_{CO} is more specific for pulmonary haemorrhage than a single high value. After an episode of pulmonary haemorrhage, the K_{CO} usually declines over a few days.[42]

REFERENCES

1 Stanescu DC, Veriter C, De Plaen JF, et al. Lung function in chronic uraemia before and after removal of excess fluid by haemodialysis. *Clin Sci* 1974; **47**: 143–51.
2 Bush A, Gabriel R. Pulmonary function in chronic renal failure: effects of dialysis and transplantation. *Thorax* 1991; **46**: 424–8.
3 Chan CH, Lai CK, Li PK, et al. Effect of renal transplantation on pulmonary function in patients with end-stage renal failure. *Am J Nephrol* 1996; **16**: 144–8.
4 Markou NK, Athanasiou M, Hroni D, Myrianthefs PM. Disorders of respiration and sleep-disordered breathing in patients with chronic renal failure. *Curr Respir Med Rev* 2006; **2**: 405–17.

5   Zidulka A, Despas PH, Milic Emili J, Anthonisen NR. Pulmonary function with acute loss of excess lung water by haemodialysis in patients with chronic uraemia. *Am J Med* 1973; **55**: 134–41.

6   Lee HY, Stretton TB, Barnes AB. The lungs in renal failure. *Thorax* 1975; **30**: 46–53.

7   Cowie J, Lambie AT, Robson JS. The influence of extracorporeal dialysis on the acid–base composition of blood and cerebrospinal fluid. *Clin Sci* 1962; **23**: 397–404.

8   Pauli HG, Reidwil H, Reubi F, Wegmuller W. H^+ and renal failure as factors in uraemic hyperventilation. *Clin Sci* 1963; **25**: 37–41.

9   Hamilton RW, Epstein PE, Henderson LW, *et al.* Control of breathing in uraemia: ventilatory response to CO_2 after haemodialysis. *J Appl Physiol* 1976; **41**: 216–22.

10   Moinard J, Guenard H. Membrane diffusion of the lungs in patients with chronic renal failure. *Eur Respir J* 1993; **6**: 225–30.

11   Herrero JA, Alvarez-Sala JL, Coronel F, *et al.* Pulmonary diffusing capacity in chronic dialysis patients. *Respir Med* 2002; **96**: 487–92.

12   Yigla M, Nakhoul F, Sabag A, *et al.* Pulmonary hypertension in patients with end-stage renal disease. *Chest* 2003; **123**: 1577–82.

13   Bark H, Heimer D, Chaimowitz C, Mostoslowski M. Effect of chronic renal failure on respiratory muscle strength. *Respiration* 1988; **54**: 151–63.

14   Siafakas NM, Argyrakopoulos T, Andreopoulos K, *et al.* Respiratory muscle strength during continuous ambulatory peritoneal dialysis (CAPD). *Eur Respir J* 1995; **8**: 109–13.

15   Mayer G, Thum J, Graf H. Anaemia and reduced exercise capacity in patients on chronic haemodialysis. *Clin Sci* 1989; **76**: 265–8.

16   Ulubay G, Akman B, Sezer S, *et al.* Factors affecting exercise capacity in renal transplantation candidates on continuous ambulatory peritoneal dialysis therapy. *Transplant Proc* 2006; **38**: 401–5.

17   Marrades RM, Roca J, Campistol JM, *et al.* Effects of erythropoietin on muscle O_2 transport during exercise in patients with chronic renal failure. *J Clin Invest* 1996; **97**: 2092–100.

18   McMahon LP, McKenna MJ, Sangkabutra T, *et al.* Physical performance and associated electrolyte changes after haemoglobin normalisation: a comparative study in haemodialysis patients. *Nephrol Dial Transplant* 1999; **14**: 1182–7.

19   Aurigemma NM, Feldman NT, Gottlieb M, *et al.* Arterial oxygenation during haemodialysis. *N Engl J Med* 1977; **297**: 871–3.

20   De Baker WA, Heyrman RM, Withesaele WM, *et al.* Ventilation and breathing patterns during haemodialysis-induced carbon dioxide unloading. *Am Rev Respir Dis* 1987; **136**: 406–10.

21   Munger MA, Ateshkadi A, Cheung AK, *et al.* Cardiopulmonary events during hemodialysis: effects of dialysis membranes and dialysate buffers. *Am J Kidney Dis* 2000; **36**: 130–39.

22   Craddock PR, Fehr H, Brigham KL, *et al.* Complement and leucocyte–mediated pulmonary dysfunction in haemodialysis. *N Engl J Med* 1977; **296**: 769–74.

23   Patterson RW, Nissenson AR, Miller J, *et al.* Hypoxaemia and pulmonary gas exchange during haemodialysis. *J Appl Physiol* 1981; **50**: 259–64.

24   Dumler R, Levin NW. Leucopoenia and hypoxaemia unrelated effects of haemodialysis. *Arch Intern Med* 1979; **139**: 1103–6.

25   Nissenson AR. Prevention of dialysis-induced hypoxaemia by bicarbonate dialysis. *Trans Am Soc Artif Intern Organs* 1980; **26**: 339–42.

26   Romaldini H, Rodriguez-Roisin R, Lopez FA, *et al.* The mechanisms of arterial hypoxaemia during haemodialysis. *Am Rev Respir Dis* 1984; **129**: 780–84.

27   Pitcher WD, Diamond SM, Heurich WL. Pulmonary gas exchange during dialysis in patients with obstructive lung disease. *Chest* 1989; **96**: 1136–41.

28   Peres-Serrano A, Fernandez-Vega F, Alvarez-Grande J. Hypoxaemia during haemodialysis in patients with impairment in pulmonary function. *Nephron* 1986; **42**: 14–18.

29   Singh S, Dale A, Morgan B, Salebjami H. Serial studies of pulmonary function in continuous ambulatory peritoneal dialysis. *Chest* 1984; **86**: 874–7.

30   Bush A, Miller J, Peacock AJ, *et al.* Some observations on the role of the abdomen in breathing in patients on peritoneal dialysis. *Clin Sci* 1985; **68**: 401–6.

31   Prezant DJ, Aldrich TK, Karpel JP, Lynn RI. Adaptations in the diaphragm's *in vivo* force–length relationship in patients on continuous ambulatory peritoneal dialysis. *Am Rev Respir Dis* 1990; **141**: 1342–9.

32   Mendelson WB, Wadhura NK, Greenberg HE, Gujavarty K, Bergofsky E. Effects of haemodialysis on sleep apnoea syndrome in end stage renal disease. *Clin Nephrol* 1990; **33**: 247–51.

33   Kuhlmann U, Becker HF, Birkhaun M, *et al.* Sleep-apnea in patients with end-stage renal disease and objective results. *Clin Nephrol* 2000; **53**: 460–66.

34   Unruh ML, Sanders MH, Redline S, *et al.* Sleep apnea in patients on conventional thrice-weekly hemodialysis: comparison with matched controls from the Sleep Heart Health Study. *J Am Soc Nephrol* 2006; **17**: 3503–9.

35 Kimmel PL, Miller G, Mendelson WB. Sleep apnoea syndrome in chronic renal disease. *Am J Med* 1989; **86**: 308–14.

36 Markou N, Kanakaki M, Myrianthefs P, *et al*. Sleep-disordered breathing in nondialyzed patients with chronic renal failure. *Lung* 2006; **184**: 43–9.

37 Tada T, Kusano KF, Ogawa A, *et al*. The predictors of central and obstructive sleep apnoea in haemodialysis patients. *Nephrol Dial Transplant* 2007; **22**: 1190–97.

38 Hanly PJ, Pierratos A. Improvement of sleep apnea in patients with chronic renal failure who undergo nocturnal hemodialysis. *N Engl J Med* 2001; **344**: 102–7.

39 Beecroft J, Duffin J, Pierratos A, *et al*. Enhanced chemo-responsiveness in patients with sleep apnoea and end-stage renal disease. *Eur Respir J* 2006; **28**: 151–8.

40 Langevin B, Fonque D, Léger P, Robert D. Sleep apnoea syndrome and end-stage renal disease: cure after transplantation. *Chest* 1993; **103**: 1330–35.

41 Ewan PW, Jones HA, Rhodes CG, Hughes JMB. Detection of intrapulmonary haemorrhage with carbon monoxide uptake. *N Engl J Med* 1976; **295**: 1391–6.

42 Greening AP, Hughes JMB. Serial estimations of carbon monoxide diffusing capacity in intrapulmonary haemorrhage. *Clin Sci* 1981; **60**: 507–12.

43 Lazor R, Bigay-Game L, Cottin V, *et al*. Alveolar hemorrhage in anti-basement membrane antibody disease: a series of 28 cases. *Medicine* 2007; **86**: 181–93.

23

Hepatic and Bowel Disease

23.1 HEPATIC DISEASE

Evaluation of respiratory function in patients with liver disease is often complicated by confounding factors, in particular the strong association between alcoholic cirrhosis and smoking. Consequently airway obstruction in a patient with liver disease is likely to be due to smoking and not to liver disease. However, epidemiological evidence suggests that alcohol consumption per se can affect spirometric volumes, and it is associated with accelerated decline of FEV_1 and VC even after allowing for the effects of smoking.[1,2]

23.1.1 Effects of ascites

The presence of ascites can restrict lung expansion and thus reduce lung volumes; in particular, functional residual capacity (FRC) is likely to be reduced.[3–5] However, the overall restrictive defect may be only modest as the net effect of abdominal fluid depends on a balance between the deflationary effect on the lungs and an inflationary effect on the lower ribs due to stretching of the diaphragm.[6] The pressure-generating capacity of the diaphragm and other inspiratory muscles is usually preserved, although the load on the inspiratory muscles is increased, with greater than normal tidal swings of pleural and transdiaphragmatic pressures.[7]

After removal of abdominal fluid, by either paracentesis or intensive diuretic treatment, lung volumes increase[3–5] and tidal pleural pressure swings are reduced.[7] There may be an accompanying small increase in arterial P_{O_2}.[8] The carbon

monoxide diffusing capacity (D_LCO) increases a little, while KCO shows a decrease,[4] as might be expected after removing an extrapulmonary cause of volume restriction.

23.1.2 Chronic liver disease

The most frequent abnormality of respiratory function in patients with chronic liver disease is a reduction in D_LCO, which is present in the majority of patients with advanced disease even after correction for haemoglobin concentration.[9,10] Typically, KCO is also reduced.

Most interest in the respiratory function of patients with chronic liver disease has centred on hypoxaemia, which can be profound. The 'cyanosed cirrhotic' was first described in 1884, and the mechanisms of hypoxaemia have been a topic of considerable interest and research. Most patients with hepatic cirrhosis have values of PaO_2 within the normal range[11,12] but, because arterial P_{CO_2} is usually reduced with advanced liver disease,[13] the alveolar–arterial oxygen gradient ($AaPO_2$) is abnormally increased in many more[14,15] – up to 60 per cent of patients with severe cirrhosis in one series.[14] The stimulus to ventilation that results in the characteristic hypocapnia and respiratory alkalosis is uncertain.[11] Overall there is a weak correlation between reduction in PaO_2 and more severe cirrhosis as assessed using standard histological criteria.[15,16]

Hypoxaemia in liver disease results essentially from abnormal function of the pulmonary vasculature, and two distinct syndromes have been described: the hepatopulmonary syndrome (HPS) associated with vascular dilatation, and the less common portopulmonary hypertension with vaso-constriction.

23.1.2.1 Hepatopulmonary syndrome

Definition

Hepatopulmonary syndrome is defined as impaired arterial oxygenation resulting from intrapulmonary vascular dilatation associated with hepatic disease.[17] It is seen with hepatic cirrhosis, irrespective of cause, and, less commonly, with chronic viral hepatitis.[18] Estimates of the prevalence of HPS vary with the population studied and with the precise quantitative criteria used to define hypoxaemia. For example, if $AaPO_2$ is used as the functional criterion, the proportion affected is appreciably greater than when arterial PO_2 alone is used.[15] A taskforce of the European Respiratory Society recommended as the criterion an $AaPO_2$ greater than 15 mmHg (2 kPa), or greater than 20 mmHg (2.7 kPa) in elderly people. In most series of advanced liver disease, e.g. among patients awaiting transplantation, a prevalence of HPS around 20 per cent is quoted but values as high as 50 per cent are found if the $AaPO_2$ criterion is used.[13] Similarly, in chronic viral hepatitis the prevalence is between 1 per cent and 10 per cent, depending on the precise definition.[18] Not surprisingly, clinically significant symptoms such as breathlessness are more likely if stricter criteria are applied. It seems likely that the milder degrees of hypoxaemia seen in patients without respiratory symptoms result from similar, but less marked, changes in the small pulmonary vessels to those in the full-blown syndrome.

Pathogenesis

The fundamental pathological abnormality associated with hypoxaemia and HPS is abnormal vascular dilatation, affecting mainly the pulmonary capillaries. Gross dilatation has sometimes been found, with capillary diameters up to 100 μm compared with the normal 7–15 μm.[19] Vasodilatation is not attributable to the passive effect of increased blood flow; it is presumably mediated chemically, although the mechanism has not been clarified. It probably results from failure of production of or metabolism by the liver of one or more vasoactive substances.

Functional mechanisms

Three main, interrelated functional mechanisms contribute to hypoxaemia in chronic liver disease. These comprise ventilation/perfusion ($\dot{V}_A/\dot{Q}$) mismatching, intrapulmonary shunt (which may be either 'anatomical' or 'physiological') and limitation of diffusion of oxygen. Portopulmonary shunts are also recognized in cirrhosis, but the relatively high oxygen content of portal venous blood makes it unlikely that they would contribute significantly to arterial desaturation. Studies using the multiple inert gas elimination technique (MIGET) have shown mild to moderate $\dot{V}_A/\dot{Q}$ inequality due to increased perfusion of lung units with low $\dot{V}_A/\dot{Q}$ ratios.[20] Shunts have been demonstrated by three different techniques: (i) bubble contrast echocardiography; (ii) macroaggregate perfusion scanning showing uptake in other organs such as the kidneys; and (iii) the classic physiological method with arterial blood sampling after a period of breathing 100 per cent oxygen. Contrast echocardiography is the most sensitive, but is essentially qualitative rather than quantitative.[21] It may show evidence of right-to-left shunting even in patients with early cirrhosis and normoxaemia.[22] Unlike the situation with a direct right-to-left shunt (such as atrial septal defect), bubbles do not appear immediately in the left ventricle after peripheral venous injection but in HPS are delayed for about three cardiac cycles.

Perfusion scanning with counting over the kidneys (assuming a normal proportion of the cardiac output perfuses the kidneys) is less sensitive but allows the severity of the shunt to be quantified.[23] The perfusion scan image of the lungs in cirrhosis is often unusually faint because the shunted macroaggregate particles bypass the lungs and are deposited in other organs. An unusual pattern of pulmonary activity accumulating gradually over several minutes has also been noted and is due to recirculation of the isotope after passage through anastomoses in other organs. The perfusion scanning method consistently gives larger shunt values than the classic 100 per cent oxygen breathing technique.[19,23–25] In this respect the pattern is different from that seen in individuals with large pulmonary arteriovenous malformations (AVMs), where the two techniques agree well (see Chapter 15, Section 15.5.2). The apparent discrepancy tends to increase with size of the shunt (Fig. 23.1).

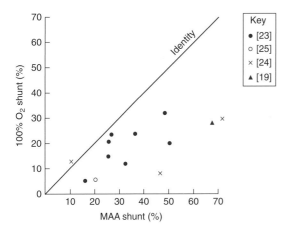

Figure 23.1 Comparison of estimates of per cent shunt using 100 per cent oxygen and radiolabelled albumin macroaggregates (MAA shunt) in individuals with hepatopulmonary syndrome from four published studies.[19,23–25] The shunt estimated by MAA infusion is generally larger than that calculated by breathing 100 per cent oxygen and the difference tends to increase with size of the shunt.

It has been suggested that the difference relates to the size of the dilated vessels, as, when these are very large, as with AVMs, the 'path length' for oxygen diffusion is increased sufficiently to limit complete equilibration. In this situation, both techniques would give similar estimates of the shunt. On the other hand, with less severe dilatation, the vessels may still be sufficiently large to allow passage of the macroaggregates into the systemic circulation, but not too large to prevent equilibration when breathing 100 per cent oxygen; consequently an 'anatomical' shunt will be recognized by the former method but not by the latter.[23]

A characteristic feature of patients with hepatic cirrhosis is an increased cardiac output and therefore a high total pulmonary blood flow. This tends to mitigate the effects of $\dot{V}_A/\dot{Q}$ mismatching, but at the same time it exaggerates 'anatomical' shunting due to more rapid passage of red blood cells through the dilated pulmonary capillaries, allowing less time for equilibration with alveolar gas. Orthodeoxia is very common in patients with HPS and falls in oxygen saturation of 10 per cent or more are not unusual.[23,26] This results from worsening matching of ventilation to perfusion (and to diffusion) when blood flow to the basal regions of the lungs increases in the upright position due to the effects of gravity amplified by the reduced pulmonary vascular tone.[26]

Effects of hepatic transplantation

Several studies have investigated the effects of hepatic transplantation on respiratory function and in particular on HPS. Indeed, severe hypoxaemia itself is an indication for transplantation, although a very low arterial P_{O_2} increases the mortality of the procedure.[27] The abnormal pulmonary gas exchange appears to be completely reversible after transplantation with normalization of oxygenation[13] and an increase in Pa_{CO_2}; the latter is seen even in individuals with normal oxygenation pre-transplantation.[28] On the other hand, the reduction of $D_L{CO}$ persists after transplantation.[13,29] The reduced CO uptake is not understood fully; it is not, in general, attributable to interstitial lung disease.[29] Although lower on average in patients with HPS compared with other severe liver disease, it is too frequently abnormal for use as a screening method to exclude HPS.[30]

23.1.2.2 Exercise in chronic liver disease

Exercise capacity is frequently limited in patients with advanced cirrhosis. The most marked effects are seen in patients with HPS in whom desaturation during exercise is characteristic, probably reflecting greater impairment of oxygen diffusion due to the combination of lower mixed venous (pulmonary arterial) P_{O_2} and more rapid transit through the pulmonary capillaries.[23] Myopathy and cardiac dysfunction may contribute in some individuals, but these are generally insufficient to account for the reduction in $\dot{V}_{O_2}$max and the abnormal pulmonary circulation is of greater relevance.[31]

23.1.2.3 Breathing during sleep in chronic liver disease

Obstructive sleep apnoea has been reported in more advanced cirrhosis and appears to be particularly associated with autonomic dysfunction.[32] Although hypocapnia is frequent in chronic liver disease, it is much less likely to provoke unstable respiratory control and central sleep apnoea than in patients with cardiac failure.[33]

23.1.2.4 Portopulmonary hypertension

The combination of pulmonary hypertension with portal hypertension is well recognized in patients with advanced liver disease but is less common than HPS.[27] As with pulmonary hypertension of other aetiology, it is associated with a reduced D_LCO, hyperventilation with a low $PaCO_2$, and mild or moderate hypoxaemia with an increased $AaPO_2$ gradient. The severity of hypoxaemia is usually much less than in the HPS, but occasionally more severe hypoxaemia due to right-to-left shunting via a patent foramen ovale is seen and can cause diagnostic confusion.[34]

23.2 INFLAMMATORY BOWEL DISEASE

Mild abnormalities of respiratory function have been described in many series of patients with inflammatory bowel disease. In general, the functional abnormalities are similar in ulcerative colitis and Crohn's disease.[35] Clinically, the most frequently encountered respiratory syndrome is a chronic productive cough, sometimes with demonstrable bronchiectasis. Airway inflammation, with appearances similar to those found in the large bowel, has often been described on bronchial biopsy. Although airway obstruction is sometimes present in patients with frank bronchiectasis,[36] there is often little evidence of airway obstruction on conventional spirometric criteria. More specific assessment of small airway function, comparing maximum flow–volume curves while breathing air and a helium oxygen mixture, has been reported to show some evidence of small airway dysfunction.[37]

The most frequent abnormality of respiratory function is a reduction in D_LCO and sometimes also in KCO, features found in several unselected case control studies.[38,39] The frequency of abnormality tends to be greater in individuals with more active bowel disease.[35,40] The mechanism has not been clarified; it is not generally attributable to interstitial lung disease, at least as demonstrable on high-resolution computed tomography (CT) scanning,[40] nor to the drugs used to treat the bowel disease.[41]

In group comparisons between patients and control subjects small reductions in both FEV_1 and VC have sometimes been found,[39,41] but these are less consistent than the reduction in D_LCO. In one study the VC correlated with body mass index,[41] suggesting that a degree of respiratory muscle weakness may be contributory in some individuals.

REFERENCES

1 Lange P, Groth S, Mortensen J, et al. Pulmonary function is influenced by heavy alcohol consumption. Am Rev Respir Dis 1988; **137**: 1119–23.

2 Garshick E, Segal MR, Worobec TG, Salekin CMS, Miller MJ. Alcohol consumption and chronic obstructive pulmonary disease. Am Rev Respir Dis 1989; **140**: 373–8.

3 Angueira CE, Kadakia SC. Effects of large-volume paracentesis on pulmonary function in patients with tense cirrhotic ascites. Hepatology 1994; **20**: 825–8.

4 Chao Y, Wang SS, Lee SD, et al. Effect of large-volume paracentesis on pulmonary function in patients with cirrhosis and tense ascites. J Hepatol 1994; **20**: 101–5.

5 Chang SC, Chang HI, Chen FJ, et al. Therapeutic effects of diuretics and paracentesis on lung function in patients with non-alcoholic cirrhosis and tense ascites. J Hepatol 1997; **26**: 833–8.

6 Hanson CA, Ritter AB, Duran W, Lavietes MH. Ascites: its effect upon static inflation of the respiratory system. Am Rev Respir Dis 1990; **142**: 39–42.

7 Duranti R, Laffi G, Misuri G, et al. Respiratory mechanics in patients with tense cirrhotic ascites. Eur Respir J 1997; **10**: 1622–30.

8 Gupta D, Lalrothuama, Agrawal PN, et al. Pulmonary function changes after large volume paracentesis. Trop Gastroenterol 2000; **21**: 68–70.

9 Hourani JM, Bellamy PE, Tashkin DP, Batra P, Simmons MS. Pulmonary dysfunction in advanced liver disease: frequent occurrence of an abnormal diffusing capacity. Am J Med 1991; **90**: 693–700.

10 Mohamed R, Freeman JW, Guest PJ, Davies MK, Neuberger JM. Pulmonary gas exchange abnormalities in liver transplant candidates. Liver Transplant 2002; **8**: 802–8.

11 Krowka MJ, Dickson ER, Wiesner RH, et al. A prospective study of pulmonary function and gas exchange following liver transplantation. Chest 1992; **102**: 1161–6.

12 Rodriguez-Roisin R, Agusti AGN, Roca J. The hepatopulmonary syndrome: new name, old complexities. Thorax 1992; **47**: 897–902.

13 Battaglia SE, Pretto JJ, Irving LB, Jones RM, Angus PW. Resolution of gas exchange abnormalities and intrapulmonary shunting following liver transplantation. Hepatology 1997; **25**: 1228–32.

14 Colle I, Langlet P, Barriere E, *et al*. Evolution of hypoxemia in patients with severe cirrhosis. *J Gastroenterol Hepatol* 2002; **17**: 1106–9.

15 Schenk P, Fuhrmann V, Madi C, *et al*. Hepatopulmonary syndrome: prevalence and predictive value of various cut offs for arterial oxygenation and their clinical consequences. *Gut* 2002; **51**: 853–9.

16 Vachiery F, Moreau R, Hadengue A, *et al*. Hypoxaemia in patients with cirrhosis: relationship with liver failure and haemodynamic alterations. *J Hepatol* 1997; **27**: 492–5.

17 Rodriguez-Roisin R, Krowka MJ, Herve P, *et al*. Pulmonary–hepatic vascular disorders (PHD). *Eur Respir J* 2004; **24**: 861–80.

18 Teuber G, Teupe C, Dietrich CF, *et al*. Pulmonary dysfunction in non-cirrhotic patients with chronic viral hepatitis. *Eur J Intern Med* 2002; **13**: 311–18.

19 Davis HH, Schwartz DJ, Lefrak SS, Susman N, Schainker BA. Alveolar–capillary oxygen dysequilibrium in hepatic cirrhosis. *Chest* 1978; **73**: 507–11.

20 Rodriguez-Roisin R, Roca J, Agusti AG, *et al*. Gas exchange and pulmonary vascular reactivity in patients with liver cirrhosis. *Am Rev Respir Dis* 1987; **135**: 1085–92.

21 Abrams GA, Jaffe CC, Hoffer PB, Binder HJ, Fallon MB. Diagnostic utility of contrast echocardiography and lung perfusion scan in patients with hepatopulmonary syndrome. *Gastroenterology* 1995; **109**: 1283–8.

22 Mimidis KP, Karatza C, Spiropoulos KV, *et al*. Prevalence of intrapulmonary vascular dilatations in normoxaemic patients with early liver cirrhosis. *Scand J Gastroenterol* 1998; **33**: 988–92.

23 Whyte MK, Hughes JM, Peters AM, *et al*. Analysis of intrapulmonary right to left shunt in the hepatopulmonary syndrome. *J Hepatol* 1998; **29**: 85–93.

24 Wolfe JD, Tashkin DP, Holly FE, Brachman MB, Genovesi MG. Hypoxemia of cirrhosis. *Am J Med* 1977; **83**: 746–54.

25 Kalra S, Pandit A, Taylor PM, Prescott MC, Woodcock AA. Concealed intrapulmonary shunting in liver disease. *Respir Med* 1994; **88**: 545–7.

26 Gomez FP, Martinez-Palli G, Barbera JA, *et al*. Gas exchange mechanism of orthodeoxia in hepatopulmonary syndrome. *Hepatology* 2004; **40**: 660–66.

27 Krowka MJ. Hepatopulmonary syndrome versus portopulmonary hypertension: distinctions and dilemmas. *Hepatology* 1997; **25**: 1282–4.

28 Rassiat E, Barriere E, Durand F, *et al*. Pulmonary hemodynamics and gas exchange after liver transplantation in patients with cirrhosis. *Dig Dis Sci* 2002; **47**: 746–9.

29 Ewert R, Mutze S, Schachschal G, Lochs H, Plauth M. High prevalence of pulmonary diffusion abnormalities without interstitial changes in long-term survivors of liver transplantation. *Transplant Intern* 1999; **12**: 222–8.

30 Lima BL, Franca AV, Pazin-Filho A, *et al*. Frequency, clinical characteristics, respiratory parameters of hepatopulmonary syndrome. *Mayo Clin Proc* 2004; **79**: 42–8.

31 Epstein SK, Zilberberg MD, Jacoby C, *et al*. Response to symptom-limited exercise in patients with the hepatopulmonary syndrome. *Chest* 1998; **114**: 736–41.

32 Ogata T, Nomura M, Nakaya Y, Ito S. Evaluation of episodes of sleep apnea in patients with liver cirrhosis. *J Med Invest* 2006; **53**: 159–66.

33 Javaheri S, Almoosa KF, Saleh K, Mendenhall CL. Hypocapnia is not a predictor of central sleep apnea in patients with cirrhosis. *Am J Respir Crit Care Med* 2005; **171**: 908–11.

34 Raffy O, Sleiman C, Vachiery F, *et al*. Refractory hypoxemia during liver cirrhosis. Hepatopulmonary syndrome or 'primary' pulmonary hypertension? *Am J Respir Crit Care Med* 1996; **153**: 1169–71.

35 Tzanakis N, Bouros D, Samiou M, *et al*. Lung function in patients with inflammatory bowel disease. *Respir Med* 1998; **92**: 516–22.

36 Butland RJA, Cole P, Citron KM, Turner-Warwick M. Chronic bronchial suppuration and inflammatory bowel disease. *Q J Med* 1981; **50**: 63–75.

37 Tzanakis N, Samiou M, Bouros D, *et al*. Small airways function in patients with inflammatory bowel disease. *Am J Respir Crit Care Med* 1998; **157**: 382–6.

38 Kuzela L, Vavrecka A, Prikazska M, *et al*. Pulmonary complications in patients with inflammatory bowel disease. *Hepatogastroenterology* 1999; **46**: 1714–19.

39 Herrlinger KR, Noftz MK, Dalhoff K, *et al*. Alterations in pulmonary function in inflammatory bowel disease are frequent and persist during remission. *Am J Gastroenterol* 2002; **97**: 377–81.

40 Marvisi M, Borrello PD, Brianti M, *et al*. Changes in the carbon monoxide diffusing capacity of the lung in ulcerative colitis. *Eur Respir J* 2000; **16**: 965–8.

41 Mohamed-Hussein AAR, Mohamed NAS, Ibrahim ME. Changes in pulmonary function in patients with ulcerative colitis. *Respir Med* 2007; **101**: 977–82.

24

Metabolic and Endocrine Disorders

24.1 OBESITY

The rapidly increasing prevalence of obesity in many countries has increased our appreciation of its effects on respiratory function. Although in the majority of obese individuals the results of conventional tests are within normal limits, epidemiological studies and sequential data in patients who have undergone weight-reduction (bariatric) surgery show that obesity can have more marked effects than previously appreciated.

24.1.1 Effects on respiratory mechanics and lung volumes

Obesity is associated with an overall reduction in the compliance of the respiratory system due to reduced distensibility of both the lungs and chest wall.[1] In addition, respiratory muscle function may be compromised, with a modest reduction of strength, as assessed by maximum respiratory pressures, and a more marked effect on respiratory muscle endurance.[2] Consequently, in obese individuals, the mechanical load imposed on the muscles is increased in the face of some impairment of their capacity.

Severe obesity causes a typical restrictive ventilatory defect. In general, VC, TLC and RV decrease progressively and in approximately linear fashion across the range of body mass index (BMI) from 20

to 40+, even though most individual values remain within the conventional normal ranges until BMI exceeds $40 \, \mathrm{kg \, m^{-2}}$ (Fig. 24.1).[3] The effects of obesity on functional residual capacity (FRC) and expiratory reserve volume (ERV) are, however, more profound and are evident even with milder degrees of obesity. The relations of FRC and ERV

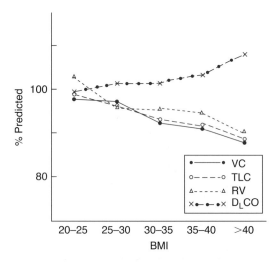

Figure 24.1 Average effects of body mass index (BMI) on lung volumes and carbon monoxide diffusing capacity ($D_L{\small CO}$) in individuals with no evidence of cardiopulmonary disease. Data from ref. 3.

Source: RV, residual volume; TLC, total lung capacity; VC, vital capacity.

to BMI are exponential[3] rather than linear, with a relatively greater effect seen with only mild or moderate obesity (Fig. 24.2).

Obesity affects the relaxation volume of the respiratory system because of the effects of abdominal weight on the position of the diaphragm. Consequently, FRC is reduced and ERV falls markedly as, with increasing weight, FRC approaches RV. Tidal breathing therefore takes place over a lower operational volume range than in non-obese individuals; this has important consequences for both airway function and pulmonary gas exchange (see below). The reduced compliance of the respiratory system also constrains the tidal volume, resulting in the relatively inefficient breathing pattern for gas exchange of a rapid respiratory frequency, with consequent disproportionate ventilation of the irreducible anatomical dead space.

Epidemiological studies show that the effect of increasing weight on VC is greater in men than in women. This is likely to reflect the different patterns of distribution of fat in the two sexes, with accumulation of abdominal fat having a greater effect than fat elsewhere and tending to be greater in men than in women.[4–6] The relatively crude measurement of BMI also fails to distinguish between increases in fat mass and in fat-free mass. Potentially these have opposing effects on VC, as increasing fat-free mass is associated with greater

muscle bulk and the consequent greater strength tends to increase VC, whereas increasing percentage of body fat is associated with progressive reduction in VC.[7] Thus, for example, subscapular skin fold thickness (an index of percentage body fat) has been shown to correlate inversely with VC after adjusting for BMI.[8]

In non-obese people, FRC falls markedly with changing position from upright to supine. In obesity, however, the ERV is already greatly diminished in the upright position and, although FRC is lower when supine, the postural fall is less than in non-obese people.[9]

24.1.2 Airway function

Routine tests of airway function are usually normal in patients with obesity. In particular, the FEV_1/VC ratio is not reduced; on the contrary, because weight has a relatively greater effect on VC than on FEV_1,[4] FEV_1/VC tends to increase in proportion to the severity of obesity as reflected by the BMI.[8] Maximum expiratory flow at lower lung volumes, FEF_{25-75} and peak flow are all usually normal.[10,11]

Nevertheless, during tidal breathing, the airways of an obese individual are narrower than in non-obese people, simply due to the lower volume range employed. Shortness of breath and wheezing

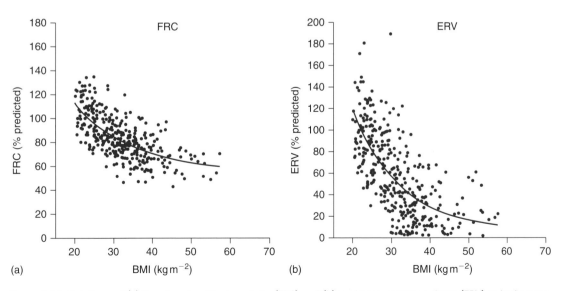

(a)   (b)

Figure 24.2 Relations of (a) functional residual capacity (FRC) and (b) expiratory reserve volume (ERV) to body mass index (BMI) in individuals with no evidence of cardiopulmonary disease. Modified from ref. 3 with permission from the American College of Chest Physicians.

are very common complaints of individuals with obesity, and obesity is recognized as a risk factor for self-reported asthma.[12] It is, however, likely that in many individuals the wheezing merely reflects breathing at low lung volumes[11] rather than asthma. Measurements of airway resistance/conductance have given somewhat variable results in obesity: some reports of specific airway conductance have shown normal values, i.e. conductance reduced (resistance increased) in proportion to the reduction in lung volume,[10] while others have suggested that airway conductance is low even in relation to the lower FRC, particularly in men.[13] Also, increased total respiratory resistance measured by forced oscillation in obese people is explained only partly by the lower operational (tidal) volume range.[9] The cause of these discrepancies is not known.

Breathing over a low operational lung volume range implies that the reserve of expiratory flow, i.e. the difference between tidal and maximal flow, is less than normal, which sets up the potential for expiratory flow limitation (EFL; see Chapter 1, Section 1.6.5.8). Expiratory flow limitation has been demonstrated using the negative pressure technique in some individuals with very severe obesity, particularly in the supine position (where the absolute volume range during tidal breathing is even lower), but also in a minority while seated at rest.[14] This phenomenon may be a contributor to the symptom of orthopnoea that is reported by many patients with severe obesity.

24.1.3 Pulmonary gas exchange and diffusing capacity

Obesity is associated with a high resting oxygen consumption out of proportion to the increased body weight.[15] In part, the disproportionately high $\dot{V}O_2$ is due to the increased oxygen cost of breathing resulting from the mechanical abnormalities, but it may also reflect inefficiency of the respiratory muscles due to the adiposity of the chest wall.[16] A reduced resting PaO_2 and widening of the alveolar–arterial PO_2 difference ($AaPO_2$) are commonly found.[17] Both the physiological shunt and the dead space/tidal volume ratio (V_D/V_T) are increased consistent with ventilation/perfusion $\dot{V}_A/\dot{Q}$ mismatching. The increased V_D/V_T also reflects the constrained tidal volume and hence

relatively larger fraction of the tidal volume ventilating the anatomical dead space. The $\dot{V}_A/\dot{Q}$ disturbance is demonstrable on a regional basis as basal ventilation is reduced, especially in those with a small ERV;[18] $\dot{V}_A/\dot{Q}$ mismatching within lung regions probably also contributes.[19] In the supine posture PaO_2 falls further and $AaPO_2$ increases in association with an increase in closing volume.[20]

The pulmonary capillary blood volume is increased in obesity[21] and, although the carbon monoxide diffusing capacity (D_LCO) is normal in the majority of subjects, it increases progressively with BMI (see Fig. 24.1).[3] Among the general population of patients undergoing pulmonary function tests, obesity is one of the commoner causes of a high D_LCO.[22] The KCO is more consistently increased,[19,23] as would be expected in the face of a potentially elevated overall D_LCO plus the effect of extrapulmonary volume restriction.

24.1.4 Ventilatory control and exercise

Ventilatory responses to both hypercapnia and hypoxia are often increased in obese individuals although, unusually, this is seen more consistently in obese women than in obese men.[24,25] Maximum work capacity and $\dot{V}O_2max$ are related inversely to BMI; with severe obesity, exercise may be markedly impaired, with values of $\dot{V}O_2max$ sometimes as low as those found in chronic congestive heart failure.[26]

24.1.5 Effects of bariatric surgery

In essence, successful bariatric surgery restores a more favourable ventilatory load/capacity ratio and leads to regression of most of the abnormalities described above towards normal values. In approximate proportion to the weight loss achieved, there are consistent increases in lung volumes, especially in FRC and ERV[23,27,28] and improvements in respiratory muscle function, both strength and endurance.[2] Arterial PO_2 increases,[27,28] and D_LCO and KCO both decline towards average normal values.[23] Ventilatory drive is reduced and responsiveness to chemical stimuli becomes more normal.[29] The frequency of apnoeas and hypopnoeas during sleep declines even in subjects without a frank sleep apnoea syndrome.[30]

24.2 OBESITY–HYPOVENTILATION SYNDROME

The obesity–hypoventilation syndrome (OHS) was first described 50 years ago as the 'Pickwickian syndrome', which identified an apparently rare condition in which extreme obesity was associated with chronic hypercapnic respiratory failure and cor pulmonale. This condition is no longer a rare curiosity but a common problem, the prevalence of which is inevitably increasing further in parallel with severe obesity in the general population. The current prevalence of OHS is not known but may be much greater than appreciated. In one study of unselected hospitalized patients with BMI greater than 35, otherwise unexplained hypercapnia was found in 31 per cent.[31]

The condition essentially defines a group of obese patients with chronic hypercapnia but no evidence of any primary disease of the lungs or thorax. Typically, patients tend to be more obese than most of those with the obstructive sleep apnoea syndrome (OSAS) alone (see Chapter 18, Section 18.2.1.1), who usually have a normal awake $PaCO_2$, although there is appreciable overlap between the two conditions. The BMI of patients with OHS usually (though not invariably) exceeds $40\,kg\,m^{-2}$, which puts affected individuals into the category of severe or morbid obesity. Chronic hypoxaemia and hypercapnia can lead to pulmonary hypertension, cor pulmonale and polycythaemia, which may further impair respiratory function and complicate the interpretation of test results.

24.2.1 Pathophysiology of obesity–hypoventilation syndrome

Obstructive sleep apnoea was first documented in patients with what would now be called OHS, and it was only subsequently appreciated that OSAS with normal daytime blood gases is much more common than OHS.

Three main patterns of sleep disordered breathing have been described in patients with OHS: (i) recurrent obstructive apnoeas and hypopnoeas; (ii) persistently increased upper airway resistance resulting in inspiratory flow limitation; and (iii) 'central' hypoventilation, i.e. a sustained reduction in ventilation unrelated to narrowing of the upper airway.[32] These types of sleep-disordered breathing are present to varying degrees in different individuals. The great majority (85–90%) of individuals with OHS have obstructive sleep apnoeas and/or hypopnoeas with an apnoea/hypopnoea index (AHI) of more than five events per hour of sleep, but a minority have apparently 'pure' hypoventilation without discrete events.[32,33] The prevalence of OHS among populations of patients with OSAS is usually between 10 per cent and 20 per cent, increasing to about 25 per cent in severe obesity.[34]

In a study of patients with OHS with no evidence of upper airway narrowing during sleep, average reductions in ventilation compared with the awake state were 25 per cent and 41 per cent in non-rapid-eye-movement (REM) and REM sleep respectively. The reduced ventilation was accompanied by a fall in oxygen saturation and an increase in transcutaneously measured PCO_2. This pattern is similar to the REM sleep-related desaturation seen in other conditions such as severe chronic obstructive pulmonary disease (COPD) or chest wall disease. In this series, the reduced ventilation was due entirely to a reduction in tidal volume.[35] Consequently alveolar ventilation would be reduced to a relatively greater extent because of the irreducible dead space.

The characteristic finding in patients with OHS that distinguishes them from individuals with uncomplicated OSAS is that the hypercapnia persists when awake. This implies that 'alveolar' ventilation (in the sense of the three-compartment model of gas exchange – see Chapter 2, Section 2.3.4) is reduced, although the limited measurements available[35] suggest that total awake ventilation is not necessarily reduced. Three mechanisms have been proposed as potential contributors to the sustained hypercapnia in these patients: (i) adverse respiratory mechanics due to the greatly increased mechanical load, with or without a reduction in capacity; (ii) a reduction in the central drive to breathe; and (iii) a consequence of the sleep-disordered breathing carried over into the awake state. In relation to the mechanics, apart from the load imposed by obesity per se (see Section 24.1.1), some data show that patients with OHS also have an unusually high upper airway resistance, not only when supine (as is seen in other patients with obesity and normocapnic OSAS) but also in the upright position.[36] Some patients with

OHS also have impaired respiratory muscle function as assessed by maximum inspiratory pressure,[35] but whether this is more marked than in eucapnic, similarly obese individuals is not clear.

Assessment of innate ventilatory responsiveness is difficult as measurements of the chemical drive to breathe are inevitably influenced by the prevailing P_{CO_2}. The slope of the response to CO_2, whether evaluated in terms of ventilation or mouth occlusion pressure ($P_{0.1}$), is less than normal and less than in eucapnic obese individuals. Also, responsiveness to CO_2 improves with treatment that corrects the hypercapnia.[37] However, it is not possible to draw firm conclusions about the causal direction of this relationship, as a chronically raised arterial P_{CO_2} inevitably reduces the ventilatory response to further increases in P_{CO_2}, due to attenuation of the stimulus (i.e. a smaller increase in hydrogen ion concentration for a given change in P_{CO_2}) in the face of a raised blood concentration of bicarbonate ions (see Chapter 5, Section 5.2.1). Consequently, whether hypercapnia results in reduced CO_2 responsiveness or vice versa becomes a circular argument, and imputation of cause and effect is not possible. The drive to breathe at rest, however, is greater than normal and similar to that found in other obese subjects without hypercapnia.[37]

During sleep, each apnoea is accompanied by a transient rise in arterial P_{CO_2}, which, over a period of time, may lead to gradual accumulation of bicarbonate ions in the blood. These would tend to blunt the ventilatory response to CO_2 and potentially, therefore, could result in sustained hypercapnia. Computer modelling of the situation suggests that this putative mechanism is a likely contributor to the development of chronic hypercapnia.[38]

24.2.2 Respiratory function awake and asleep

Lung volumes are reduced commensurate with the (usually severe) obesity. By definition, Pa_{CO_2} is elevated and therefore Pa_{O_2} breathing air is reduced. Arterial bicarbonate is increased and, in the chronic stable situation, the arterial pH is near normal. Acute presentation of patients with OHS is relatively common when a hitherto unrecognized situation has, for whatever reason, become unstable and patients present with acute decompensation of chronic hypercapnic respiratory failure.[39]

The clue to the diagnosis is often given by measurements of oxygenation during sleep, which show a low baseline saturation, on which is superimposed a variable rate of dips in Sa_{O_2}, depending on the AHI. In patients without significant upper airway obstruction there is more persistent desaturation, typically during REM sleep, when it may be profound. Inevitably, because of the shape of the haemoglobin–oxygen desaturation curve, the low awake Sa_{O_2} amplifies the reductions in Sa_{O_2} during sleep.

24.2.3 Treatment of obesity–hypoventilation syndrome

As with other extrapulmonary causes of hypercapnic respiratory failure, nocturnal non-invasive ventilation (NIV) is very effective and leads to correction of daytime arterial blood gases.[40] However, in many patients effective control of the problem can be achieved with the simpler technology of continuous positive airway pressure (CPAP), as used in non-hypercapnic individuals with OSAS. The majority of stable patients with a combination of OHS and OSAS are adequately treated using CPAP ab initio,[40,41] although some may require supplementary oxygen at night at first in order to raise Sa_{O_2} consistently above 90 per cent. When patients present with acute decompensation, NIV is often used initially, with or without oxygen, but oxygen can sometimes be withdrawn later and transition to CPAP is often sufficient to maintain control.[39] Whether, in the minority of patients without significant obstructive events, long-term NIV is necessary is not clear; even in the absence of upper airway obstruction, treatment with CPAP may aid oxygenation in such individuals by its inflationary effect on lung volume.

24.3 MALNUTRITION

The effects of malnutrition on respiratory function have been relatively little studied but they can be significant and the importance of poor nutritional status is doubtless underestimated or ignored in many patients. Malnutrition may exacerbate the functional effects of other conditions, particularly COPD[42] and cystic fibrosis.[43] One study that included many malnourished patients with malignant disease showed pronounced respiratory muscle weakness causing significant volume restriction.[44] The diameter of the respiratory muscle fibres is proportional to the severity of malnutrition, as assessed by body weight as a percentage of the ideal value,[45] but some evidence suggests that, in more severe undernutrition, respiratory muscle strength may be reduced disproportionately, perhaps due to an additional myopathic process.[44]

In malnutrition due to anorexia nervosa, maximum respiratory pressures are impaired,[46] although lung volumes are relatively normal, apart from an increase in residual volume,[46,47] which may be due to expiratory muscle weakness. $D_L CO$ is well preserved.[46] The ventilatory and mouth occlusion pressure responses to CO_2 stimulation are decreased.[47] Interestingly, even short periods of semi-starvation of healthy subjects can lead to reduction in the ventilatory response to hypoxia.[48] Whether these findings are related to respiratory muscle weakness or whether central respiratory control is depressed in malnourished patients is not clear. In either case there might be important clinical implications in relation to the consequences of intercurrent infections or other insults in malnourished individuals. Improvements in respiratory muscle function are demonstrable in critically ill malnourished individuals[49] and in COPD[50] after short-term parenteral nutrition.

More specific depletion of electrolytes may occur in some clinical situations: hypokalaemia is a well-recognized cause of generalized muscle weakness, but no specific studies of its effects on respiratory function are available. On the other hand, repletion of magnesium, another cation important for muscle contraction, in deficient individuals produces potentially significant improvements in maximum respiratory pressures.[51]

24.4 THYROID DISEASE

The most important link between thyroid disease and respiratory function is the influence of excess or lack of thyroid hormone on tissue metabolism and oxygen consumption. Classically, measurement of resting $\dot{V}O_2$ (basal metabolic rate) was the main diagnostic test for hyper- and hypothyroid states, but it fell into disuse with the advent of specific tests of thyroid function. A more relevant

modern application of respiratory function testing in thyroid disease is in recognition of compression of the central airway by a large goitre, especially when this extends retrosternally. Depending on the site of airway narrowing, a goitre may produce the characteristic maximum flow–volume curves of either extrathoracic or central intrathoracic airway narrowing (see Chapter 12, Section 12.1.2). Automated analysis of flow–volume curves may improve recognition of upper airway narrowing caused by a goitre.[52] More subtle abnormalities of pulmonary function are also associated with both hyper- and hypothyroidism.

24.4.1 Hyperthyroidism

24.4.1.1 Effects on respiratory mechanics

A reduced VC in thyrotoxicosis was first reported as long ago as 1917, and mild reductions, with average values in most series around 80 per cent of predicted, are found regularly.[53,54] The residual volume is usually somewhat increased, such that TLC is normal. The balance of evidence favours weakness of the respiratory muscles as the main mechanism of these abnormalities. Reductions in maximum respiratory pressures with improvements after treatment are regularly demonstrable.[54–57] The impairment of maximum pressures correlates with the level of circulating thyroid hormones[54] and with the strength of non-respiratory muscles.[55] Another possible contributor to the abnormal pulmonary mechanics in some patients is pulmonary vascular congestion. A reduction in lung compliance is demonstrable in many patients, with improvement after treatment,[53] but this would be compatible with either mechanism of volume reduction. The reduced lung distensibility may explain the well-recognized breathing pattern of hyperthyroid patients with small tidal volume and rapid frequency.

24.4.1.2 Effects on gas exchange

The $D_L CO$ is usually normal at rest, despite an increased pulmonary blood flow; the membrane (D_m) and capillary volume (V_c) components of $D_L CO$ have also been reported as normal.[58] The normal V_c has been quoted as evidence against vascular congestion as the main explanation of the abnormal mechanics, as also has the inability to influence V_c by the application of peripheral tourniquets with the aim of reducing the central blood volume.[58] The mechanical abnormalities are generally not sufficient to disturb gas exchange, so that arterial blood gases at rest are usually normal.

24.4.1.3 Resting ventilation and exercise performance

Resting ventilation is increased, partly because of the requirements of increased tissue metabolism and partly because of the inefficient breathing pattern, which, because of a small tidal volume, results in an abnormally large V_D/V_T ratio. Breathlessness on exertion is a common early complaint of patients with hyperthyroidism, and exercise ventilation is increased for several reasons (Fig. 24.3): first, the oxygen consumption at a given workload on exercise is increased; second, the inefficient breathing pattern is maintained on exercise and, because of the increased dead space ventilation, the total ventilation is excessive for the $\dot{V}_{O_2}$; and third, in some patients there is alveolar hyperventilation in addition, which results in a fall in Pa_{CO_2}.[59] Tachypnoea on exertion is particularly marked, but the relation of breathlessness to ventilation is similar to normal.[56,60] Exercise capacity and $\dot{V}_{O_2}$max are reduced, and the anaerobic threshold is reached at a lower-than-normal level of $\dot{V}_{O_2}$.[61] All aspects of exercise performance improve with restoration of the euthyroid state.[61]

24.4.1.4 Ventilatory drive

The ventilatory responses to CO_2 and hypoxia tend to be high and fall after treatment of hyperthyroidism.[62] On exercise in untreated patients the mouth occlusion pressure $(P_{0.1})$ for a given metabolic load is increased in proportion to the concentration of circulating thyroid hormone. The increased ventilatory drive is also reduced after treatment by β-receptor blockade, even without specific anti-thyroid treatment, suggesting that the effect is mediated by β-adrenergic stimulation.[60]

24.4.2 Hypothyroidism

24.4.2.1 Effects on respiratory mechanics

In many patients the effects of hypothyroidism are compounded by those of obesity, which often contributes to reduction in lung volumes. In the absence of severe obesity, VC is usually in the low normal range; respiratory muscle weakness is, however, often demonstrable, with reduced maximum respiratory pressures and marked improvement after treatment.[63] The reduction in maximum pressures is related to the severity of hypothyroidism, as assessed by measurement of circulating thyroid stimulating hormone.[63] It is not clear whether the weakness, which appears to be common, is primarily myopathic or neuropathic. Impaired phrenic nerve conduction velocity and slow maximum relaxation rate of the diaphragm have both been demonstrated.[64]

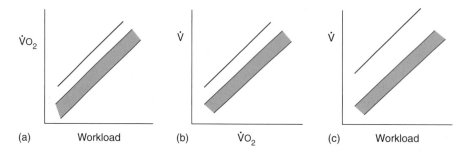

Figure 24.3 Schematic diagram of ventilation on exercise in hyperthyroidism compared with normal (shaded area). At any given workload, the oxygen consumption is greater than normal (a). At any given oxygen consumption, the ventilation is excessive (b), so that in relation to workload (c) the ventilation is greatly increased. Based on data from ref. 59.

The latter corresponds to the well-recognized clinical sign of slowly relaxing tendon reflexes.

24.4.2.2 Effects of gas exchange

Hypercapnia is well recognized in severe myxoedema,[65] and reduced ventilatory responsiveness may contribute to the development of respiratory failure.[66] With treatment of hypothyroidism, the $PaCO_2$ returns to normal rapidly, whereas respiratory muscle weakness recovers only slowly over several months.[64,65]

Some hypothyroid patients show a widened $AaPO_2$ that worsens on exercise, probably due to a combination of a reduced cardiac output and ventilation/perfusion mismatching.[67] The $\dot{V}O_2$max is reduced, even in individuals with subclinical hypothyroidism, and blood lactate on exercise is abnormally high.[68,69]

24.4.2.3 Hypothyroidism and sleep-disordered breathing

An association of hypothyroidism with OSAS is well recognized, but estimates of the strength of the association vary. Obstructive sleep apnoea, defined as AHI >5 and reversible by anti-thyroid treatment, has been reported in as many as 30 per cent of hypothyroid individuals.[70] On the other hand, in populations with OSAS, screening for hypothyroidism is reported positive in between 1 per cent and 9 per cent,[71–73] which may be little more than the prevalence in the non-apnoeic population.[73] Individuals with hypothyroidism and OSA tend to be older and heavier than the average hypothyroid patient. Improvement in the apnoea frequency with treatment of hypothyroidism can occur before significant loss of weight,[74] but resolution after control of thyroid function is not universal and some need continued treatment with CPAP.[75] The low oxygen consumption of patients with hypothyroidism may attenuate the falls in SaO_2 that result from apnoea; for this reason, correction of metabolic rate by thyroxine might initially exacerbate desaturation.[75] The potential mechanisms of OSA in hypothyroidism include deposition of mucoprotein in the tongue or upper airway wall and myopathy of the upper airway dilator muscles;[75] reduced central respiratory drive may also contribute.

24.5 PITUITARY DISEASE

Both excess and deficiency of growth hormone affect the size of many visceral organs, and the lungs are no exception. Both conditions may also be associated with sleep-disordered breathing.

24.5.1 Acromegaly

Increased lung volumes are often found in patients with acromegaly,[76–81] with values of TLC as large as 150 per cent predicted, especially in men. In general, increases are relatively less in affected females.[77,78] The subdivisions of lung volume are, in general, increased by a similar proportional amount. Anthropometry confirms increases in the anteroposterior diameter and circumference of the ribcage, which accommodates the enlarged lungs.[76]

Is the increase in lung volume mainly in alveolar number or size? Attempts have been made to answer this question by detailed analysis of the pressure–volume (PV) curve of the lungs using the index K obtained by fitting a monoexponential curve to the PV relationship (see Chapter 1, Section 1.2.2). K in effect represents a volume-independent index of alveolar distensibility and would be expected to increase with larger alveolar size. The results of different studies have, however, been conflicting, with one study reporting normal values (and therefore favouring an increased alveolar number)[79] and another showed abnormally high values (which would favour larger alveoli).[81]

Maximum respiratory pressures are reduced in many patients with acromegaly.[80] Although the reduction in $P_I$max might be attributable to the hyperinflation caused by large lungs, this would not account for a reduction in $P_E$max, which suggests a degree of muscle weakness.

Patients with acromegaly sometimes develop upper airway obstruction as a result of soft tissue enlargement in the pharynx or larynx or, less commonly, an enlarged goitre. Comparison of maximum mid-inspiratory and mid-expiratory flows suggested upper airway narrowing in half the patients in one series.[78] A reduction in maximum expiratory flow at small lung volumes has also been reported. However, this may not necessarily imply narrowing of the smaller airways, as it could result from disproportionate growth of the alveoli in relation to the bronchial tree.[82]

Arterial blood gases at rest are usually normal.[80] The $D_L CO$ is normal[79,81] or sometimes increased,[78] while $K CO$ is related inversely to TLC.[79]

An additional consequence of narrowing of the upper airway is the propensity to develop obstructive sleep apnoea, which is common in patients with acromegaly.[83–85] Not only is the pharyngeal lumen reduced in size when awake, but also it is abnormally collapsible.[84] Several factors contribute, including abnormal craniofacial bony structure[83] and enlargement of the tongue[85] and pharyngeal soft tissue. Successful treatment of growth hormone excess with octreotide has been shown to improve OSA, with a corresponding reduction in tongue volume demonstrable by magnetic resonance imaging (MRI).[85]

24.5.2 Hypopituitarism

Acquired deficiency of growth hormone in adults has been reported to produce a restrictive ventilatory defect with reductions in all the subdivisions of lung volume,[77,86] although some data show little effect.[87] Measurements of maximum pressures show no evidence of respiratory muscle weakness in patients with adult-onset growth hormone deficiency,[77,86] although this is demonstrable in adults who developed deficiency in childhood.[88] The single-breath $D_L CO$ is mildly reduced and pulmonary gas exchange is normal.[86] It appears likely, therefore, that the lungs may atrophy with deficiency of growth hormone in a manner complementary to the hypertrophy with its excess. Growth hormone replacement in deficient adults increases $\dot{V}O_2 max$ measured by progressive exercise testing, the improvement being attributed to increased lean body mass and perhaps to improved cardiac function.[89] One report found OSA to be common with growth hormone deficiency,[90] but the mechanism is not clear. Of potential therapeutic importance, growth hormone replacement was not associated with exacerbation of the OSA.[90]

24.6 DIABETES MELLITUS

Abnormal respiratory function in diabetes might be expected due to its consequences of glycosylation of connective tissue proteins and microangiopathy. Factors that influence respiratory function in diabetes include age, duration of disease, and the presence or absence of generalized microvascular disease or autonomic neuropathy. In general, the effects of diabetes on simple respiratory function tests are modest,[91] although their potential importance has been highlighted by the development of inhaled insulin as potential long-term treatment for some diabetic patients. Also of likely clinical relevance are the effects of diabetes on exercise function and breathing during sleep. Qualitatively the effects of type 1 and type 2 diabetes on respiratory function are similar, but the additional effects of coexisting obesity are more likely in the latter.

24.6.1 Effects on respiratory mechanics

Several recent large epidemiological studies have confirmed earlier data from small series suggesting mild reductions in FEV_1 and VC. Average reductions are of the order of only 10 per cent predicted but the effect is more marked in individuals with diabetes of long duration.[92] Overall, the rate of decline of spirometric volumes appears similar to that in the non-diabetic population,[93] but it is faster in those with less well-controlled diabetes.[94] Even among individuals not diagnosed with frank diabetes, epidemiological studies show inverse correlations between FEV_1 or VC and glucose intolerance,[95] raised blood insulin and insulin resistance.[96,97] These associations persist after adjusting for potential confounders, particularly age, BMI, the ratio of waist to hip circumference (an indirect estimate of abdominal obesity) and the level of habitual physical activity.[96]

The mechanism of the generally mild reductions in FEV_1 and VC is unclear. Respiratory muscle weakness does not appear to be an adequate explanation.[98] Changes in the elastic behaviour of the lungs have been suggested, possibly related to glycosylation of connective tissue proteins in the alveolar wall.[99] The shape factor, K, of the static PV curve has been reported variously to be increased[99] or normal,[100] implying that lung distensibility is normal or increased rather than reduced. Another proposed explanation relates to the elastic behaviour of the ribcage, as in one series the reduction of lung volumes was confined to subjects with general limitation of joint mobility.[101]

Airway function, at least as assessed by the ratio of FEV_1/VC, is usually normal in non-smoking diabetic individuals, but one study investigating small airway function by measurement of dynamic compliance suggested that this may be abnormal in some individuals.[102] In patients with complicating autonomic neuropathy, the bronchodilator response to an anticholinergic agent is less than in patients without neuropathy, suggesting diminished vagal tone in the former.[103]

24.6.2 Effects on carbon monoxide uptake

The $D_L CO$ has been reported variously to be either normal[104,105] or modestly reduced.[104,106,107] Similarly, measurements of $K CO$ have varied, with low,[99,108] normal[109] and raised[104] values reported. The last was in individuals with mildly reduced TLC and there was an inverse correlation between TLC and $K CO$, suggesting that the increase resulted from extrapulmonary restriction. Reductions in $D_L CO$ and/or $K CO$ have been shown to relate consistently to evidence of diabetic microangiopathy elsewhere, particularly in the retina or the kidneys.[105,106,108,110] Impairment of CO uptake is therefore likely to imply pulmonary diabetic microangiopathy, which has been demonstrated in post-mortem studies of diabetes.[111]

24.6.3 Ventilatory control and exercise performance

The presence of autonomic neuropathy in many patients with longstanding diabetes is likely to influence ventilatory control, but the available data are somewhat inconsistent, with both reduced[112] and increased[113] ventilatory responses to CO_2 described. The discrepancies in the literature may potentially be explained by divergent effects on central and peripheral chemical control of breathing, as one study of diabetic subjects with autonomic neuropathy has shown increased central chemosensitivity but reduced peripheral sensitivity.[114]

Exercise performance is impaired in many individuals, particularly those with poor diabetic control and/or evidence of microangiopathy (e.g. microalbuminuria). Such individuals show consistent reductions in $\dot{V}O_2$max and maximum workload on progressive exercise testing.[105,115,116] Correspondingly, the ventilatory response to exercise is high with an increased slope of the relationship of ventilation to $\dot{V}CO_2$, while abnormal cardiac function may also contribute in those with microangiopathy.[116]

24.6.4 Diabetes and sleep apnoea

Patients with diabetes have a high prevalence of sleep-disordered breathing and especially obstructive sleep apnoea; in one study an AHI greater than 15 was found in 36 per cent of a large diabetes clinic population.[117] Inevitably, particularly in type 2 diabetes, obesity confounds this association, but in epidemiological studies sleep-disordered breathing is associated with both glucose intolerance[118] and frank diabetes[119] independently of BMI. If this represents a true cause and effect relationship, the direction of causality, i.e. whether diabetes causes sleep apnoea or vice versa, is uncertain.[119]

Among individuals with frank diabetes, sleep apnoea is associated particularly with the presence of autonomic neuropathy,[114,120] and there appears to be no association in individuals without this complication. The apnoeas are characteristically obstructive rather than central. It has been argued that reduced peripheral chemosensitivity associated with autonomic neuropathy may 'protect' against the development of central apnoea by preventing the usual destabilization of respiratory control that results from post-apnoea hyperventilation.[114]

REFERENCES

1 Pelosi P, Croci M, Ravagnan I, Vicardi P, Gattinoni L. Total respiratory system, lung, and chest wall mechanics in sedated-paralysed postoperative morbidly obese patients. *Chest* 1996; **109**: 144–51.

2 Weiner P, Waizman J, Weiner M, *et al*. Influence of excessive weight loss after gastroplasty for morbid obesity on respiratory muscle performance. *Thorax* 1998; **53**: 39–42.

3 Jones RL, Nzekwu M-MU. The effects of body mass index on lung volumes. *Chest* 2006; **130**: 827–33.

4 Wise RA, Enright PL, Connett JE, *et al*. Effect of weight gain on pulmonary function after smoking cessation in the lung health study. *Am J Respir Crit Care Med* 1998; **157**: 866–72.

5 Canoy D, Luben R, Welch A, *et al*. Abdominal obesity and respiratory function in men and women in the EPIC-Norfolk study, United Kingdom. *Am J Epidemiol* 2004; **159**: 1140–49.

6 Ochs-Balcom HM, Grant BJB, Muti P, *et al.* Pulmonary function and abdominal adiposity in the general population. *Chest* 2006; **129**: 853–62.

7 Lazarus R, Gore CJ, Booth M, Owen N. Effects of body composition and fat distribution on ventilatory function in adults. *Am J Clin Nutr* 1998; **68**: 35–41.

8 Lazarus R, Sparrow D, Weiss ST. Effects of obesity and fat distribution on ventilatory function: the normative aging study. *Chest* 1997; **111**: 891–8.

9 Watson RA, Pride NB. Postural changes in lung volumes and respiratory resistance in subjects with obesity. *J Appl Physiol* 2005; **98**: 512–17.

10 Zerah F, Harf A, Perlemuter L, *et al.* Effects of obesity on respiratory resistance. *Chest* 1993; **103**: 1470–76.

11 Schachter LM, Salome CM, Peat JK, Woolcock AJ. Obesity is a risk for asthma and wheeze but not airway hyperresponsiveness. *Thorax* 2001; **56**: 4–8.

12 Sin DD, Jones RL, Man SF. Obesity is a risk factor for dyspnea but not for airflow obstruction. *Arch Intern Med* 2002; **162**: 1477–81.

13 King GG, Brown NJ, Diba C, *et al.* The effects of body weight on airway calibre. *Eur Respir J* 2005; **25**: 896–901.

14 Ferretti A, Giampiccolo P, Cavalli A, Milic-Emili J, Tantucci C. Expiratory flow limitation and orthopnea in massively obese subjects. *Chest* 2001; **119**: 1401–8.

15 Kress JP, Pohlman AS, Alverdy J, Hall JB. The impact of morbid obesity on oxygen cost of breathing at rest. *Am J Respir Crit Care Med* 1999; **160**: 883–6.

16 Cherniack RW, Guenter CA. The efficiency of the respiratory muscles in obesity. *Can J Biochem Physiol* 1961; **39**: 1215–22.

17 Jenkins SC, Moxham J. The effects of mild obesity on lung function. *Respir Med* 1991; **85**: 309–12.

18 Holley HS, Milic Emili J, Becklake MR, Bates DV. Regional distribution of pulmonary ventilation and perfusion in obesity. *J Clin Invest* 1967; **46**: 475–81.

19 Partridge MR, Ciofetta G, Hughes JMB. Topography of ventilation–perfusion ratios in obesity. *Bull Eur Physiopathol Respir* 1978; **14**: 765–73.

20 Hakala K, Maasilta P, Sovijarvi AR. Upright body position and weight loss improve respiratory mechanics and daytime oxygenation in obese patients with obstructive sleep apnoea. *Clin Physiol* 2000; **20**: 50–55.

21 Oppenheimer BW, Berger KI, Rennert DA, *et al.* Effect of circulatory congestion on the components of pulmonary diffusing capacity in morbid obesity. *Obesity* 2006; **14**: 1172–80.

22 Saydain G, Beck KC, Decker PA, Cowl CT, Scanlon PD. Clinical significance of elevated diffusing capacity. *Chest* 2004; **125**: 446–52.

23 Ray CS, Sue DY, Bray G, Hansen JE, Wasserman K. Effects of obesity on respiratory function. *Am Rev Respir Dis* 1983; **128**: 501–6.

24 Kunitomo F, Kimura H, Tatsumi K, *et al.* Sex differences in awake ventilatory drive and abnormal breathing during sleep in eucapnic obesity. *Chest* 1988; **93**: 968–76.

25 Buyse B, Markous N, Cauberghs M, *et al.* Effect of obesity and/or sleep apnea on chemosensitivity: differences between men and women. *Respir Physiol Neurobiol* 2003; **134**: 13–22.

26 Gallagher MJ, Franklin BA, Ehrman JK, *et al.* Comparative impact of morbid obesity vs. heart failure on cardiorespiratory fitness. *Chest* 2005; **127**: 2197–203.

27 Thomas PS, Coiwen ER, Hulands G, Milledge JS. Respiratory function in the morbidly obese before and after weight loss. *Thorax* 1989; **44**: 382–6.

28 Refsum HE, Holter PH, Lovig T, Haffner JF, Stadaas JO. Pulmonary function and energy expenditure after marked weight loss in obese women: observations before and one year after gastric banding. *Int J Obes* 1990; **14**: 175–83.

29 El-Gamal H, Khayat A, Shikora S, Unterborn JN. Relationship of dyspnea to respiratory drive and pulmonary function tests in obese patients before and after weight loss. *Chest* 2005; **128**: 3870–974.

30 Karason K, Lindroos AK, Stenlof K, Sjostrom L. Relief of cardiorespiratory symptoms and increased physical activity after surgically induced weight loss: results from the Swedish Obese Subjects Study. *Arch Intern Med* 2000; **160**: 1797–802.

31 Nowbar S, Burkart KM, Gonzales R, *et al.* Obesity-associated hypoventilation in hospitalized patients: prevalence, effects, and outcome. *Am J Med* 2004; **116**: 1–7.

32 Berger KI, Ayappa I, Chatr-Amontri B, *et al.* Obesity hypoventilation syndrome as a spectrum of respiratory disturbances during sleep. *Chest* 2001; **120**: 1231–8.

33 Kessler R, Chaouat A, Schinkewitch P, *et al.* The obesity–hypoventilation syndrome revisited: a prospective study of 34 consecutive cases. *Chest* 2001; **120**: 369–76.

34 Mokhlesi B, Tulaimat A. Recent advances in obesity hypoventilation syndrome. *Chest* 2007; **132**: 1322–36.

35 Becker HF, Piper AJ, Flynn WE, *et al.* Breathing during sleep in patients with nocturnal desaturation. *Am J Respir Crit Care Med* 1999; **159**: 112–18.

36 Lin CC, Wu KM, Chou CS, Liaw SF. Oral airway resistance during wakefulness in eucapnic and hypercapnic sleep apnea syndrome. *Respir Physiol Neurobiol* 2004; **139**: 215–24.

37 Han F, Chen E, Wei H, *et al.* Treatment effects on carbon dioxide retention in patients with obstructive

sleep apnea–hypopnea syndrome. *Chest* 2001; **119**: 1814–19.

38 Norman RG, Goldring RM, Clain JM, *et al.* Transition from acute to chronic hypercapnia in patients with periodic breathing: predictions from a computer model. *J Appl Physiol* 2006; **100**: 1733–41.

39 De Llano LAP, Golpe R, Piquer MO, *et al.* Short-term and long-term effects of nasal intermittent positive pressure ventilation in patients with obesity–hypoventilation syndrome. *Chest* 2005; **128**: 587–94.

40 Banerjee D, Yee BJ, Piper AJ, Zwillich CW, Grunstein RR. Obesity hypoventilation syndrome: hypoxemia during continuous positive airway pressure. *Chest* 2007; **131**: 1678–84.

41 Piper AJ, Wang D, Yee BJ, Barnes DJ, Grunstein RR. Randomised trial of CPAP vs bilevel support in the treatment of obesity hypoventilation syndrome without severe nocturnal desaturation. *Thorax* 2008; **63**: 395–401.

42 Schwartz DB. Malnutrition in chronic obstructive pulmonary disease. *Respir Care Clin North Am* 2006; **12**: 521–31.

43 Dray X, Kanaan R, Bienvenu T, *et al.* Malnutrition in adults with cystic fibrosis. *Eur J Clin Nutr* 2005; **59**: 152–4.

44 Arora NS, Rochester DF. Respiratory muscle strength and maximal voluntary ventilation in undernourished patients. *Am Rev Respir Dis* 1982; **126**: 5–8.

45 Hards JM, Reid WD, Pardy RI, Paré PE. Respiratory muscle fiber morphometry: correlation with pulmonary function and nutrition. *Chest* 1990; **97**: 1037–44.

46 Pieters T, Boland B, Beguin C, *et al.* Lung function study and diffusion capacity in anorexia nervosa. *J Intern Med* 2000; **248**: 137–42.

47 Gonzalez-Moro JM, De Miguel-Diez J, Paz-Gonzalez L, *et al.* Abnormalities of the respiratory function and control of ventilation in patients with anorexia nervosa. *Respiration* 2003; **70**: 490–95.

48 Doekel RC, Zwillich CW, Scoggin CH, *et al.* Clinical semi-starvation, depression of hypoxic ventilatory response. *N Engl J Med* 1976; **295**: 358–61.

49 Kelly SM, Rosa A, Field S, *et al.* Inspiratory muscle strength and body composition in patients receiving total parenteral nutrition therapy. *Am Rev Respir Dis* 1984; **130**: 33–7.

50 Creutzberg EC, Wouters EF, Mostert R, Weling-Scheepers CA, Schols AM. Efficacy of nutritional supplementation therapy in depleted patients with chronic obstructive pulmonary disease. *Nutrition* 2003; **19**: 120–27.

51 Molloy DW, Dhingra S, Solven F, Wilson A, McCarthy DS. Hypomagnesemia and respiratory muscle power. *Am Rev Respir Dis* 1984; **129**: 497–8.

52 Bright P, Miller MR, Franklyn JA, Sheppard MC. The use of a neural network to detect upper airway obstruction caused by goiter. *Am J Respir Crit Care Med* 1998; **157**: 1885–91.

53 Freedman S. Lung volumes and distensibility and maximum respiratory pressures in thyroid disease before and after treatment. *Thorax* 1978; **33**: 785–90.

54 Siafakas NM, Milona I, Salesiotou V, *et al.* Respiratory muscle strength in hyperthyroidism before and after treatment. *Am Rev Respir Dis* 1992; **146**: 1025–9.

55 Mier A, Brophy C, Wass JAH, Besser GM, Green M. Reversible respiratory muscle weakness in hyperthyroidism. *Am Rev Respir Dis* 1989; **139**: 529–33.

56 McElvaney GN, Wilcox PG, Fairbarn MS, *et al.* Respiratory muscle weakness and dyspnea in thyrotoxic patients. *Am Rev Respir Dis* 1990; **141**: 1221–7.

57 Goswami R, Guleria R, Gupta AK, *et al.* Prevalence of diaphragmatic muscle weakness and dyspnoea in Graves' disease and their reversibility with carbimazole therapy. *Eur J Endocrinol* 2002; **147**: 299–303.

58 Stein M, Kimbel P, Johnson RL. Pulmonary function in hyperthyroidism. *J Clin Invest* 1961; **40**: 348–63.

59 Massey DG, Becklake MR, McKenzie JM, Bates DV. Circulatory and ventilatory response to exercise in thyrotoxicosis. *N Engl J Med* 1967; **276**: 1104–12.

60 Small D, Gibbons W, Levy RD, *et al.* Exertional dyspnoea and ventilation in hyperthyroidism. *Chest* 1992; **101**: 1268–73.

61 Irace L, Pergola V, Di Salvo G, *et al.* Work capacity and oxygen uptake abnormalities in hyperthyroidism. *Minerva Cardioangiol* 2006; **54**: 355–62.

62 Zwillich CW, Weil JV. Increased ventilatory response to hypoxia and hypercapnia during thyrotoxicosis. *Am Rev Respir Dis* 1976; **113**: 254.

63 Siafakas NM, Salesiotou V, Filaditaki V, *et al.* Respiratory muscle strength in hypothyroidism. *Chest* 1992; **102**: 189–94.

64 Laroche CM, Cairns T, Moxham J, Green M. Hypothyroidism presenting with respiratory muscle weakness. *Am Rev Respir Dis* 1988; **138**: 472–4.

65 Weiner M, Chausow A, Szidon P. Reversible respiratory muscle weakness in hypothyroidism. *Br J Dis Chest* 1986; **80**: 391–5.

66 Zwillich CW, Pierson DJ, Hofeldt FD. Ventilatory control in myxedema and hypothyroidism. *N Engl J Med* 1975; **292**: 662–5.

67 Burack R, Edwards RHT, Green M, Jones NL. The response to exercise before and after treatment of myxoedema with thyroxine. *J Pharmacol Exp Ther* 1971; **176**: 212–19.

68 Monzani F, Caraccio N, Siciliano G, *et al.* Clinical and biochemical features of muscle dysfunction in subclinical hypothyroidism. *J Clin Endocrinol Metab* 1997; **82**: 3315–18.

69 Caraccio N, Natali A, Sironi A, et al. Muscle metabolism and exercise tolerance in subclinical hypothyroidism: a controlled trial of levothyroxine. *J Clin Endocrinol Metab* 2005; **90**: 4057–62.

70 Jha A, Sharma SK, Tandon N, et al. Thyroxine replacement therapy reverses sleep-disordered breathing in patients with primary hypothyroidism. *Sleep Med* 2006; **7**: 55–61.

71 Kapur VK, Koepsell TD, deMaine J, et al. Association of hypothyroidism and obstructive sleep apnea. *Am J Respir Crit Care Med* 1998; **158**: 1379–83.

72 Skjodt NM, Atkar R, Easton PA. Screening for hypothyroidism in sleep apnea. *Am J Crit Care Med* 1999; **160**: 732–5.

73 Miller CM, Husain AM. Should women with obstructive sleep apnea syndrome be screened for hypothyroidism? *Sleep Breathing* 2003; **7**: 185–8.

74 Lin C-C, Tsan K-W, Chen P-J. The relationship between sleep apnoea syndrome and hypothyroidism. *Chest* 1992; **102**: 1663–7.

75 Grunstein RR, Sullivan CE. Sleep apnoea and hypothyroidism: mechanisms and management. *Am J Med* 1988; **85**: 775–9.

76 Brody JS, Fisher AB, Gocmen A, DuBois AB. Acromegalic pneumomegaly: lung growth in the adult. *J Clin Invest* 1970; **49**: 1051–60.

77 De Troyer A, Desir D, Copinschi G. Regression of lung size in adults with growth hormone deficiency. *Q J Med* 1980; **49**: 329–40.

78 Trotman-Dickenson B, Weetman AP, Hughes JMB. Upper airway obstruction and pulmonary function in acromegaly: relationship to disease activity. *Q J Med* 1991; **79**: 527–38.

79 Donnelly PM, Grunstein RR, Peat JK, Woodcock AJ, Bye PT. Large lungs and growth hormone: an increased alveolar number? *Eur Respir J* 1995; **8**: 938–47.

80 Iandelli I, Gorini M, Duranti R, et al. Respiratory muscle function and control of breathing in patients with acromegaly. *Eur Respir J* 1997; **10**: 977–82.

81 Garcia-Rio F, Pino JM, Diez JJ, et al. Reduction of lung distensibility in acromegaly after suppression of growth hormone hypersecretion. *Am J Respir Crit Care Med* 2001; **164**: 852–7.

82 Siafakas NM, Sigales J, Filaditaki B, Tsirogiannis K. Small airway function in acromegaly. *Bull Eur Physiopathol Respir* 1987; **23**: 329–34.

83 Hochban W, Ehlenz K, Conradt R, Brandenburg U. Obstructive sleep apnoea in acromegaly: the role of craniofacial changes. *Eur Resp J* 1999; **14**: 196–202.

84 Isono S, Saeki N, Tanaka A, Nishino T. Collapsibility of passive pharynx in patients with acromegaly. *Am J Respir Crit Care Med* 1999; **160**: 64–8.

85 Herrmann BL, Wessendorf TE, Ajaj W, et al. Effects of octreotide on sleep apnoea and tongue volume (magnetic resonance imaging) in patients with acromegaly. *Eur J Endocrinol* 2004; **151**: 309–15.

86 Jain BP, Brody JS, Fisher AB. The small lung of hypopituitarism. *Am Rev Respir Dis* 1973; **108**: 49–55.

87 Meineri I, Andreani O, Sanna R, et al. Effect of low-dosage recombinant human growth hormone therapy on pulmonary function in hypopituitary patients with adult-onset growth hormone deficiency. *J Endocrinol Invest* 1998; **21**: 423–7.

88 Merola B, Sofia M, Longobardi S, et al. Impairment of lung volumes and respiratory muscle strength in adult patients with growth hormone deficiency. *Eur J Endocrinol* 1995; **133**: 680–85.

89 Cuneo RC, Salomon F, Wiles CM, Hesp R, Sonksen PH. Growth hormone treatment in growth-hormone deficient adults: II. Effects on exercise performance. *J Appl Physiol* 1991; **70**: 695–700.

90 Peker Y, Svensson J, Hedner J, Grote L, Johannsson G. Sleep apnoea and quality of life in growth hormone (GH)-deficient adults before and after 6 months of GH replacement therapy. *Clin Endocrinol* 2006; **65**: 98–105.

91 Goldman MD. Lung dysfunction in diabetes. *Diabetes Care* 2003; **26**: 1915–18.

92 Davis TM, Knuiman M, Kendall P, Vu H, Davis WA. Reduced pulmonary function and its association in type 2 diabetes: the Fremantle Diabetes Study. *Diabetes Res Clin Pract* 2000; **50**: 153–9.

93 Lange P, Parner J, Schnohr P, Jensen G. Copenhagen City Heart Study: longitudinal analysis of ventilatory capacity in diabetic and nondiabetic adults. *Eur Respir J* 2002; **20**: 1406–12.

94 Davis WA, Knulman M, Kendall P, et al. Glycemic exposure is associated with reduced pulmonary function in type 2 diabetes: the Fremantle Diabetes Study. *Diabetes Care* 2004; **27**: 752–7.

95 McKeever TM, Weston PJ, Hubbard R, Fogarty A. Lung function and glucose metabolism: an analysis of data from the Third National Health and Nutrition Examination Survey. *Am J Epidemiol* 2005; **161**: 546–56.

96 Lazarus R, Sparrow D, Weiss ST. Impaired ventilatory function and elevated insulin levels in non-diabetic males: the Normative Aging Study. *Eur Respir J* 1998; **12**: 635–40.

97 Lawlor DA, Ebrahim S, Smith GD. Associations of measures of lung function with insulin resistance and type 2 diabetes: findings from the British Women's Heart and Health Study. *Diabetologia* 2004; **47**: 195–203.

98 Wanke T, Formanek D, Aninger M, et al. Inspiratory muscle performance and pulmonary function

changes in insulin-dependent diabetes mellitus. *Am Rev Respir Dis* 1991; **143**: 97–100.

99 Sandler M, Bunn AE, Stewart RI. Cross-sectional study of pulmonary function in patients with insulin-dependent diabetes mellitus. *Am Rev Respir Dis* 1987; **135**: 223–9.

100 Maccioni FJ, Colebatch HJH. Lung volume and distensibility in insulin-dependent diabetes mellitus. *Am Rev Respir Dis* 1991; **143**: 1253–6.

101 Schnapf BM, Banks RA, Silverstein JH, *et al.* Pulmonary function in insulin dependent diabetes mellitus with limited joint mobility. *Am Rev Respir Dis* 1984; **130**: 930–32.

102 Mancini M Filippelli M, Seghieri G, *et al.* Respiratory muscle function and hypoxic ventilatory control in patients with type 1 diabetes. *Chest* 1999; **115**: 1553–62.

103 Douglas NJ, Campbell IW, Ewing DJ, Clarke DB, Flenley DC. Reduced airway vagal tone in diabetic patients with autonomic neuropathy. *Clin Sci* 1981; **61**: 581–4.

104 Cooper BG, Taylor R, Alberti KGMM, Gibson GJ. Lung function in patients with diabetes mellitus. *Respir Med* 1990; **84**: 235–9.

105 Benbassat CA, Stern E, Kramer M, *et al.* Pulmonary function in patients with diabetes mellitus. *Am J Med Sci* 2001; **322**: 127–32.

106 Marvisi M, Bartolini L, del Borrello P, *et al.* Pulmonary function in non-insulin-dependent diabetes mellitus. *Respiration* 2001; **68**: 268–72.

107 Guazzi M, Brambilla R, De Vita S, Guazzi MD. Diabetes worsens pulmonary diffusion in heart failure, and insulin counteracts this effect. *Am J Respir Crit Care Med* 2002; **166**: 978–82.

108 Weir DC, Jennings PE, Hendy MS, Barnett AH, Burge PS. Transfer factor for carbon monoxide in patients with diabetes with and without microangiopathy. *Thorax* 1988; **43**: 725–6.

109 Britton J. Is the carbon monoxide transfer factor diminished in the presence of diabetic retinopathy in patients with insulin-dependent diabetes mellitus? *Eur Respir J* 1988; **1**: 403–6.

110 Ljubic S, Metelko Z, Car N, Roglic G, Drazic Z. Reduction of diffusion capacity for carbon monoxide in diabetic patients. *Chest* 1998; **114**: 1033–5.

111 Matsubara T, Hara F. The pulmonary function and histopathological studies of the lung in diabetes mellitus. *J Nippon Med School* 1991; **58**: 528–36.

112 Homma I, Kageyama S, Nagai T, *et al.* Chemosensitivity in patients with diabetic neuropathy. *Clin Sci* 1981; **61**: 599–603.

113 Nishimura M, Miyamoto K, Suzuki A, *et al.* Ventilatory and heart rate responses to hypoxia and hypercapnia in patients with diabetes mellitus. *Thorax* 1989; **44**: 251–7.

114 Bottini P, Dottorini ML, Cristina Cordoni M, Casucci G, Tantucci C. Sleep-disordered breathing in nonobese diabetic subjects with autonomic neuropathy. *Eur Respir J* 2003; **22**: 654–60.

115 Niranjan V, McBrayer DG, Ramirez LC, Raskin P, Hsia CC. Glycemic control and cardiopulmonary function in patients with insulin-dependent diabetes mellitus. *Am J Med* 1997; **103**: 504–13.

116 Lau AC, Lo MK, Leung GT, *et al.* Altered exercise gas exchange as related to microalbuminuria in type 2 diabetic patients. *Chest* 2004; **125**: 1292–8.

117 Einhorn D, Stewart DA, Erman MK, *et al.* Prevalence of sleep apnea in a population of adults with type 2 diabetes mellitus. *Endocr Pract* 2007; **13**: 355–62.

118 Punjabi NM, Shahar E, Redline S, *et al.* Sleep Heart Health Study Investigators. Sleep-disordered breathing, glucose intolerance, and insulin resistance: the Sleep Heart Health Study. *Am J Epidemiol* 2004; **160**: 521–30.

119 Reichmuth KJ, Austin D, Skatrud JB, Young T. Association of sleep apnea and type II diabetes: a population-based study. *Am J Respir Crit Care Med* 2005; **172**: 1590–95.

120 Ficker JH, Dertinger SH, Siegfried W, *et al.* Obstructive sleep apnoea and diabetes mellitus: the role of cardiovascular autonomic neuropathy. *Eur Respir J* 1998; **11**: 14–19.

25

Rheumatic and Connective Tissue Disorders

25.1 GENERAL PATTERN OF RESPIRATORY DYSFUNCTION

Studies of respiratory function in the rheumatic and collagen-vascular diseases (CVD) emphasize the frequency with which the lungs are affected even in the absence of respiratory symptoms. In many cases the precise pathological correlates of the functional changes are uncertain. Pathological information is available from autopsy studies on a few cases, but the abnormalities observed in such highly selected groups are not necessarily responsible for the abnormal function described in other patients.

The pattern of a restrictive ventilatory defect with disproportionate reduction in the carbon monoxide diffusing capacity (D_LCO) is common to several conditions; in many it reflects interstitial lung disease, but pulmonary vascular abnormalities, respiratory muscle weakness, and pleural and ribcage abnormalities in varying combinations may also contribute. Comparisons of interstitial lung disease in CVD with idiopathic pulmonary fibrosis (IPF) generally show a better prognosis in the former, even when respiratory function at presentation is similar.[1] Unlike the progressive decline seen in most individuals with IPF, respiratory function in CVD-associated interstitial disease often improves with treatment or remains stable for prolonged periods. No specific functional features distinguish these two groups of patients, but the distribution of histopathological type does differ, with a relatively higher prevalence of non-specific interstitial pneumonia (NSIP) than usual interstitial pneumonia (UIP), at least in systemic sclerosis, Sjögren's syndrome and dermatomyositis/polymyositis; data on the distribution of pathological pattern in rheumatoid arthritis are less consistent. However, the generally better prognosis of CVD-associated interstitial lung disease is not simply attributable to a greater proportion of NSIP, as UIP in association with CVD has a better prognosis than a similar histopathological pattern in patients with IPF.[2] Across the range of conditions and pathological appearances, lung function (especially VC) is, along with age, one of the strongest independent predictors of survival. The D_LCO also predicts survival, particularly in patients with the UIP histopathological pattern.[2]

25.2 RHEUMATOID ARTHRITIS

The frequency and pattern of abnormal lung function in patients with rheumatoid arthritis (RA) vary considerably between different series. Several factors are likely to contribute in varying proportions in different individuals. Pleural effusions and pleural thickening are common in RA, while interstitial lung disease is recognizable by high-resolution computed tomography (HRCT) scanning in as many as 19 per cent of patients.[3] Unlike the other diseases in this group, the histopathological pattern of interstitial disease in RA is commonly UIP.[2] This produces the expected functional pattern of a restrictive ventilatory defect with disproportionately reduced D_LCO and low KCO.[3,4]

Abnormal function is also reported frequently in patients without overt respiratory disease. In some series, a reduced D_LCO is the most common abnormality described,[4,5] although others report a mildly reduced VC more commonly.[6] It seems likely that mild volume restriction in patients with normal lungs on CT scanning is attributable to either musculoskeletal abnormalities or pleural thickening, with the relative contributions of each varying between patients. Impaired respiratory muscle strength has also been described.[7,8] In one study, $P_I$max was related inversely to the duration of treatment with corticosteroids,[7] but whether this association represents cause and effect or whether the duration of therapy merely implies more severe rheumatoid disease is not clear.

Several studies have reported an association of abnormal lung function with smoking in RA, sufficiently strong to suggest a synergistic effect. This applies not only to airway obstruction but also to D_LCO and the presence of interstitial lung disease.[4] Functional evidence of airway obstruction is relatively common, even among non-smoking patients, with a prevalence of 16 per cent in one controlled study of non-smokers.[9] The severity of functional airway obstruction correlates with CT-demonstrated bronchial wall thickening[10] and with the presence of bronchiectasis.[9,10]

In patients with neither respiratory symptoms nor overt lung disease, a reduced D_LCO can remain stable for several years and does not necessarily presage the development of clinical disease.[5]

25.3 SYSTEMIC SCLEROSIS (SCLERODERMA)

Interstitial lung disease and pulmonary hypertension are common in systemic sclerosis, and many patients have both.[11] Both CT-demonstrable fibrosis and a low VC correlate independently with pulmonary hypertension.[12] A reduced D_LCO is found in the majority of patients[13] and may relate to either interstitial lung disease or pulmonary vascular disease, or both. A restrictive ventilatory defect is also very common.[14]

Qualitatively, the functional abnormalities in patients with systemic sclerosis-associated interstitial lung disease are similar to those of IPF, but, for a given CT extent, the former have less severe impairment with better preserved PaO_2 and less oxygen desaturation on exercise.[15] The severity of reduction of D_LCO correlates with the extent of honeycombing on CT scanning,[16] but the overall histopathological pattern is more likely to be fibrotic NSIP than UIP. The mortality of patients from systemic sclerosis with interstitial lung disease is much better related to respiratory function than to the histological appearances.[17] In particular, higher mortality correlates with lower initial D_LCO and VC and also with the rate of deterioration of D_LCO.[17]

Abnormal function is related neither to the extent of skin changes nor to the presence or absence of the ScL-70 antibody; however, function tends to be better preserved in patients without anticentromere antibody (who also have less interstitial lung disease).[18]

Although airway obstruction has been described in occasional non-smoking patients, this is not generally a feature of systemic sclerosis.[14,19] In patients with evidence of lung disease, the expected ventilation/perfusion disturbances and desaturation on exercise are commonly present. The reduction in oxygen saturation during a 6-min walk is greater in patients with a lower VC.[20] Detailed exercise testing shows reductions in maximum exercise capacity and symptom-limited $\dot{V}O_2$max, with widening of the alveolar–arterial PO_2 gradient ($AaPO_2$) and a high dead space/tidal volume ratio (V_D/V_T); these abnormalities are most marked in patients with reduced D_LCO but are also demonstrable in some with relatively normal D_LCO.[21] The anaerobic threshold is low and $\dot{V}O_2$ max is inversely proportional to the resting pulmonary artery pressure.[22]

Treatment of patients with systemic sclerosis-related interstitial lung disease with cyclophosphamide has been shown in a randomized controlled trial to produce a modest increase in VC.[23]

As long ago as 1892 it was suggested that extensive scleroderma of the skin of the thorax might impair breathing. However, to impede lung expansion significantly, superficial involvement would have to be very extensive and probably would need to include the abdominal wall in addition, since abdominal displacement represents an important pathway of lung expansion. The later appreciation that pulmonary fibrosis is very common reduced emphasis on this mechanism of volume restriction, but occasional patients have been reported in whom extrapulmonary restriction may be a factor, due to either involvement of the chest wall by sclerodermatous changes[24,25] or weakness of the respiratory muscles.[26]

In patients with Raynaud's phenomenon but without other features of scleroderma, a transient reduction in $D_L CO$ is demonstrable following immersion of the hands in cold water. This results from reduction in the pulmonary capillary blood volume and implies that the abnormal reactivity of the digital vessels is shared by the small pulmonary vessels. However, the effect is not apparent in patients with overt systemic sclerosis, presumably because the small pulmonary vessels are then less reactive.[27]

25.4 SYSTEMIC LUPUS ERYTHEMATOSUS

Abnormal lung function is very common in patients with systemic lupus erythematosus (SLE), but the pathological changes responsible are less clearly established than in systemic sclerosis. Overt interstitial lung disease is uncommon in SLE but is seen in some individuals with more severe respiratory symptoms.[28] High-resolution CT scanning shows evidence of mild subclinical interstitial disease in a larger proportion.[29] Pleural effusions and subsequent pleural thickening are also common, although extensive pleural thickening is unusual; a large pericardial effusion may occasionally contribute to the reduction of lung volumes. Less common respiratory manifestations include acute lupus pneumonitis, alveolar haemorrhage, pulmonary vascular disease, and pulmonary hypertension and the 'shrinking lung syndrome' (see below). Even among patients without overt lung disease, reduction of VC[30,31] and, more commonly, of $D_L CO$ is frequent.[31,32] A reduced $D_L CO$ has been reported in up to 80 per cent of unselected patients in some series[33,34] and is often seen without clinical evidence of respiratory involvement.[32,35] The KCO was shown to correlate inversely with disease activity in one study.[30] Paradoxically, KCO may be relatively more normal in patients with more severe volume restriction, suggesting that the smallest lung volumes are due to extrapulmonary restriction (e.g. as in the 'shrinking lung syndrome' – see below).

Airway function in non-smoking patients with SLE is generally normal.[36] Exercise testing, even in patients with relatively quiescent disease and normal resting lung function, is likely to show a reduction in capacity and $\dot{V}O_2$max, with a low anaerobic threshold, features compatible with peripheral deconditioning.[36,37]

25.4.1 Shrinking lung syndrome

This unusual clinical and functional picture of SLE is characterized by breathlessness with orthopnoea, a restrictive ventilatory defect that can be severe, radiographically clear lung fields and high diaphragms. A proportion of such patients have a concurrent or previous history of myopathy or myositis,[38,39] and a previous history of pleurisy is very common.[32,39] CT scanning typically shows relatively minor abnormalities, insufficient to account for severe volume restriction: although a history of pleurisy is common, residual pleural thickening is usually trivial or absent; basal atelectasis may be present, but there is no evidence of either interstitial or severe pleural disease.[38,39]

The aetiology of the syndrome is unclear and has been a matter of some controversy. Several studies have shown evidence of respiratory muscle weakness on volitional testing, with impaired maximum respiratory pressures or maximum transdiaphragmatic pressure.[33,39–42] One clinicopathological study of a single case at autopsy showed evidence of fibrosis and atrophy of the diaphragmatic muscle,[40] while another showed a severe demyelinating neuropathy.[43] On the other hand, a study of diaphragmatic function using phrenic stimulation in patients in whom a generalized myopathy had been excluded reported normal results.[44] Also, in one patient with acute SLE and impaired $P_I$max, normal diaphragmatic strength was demonstrated on magnetic stimulation, even though paradoxical motion of the abdomen was evident.[45] It seems, therefore, that although the 'shrinking lung syndrome' results from diaphragmatic dysfunction, impaired muscle strength is not the explanation in all cases. The frequent association with previous pleurisy may be relevant, in that, possibly, in the acute phase some patients develop inhibition of diaphragm movement due to pain, with a pattern of breathing that is protective and that persists even after the acute inflammation has resolved.

Lung perfusion scans in patients with the 'shrinking lung syndrome' are notable for their normality.[33,39] Respiratory function in this syndrome can improve with treatment and then remain stable for many years,[39] although further decrements may accompany acute exacerbations of the disease (Fig. 25.1).

25.5 DERMATOMYOSITIS AND POLYMYOSITIS

Interstitial lung disease is common in patients with dermatomyositis or polymyositis, particularly in those with anti-Jo-1 (anti-synthetase) antibodies.[46] The histological pattern is usually NSIP and respiratory function shows a typical restrictive ventilatory defect, disproportionate reduction of $D_L CO$ and disturbed gas exchange.[47] A degree of respiratory muscle weakness commonly accompanies the

generalized weakness; its functional pattern is similar to that in other proximal myopathies (see Chapter 20, Section 20.2.1). It can be of sufficient severity to produce hypercapnia and to require assisted ventilation.[48] The generalized muscle weakness impairs exercise capacity, with reduced $\dot{V}O_2$max, but there is no clear relationship between exercise capacity and the blood level of the muscle enzyme creatine kinase.[49]

Interstitial lung disease usually responds well to treatment with corticosteroids, and the resulting improvement in HRCT appearances correlates with increasing VC and $D_L CO$.[47]

25.6 MIXED CONNECTIVE TISSUE DISEASE

Mixed connective tissue disease shares certain features with scleroderma, SLE and polymyositis but is classified separately because of its different immunological features. As with SLE and scleroderma, there is a high frequency of abnormal respiratory function, and again the $D_L CO$ usually shows the most severe abnormality.[50] The 'shrinking lung syndrome' has been reported, as in SLE.[51]

25.7 SJÖGREN'S SYNDROME

In primary Sjögren's syndrome (i.e. unassociated with another connective tissue disorder) abnormalities of both the alveoli and the airways are well recognized. Clinical and CT evidence suggests that airway disease is more common than interstitial lung disease[52] and, functionally, airway abnormalities are more frequent, although usually not severe.[53] A reduced FEV_1 and FEV_1/VC ratio are sometimes seen, but, more commonly, abnormalities suggesting peripheral airway narrowing are found, e.g. a raised RV/TLC ratio[54] or reduced maximum expiratory flow at low lung volumes.[53] In patients with interstitial lung disease, the typical restrictive defect with disproportionate reduction of $D_L CO$ is seen, and correlations between CT and functional abnormalities have been reported.[52] Some authors have also found a relation between CT evidence of airway disease and impaired function,[52] but others report no such correlation.[55]

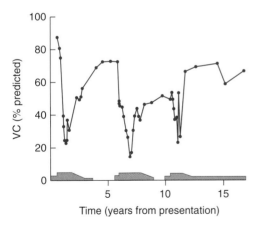

Figure 25.1 Sequential measurements of vital capacity (VC) (% predicted) over 17 years in a young woman with 'shrinking lungs' due to systemic lupus erythematosus (SLE). Shaded areas indicate prednisolone treatment. Three major 'crises' are seen, followed in each case by gradual recovery of VC.

25.8 RELAPSING POLYCHONDRITIS

Relapsing polychondritis is a rare inflammatory disease of cartilage-containing tissue, including the cartilage of the nose, larynx, airways and ribs. The functional abnormalities result from varying combinations of structural narrowing of the airway lumen and loss of rigidity (increased compliance) due to inflammation and destruction of airway cartilage and consequent abnormally large dynamic variation in calibre during breathing. The narrowing may be localized to the larynx or to a short segment of trachea, or it can extend more distally along the cartilage containing airways. The most useful functional information is obtained by examining maximum expiratory and inspiratory flow volume curves (see Fig. 12.5b in Chapter 12). Varying combinations of limitation of maximum expiratory and inspiratory flow have been reported.[56-59] The exact pattern depends on the main sites and the nature of the narrowing, in particular whether it is predominantly intrathoracic (mainly expiratory flow limitation) or extrathoracic (mainly inspiratory limitation) or both. Abnormal function is more sensitive than bronchoscopy or radiographic imaging in assessing the severity, extent and nature of airway narrowing as it gives an overall picture of airway function, with assessment of dynamic changes as well as any fixed structural narrowing. Marked oscillations of flow are characteristic of dynamic changes due to instability of the airway during forceful breathing manoeuvres. If airway obstruction becomes very severe, resting ventilation may be compromised and hypercapnia can develop.[56]

25.9 INHERITED DISORDERS

25.9.1 Marfan's syndrome

Marfan's syndrome is an inherited defect of fibrillin, a major component of the microfibrils in all connective tissue. Consequently, both the lungs and the chest wall are likely to be affected. The unusual height of individuals with Marfan's syndrome results mainly from disproportionate length of the limbs. One study reported that lung volumes were smaller than predicted from the standing height but normal when related to sitting height.[60] However, this was not confirmed in a more recent study, which showed that VC was close to that predicted from overall height while RV (and consequently TLC) was significantly greater than predicted.[61] The cause of the discrepancy is unresolved. Although emphysema is a suspected association of Marfan's syndrome, D_LCO values are usually in the low normal range.[61] Exercise capacity and $\dot{V}O_2$max are reduced, probably due in most cases to deconditioning rather than to cardiopulmonary dysfunction.[61] A high prevalence of obstructive sleep apnoea has been reported and may be due to either abnormal compliance of the larynx[62] or maxillary constriction related to the high hard palate.[63]

25.9.2 Ehlers–Danlos syndrome and cutis laxa

Ehlers–Danlos syndrome is a disorder of connective tissue associated with various biochemical abnormalities of collagen. Scoliosis and pectus excavatum are common, and a mild restrictive ventilatory defect may be present, associated with a raised KCO consistent with extrapulmonary volume restriction.[64] However, other individuals have been reported to have increased lung volumes, impaired gas exchange and a heightened tendency of both the lower and upper airways to collapse.[65] Cutis laxa is an inherited disorder of elastin that is associated with premature emphysema and severe airway obstruction.[66]

25.9.3 Fibrodysplasia ossificans progressiva

In this rare condition, calcification and ossification develop in soft tissues, leading to ankylosis of the costovertebral joints, with fixation and impaired expansion of the ribcage. The functional effects resemble those of ankylosing spondylitis (see Chapter 16, Section 16.5), but the restrictive ventilatory pattern is usually more severe.[67]

25.9.4 Achondroplasia

Conventional prediction of lung volumes from standing height is clearly inappropriate in achondroplasia. Although sitting height is more relevant, this overestimates trunk height, as the head is disproportionately large and consequently lung volumes appear reduced.[68] The lungs are otherwise functionally normal and maximum respiratory pressures are similarly normal.[68] However, abnormal breathing during sleep is common, with mainly obstructive apnoeas and hypopnoeas described, but also central hypopnoeas and disproportionate hypoxaemia.[69] Apneustic breathing (see Chapter 20, Section 20.1.1) has also been reported.[70] Many of these abnormalities appear related to cervicomedullary compression and can improve after decompressive surgery[69] or can be controlled by continuous positive airway pressure (CPAP) treatment.[71]

REFERENCES

1 Agusti C, Xaubet A, Roca J, Agusti AG, Rodriguez-Roisin R. Interstitial pulmonary fibrosis with and without associated collagen vascular disease: results of a two year follow up. *Thorax* 1992; **47**: 1035–40.

2 Park JH, Kim DS, Park IN, *et al.* Prognosis of fibrotic interstitial pneumonia: idiopathic versus collagen vascular disease-related subtypes. *Am J Respir Crit Care Med* 2007; **175**: 705–11.

3 Dawson JK, Fewins HE, Desmond J, Lynch MP, Graham DR. Fibrosing alveolitis in patients with rheumatoid arthritis as assessed by high resolution computed tomography, chest radiography, and pulmonary function tests. *Thorax* 2001; **56**: 622–7.

4 Saag KG, Kolluri S Koehnke RK, *et al.* Rheumatoid arthritis lung disease: determinants of radiographic and physiologic abnormalities. *Arthritis Rheum* 1996; **39**: 1711–19.

5 Fuld JP, Johnson MK, Cotton MM, *et al.* A longitudinal study of lung function in non-smoking patients with rheumatoid arthritis. *Chest* 2003; **124**: 1224–31.

6 Banks J, Banks C, Cheong B, *et al.* An epidemiological and clinical investigation of pulmonary function and respiratory symptoms in patients with rheumatoid arthritis. *Q J Med* 1992; **85**: 795–806.

7 Gorini M, Ginanni R, Spinelli A, *et al.* Inspiratory muscle strength and respiratory drive in patients with rheumatoid arthritis. *Am Rev Respir Dis* 1990; **142**: 289–94.

8 Cimen B, Deviren SD, Yorgancloglu ZR. Pulmonary function tests, aerobic capacity, respiratory muscle strength and endurance of patients with rheumatoid arthritis. *Clin Rhematol* 2001; **20**: 168–73.

9 Vergnenegre A, Pugnere N, Antonini MT, *et al.* Airway obstruction and rheumatoid arthritis. *Eur Respir J* 1997; **10**: 1072–8.

10 Terasaki H, Fujimoto K, Hayabuchi N, *et al.* Respiratory symptoms in rheumatoid arthritis: relation between high resolution CT findings and functional impairment. *Radiat Med* 2004; **22**: 179–85.

11 Chang B, Wigley FM, White B, Wise RA. Scleroderma patients with combined pulmonary hypertension and interstitial lung disease. *J Rheumatol* 2003; **30**: 2398–405.

12 Plastiras SC, Karadimitrakis SP, Kampolis C, Moutsopoulos HM, Tzelepis GE. Determinants of pulmonary arterial hypertension in scleroderma. *Semin Arthritis Rheum* 2007; **36**: 392–6.

13 Tashkin DP, Clements PJ, Wright RS, *et al.* Interrelationships between pulmonary and extrapulmonary involvement in systemic sclerosis: a longitudinal analysis. *Chest* 1994; **105**: 489–95.

14 Spagnolatti L, Zola MC, Volpini E, *et al.* Pulmonary function in patients with systemic sclerosis. *Monaldi Arch Chest Dis* 1997; **52**: 4–8.

15 Wells AU, Hansell DM, Rubens MB, *et al.* Functional impairment in lone cryptogenic fibrosing alveolitis and fibrosing alveolitis associated with systemic sclerosis: a comparison. *Am J Respir Crit Care Med* 1997; **155**: 1657–64.

16 Kim EA, Johkoh T, Lee KS, *et al.* Interstitial pneumonia in progressive systemic sclerosis: serial high-resolution CT findings with functional correlation. *J Comput Assist Tomogr* 2001; **25**: 757–63.

17 Bouros C, Wells AU, Nicholson AG, *et al.* Histopathologic subsets of fibrosing alveolitis in patients with systemic sclerosis and their relationship to outcome. *Am J Respir Crit Care Med* 2002; **165**: 1581–6.

18 Kane GC, Varga J, Conant EF, *et al.* Lung involvement in systemic sclerosis (scleroderma): relation to classification based on extent of skin involvement or autoantibody status. *Respir Med* 1996; **90**: 223–30.

19 Kostopoulos C, Rassidakis A, Sfikakis PP, Antoniades L, Maurikakis M. Small airways dysfunction in systemic sclerosis: a controlled study. *Chest* 1992; **102**: 875–81.

20 Villalba WO, Sampaio-Barros PD, Pereita MC, *et al.* Six-minute walk test for the evaluation of pulmonary disease severity in scleroderma patients. *Chest* 2007; **131**: 217–22.

21 Schwaiblmair M, Behr J, Fruhmann G. Cardio-respiratory responses to incremental exercise in patients with systemic sclerosis. *Chest* 1996; **110**: 1520–25.

22 Morelli, S, Ferrante L, Sgreccia A, *et al.* Pulmonary hypertension is associated with impaired exercise

performance in patients with systemic sclerosis. *Scand J Rheumatol* 2000; **29**: 236–42.

23 Tashkin DP, Elashoff R, Clements PJ, *et al.* Cyclophosphamide versus placebo in scleroderma lung disease. *N Engl J Med* 2006; **354**: 2655–66.

24 Russell DC, Maloney A, Muir AL. Progressive generalised scleroderma: respiratory failure from primary chest wall involvement. *Thorax* 1981; **36**: 219–20.

25 Iliffe GD, Pettigrew NM. Hypoventilatory respiratory failure in generalised scleroderma. *Br Med J* 1983; **286**: 337–8.

26 Chausow AM, Kane T, Levinson D, Szidon JP. Reversible hypercapnic respiratory insufficiency in scleroderma caused by respiratory muscle weakness. *Am Rev Respir Dis* 1984; **130**: 142–4.

27 Barr WG, Fahey PJ. Reduction of pulmonary capillary blood volume following cold exposure in patients with Raynaud's phenomenon. *Chest* 1988; **24**: 1195–9.

28 Ooi GC, Ngan H, Peh WC, Mok MY, Ip M. Systemic lupus erythematosus patients with respiratory symptoms: the value of HRCT. *Clin Radiol* 1997; **52**: 775–81.

29 Sant SM, Doran M, Fenelon HM, Breatnach ES. Pleuropulmonary abnormalities in patients with systemic lupus erythematosus: assessment with high resolution computed tomography, chest radiography and pulmonary function tests. *Clin Exp Rheumatol* 1997; **15**: 507–13.

30 Rolla G, Brussino L, Bertero MT, *et al.* Respiratory function in systemic lupus erythematosus: relation with activity and severity. *Lupus* 1996; **5**: 38–43.

31 Paran D, Fireman E, Levartovsky D, *et al.* Pulmonary dysfunction in systemic lupus erythematosus and anti-phospholipid syndrome patients. *Scand J Rheumatol* 2007; **36**: 285–90.

32 Nakano M, Hasegawa H, Takada T, *et al.* Pulmonary diffusion capacity in patients with systemic lupus erythematosus. *Respirology* 2002; **7**: 45–9.

33 Gibson GJ, Edmonds JP, Hughes GRV. Diaphragm function and lung involvement in systemic lupus erythematosus. *Am J Med* 1977; **63**: 926–32.

34 Andonopoulos AP, Constantopoulos SH, Galanopolou V, *et al.* Pulmonary function of non-smoking patients with systemic lupus erythematosus. *Chest* 1988; **94**: 312–15.

35 Traynor AE, Corbridge TC, Eagan AE, *et al.* Prevalence and reversibility of pulmonary dysfunction in refractory systemic lupus: improvement correlates with disease remission following hematopoietic stem cell transplantation. *Chest* 2005; **127**: 1680–89.

36 Forte S, Carlone S, Vaccaro F, *et al.* Pulmonary gas exchange and exercise capacity in patients with systemic lupus erythematosus. *J Rheumatol* 1999; **26**: 2591–4.

37 Keyser RE, Rus V, Cade WT, *et al.* Evidence for aerobic insufficiency in women with systemic lupus erythematosus. *Arthritis Rheum* 2003; **49**: 16–22.

38 Warrington KJ, Moder KG, Brutinel WM. The shrinking lungs syndrome in systemic lupus erythematosus. *Mayo Clin Proc* 2000; **75**: 467–72.

39 Karim MY, Miranda LC, Tench CM, *et al.* Presentation and prognosis of the shrinking lung syndrome in systemic lupus erythematosus. *Semin Arthritis Rheum* 2002; **31**: 289–98.

40 Rubin LA, Urowitz MB. Shrinking lung syndrome in SLE: a clinical pathological study. *J Rheumatol* 1983; **10**: 973–6.

41 Wilcox PG, Stein HM, Clarke SD, Paré PD, Pardy RL. Phrenic nerve function in patients with diaphragmatic weakness and systemic lupus erythematosus. *Chest* 1988; **93**: 352–8.

42 Evans SA, Hopkinson ND, Kinnear WJM, *et al.* Respiratory disease in systemic lupus erythematosus: correlation with results of laboratory tests and histological appearance of muscle biopsy specimens. *Thorax* 1992; **47**: 957–60.

43 Hardy K, Herry I, Attali V, Cadranel J, Similowski T. Bilateral phrenic paralysis in a patient with systemic lupus erythematosus. *Chest* 2001; **119**: 1274–7.

44 Laroche CM, Mulvey DA, Hawkins P, *et al.* Diaphragm strength in the 'shrinking lung' syndrome of systemic lupus erythematosus. *Q J Med* 1989; **71**: 429–39.

45 Hawkins P, Davison AG, Dasgupta B, Moxham J. Diaphragm strength in acute systemic erythematosus in a patient with paradoxical abdominal motion and reduced lung volumes. *Thorax* 2001; **56**: 329–30.

46 Fathi M, Dastmalchi M, Rasmussen E, Lundberg IE, Tornling G. Interstitial lung disease, a common manifestation of newly diagnosed polymyositis and dermatomyositis. *Ann Rheum Dis* 2004; **63**: 297–301.

47 Arakawa H, Yamada H, Kurihara Y, *et al.* Nonspecific interstitial pneumonia associated with polymyositis and dermatomyositis: serial high-resolution CT findings and functional correlation. *Chest* 2003; **123**: 1096–103.

48 Braun NMT, Arora NS, Rochester DF. Respiratory muscle and pulmonary function in polymyositis and other proximal myopathies. *Thorax* 1983; **38**: 616–23.

49 Wiesinger GF, Quittan M, Nuhr M, *et al.* Aerobic capacity in adult dermatomyositis/polymyositis patients and healthy controls. *Arch Phys Med Rehabil* 2000; **81**: 1–5.

50 Bodolay E, Szekanecz A, Devenyl K, *et al.* Evaluation of interstitial lung disease in mixed connective tissue disease. *Rheumatology* 2005; **44**: 656–61.

51 Martens J, Demedts M. Diaphragm dysfunction in mixed connective tissue disease. *Scand J Rheumatol* **11**: 1982; 165–7.

52 Taouli B, Brauner MW, Mourey I, Lemouchi D, Grenier PA. Thin-section chest CT findings of primary Sjögren's syndrome: correlation with pulmonary function. *Eur Radiol* 2002; **12**: 1504–11.

53 Papiris SA, Maniati M, Constantopoulos SH, *et al.* Lung involvement in primary Sjögren's syndrome is mainly related to the small airway disease. *Ann Rheum Dis* 1999; **58**: 61–4.

54 Lahdensuo A, Korpela M. Pulmonary findings in patients with primary Sjögren's syndrome. *Chest* 1995; **108**: 316–19.

55 Uffmann M, Kiener HP, Bankier AA, *et al.* Lung manifestation in asymptomatic patients with primary Sjögren syndrome: assessment with high resolution CT and pulmonary function tests. *J Thorac Imaging* 2001; **16**: 282–9.

56 Gibson GJ, Davis P. Respiratory complications of relapsing polychondritis. *Thorax* 1974; **29**: 726–31.

57 Mohsenifar Z, Taskin DP, Carson SA, Bellamy BE. Pulmonary function in patients with relapsing polychondritis. *Chest* 1982; **81**: 711–17.

58 Krell WS, Staats BA, Hyatt RE. Pulmonary function in relapsing polychondritis. *Am Rev Respir Dis* 1986; **133**: 1120–23.

59 Sarodia BD, Dasgupta A, Mehta AC. Management of airway manifestations of relapsing polychondritis: case reports and review of literature. *Chest* 1999; **116**: 1669–75.

60 Streeten EA, Murphy EA, Pyeritz RE. Pulmonary function in the Marfan syndrome. *Chest* 1987; **91**: 408–12.

61 Giske I, Stanghelle JK, Rand-Hendrikssen S, *et al.* Pulmonary function, working capacity and strength in young adults with Marfan syndrome. *J Rehabil Med* 2003; **35**: 221–8.

62 Cistulli PA, Sullivan CE. Sleep-disordered breathing in Marfan's syndrome. *Am Rev Respir Dis* 1993; **147**: 645–8.

63 Cistulli PA, Richards GN, Palmisano RG, *et al.* Influence of maxillary constriction on nasal resistance and sleep apnoea severity in patients with Marfan's syndrome. *Chest* 1996; **110**: 1184–8.

64 Ayres JG, Pope FM, Reidy JF, Clark TJH. Abnormalities of the lungs and thoracic cage in Ehlers–Danlos syndrome. *Thorax* 1985; **40**: 300–305.

65 Morgan AW, Pearson SB, Davies S, Gooi HC, Bird HA. Asthma and airways collapse in two heritable disorders of connective tissue. *Ann Rheum Dis* 2007; **66**: 1369–73.

66 Turner-Stokes L, Turton C, Pope FM, Green M. Emphysema and cutis laxa. *Thorax* 1983; **38**: 790–92.

67 Kussmaul WG, Esmail AN, Sagar Y, *et al.* Pulmonary and cardiac function in advanced fibrodysplasia ossificans progressiva. *Clin Orthop Relat Res* 1998; **346**: 104–9.

68 Stokes DC, Wohl MEB, Wise RA, Pyeritz RE, Fairclough DL. The lungs and airways in achondroplasia. *Chest* 1990; **98**: 145–52.

69 Nelson FW, Hecht JT, Horton WA, *et al.* Neurological basis of respiratory complications in achondroplasia. *Ann Neurol* 1988; **24**: 89–93.

70 Mador MJ, Tobin MJ. Apneustic breathing: a characteristic feature of brainstem compression in achondroplasia? *Chest* 1990; **97**: 877–83.

71 Waters KA, Everett F, Silence DO, Fagan ER, Sullivan CE. Treatment of obstructive sleep apnea in achondroplasia: evaluation of sleep, breathing, and somatosensory-evoked potentials. *Am J Med Genet* 1995; **59**: 460–66.

26

Psychogenic Dyspnoea

Respiratory physicians are often presented with patients who complain of breathlessness with little or no evidence of organic cardiopulmonary disease. Some have significant psychopathology, which may be clinically overt or may be revealed only by detailed psychiatric assessment. The underlying psychiatric conditions include anxiety, depression, and obsessional and hysterical disorders, while other patients present following bereavement or with concern about the presence of a life-threatening illness.[1] Sometimes there is evidence of mild organic disease, such as asthma, but with incapacitating symptoms disproportionate to any objective functional abnormality. Some individuals develop disabling breathlessness after occupational exposure to possibly harmful agents, but with no evidence of any adverse physical effect; in some a compensation claim and/or legal proceedings are pending. These overlapping syndromes go under various names, of which 'hyperventilation syndrome'[2] and 'idiopathic hyperventilation' are the most commonly used.

Another condition that may be a manifestation of underlying psychopathology is vocal cord dysfunction, also known as 'emotional laryngeal wheezing', in which there is abnormal adduction of the vocal cords, predominantly during inspiration but also sometimes during expiration. Both of these conditions can cause diagnostic confusion, particularly with asthma. Indeed, either may coexist with mild asthma and such individuals make up a significant proportion of those attending 'difficult asthma' clinics, often with apparently 'steroid-resistant asthma'.[3]

26.1 HYPERVENTILATION SYNDROME

Hyperventilation, in general, implies ventilation in excess of the metabolic requirement and it has many causes. A large physiological dead space occurs in many lung diseases, necessitating excessive total ventilation if a normal arterial P_{CO_2} is to be maintained. Hyperventilation with a low Pa_{CO_2} implies alveolar hyperventilation and also has many organic causes, such as pulmonary vascular disease, asthma and metabolic acidosis. The term 'hyperventilation syndrome', however, is usually confined to individuals in whom overt organic causes have been excluded and in whom the hyperventilation is physiologically inappropriate. Patients with the condition complain of exertional breathlessness, which can be severely incapacitating and they may also be breathless at rest.[4] Some describe the sensation as a difficulty in taking a full satisfying inspiration ('air hunger'),[5] and the discomfort may be relieved if a deep breath can be achieved. Correspondingly, resting tidal breathing may be punctuated by frequent sighing, a feature that can be demonstrated by a simple recording of tidal breathing against time.[6] Other common symptoms include chest pain, vertigo, paraesthesiae and, occasionally, syncope. It is usually assumed that these result from the hypocapnic alkalosis induced by hyperventilation and the symptoms can often be reproduced by voluntary deep breathing.[1] Monitoring end tidal P_{CO_2} ($P_{ET}CO_2$) during wakefulness shows that it is low, either intermittently or persistently, but typically it rises gradually to normal during sleep.[7] This pattern is consistent with abnormal behavioural influences on respiratory control during wakefulness, presumably of largely emotional origin; during sleep these influences are greatly diminished and a more normal situation is regained under the influence of the metabolic control system, whereas during wakefulness behavioural influences can override and drive ventilation. The ventilatory response to rebreathing CO_2 is normal, while the response to hypoxia is less than normal. However, the hypoxic response increases to normal if, during rebreathing, CO_2 is added to the system to raise $PaCO_2$ to a normal value; this finding is consistent with the normal attenuation by hypocapnia of peripheral chemoreceptor hypoxic drive.[4]

The relevance of hypocapnia to the symptoms of the syndrome has been questioned by finding that, in some individuals, they can be reproduced by voluntary hyperventilation of air containing a small concentration of CO_2 sufficient to prevent hypocapnia.[8] Furthermore, the development of symptoms may precede hyperventilation, i.e. hyperventilation may be a reaction to stress rather than necessarily the cause of it.[8] These observations have cast doubt on the validity of the traditional hyperventilation provocation test, although, at a pragmatic level, the test still has clinical value if it is positive and reproduces the patient's symptoms.[1]

A useful finding on simple respiratory function testing is that many subjects with hyperventilation syndrome experience considerable difficulty in performing simple tests in a reproducible manner. An experienced clinical physiologist may suspect the aetiology simply from the forced expiratory spirogram, which may show the consequences of incomplete and inconsistent efforts during the forced manoeuvre or during the preceding full inspiration (Fig. 26.1). Individuals with 'sighing breathing' have been reported to have a smaller VC and consequently larger RV than those with a more normal breathing pattern,[6] but overall the results of spirometry, lung volumes and carbon monoxide diffusing capacity (D_LCO) are within normal limits,[4] provided that the subject is able to perform the tests adequately. Arterial PO_2 is characteristically higher than normal due to the alveolar hyperventilation.

Hyperventilation and/or hypocapnia may not be present continuously. One study showed a large

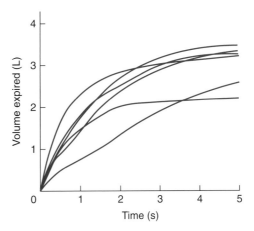

Figure 26.1 Characteristic forced expiratory spirograms of a patient with psychogenic dyspnoea showing poor consistency on repeated measurement.

effect of posture, with normal $P_{ET}CO_2$ supine but a marked increase in ventilation and reduction in PCO_2 within 5 min of standing upright.[9] In individuals with hyperventilation syndrome and chronic resting hypocapnia, the low $PaCO_2$ remains largely unchanged during exercise, with excessive ventilation in relation to the metabolic load, i.e. a high slope of the relationship between ventilation and CO_2 output. Unlike normal subjects, in whom progressive exercise is usually terminated by leg discomfort, these patients are limited by severe breathlessness, which causes them to cease exercise at a lower-than-normal maximum (peak) oxygen consumption.[4]

26.2 VOCAL CORD DYSFUNCTION

Vocal cord dysfunction is characterized by paradoxical narrowing or closure of the vocal cords. It occurs most commonly during inspiration, but it may also be present intermittently during expiration. The consequent limitation of airflow may be accompanied by wheezing, stridor or shortness of breath. Organic causes of vocal cord dysfunction are increasingly recognized, most commonly in association with oesophageal reflux and, more rarely, in dystonias or other neurological conditions affecting control of the vocal cords.

In the absence of an overt organic cause, the condition is more common in young or middle-aged

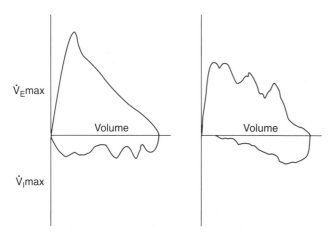

$\dot{V}_E$max

Volume

Volume

$\dot{V}_I$max

Figure 26.2 Appearances of maximum expiratory flow–volume (MEFV) and maximum inspiratory flow–volume (MIFV) curves with vocal cord dysfunction. Note the disproportionately reduced and varying maximum inspiratory flow ($\dot{V}_I$max); maximum expiratory flow may be normal or may also show irregular reduction.

females than in other groups; many patients are overweight and a previous psychiatric history is common. Vocal cord dysfunction is best diagnosed by laryngoscopy or fibre-optic bronchoscopy, which allows direct visualization of vocal cord adduction on inspiration. The condition often masquerades as, or coexists with, asthma. Indeed, up to one-half of affected individuals have other features consistent with asthma,[10] although this is usually mild. Patients may present acutely with symptoms sufficiently severe to warrant bronchial intubation and ventilation, when it is noteworthy that, unlike the situation with acute asthma, the inflation pressure is unusually low.

Vocal cord dysfunction can also present as breathlessness on exercise, often with a sensation of 'choking', when it may cause diagnostic confusion with exercise-induced asthma.[11] Challenge tests aimed at distinguishing the condition from asthma can mislead as vocal cord dysfunction may be provoked by exercise or chemical agents such as methacholine.[11,12] In individuals without coexistent asthma FEV_1 and VC between episodes may be normal, provided they are obtained with maximum cooperation, but patients often require encouragement as performance is often notably inconsistent. The most useful functional information is obtained from maximum flow–volume curves, which, in addition to variable performance, typically show low maximum inspiratory flow and/or premature

truncation of the inspiratory curve (Fig. 26.2). There may be oscillations of expiratory or inspiratory flow associated with varying patency of the larynx. Although relatively insensitive between acute attacks, maximum flow volume curves even in remission may show truncation of inspiratory flow or an increase in the mid-VC flow ratio $\dot{V}_E$max/$\dot{V}_I$max.[10]

Airway resistance measured by plethysmography is characteristically normal in the face of reductions in maximum flow,[3] although a modest increase in resistance, presumably associated with persistent adduction of the cords, has also been described.[13]

Blood gases during an acute episode may show hypoxaemia, usually with hypocapnia although, occasionally, hypercapnia may supervene if laryngeal narrowing is very severe.[14]

REFERENCES

1 Howell JBL. The hyperventilation syndrome: a syndrome under threat? *Thorax* 1997; **52** (suppl. 3): S30–34.

2 Kerr WJ, Gliebe PA, Dalton JW. Physical phenomena associated with anxiety states: the hyperventilation syndrome. *Cal West Med* 1938; **48**: 12–16.

3 Thomas PS, Geddes DM, Barnes PJ. Pseudo-steroid resistant asthma. *Thorax* 1999; **54**: 352–6.

4 Jack S, Rossiter HB, Pearson MG, *et al.* Ventilatory responses to inhaled carbon dioxide, hypoxia and

exercise in idiopathic hyperventilation. *Am J Respir Crit Care Med* 2004; **170**: 118–25.

5 Gardner WN. The pathophysiology of hyperventilation disorders. *Chest* 1996; **109**: 516–34.

6 Alijadeff G, Molho M, Katz I, *et al.* Pattern of lung volumes in patients with sighing breathing. *Thorax* 1993; **48**: 809–11.

7 Gardner WN, Meah MS, Bass C. Controlled study of respiratory responses during prolonged measurement in patients with chronic hyperventilation. *Lancet* 1986; **ii**: 826–30

8 Hornsveld HK, Garssen B, Dop MJC, *et al.* Double-blind placebo-controlled study of the hyperventilation provocation test and the validity of the hyperventilation syndrome. *Lancet* 1996; **348**: 154–8.

9 Malmberg LP, Tamminen K, Sovijarvi ARA. Orthostatic increase of respiratory gas exchange in the hyperventilation syndrome. *Thorax* 2000; **55**: 295–301.

10 Newman KB, Mason UG, Schmaling KB. Clinical features of vocal cord dysfunction. *Am J Respir Crit Care Med* 1995; **152**: 1382–6.

11 McFadden ER, Zawadski DK. Vocal cord dysfunction masquerading as exercise induced asthma. *Am J Respir Crit Care Med* 1996; **153**: 942–7.

12 Morris MJ, Deal LE, Bean DR, Grbach VX, Morgan JA. Vocal cord dysfunction in patients with exertional dyspnoea. *Chest* 1999; **116**: 1676–82.

13 Vlahakis NE, Patel AM, Maragos NE, Beck KC. Diagnosis of vocal cord dysfunction. *Chest* 2002; **122**: 2246–9.

14 Niven RM, Roberts T, Pickering CAC, Webb AK. Functional upper airway obstruction presenting as asthma. *Respir Med* 1992; **86**: 513–16.

INTERPRETATION OF RESPIRATORY FUNCTION TESTS

27

Use of Respiratory Function Tests

27.1 ROLES OF RESPIRATORY FUNCTION TESTS

See Table 27.1.

Tests of function alone rarely produce specific clinical diagnoses. In this respect, respiratory function tests are similar to tests of function of other organs such as the liver or kidneys. One obvious exception to this generalization is asthma, which is defined in terms of variability of function. Otherwise, the role of the tests in diagnosis is essentially supportive, with a pattern of abnormality suggesting or supporting the diagnosis of a group of conditions with similar functional effects. When determining the likelihood of a particular diagnosis, the functional abnormalities need to be considered in the context of clinical features, imaging and, sometimes, histopathological information. Ideally, the results would be interpreted in light of the pre-test probability of a condition: as with any investigation used to support or refute a diagnosis, the value in a particular case varies with the likelihood of the diagnosis in question,[1] but, in practice, precise quantitative evaluation is rarely possible.

Respiratory function tests have a major role in locating the sites of dysfunction, e.g. whether the abnormality is predominantly in the airways, alveoli or chest wall and, in the context of airway narrowing, whether the pattern is of diffuse intrathoracic airway obstruction or localized narrowing of the central airway.

Objective measurements are essential for quantifying the severity of a functional disturbance,

Table 27.1 Roles of respiratory function tests

Diagnosis	Supporting or excluding
	Pattern recognition
Locating site of abnormality	Airways, alveoli, pulmonary vasculature, chest wall, respiratory muscles
	Diffuse vs. localized airway narrowing
Quantifying severity	
Monitoring	Natural history/progression
	Effects of treatment
	Effects of occupational hazards
Assessing prognosis	

whether it be using FEV_1 to grade airway obstruction or carbon monoxide diffusing capacity (D_LCO) or blood gases to assess the severity of gas exchange disturbance. The relation between a single measurement at rest and an individual's symptoms is often rather weak, partly because a single measurement gives incomplete evaluation of respiratory function and partly because symptoms, particularly breathlessness, depend on several other factors, including habitual activity, expectations and personality. Nevertheless, a major discrepancy between symptoms and objective measurements can aid decisions about likely cause and effect. This applies, for example, in the common situation of a breathless patient whose symptoms may relate to either cardiac or pulmonary disease, in whom relatively normal spirometric volumes may favour the former.

Sequential measurements of respiratory function are of considerable value in monitoring the progress of a patient, in relation to both the natural

Table 27.2 Forced expiratory volume in 1s (FEV$_1$) and/or vital capacity (VC) as independent predictors of mortality or survival

Condition	Ref.
COPD	2
Asthma	2
Cystic fibrosis	3
Post-pneumonectomy	4
Idiopathic pulmonary fibrosis	5
Systemic sclerosis	6
Ischaemic heart disease	7
Motor neuron disease	8
Duchenne muscular dystrophy	9

COPD, chronic obstructive pulmonary disease.

Table 27.3 What is the question?

Are the results compatible with a particular diagnosis or diagnoses?
How severe is the functional defect?
What is the cause of breathlessness?
Has there been improvement/deterioration?
Is a particular treatment indicated (e.g. oxygen)?
Is the patient fit to fly?

history of the condition and the effects of treatment. Simple spirometric measurements of FEV$_1$ and/or VC are very powerful prognostic indicators in a remarkably wide range of conditions, not only respiratory such as chronic obstructive pulmonary disease (COPD) and cystic fibrosis, but also cardiac and neuromuscular diseases (Table 27.2). Serial measurements of the rate of decline of FEV$_1$ or VC give even stronger prognostic information. In most situations spirometric measurements retain their prognostic value even after account is taken of the likely confounding factors.

Routine monitoring of respiratory function has a major role in surveillance of workers exposed to potential industrial hazards, both in recognizing specific occupational causes of asthma and in identifying adverse effects of the increasing number of chemical agents that are potentially injurious to the lungs.

27.2 CLINICAL APPLICATION

27.2.1 What is the question?

In clinical testing it is always helpful to know the reason for requesting the tests. This determines which tests are most appropriate and how to interpret the results in the most useful fashion. Examples of possible questions are listed in Table 27.3.

27.2.2 Technical aspects

The technical requirements of the commoner respiratory function tests are covered in detail by the

reports of an American Thoracic Society/European Respiratory Society (ATS/ERS) Task Force on standardization of lung function testing.[10–14] The tests require the cooperation of the subjects to varying degrees, with some much more dependent on effort than others. At least three measurements are usually obtained with the common tests of spirometry, D$_L$CO and plethysmographic lung volumes, and more may be required if the results are inconsistent. With maximum respiratory pressures, which by definition involve maximum effort, a larger number is desirable as several practice manoeuvres may be needed to produce consistency. With helium dilution measurements of lung volume, a single estimate is recommended,[12] but this is a counsel of convenience and practicability rather than the ideal. Because of dynamic airway compression, measurements during forced expiration have the advantage of being relatively independent of the expiratory effort (and even more so in patients with airway disease than in healthy subjects) but, in order to generate valid results, the preceding inspiration needs to be maximal. The comments of an experienced technician or clinical physiologist supervising the tests are particularly helpful when performance appears inconsistent. It is, for example, important to distinguish a progressively declining FEV$_1$ seen on repeat testing in some asthmatic patients with very hyperresponsive airways from inadequate preceding inspiratory effort.

Computerization has brought considerable benefits to lung function laboratories in terms of greater efficiency and avoiding mathematical or transcription errors. Nevertheless, caution is required with modern automated systems as a patient may be 'plugged in' at one end, with a series of 'magic numbers' appearing at the other and the intermediate stages hidden from the eye. It should at least be possible to retrieve the raw data from which the results were calculated so that any apparent discrepancies can be resolved and periodic checks made.

Routine calibration of individual equipment components is standard procedure, but 'biological calibration' with regular measurements on healthy individuals with known respiratory function is also good practice for checking on the performance of a complete system.

27.2.3 Choice of tests

The tests described in this book are mainly everyday tests available in most large general hospitals. The choice of the test or tests in an individual patient should, where possible, be determined by the information being sought, as the appropriateness depends on the clinical context. Other important factors in the choice of a test are (i) its acceptability to, and ease of performance by, the patient (e.g. arterial blood gases vs. oximetry); (ii) its signal-to-noise ratio (e.g. FEV_1 vs. airway resistance measurements); and (iii) its cost-effectiveness, which includes consideration of the capital cost of equipment, cost of consumable items, staff time, etc. in proportion to the value of the information likely to be obtained.

In general, the simpler and longer established tests score highest on all three counts. There is an understandable tendency to regard more complex or more recently introduced tests as more informative, but this is often misguided. For example, there is little evidence that measurements of airway resistance are more useful than tests of forced expiration in assessing airway obstruction, at least in cooperative subjects, or that pulmonary compliance is superior to VC for following patients with pulmonary fibrosis. Furthermore, 'sensitive' tests, which have an epidemiological role in detection of abnormality at a presymptomatic stage, do not necessarily have an advantage when used in symptomatic patients. Unfortunately, many of the sensitive tests introduced particularly for detecting early 'small airway' disease have not stood the test of time.

There is a danger in making too many measurements, a problem that has been exacerbated by the large number of indices available with computerization of results. For example, a single forced expiration and inspiration can generate between 20 and 30 different indices in the various domains of volume, time and flow. Superficially, this multiplicity of information may appear impressive, but it is likely not only to discourage the novice but also to confuse the non-specialist. For most tests it has become conventional to set the lower limit of the 'normal' range at the fifth percentile (see Chapter 8, Section 8.9). For a single test, this implies that if measurements are made in 20 healthy subjects, one is likely to be below the normal range by chance. If more than one test or measurement is used, the proportion of apparently abnormal results (false positives) increases, the size of the effect depending on the degree to which the measurements are independent of each other. For example, if two completely independent functional measurements are made, the proportion of healthy subjects with both measurements above the lower limit of normal would be expected to fall from 0.95 to 0.95^2 (i.e. 0.903); with three independent measurements the proportion with all three above the fifth percentile would be 0.95^3 (i.e. 0.857), and so on, and thus the false positive rate increases progressively. If multiple indices are derived from forced expiration and inspiration, the situation is different as, clearly, they are not completely independent of each other (e.g. FEV_1 is likely to be low if FVC is low), but nevertheless the greater the number of indices measured, the higher the false positive rate.[15] These considerations reinforce the argument to use only FEV_1, (F)VC and their ratio as the primary measurements for interpretation of forced expiration,[14] at least in patients with diffuse airway obstruction, e.g. COPD or asthma. Of course, other indices come into their own for recognition and assessment of central airway narrowing (see Chapter 12, Section 12.1.1).

Suggested approaches to the use of respiratory function tests in some common clinical situations are given below.

27.2.3.1 The patient with suspected asthma

The functional hallmark of airway obstruction in asthma is its variability rather than 'reversibility'. Even in healthy subjects, a reduction in airway resistance is measurable after inhalation of a bronchodilator and, in general, the distinction of 'reversible' from 'irreversible' airway obstruction is simplistic. Although various limits for the increase in FEV_1 regarded as 'significant' bronchodilatation have been proposed (see Chapter 11, Section 11.2.3), these are aimed mainly at detecting changes that exceed random variation of the measurement rather than at diagnosing asthma. As a group, patients with asthma show a larger increase in FEV_1 after bronchodilator than those with COPD, but, in an individual, the response is valuable diagnostically only if it is large (e.g. increase in FEV_1 >400 mL). As discussed in Chapter 9, Section 9.5.1, with more severe airway obstruction a larger bronchodilator 'signal' may be given by measurements other than those obtained during forced expiration, such as a reduction in the extent of dynamic hyperinflation due to less expiratory flow limitation.

The choice of tests to demonstrate the presence of airway obstruction in asthma is not critical, but, for documenting variability, self-monitoring of peak expiratory flow (PEF) has obvious advantages (see Chapter 11, Section 11.2.2). For single measurements in the outpatient clinic, FEV_1 and VC are preferable as they give more discriminatory information.

The diagnosis of asthma presents greater difficulty in older subjects, especially in those with a marked degree of persistent airway narrowing. More detailed assessment including lung volumes and D_LCO is useful as supporting evidence, with the D_LCO and KCO expected to be normal or even increased (see Chapter 11, Section 11.6), while in COPD, and especially emphysema, they are reduced (see Chapter 9, Section 9.7). It should, however, be noted that the diagnoses of emphysema and asthma are not mutually exclusive and, although there is no good evidence that asthma causes emphysema, each is sufficiently common for them to coexist in many individuals.

A specific area of diagnostic difficulty is presented by the patient with so-called 'cough-variant asthma', in whom cough rather than breathlessness and wheezing is the main symptom, and function is normal or near-normal. In this situation, a provocation test is of particular clinical value, using exercise (in younger, fitter subjects), cold air or a nonspecific chemical stimulus such as methacholine.

27.2.3.2 The patient with 'unexplained' breathlessness

In many patients with previously unexplained breathlessness, the cause becomes obvious once spirometry is performed, as assessment of the severity of airway narrowing on clinical grounds alone is notoriously poor. Oximetry showing a normal resting oxygen saturation will exclude significant hypoxaemia as a contributory factor in the great majority of cases. If the explanation is not forthcoming after spirometry and measurement of SaO_2, then several possible options are open: of the more readily available tests, the D_LCO is the next most useful 'screening' test in view of its relative sensitivity (see Table 3.1 in Chapter 3). If D_LCO, spirometry and SaO_2 are all unequivocally normal, most respiratory causes of breathlessness are excluded, provided the spirometric measurements are made at a time when the patient is symptomatic, as it is all too common for the severity of asthma to be underestimated if measurements are made only in the middle of the day.

The role of other tests depends on the clinical suspicions and on the results of the simpler tests. Measurement of lung volumes identifies a restrictive ventilatory defect, without indicating whether the abnormality is within or without the lungs; if the lung fields are clear radiographically and if D_LCO is relatively normal, perhaps with a high KCO, attention turns to extrapulmonary disease: pleural thickening, skeletal abnormality or muscle weakness. Respiratory muscle weakness can usually be identified by measurement of maximum static pressures, but the normal range is wide and false positive results are not infrequent, as true maximum effort requires encouragement and practice. If, on the other hand, TLC is increased with relatively normal spirometry, then asthma or early emphysema are possibilities: the D_LCO and KCO should be discriminatory in this situation. If spirometric volumes suggest a 'restrictive' pattern but TLC is normal (i.e. residual volume is increased), possibilities include cardiac disease (e.g. mitral valve disease), skeletal deformities and muscle weakness.

If SaO_2 is low or borderline, then arterial blood gases with calculation of the alveolar–arterial PO_2 gradient $(AaPO_2)$ are useful for evaluating the severity and possible causes of gas exchange disturbance. Measurement on exercise is more sensitive and desaturation during a simple corridor walk may point to the likely cause(s). A progressive exercise test may be revealing as it allows direct observation of the patient at the time of symptoms, objective evaluation of capacity and assessment of motivation, and the physiological pattern may point to the likely cause of breathlessness. Occasionally, ischaemic changes become obvious on the electrocardiogram (ECG) and offer a sufficient explanation for impaired effort tolerance and breathlessness.

Chronic pulmonary embolism can be difficult to exclude by conventional respiratory function tests, as respiratory mechanics are usually normal and D_LCO is relatively insensitive unless widespread disease of the small pulmonary vessels is present. Perfusion lung scanning or more definitive investigation by computed tomography (CT) pulmonary angiography is indicated if this remains a possible explanation of the symptoms.

27.2.3.3 Suspected upper airway obstruction

The common spirometric measurements of FEV_1 and VC are relatively insensitive to narrowing of the central airway, although FEV_1 falls with more severe narrowing. Detection of upper airway obstruction represents the single most important clinical use of maximum flow volume curves (see Chapter 12, Section 12.1.2). The 'straight' spirogram (see Fig. 12.6a in Chapter 12), disproportionate reduction of PEF or, if measured, of forced inspiratory volume in 1 s (FIV_1) or specific airway conductance (SG_{AW}) are all useful clues, but the overall contour of the maximum expiratory flow–volume (MEFV) and maximum inspiratory flow–volume (MIFV) curves usually gives the most revealing evidence (see Figs 12.2–12.5). It should, however, be noted that the sensitivity of the MEFV curve to upper airway narrowing is reduced in patients with coexisting diffuse intrathoracic airway obstruction due to COPD or asthma (see Chapter 12, Section 12.1.2.4).

27.2.3.4 Responses to treatment

For evaluating the response of patients with airway obstruction to treatment, simple spirometry usually suffices. Although measurement of dynamic hyperinflation at rest or on exercise is more sensitive in advanced disease, it has been used mainly in the context of large clinical trials and the methodology is insufficiently well standardized for routine clinical application. In some patients with COPD the VC increases relatively more after bronchodilatation than FEV_1 or FVC, implying

a reduction in the ratio FEV_1/VC despite obvious improvement, and the ratio is thus unhelpful as a guide to either severity or improvement with treatment. Simple exercise tests such as the 6-min walk distance, together with subjective grading of breathlessness during the test, are useful adjuncts in patients with more severe disease.

In alveolar disease such as sarcoidosis or interstitial pulmonary fibrosis, progress and response to treatment such as corticosteroids can usually be monitored successfully by sequential measurements of VC, sometimes with the addition of D_LCO, which may occasionally show an increase without definite improvement in VC. Some advocate measurements on exercise, particularly of the $AaPO_2$ gradient, but the criteria for improvement are not well standardized and the measurement has poor cost-effectiveness in routine clinical use.

27.2.3.5 Preoperative assessment

The particular problem of thoracic surgery for bronchial carcinoma is considered in detail in Chapter 12, Section 12.2. With both abdominal and thoracic surgery the frequency of postoperative complications is related to preoperative respiratory function, which should be assessed in any patient with respiratory symptoms and probably in all over the age of 50 years. Usually, spirometry and oxygen saturation by oximetry suffice, with further investigation if these are abnormal. General anaesthesia inevitably results in deterioration of pulmonary gas exchange, and preoperative hypercapnia, in particular, predicts a high risk of complications. Peak expiratory flow has been suggested as a particularly useful predictor because of the similarity of the manoeuvre to the production of an adequate cough. The identification of airway obstruction preoperatively not only warns of possible postoperative problems but also directs attention to the need for treatment to optimize respiratory function.

27.3 INTERPRETATION OF RESPIRATORY FUNCTION TESTS

27.3.1 General considerations

Account should always be taken of any technical comments on the performance of the tests as, self-evidently, interpretation needs to be more cautious if the results were poorly reproducible or performance was noted to be inconsistent. For most tests, including forced expiration, maximum respiratory pressures, lung volumes and diffusing capacity, errors due to poor cooperation are likely to be in the direction of abnormally low values, so that in this sense the results are 'fail-safe'. Note, however, that the converse applies to Kco, because, if the subject fails to take a full inspiration, a high value (similar to that seen with extrapulmonary volume restriction) results.

27.3.2 Reference values

The choice of appropriate reference values presents a problem that is not completely resolved. Most laboratories in Europe continue to use the 'summary equations' originally published by the European Coal and Steel Community and subsequently endorsed by the European Respiratory Society.[16,17] These are, however, far from ideal as they were derived from many different populations and most of the data are more than 20 years old, so the normal standards may not reflect the current performance of healthy individuals in the community. The ATS/ERS Task Force recommended using the more recent National Health and Nutrition Examination Survey (NHANES) data for North America,[14] but the Task Force made no firm recommendations for the rest of the world. As discussed in Chapter 8, Section 8.3, a large number of sources of reference data are now available for various ethnic groups in many countries,[14] and the general advice remains to choose equations that give values close to the mean predicted in a group of healthy subjects studied in the laboratory concerned.

When determining ranges of normality, most authorities adopt the range ±1.645 standard deviations (SD) of the reference population (i.e. z score between +1.645 and −1.645), as described in Chapter 8, Section 8.9. In principle, this range encompasses 90 per cent of the healthy population, provided that the measurements are distributed normally, with 5 per cent of normal subjects having values below and 5 per cent above these limits. It should be remembered that not only will a small proportion of healthy subjects have values outwith these limits (false positives), but also a number of patients with undoubted disease will have values within the 'normal' ranges (false negatives). For this reason, pattern recognition, with consistency across several different measurements, is often more helpful than an isolated apparently abnormal result.

27.3.3 Patterns of abnormality

The common patterns of abnormality of spirometry, lung volumes and CO diffusing capacity are summarized in Table 27.4.

Most modern spirometers generate MEFV and MIFV curves at the same time as the simpler volume measurements of FEV_1 and (F)VC. Nevertheless, apart from the particular case of identifying narrowing of the central airway, the simpler indices generally suffice in the assessment of airway disease. In particular, if the FEV_1 and FEV_1/VC are normal, then the clinical significance of apparent abnormalities of flow towards the end of forced expiration is doubtful, particularly as such measurements have a very wide normal range. MEFV curves are helpful for visualizing the effort applied, as the early part of forced expiration, including PEF, is the most effort-dependent. Other measurements from flow–volume curves

Table 27.4 Common patterns of respiratory function (alternative findings in brackets)

Condition	FEV_1	VC	FEV_1/VC	RV	TLC	D_Lco	Kco
COPD	↓↓	↓	↓	↑↑	↑	↓↓	↓
Asthma	↓↓	↓	↓	↑↑	↑	→(↑)*	→(↑)
Interstitial fibrosis	↓	↓	→	→	↓	↓↓	↓(→)
Extrapulmonary restriction	↓	↓	→	↑(→)	↓	→	↑
Pulmonary vascular disease	→	→	→	→	→	↓↓	↓↓

COPD, chronic obstructive pulmonary disease; FEV_1, forced expiratory volume in 1 s; Kco, transfer coefficient; RV, residual volume; TLC, total lung capacity; D_Lco, carbon monoxide diffusing capacity; VC, vital capacity.

*May be reduced if airway obstruction severe.

are more useful when longitudinal changes are being monitored within a subject, but cross-sectional one-off measurements are much less useful. The appearance of the MEFV curve can be seductive and it is easily overinterpreted, particularly in relation to the shape of the curve at lower lung volumes. Concavity (convexity towards the volume axis) is a characteristic feature of diffuse airway obstruction, but it is also a feature of normal ageing. The appearances are qualitatively similar and the difference is simply one of degree. Although such concavity would definitely be abnormal in a 20-year-old, it is the usual finding in a healthy middle-aged or elderly subject.

The forced expiratory flow between 25 per cent and 75 per cent of FVC expired (FEF_{25-75}), formerly known as maximal mid-expiratory flow (MMEF) is often derived from the MEFV curve, although its introduction actually predated that of flow–volume curves as it is easily obtained from a spirogram of volume against time (see Fig. 1.39a in Chapter 1). Traditionally this measurement is more favoured in North American than in European laboratories; initially considered to be a test of 'small airway disease', it suffers from a lack of specificity as it is reduced not only in patients with airway disease but also in those with a restrictive ventilatory pattern, and the interpretation of sequential measurements is confounded by even small differences in FVC.

27.3.4 Reporting respiratory function tests

Ideally, the reason for requesting respiratory function tests should have been defined, but if, as is often the case, this is not stated, the reporter may need to try and interpret what the question was. All available information should be used when reporting the results. As well as clinical details, it is often advisable to take account of the plain radiographic or CT appearances of the lungs, body mass index, smoking history and haemoglobin concentration. Rather than simply restating the numerical results in terms of whether values are normal, increased or reduced, the overall pattern should be reviewed and interpreted in the clinical context. Equally, however, there is a danger of overinterpretation, and caution may be required, particularly if some of the collateral information is not available.

27.3.5 Interpreting arterial blood gas data

An approach to the interpretation of blood gas and acid–base data is illustrated in Boxes 27.1–27.4.

Box 27.1 Interpretation of arterial blood gases 1

Pao_2	13.4 kPa	100 mmHg
$Paco_2$	2.9 kPa	22 mmHg
pH	7.25	
$[HCO_3^-]$	9.4×10^{-3} M	

1 Calculation of alveolar Po_2 (assumed $F_IO_2 = 0.21$):

$$P_AO_2 = P_IO_2 - Paco_2/0.8$$
$$= 20 - 2.9/0.8$$
$$= 16.4 \text{ kPa (123 mmHg)}$$

2 Calculation of alveolar–arterial Po_2 difference:

$$AaPo_2 = 16.4 - 13.4 = 3.0 \text{ kPa (23 mmHg)}$$

3 Interpretation of gas exchange:
   - $AaPo_2$ appears to be greater than normal but attributable to high P_AO_2
   - gas exchange normal

4 Interpretation of acid–base status: typical metabolic acidosis.

Clinical scenario: diabetic ketoacidosis.

Box 27.2 Interpretation of arterial blood gases 2

Pao_2	5.8 kPa	44 mmHg
$Paco_2$	9.5 kPa	71 mmHg
pH	7.37	
$[HCO_3^-]$	40×10^{-3} M	

1 Calculation of alveolar Po_2 (assumed $F_IO_2 = 0.21$):

$$P_AO_2 = P_IO_2 - Paco_2/0.8$$
$$= 20 - 9.5/0.8$$
$$= 8.1 \text{ kPa (61 mmHg)}$$

2 Calculation of alveolar–arterial Po_2 difference:

$$AaPo_2 = 8.1 - 5.8 = 2.3 \text{ kPa (17 mmHg)}$$

3 Interpretation of gas exchange:
   - severe hypercapnia and hypoxaemia
   - $AaPo_2$ appears only mildly ↑, but very abnormal in context of ↓ P_AO_2
   - likely severe $\dot{V}_A/\dot{Q}$ mismatching with ↓ (ideal) alveolar ventilation (other mechanisms of hypoxaemia not excluded)

4 Interpretation of acid–base status: typical chronic respiratory acidosis.

Clinical scenario: severe chronic obstructive pulmonary disease (COPD) with chronic respiratory failure.

Box 27.3 Interpretation of arterial blood gases 3

Pao_2	4.5 kPa	34 mmHg
$Paco_2$	8.0 kPa	60 mmHg
pH	7.04	
$[HCO_3^-]$	15×10^{-3} M	

1 Calculation of alveolar Po_2 (assumed $F_{I}O_2 = 0.21$):

$$P_{A}O_2 = P_{I}O_2 - Paco_2/0.8$$
$$= 20 - 8.0/0.8$$
$$= 10\ kPa\ (75\ mmHg)$$

2 Calculation of alveolar–arterial Po_2 difference:

$$AaPo_2 = 10 - 4.5 = 5.5\ kPa\ (41\ mmHg)$$

3 Interpretation of gas exchange:
 • severe hypercapnia and hypoxaemia
 • $AaPo_2$ markedly ↑, especially in context of low $P_{A}O_2$
 • likely severe $\dot{V}_A/\dot{Q}$ mismatching with ↓ (ideal) alveolar ventilation (other contributory mechanisms to hypoxaemia not excluded)

4 Interpretation of acid–base status: severe acidaemia: not solely respiratory (↓ $[HCO_3^-]$) and not solely metabolic (↑ $Paco_2$), i.e. combined respiratory and metabolic acidosis.

Clinical scenario: post-cardiac arrest with respiratory and circulatory failure.

Box 27.4 Interpretation of arterial blood gases 4

Pao_2	10.8 kPa	81 mmHg
$Paco_2$	11.2 kPa	84 mmHg
pH	7.24	
$[HCO_3^-]$	35×10^{-3} M	

1 Calculation of alveolar Po_2 (assumed $F_{I}O_2 = 0.21$):

$$P_{A}O_2 = P_{I}O_2 - Paco_2/0.8$$
$$= 20 - 11.2/0.8$$
$$= 6.0\ kPa\ (45\ mmHg)$$

2 Calculation of alveolar–arterial Po_2 difference:
$$AaPo_2 = 6.0 - 10.8 = -4.8\ kPa\ (?)$$

3 Interpretation of gas exchange:
 • severe hypercapnia but only mild hypoxaemia
 • negative $AaPo_2$ not possible – therefore patient must have been breathing oxygen

4 Interpretation of acid–base status: typical acute-on-chronic respiratory acidosis.

Clinical scenario: acute exacerbation of severe chronically hypercapnic chronic obstructive pulmonary disease (COPD).

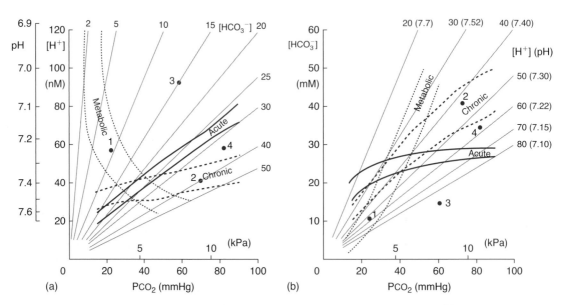

Figure 27.1 Acid–base data of examples 1–4 plotted on the graphs illustrated in Fig. 4.11 of (a) hydrogen ion activity, $[H^+]$ and pH against Pco_2 (isopleths represent constant $[HCO_3^-]$) and (b) $[HCO_3^-]$ against Pco_2 (isopleths of constant $[H^+]$ (pH)). Solid lines indicate the ranges for uncomplicated acute respiratory acidosis and alkalosis, broken lines for chronic respiratory acidosis and alkalosis, and dotted lines for metabolic acidosis and alkalosis. Examples 1 and 2 fall within the bands for metabolic acidosis and chronic respiratory acidosis respectively; example 3 lies between bands for acute respiratory and metabolic acidosis as it reflects a combination of the two; similarly, example 4, showing acute plus chronic acidosis lies between the relevant bands.

In each, pulmonary gas exchange is evaluated by calculation of the $AaPO_2$ using the alveolar air equation and the concept of 'ideal' alveolar gas (see Chapter 2, Section 2.3.3) and acid–base status is analysed in terms of the four traditional types of disturbance as illustrated by plotting the data on acid–base 'maps' (Fig. 27.1). The examples cover four of the common clinical situations where blood gases may be measured, and the approach is only one of many possible methods of analysis. One point that these examples illustrate particularly well is how interpretation of $AaPO_2$ depends on the prevailing alveolar PO_2 (see Fig. 4.10 in Chapter 4).

27.4 CONCLUDING REMARKS

The foregoing outlines only a few of the clinical situations where respiratory function testing is useful. The tests are of major importance in common clinical situations such as the management of respiratory failure and asthma, and in a wider context they have proved of immense value in industrial medicine, epidemiology and clinical research. Detailed measurements in the lung function laboratory should not be decried when there are clear indications, but for tests of respiratory function to be of greatest value in everyday clinical practice the emphasis should be on frequent use of simple measurements in the hospital ward, outpatient clinic and primary care setting.

REFERENCES

1 Griner PF, Mayewski RJ, Mushlin AI, Greenland P. Selection and interpretation of diagnostic tests and procedures: principles and applications. *Ann Intern Med* 1981; **94**: 557–92.

2 Hansen EF, Phanareth K, Laursen LC, Kok-Jensen A, Dirksen A. Reversible and irreversible airflow obstruction as predictor of overall mortality in asthma and chronic obstructive pulmonary disease. *Am J Respir Crit Care Med* 1999; **159**: 1267–71.

3 Kerem E, Risman J, Corey M, Canny GJ, Levison H. Prediction of mortality in patients with cystic fibrosis. *N Engl J Med* 1992; **326**: 1187–91.

4 Putnam JB, Lammermeier DE, Colon R, *et al.* Predicted pulmonary function and survival after pneumonectomy for primary lung carcinoma. *Ann Thorac Surg* 1990; **49**: 909–15.

5 Mapel DW, Hunt WC, Utton R, *et al.* Idiopathic pulmonary fibrosis: survival in population based cohorts. *Thorax* 1998; **53**: 469–76.

6 Simeon C-P, Armadans L, Fonollosa V, *et al.* Survival prognostic factors and markers of morbidity in Spanish patients with systemic sclerosis. *Ann Rheum Dis* 1997; **56**: 723–8.

7 Tockman MS, Pearson JD, Fleg JL, *et al.* Rapid decline in FEV_1: a new risk factor for coronary heart disease mortality. *Am J Respir Crit Care Med* 1995; **151**: 390–98.

8 Fallat RJ, Jesitt B, Bass M, Kamm, B, Norris FH. Spirometry in amyotrophic lateral sclerosis. *Arch Neurol* 1979; **36**: 74–80.

9 Phillips MF, Smith PE, Carroll N, Edwards RHT, Calverley PMA. Nocturnal oxygenation and prognosis in Duchenne muscular dystrophy. *Am J. Respir Crit Care Med* 1999; **160**: 198–202.

10 Miller MR, Crapo R, Hankinson J, *et al.* General considerations for lung function testing. *Eur Respir J* 2005; **26**: 153–61.

11 Miller MR, Hankinson J, Brusasco V, *et al.* Standardisation of spirometry. *Eur Respir J* 2005; **26**: 319–38.

12 Wanger J, Clausen JL, Coates A, *et al.* Standardisation of the measurement of lung volumes. *Eur Respir J* 2005; **26**: 511–22.

13 MacIntyre N, Crapo RO, Viegi G, *et al.* Standardisation of the single breath determination of carbon monoxide uptake in the lung. *Eur Respir J* 2005; **26**: 720–35.

14 Pellegrino R, Viegi G, Brusasco V, *et al.* Interpretative strategies for lung function tests. *Eur Respir J* 2005; **26**: 948–68.

15 Vedal S, Crapo RO. False positive rates of multiple pulmonary function tests in healthy subjects. *Bull Eur Physiopathol Respir* 1983; **19**: 263–6.

16 Quanjer PH. Standardised lung function testing. *Bull Eur Physiopathol Respir* 1983; **19** (suppl. 5).

17 European Respiratory Society. Standardised lung function testing. *Eur Respir J* 1993; **6** (suppl. 16).

18 Hankinson JL, Odencratz JR, Fedan KB. Spirometric reference values from a sample of the general US population. *Am J Respir Crit Care Med* 1999; **159**: 179–87.

Glossary of Terms, Abbreviations and Units

Abbreviation	Measurement	Units Traditional	SI	Comments
VENTILATION				
$\dot{V}$	Minute ventilation	$L\,min^{-1}$	$L\,min^{-1}$	$\dot{V}_I$ and $\dot{V}_E$ denote inspired and expired ventilation
$\dot{V}_A$	Alveolar ventilation	$L\,min^{-1}$	$L\,min^{-1}$	See Section 2.3.5 for meanings of 'alveolar'
V_T	Tidal volume	mL, L	mL, L	
f	Breathing frequency	min^{-1}	min^{-1}	
T_I	Mean inspiratory time	s	s	
T_E	Mean expiratory time	s	s	
T_{TOT}	Mean breath duration	s	s	Equals $60/f$
V_T/T_I	Mean inspiratory flow	$L\,s^{-1}$	$L\,s^{-1}$	
T_I/T_{TOT}	Inspiratory duty cycle	–	–	
V_D	Dead space	mL, L	mL, L	Usually physiological (unless anatomical is specified)
V_D/V_T	Dead space/tidal volume ratio	–	–	V_D usually physiological
MBC	Maximum breathing capacity	$L\,min^{-1}$	$L\,min^{-1}$	Indirect MBC sometimes estimated from FEV_1
MVV	Maximum voluntary ventilation	$L\,min^{-1}$	$L\,min^{-1}$	Usually measured over 15 s
VOLUMES				
TLC	Total lung capacity	L	L	
VC	Vital capacity	L	L	
FVC	Forced vital capacity	L	L	Less than VC in airway obstruction
FEV_1	Forced expiratory volume in 1 s	L	L	Other periods, e.g. $FEV_{0.75}$ now little used
FEV_6	Forced expiratory volume in 6 s	L	L	Sometimes used as surrogate for FVC
RV	Residual volume	L	L	
FRC	Functional residual capacity	L	L	
ERV	Expiratory reserve volume	L	L	Equals (FRC − RV)
IC	Inspiratory capacity	L	L	Equals (TLC − FRC)
FIV_1	Forced inspiratory volume in 1 s	L	L	
TGV	Thoracic gas volume	L	L	Used sometimes as a general term and sometimes as plethysmographic estimate of FRC

(Continued)

Abbreviation	Measurement	Units Traditional	SI	Comments
Vr	Relaxation volume	L	L	
IRV	Inspiratory reserve volume	L	L	Equals (TLC − end inspiratory tidal volume)
DH	Dynamic hyperinflation			

PRESSURES

Abbreviation	Measurement	Units Traditional	SI	Comments
P_{alv}	Alveolar gas pressure (total)	cmH_2O	kPa	
P_{pl}	Pleural surface pressure	cmH_2O	kPa	
P_L	Lung recoil pressure	cmH_2O	kPa	Also $P_{st(L)}$ and equals static transpulmonary pressure i.e. at TLC
$P_L max$	Maximum lung recoil pressure	cmH_2O	kPa	
P_w	Chest wall recoil pressure	cmH_2O	kPa	Also $P_{st(w)}$
P_{RS}	Recoil pressure of total respiratory system	cmH_2O	kPa	Also $P_{st(RS)}$
$P_I max$	Maximum (strictly minimum) static inspiratory alveolar pressure	cmH_2O	kPa	Usually measured at the mouth with closed or virtually closed airway
$P_E max$	Maximum static expiratory alveolar pressure	cmH_2O	kPa	
P_{mus}	Net pressure generated by respiratory muscles	cmH_2O	kPa	
P_{ab}	Subdiaphragmatic abdominal pressure	cmH_2O	kPa	
P_{di}	Transdiaphragmatic pressure	cmH_2O	kPa	Equals ($P_{ab} - P_{pl}$)
$P_{0.1}$	Mouth occlusion pressure 0.1 s after onset of inspiratory effort	cmH_2O	kPa	
P_{box}	Box pressure	cmH_2O	kPa	
$PEEP_i$	Intrinsic positive end expiratory pressure	cmH_2O	kPa	
SNIP	Sniff nasal inspiratory pressure	cmH_2O	kPa	

FLOW

Abbreviation	Measurement	Units Traditional	SI	Comments
PEF	Peak expiratory flow	$L\,min^{-1}, L\,s^{-1}$	$L\,min^{-1}, L\,s^{-1}$	
PIF	Peak inspiratory flow	$L\,min^{-1}, L\,s^{-1}$	$L\,min^{-1}, L\,s^{-1}$	
$\dot{V}_E max$	Maximum expiratory flow	$L\,s^{-1}$	$L\,s^{-1}$	
$\dot{V}_I max$	Maximum inspiratory flow	$L\,s^{-1}$	$L\,s^{-1}$	
FEF_{25}	Forced expiratory flow after 25% FVC expired	$L\,s^{-1}$	$L\,s^{-1}$	Formerly $\dot{V}max_{75}$, where 75 represents %FVC remaining in the lungs
FEF_{50}	Forced expiratory flow after 50% FVC expired	$L\,s^{-1}$	$L\,s^{-1}$	Formerly $\dot{V}max_{50}$, where 50 represents %FVC remaining in the lungs
FEF_{75}	Forced expiratory flow after 75% FVC expired	$L\,s^{-1}$	$L\,s^{-1}$	Formerly $\dot{V}max_{25}$, where 25 represents %FVC remaining in the lungs

Abbreviation	Measurement	Units Traditional	SI	Comments
FEF_{25-75}	Average forced expiratory flow between 25% and 75% of FVC *expired*	$L s^{-1}$	$L s^{-1}$	Formerly maximum mid-expiratory flow (MMF, MMEF)
MEFV, MIFV	Maximum expiratory (inspiratory) flow–volume curve	–	–	
IVPF	Isovolume pressure–flow relationship	–	–	
MFSR	Maximum flow static recoil relationship	–	–	
$\ddot{V}$	Acceleration	$L s^{-1}$	$L s^{-1}$	
EFL	Expiratory flow limitation			

RESISTANCE AND COMPLIANCE

Abbreviation	Measurement	Units Traditional	SI	Comments
R_{AW}	Airway resistance	$cmH_2O\ L^{-1}s$	$kPa\ L^{-1}s$	
R_{na}	Nasal airway resistance	$cmH_2O\ L^{-1}s$	$kPa\ L^{-1}s$	
G_{AW}	Airway conductance	$L s^{-1}cmH_2O^{-1}$	$L s^{-1}kPa^{-1}$	
SG_{AW}	Specific airway conductance	$s^{-1}cmH_2O^{-1}$	$s^{-1}kPa^{-1}$	Equals G_{AW}/TGV
R_{RS}	Resistance of respiratory system	$cmH_2O\ L^{-1}s$	$kPa\ L^{-1}s$	
R_{us}	Resistance of upstream airway segment	$cmH_2O\ L^{-1}s$	$kPa\ L^{-1}s$	Applicable only during forced expiration
G_{us}	Conductance of upstream airway segment	$L s^{-1}cmH_2O^{-1}$	$L s^{-1}kPa^{-1}$	Applicable only during forced expiration
C_L	Pulmonary compliance	$L cmH_2O^{-1}$	$L kPa^{-1}$	C_Lst and $C_L$dyn distinguish static and dynamic compliance
C_w	Chest wall compliance	$L cmH_2O^{-1}$	$L kPa^{-1}$	
C_{RS}	Total respiratory compliance	$L cmH_2O^{-1}$	$L kPa^{-1}$	
Z_{RS}	Respiratory impedance	$cmH_2O\ L^{-1}s$	$kPa\ L^{-1}s$	
X_{RS}	Reactance of respiratory system	$cmH_2O\ L^{-1}s$	$kPa\ L^{-1}s$	

BLOOD FLOW

Abbreviation	Measurement	Units Traditional	SI	Comments
$\dot{Q}_t$	Total pulmonary blood flow	$L min^{-1}$	$L min^{-1}$	
$Q_{va}/\dot{Q}_t$	Shunt fraction	–	–	Specify whether physiological or anatomical
SV	Stroke volume	mL	mL	
HR	Heart rate	min^{-1}	min^{-1}	Also fH

GAS EXCHANGE

Abbreviation	Measurement	Units Traditional	SI	Comments
$\dot{V}_{O_2}$	Oxygen consumption	$mL min^{-1}$, $L min^{-1}$	$mmol min^{-1}$	
$\dot{V}_{CO_2}$	CO_2 output	$mL min^{-1}$, $L min^{-1}$	$mmol min^{-1}$	
$\dot{V}_{O_2}max$	Maximum oxygen uptake	$L min^{-1}$	$mmol min^{-1}$	In clinical testing usually 'symptom limited' or 'peak' oxygen uptake
R	Respiratory exchange ratio	–	–	$\dot{V}_{CO_2}/\dot{V}_{O_2}$ measured at the mouth

(*Continued*)

Abbreviation	Measurement	Units Traditional	SI	Comments
F_EO_2, F_ECO_2	Fractional expired gas concentration	%	%	
P_ECO_2	Mixed expired P_{CO_2}	mmHg	kPa	
$P_{ET}CO_2$	End tidal P_{CO_2}	mmHg	kPa	Close to P_ACO_2 only in normal subjects
P_ACO_2, P_AO_2	Alveolar partial pressures	mmHg	kPa	See Section 2.3.5 for meanings of 'alveolar'
$Paco_2$, Pao_2	Arterial partial pressures	mmHg	kPa	
$P\bar{v}co_2$, $P\bar{v}o_2$	Mixed venous partial pressures	mmHg	kPa	$P\bar{v}co_2$ by oxygenated rebreathing method differs from $P\bar{v}co_2$ by sampling PA blood (see Section 4.3.4)
$Pc'o_2$	End pulmonary capillary P_{O_2}	mmHg	kPa	Usually assumed to equal P_AO_2
$AaPo_2$	Alveolar–arterial P_{O_2} difference	mmHg	kPa	P_AO_2 is usually the 'effective' value (see Section 2.3.5). Syn. $AaDo_2$
Cao_2, $C\bar{v}o_2$	Blood oxygen content (concentration)	mL %	mmol L^{-1}	
Sao_2, $S\bar{v}o_2$	Per cent saturation of haemoglobin with oxygen	%	%	
P_{50}	P_{O_2} at 50% saturation (with pH = 7.4 and P_{CO_2} = 40 mmHg)	mmHg	kPa	
pH	Negative logarithm to base 10 of hydrogen ion concentration	–	–	Strictly, hydrogen ion activity rather than concentration
$[H^+]$	Hydrogen ion concentration	nM (10^{-9}M)	nM	Strictly hydrogen ion activity
$[HCO_3^-]$	Bicarbonate ion concentration	mM (10^{-3}M)	mM	Arterial concentration, usually calculated from $[H^+]$ and P_{CO_2}. Venous 'bicarbonate' measures dissolved CO_2 in addition
pK_A	Negative logarithm to base-10 of apparent dissociation constant of carbonic acid	–	–	Usually assumed to equal 6.1
$P_{tc}CO_2$	Transcutaneous P_{CO_2}	mmHg	kPa	

CARBON MONOXIDE DIFFUSING CAPACITY

Abbreviation	Measurement	Units Traditional	SI	Comments
D_LCO	Carbon monoxide diffusing capacity	mL min^{-1} mmHg^{-1}	mmol min^{-1} kPa^{-1}	Otherwise T_LCO, transfer factor
V_A	Alveolar volume	L	L	Usually simultaneously estimated by inert gas dilution in single-breath manoeuvre
Kco	Krogh factor	mL min^{-1} mmHg^{-1}L^{-1}	mmol min^{-1} kPa^{-1} L^{-1}	Syn. D_L/V_A, transfer coefficient
D_m	Diffusing capacity of pulmonary membrane	mL min^{-1} mmHg^{-1}	mmol min^{-1} kPa^{-1}	
V_c	Pulmonary capillary blood volume	mL	mL	Syn. Q_c
θ	Reaction rate of CO with oxyhaemoglobin	mL CO min^{-1} mmHg^{-1} mL^{-1}	mmol min^{-1} kPa^{-1}L^{-1}	

Index

Page numbers in **bold** type refer to tables and those in *italics* refer to figures. Pages P1-P4 are found between pp. 86 and 87.

Hypoalbuminaemia 94, 195
Hypocapnia
    in acute respiratory distress syndrome 237
    after lung transplantation 282–3
    in asthma 32
    in central sleep apnoea 300
    in chronic cardiac failure 308
    in chronic liver disease 365, 367
    in chronic renal failure 359
    effects on airway resistance 32
    in hyperventilation syndrome 392–3
    in pulmonary hypertension 266–7
    in pulmonary thromboembolism 264–5
    in vocal cord dysfunction 394
Hypopituitarism 378
Hypopnoea 106, 111–12
    in achondroplasia 389
    in acid maltase deficiency 343
    after stroke 334
    in Duchenne muscular dystrophy 340
    in motor neuron disease 338
    in obesity hypoventilation syndrome 373–4
    in obstructive sleep apnoea syndrome 296, 298
    in respiratory muscle weakness 330
Hypothyroidism 376–7
Hypoventilation *87*, **106**, 325–6, *P1*
    alveolar 87, **91**
    in Arnold–Chiari malformation 335
    in central sleep apnoea 299
    in chronic obstructive pulmonary disease *109*, 166
    in Duchenne muscular dystrophy *109*
    in multisystem atrophy 335
    in non-REM sleep 325
    in post-polio syndrome 337
    in respiratory muscle weakness 329–30
    sedative drugs 87
    skeletal deformity and 87, 108
    see also Obesity–hypoventilation syndrome,
        REM-related hypoventilation
Hypoxaemia 86–9, **91**, *P1, P2, P3, P4*
    in acute respiratory distress syndrome 89, 237
    after lung transplantation 285
    after stroke 334
    after thoracoplasty 277
    in alveolar proteinosis 255–6
    in ankylosing spondylitis 276
    in bronchiectasis 193
    in bronchiolitis obliterans syndrome 287
    in chronic cardiac failure 308
    in chronic liver disease 365–8
    in chronic obstructive pulmonary disease 166–8
    in chronic renal failure 359

in congenital heart disease 317–18
    in desquamative interstitial pneumonia 249
    during haemodialysis **360**, 361
    exercise and 123
    fat embolism and 267
    in HIV infection 236
    in idiopathic pulmonary fibrosis 247
    in left ventricular failure 308
    mechanisms of **86**, 87–9, *P1, P2, P3, P4*
    in multiple sclerosis 337
    in myocardial infarction 308
    nocturnal 297, 330
    in obesity–hypoventilation syndrome 373
    in obstructive sleep apnoea syndrome 297
    in pleural effusion 274
    in pneumonia 235–6
    in polycythaemia 353
    in pulmonary arteriovenous malformations 268
    in pulmonary hypertension 266–7
    in pulmonary thromboembolism 264–5
    in sarcoidosis 252
    in scoliosis 276–7
    in sickle cell anaemia 355
    in spinal cord lesions 336
    in vocal cord dysfunction 394
    see also Arterial hypoxaemia
Hypoxia 32, 99, *100*, **106**, 297
    see also Tissue hypoxia
Hysteresis *206, 207, 239*

Iatrogenic alveolitis 256
Iatrogenic fibrosis 256
Idiopathic central sleep apnoea syndrome 300
Idiopathic interstitial pneumonias 243
Idiopathic pulmonary fibrosis 242–8, **249**, **250**, 251,
        384, **400**
Immunosuppressive treatment after lung
        transplantation, effects of 286
Inert gas method for measuring lung volume 19–21, *22*
Inflammatory bowel disease 368
Influenza 235
Inhalation challenge testing 45, **46**, 47
Inspiration, mechanics of 3–7
    see also Forced inspiration
Inspiratory capacity 16, 157–8, 170, 172
Inspiratory duty ratio 102
Inspiratory flow, *see* Maximum inspiratory flow
Inspiratory flow limitation 110
Inspiratory pressure, *see* Maximum inspiratory pressure
Inspiratory reserve volume *16*
Interrupter method, measurement of airway resistance 33
Interstitial fibrosis 87, **404**

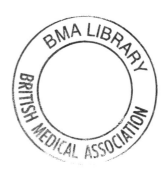